Caring for Older Adults Holistically

SEVENTH EDITION

Tamara R. Dahlkemper, MSN, RN
Associate Professor
   Annie Taylor Dee School of Nursing
   Weber State University
   Ogden, Utah

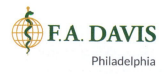

F.A. DAVIS

Philadelphia

F.A. Davis Company
1915 Arch Street
Philadelphia, PA 19103
www.fadavis.com

Copyright © 2020 by F.A. Davis Company

Printed in the United States of America

Last digit indicates print number: 10 9 8 7 6 5 4 3 2 1

Publisher: Terri Wood Allen
Senior Content Project Manager: Amy M. Romano
Illustration and Design Manager: Carolyn O'Brien

As new scientific information becomes available through basic and clinical research, recommended treatments and drug therapies undergo changes. The author(s) and publisher have done everything possible to make this book accurate, up to date, and in accord with accepted standards at the time of publication. The author(s), editors, and publisher are not responsible for errors or omissions or for consequences from application of the book, and make no warranty, expressed or implied, in regard to the contents of the book. Any practice described in this book should be applied by the reader in accordance with professional standards of care used in regard to the unique circumstances that may apply in each situation. The reader is advised always to check product information (package inserts) for changes and new information regarding dose and contraindications before administering any drug. Caution is especially urged when using new or infrequently ordered drugs.

Library of Congress Cataloging-in-Publication Data

Caring for older adults holistically / [edited by] Tamara R. Dahlkemper.
Description: Seventh edition. | Philadelphia: F.A. Davis Company, [2020] |
  Includes bibliographical references and index.
Identifiers: LCCN 2019019756 (print) | LCCN 2019021777 (ebook) | ISBN
  9781719640299 (ebook) | ISBN 9780803689923 (pbk.)
Subjects: | MESH: Geriatric Nursing—methods | Holistic Nursing—methods |
  Geriatric Assessment—methods | Aging—physiology
Classification: LCC RC954 (ebook) | LCC RC954 (print) | NLM WY 152 | DDC
  618.97/0231—dc23
LC record available at https://lccn.loc.gov/2019019756

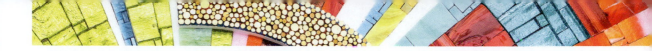

Dedication

This book is dedicated to Dr. Mary Ann Anderson, the original author of this book. She was my mentor and my friend.

Acknowledgments

I want to recognize the gerontological nurses in professional practice who exhibit their caring skills to those who have grown older. The job you do is challenging and requires your very best. Thank you for being willing to do it! I also want to acknowledge the nursing faculty who incorporate concepts related to caring for older adults in their courses. You are teaching the future generation the importance of caring for the older adults in our lives.

I wish to acknowledge F.A. Davis editors, Terri Allen and Amy Romano, for their patient assistance. Thank you also to Developmental Editor Kathleen Scogna for her editing suggestions to improve the textbook.

To my husband and family who provide constant support for my many endeavors. I love you all!

Preface

The book is designed to assist students with information to help them care for our aging population. Students will study Dr. Jean Watson's Theory of Human Caring, Maslow's Hierarchy of Needs, and other current or well-established theories that will enhance their practice. Unique to this book is information on gerotranscendence, transitions, and caring theories designed for gerontological practice.

The foundation of this book is that of critical thinking. It is full of compelling questions that illustrate what it is to be a nurse. The critical thinking assignments draw the reader into the realm of wondering, "what if … ?" rather than thinking "this is …" It is designed to be reader friendly in that it conveys a feeling of conversation with a group of wise nurses who care deeply about nursing and its participants. This book also conveys a deep respect for every person who provides the most valuable kind of care, that art of caring for those who have gone before us and made the world a better place because of their effort—older adults.

New to this edition are Key Terms, Key Points, and Cultural Considerations in every chapter.

Each chapter has a presentation on what should be the priority focus of the chapter and assignments that can be done in or out of class, if the teacher chooses to use them. Chapter Concepts are identified at the beginning of every chapter, to support use of this text in programs that teach conceptually. Each chapter also includes features to assist student learning: Evidence-Based Practice, Focused Learning Charts, Patient Education, Think Like a Nurse, and Safe, Effective Nursing Care.

Students can use the online case studies, critical thinking activities, and interactive clinical scenarios to enhance their learning. For the faculty there are PowerPoint presentations, a well-developed test bank, and a new Active Classroom Instructors Guide located online.

Registered nurses, who maintain a clinical practice and value the role of the licensed practical/vocational nurse (LPN/LVN), wrote this book. The purpose of this book is to assist the future nurse to give informed and holistic care to the growing population of older adults living today.

LPN/LVN Connections

F.A. Davis is pleased to include LPN/LVN Connections, a consistent and recognizable approach to design and content that will make it easier for students and instructors to use multiple F.A. Davis textbooks throughout the LPN/LVN curriculum.

We have increased continuity whenever possible, without erasing the authors' autonomy or changing legacy content that has been popular in past editions. This makes it easier for instructors and students to move through the textbooks and ancillary products while recognizing shared themes and featured content.

Textbook Design, Style, and Pedagogy

- All textbook chapters include the following:
  - Numbered Learning Outcomes
  - Key Terms listed on the chapter opener and boldfaced where first defined in the chapter
  - Chapter Concepts
  - Bulleted Key Points
  - NCLEX-style Review Questions, with answers right on the page for ease of reference
  - Chapter references, located online
- A reading level evaluation is performed during the manuscript development, to ensure readability.
- A uniform, space-saving internal design features special heads and colors that are shared across titles for features with similar content, to increase recognition.
- Consistent and current terminology and laboratory values across titles; the authors followed *Davis's Comprehensive Handbook of Laboratory & Diagnostic Tests with Nursing Implications* by Van Leeuwen and Bladh for all values.

Standardized Faculty Resources

- Active Classroom Instructor's Guide (ACIG) provides pre-, during-, and post-class suggestions for activities and assignments. Abundant activities to promote an active classroom are included.
- eBook
- NCLEX-style test bank
- PowerPoint presentations

F.A. Davis LPN/LVN Advisory Board

Deborah D. Brabham, PhD, RN, CNE
Professor of Nursing
Florida State College at Jacksonville
Jacksonville, FL

Jennifer Briggs, MS, RN
Clinical Instructor, Practical Nursing
Adjunct Instructor, ADRN
Idaho State University
Pocatello, ID

Charlene Cowley, MS, RN, CPNP
Pediatric Nursing Instructor
Pima Community College—Desert Vista
    Campus
Tucson, AZ

Shelley Eckvahl, RN, MSN
Professor, Nursing
Chaffey College
Chino Hills, CA

Deana I. Elkins, MSN, RN
SCC Nursing Instructor
Southeastern CC
Whiteville, NC

Cynthia Hotaling, MSN, RN
Professor—LPN and ADN Programs
Owens Community College
Findlay, OH

Dawn Johnson, DNP, RN, Ed
Practical Nurse Program Director
Great Lakes Institute of Technology
Erie, PA

Chun Hee McMahon, RN, CHPN
Instructor, Vocational Nursing Program
Clovis Adult Education
Clovis, CA

Paula K. Mundell, MSN, RN
Coordinator, Nursing Program
Delaware Technical Community College
Dover, DE

Deloris Paul, MSN, RN
Assistant Professor Facilitator, Practical Nursing
    Program
Santa Fe College
Gainesville, FL

Judith Pelletier, MSN, RN, CNE
Director, Division of Nurse Education
Upper Cape Cod Regional Technical School
Bourne, MA

Helen Rice, MSN, BSN, RN
LVN Program Director
Sacramento City College
Sacramento, CA

Linda Rogers-Antuono, MSN/ED
Nursing Program Manager
Charlotte Technical College
Port Charlotte, FL

Andrea D. Ruff, MS, RN
Coordinator of Healthcare Occupations
Cayuga-Onondaga BOCES
Auburn, NY

Mary Russo, MSN, RN
Nursing Professor
Lincoln Land CC
Jacksonville, IL

Ellen Santos, MSN, RN, CNE
Director of Practical Nursing
Assabet Valley Regional Tech
Marlborough, MA

Louise Schwabenbauer, RN, MSN, MEd
Professor of Nursing
Practical Nursing Program Lead
Lord Fairfax Community College
Middletown, VA

Rosette Strandberg, MSN, Ed, RN
Director/Professor, Vocational Nursing Program
Santa Barbara City College
Santa Barbara, CA

Amy Szoka, PhD, RN
Chair, School of Nursing
Daytona State College
Daytona Beach, FL

Patricia Taylor, MSN-Ed, RN
Practical Nursing Coordinator
Kapi'olani Community College
University of Hawaii
Honolulu, HI

Donna M. Theodore, MSN, MA, RN, LMHC
Nurse Administrator/ Director
Diman Regional Technical Institute
Fall River, MA

Loretta Vobr, MS, RN
LPN Instructor
Northwest Technical College
Bemidji, MN

Contributors

Kathleen Paco Cadman, MSN, RN, RAC-CT, CNE
Associate Professor
Annie Taylor Dee School of Nursing
Weber State University
Ogden, UT
Chapter 7 Safety

Richard Dahlkemper, PhD
Associate Professor Emeritus
Weber State University
Ogden, UT
*Chapter 5 Legal, Ethical, and Financial
   Considerations*

Rieneke Holman, PhD, RN
Associate Professor, Associate Degree Clinical
   Coordinator
Annie Taylor Dee School of Nursing
Weber State University
Ogden, UT
Chapter 20 Pharmacology

Deborah M. Judd, DNP, APRN, FNP-C
Professor
Annie Taylor Dee School of Nursing
Weber State University
Ogden, UT
Chapter 21 Laboratory Values

Diane Leggett-Fife, PhD, RN
Associate Professor
Annie Taylor Dee School of Nursing
Weber State University
Ogden, UT
Chapter 3 Supporting Life Transitions and Spirituality
Chapter 6 Promoting Wellness

Ann Rocha, PhD, FNP-BC
Assistant Professor
Annie Taylor Dee School of Nursing
Weber State University
Ogden, UT
*Chapter 12 Management and Leadership Role of
   the Licensed Practical/Vocational Nurse*

Holli Sowerby, EdD, MSN, RN, CNE
Associate Professor
Annie Taylor Dee School of Nursing
Weber State University
Ogden, UT
*Chapter 4 The Use of the Nursing Process and
   Nursing Diagnosis*
Chapter 15 Physiological Assessment
Chapter 17 Psychological Assessment

Jamie Wankier, MSN, RN
Associate Professor
Annie Taylor Dee School of Nursing
Weber State University
Ogden, UT
Chapter 10 End-of-Life Issues

Kristiann T. Williams, DNP, APRN, FNP-C
Associate Professor
Annie Taylor Dee School of Nursing
Weber State University
Ogden, UT
Chapter 14 Common Medical Diagnoses

Reviewers

Ann Black, RN, MSN
PN Faculty
Montgomery Community College
Troy, NC

Toni Stephens, MSN
Professor, PN Program Director/Instructor
Louisiana Delta Community College
Tallulah, LA

Kelly A. Stone, BSN, RN
PN Program Coordinator
University of Arkansas Community College
  at Batesville
Batesville, AR

Contents

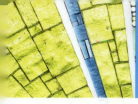

CHAPTER 1
Holistic Caring

Tamara Dahlkemper

KEY TERMS

gerontology
geriatrics
holism
holistic care
gerotranscendence
transpersonal caring

CHAPTER CONCEPTS

Advocacy
Caring

LEARNING OUTCOMES

1. Define gerontological nursing.
2. Discuss the current demographics of people older than age 65 years.
3. Write a one-sentence nursing philosophy.
4. Define the word *holism* as it relates to gerontological nursing.
5. Discuss the theory "The Science of Human Caring" by Dr. Jean Watson as it relates to clinical practice.
6. Describe five examples of how you, as a novice nurse, can use Watson's theory as you give nursing care to older adults.
7. Define the concept of "gerotranscendence."

CASE STUDY

You have been working as a licensed practical nurse (LPN) for 2 years at a skilled nursing facility on the memory care unit. You have learned to love the residents and enjoy the interactions you have with their family members when they come to visit.

Although there is a great deal of agitated behavior displayed by the residents, you understand the phrase, "There is a reason for every behavior." You take the time to observe and listen to residents carefully to understand what is going on inside their minds. Then you act on what you have seen and understood. You seem to do this naturally, based on your knowledge of holistic and caring nursing care, and have received compliments from your nurse manager on your skills.

The nurse manager has hired John, a new certified nursing assistant (CNA), and she has asked you to orient

Continued

CASE STUDY—cont'd

him to your philosophy of care for persons with dementia. You have worked with John for two shifts and are concerned about some of his behaviors. You have noticed the following:

1. He consistently calls the residents "honey," "dearie," and "sweetie," and he does not appear interested in learning their names.
2. He is impatient when the residents are slow in walking and puts them in a wheelchair to get them to the dining room more quickly.
3. He does not allow time for the residents to eat on their own and tries to spoon-feed them.
4. You noticed one resident who did not have her hair combed or her dentures in, and it was 10:00 a.m.
5. He got into an argument with an older man who was confused and wanted to leave the building.
6. He does not listen to you or treat you with respect.
7. He does not listen to family members when they ask for things their loved one needs.

Apply the principles you read in this chapter and make a narrative summary of your thinking regarding the following questions. Add more ideas and comments to your paper than what is listed in the solution.

• How does the CNA's behavior conflict with your holistic and caring philosophy?
• What will you do about the problem?

Welcome to gerontology! Perhaps in no other specialty will you learn information and skills that will assist you in being successful in all areas of nursing. "How can one class touch all segments of health care?" you may ask. "How" is answered simply by the growing number of persons older than age 65 who are living instead of dying. Caring for them is what gerontology is by definition. This ever-expanding group of older adults in the United States need, and will continue to need, health care because of the normal consequences of aging as well as the acute and chronic diseases that occur in all age groups. Older adults connect with all age groups, and because of their increasing numbers, nurses will be seeing them in more roles than ever before in our history.

GERONTOLOGICAL NURSING

It is important to understand the terminology that goes with the specialty of gerontological nursing. The word *gerontological* comes from the Greek words *gero,* meaning "related to old age," and *ology,* meaning "the study of." The word **gerontology** refers to the study of the complex topic of human aging. It includes physical, emotional, social, spiritual, and economic considerations. It is an aspect of nursing that impacts all areas of society, including health-care resources, politics, housing, education, business, and lawmaking. Another commonly used word is *geriatrics.* The Greek word *geras* means "old age," and the word *iatro* means "relating to medical treatment." The word **geriatrics** refers to the medical specialty that deals with the diagnosis and treatment of elderly adults. The word *geriatrics* is very specific; it refers to medical treatment only. *Gerontology* covers several aspects of need for older adults. This definition is appropriate because of the holistic nature of nursing practice.

Gerontological nurses are currently in demand and will likely to continue to be in the future. Older adults are the fastest growing segment of the population in the United States. There are elderly people in home health settings, hospitals, homeless shelters, assisted living centers, and nursing homes. People older than age 65 occupy approximately 65% of the beds in acute hospital settings. The percentage of people older than 65 years continues to increase in home health and hospice settings. They are also more frequently present in pediatric and neonatal care units as custodial grandparents for children whose parents are unable to provide appropriate care. You will be interacting with and caring for older people throughout your career wherever you work.

Priority Setting

As you enter your new profession of licensed practical/vocational nursing, you will be expected to determine priorities that relate to the person receiving care, the environment, and the health-care team, among other things. In each chapter of this book, there will be a box titled "Priority Setting." It will focus on your development as a professional and the management of the priorities of care for the elderly people for whom you are responsible as a nurse. Setting priorities is a challenge. When you are licensed as a practical nurse, you will come to realize that others expect you to identify and meet the demands of patient care priorities.

Thoughtfully read the Priority Setting boxes and work to incorporate the priorities identified into your nursing practice. Some may seem simple; others may seem a bit daunting. I want to assure you, though, that all of them are important in your role as an LPN.

Here is your first Priority Setting challenge.

The priority for this chapter is to develop a holistic caring framework within yourself. This type of care puts you on the cutting edge of health-care delivery and transforms you into a professional nurse.

As a nurse in the 21st century, you are expected to practice the skills of this profession on the cutting edge. Holistic approaches to care that are guided by what the literature refers to as a *caring ontology* (caring philosophy) are on the cutting edge. Historically, nurses have been very task-oriented. Such nurses carried the notorious list I refer to in the chapter. When everything was checked off the list, the nurse considered his or her work completed. There is more expected in this era of nursing. Everything on the list has to be done, as "the list" contains the critical interventions that will improve the health of the person receiving care—yet it needs to be done within the framework of holistic caring.

You will need to reread this chapter if you finish it and are unsure about the characteristics of holistic caring.

Why? Because you need to start now to incorporate them into your philosophy of nursing and daily practice.

- You must learn to listen to people both verbally and nonverbally.
- You probably need to slow down. Do not rush people or even seem to be in a hurry when with a patient or family. This is especially true of older adults, who may need to do things more slowly because of the process of aging.

- Consider family members and significant others as critical to the care you administer. They need to be involved with every stage of treatment and are a valuable source of information.
- Give your *full* attention to the individual to whom you are giving care at the moment. Consider that person's feelings, personal needs, and strong individuality while you are with him or her. Learn from the individual as you teach him or her, and respect the person for the life that he or she has lived.

These are some of the components of transpersonal caring. Learn to live this concept as you practice your art of nursing.

Gerontology is a nursing specialty comprising certified nurses, clinical specialists, and geriatric nurse practitioners who give care only to people older than 65 years. There are nurses in the specialty who have a great deal of experience and novice (or new) nurses just like you. Together, all of us, whether experienced or novice nurses, make a valuable team for the frail and vulnerable older adults who need nursing care and for the well elderly individuals who are focused on health promotion. Gerontological nursing is exciting and varied, and I compliment you for being interested in this area of health care.

Early in my more than 30 years of experience as a registered nurse, I chose to be a gerontological nurse. I made this choice at a time when gerontological nurses were thought to be lesser skilled nurses. "If they were any good, they would be working in the intensive care units (ICUs), wouldn't they?" was a common comment. Fortunately, things have changed.

Gerontological nurses have a specific body of knowledge that they must master (similar to the ICU nurse) to be effective in their practice. For example, did you know that most elderly people who have heart attacks are less likely to have chest pain? In addition, medication doses for a middle-aged person may overwhelm the systems of an elderly person with devastating results. Aging brings with it stages of life development that are different from any previous stage; gerontological nurses need to know and understand these stages. The knowledge required to give gerontological care needs to be learned, understood, and implemented for the elders in this society to have the best quality of life possible.

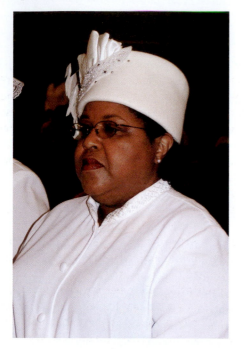

This elegant woman represents the growing number of older women in the United States who are living longer than older men.

In the current health-care environment, people respect gerontological nurses for their multiple skills and abilities. Who but a nursing home nurse can pass medications to 42 residents twice in one shift without making a mistake? Who has the skills and knowledge to calm a pacing, agitated older person with dementia by using validation therapy, a communication technique specifically for elders with dementia? I am proud to be a gerontological nurse and willingly talk to others about how wonderful my career has been because of that choice made long ago to work with older adults.

DEMOGRAPHICS OF AGING

Old age is new. I find that simple statement to be true because of my age. I actually feel the consequences of aging. I am sure many of you reading this book do not notice from week to week or month to month that you are aging. I am in my 60s, have some chronic diseases, and I feel them. Growing older is new for every person who experiences it, and it is new for our society as well. In the history of the United States, there never have been so many people older than age 65.

The composition of the American population is different today from that of any previous generation.

The numbers of old people previously were small compared with the number of older adults who are age 65 and older today. Individuals 65 and older now make up 14.9% of the population (U.S. Census Bureau, 2017). In 2010, there were almost 23 million women and 17 million men in that age group. The U.S. Census Bureau also projects that the number of people who are 85 years and older will increase from 4.6 million to 9.6 million by 2030 (U.S. Department of Commerce, 2011).

What is the makeup of this growing number of older adults? The increase in numbers is attributed to the group referred to as the "baby boomers," people born between 1946 and 1965 after World War II. In 2011, the first individuals who turned 65 began applying for Social Security and Medicare (U.S. Census Bureau, 2017). This places federal financial concerns over paying for baby boomer retirement at the forefront.

Besides the sheer number of aging baby boomers, other reasons for the increased number of older individuals in our society include better nutrition, sanitation, and overall living conditions; lower infant mortality rates; and more effective medical management of acute and chronic diseases. There are specific trends related to sex, however. Because more women reach 65 years of age than men, there are more older women than men in the older-than-85 category. This also means there are more single older women than single older men. However, the current trends show that the ratio of men to women is slowly increasing (U.S. Census Bureau, 2017).

Point of Interest

The increased numbers of elderly people in the United States have resulted in new definitions of aging. The term *young-old* is used for people 65 to 74 years old; *middle-old* is used for people 75 to 84 years old; *old-old* is used for people 85 to 100 years old; and *elite-old* is used for people older than 100 years. It is necessary to define the differences for each age group because of the health needs, medication dosages, and frailty that relate specifically to each age category.

Compare the previous numbers with the fact that, in 1776, when the Declaration of Independence was signed, a child born in the United States had a life expectancy of 35 years. In 1930, life expectancy was 59.7 years; in 1965, it was 70.2 years. Today, the average life expectancy is 81.2 years for women and 76.3 years for men (U.S. Department of Health and Human Services, 2017).

Point of Interest

The National Council on Aging (2017) lists the following 10 diseases as the leading chronic conditions affecting people older than 65 years:

1. Hypertension
2. High cholesterol
3. Arthritis
4. Ischemic heart disease
5. Diabetes
6. Chronic kidney disease
7. Heart failure
8. Depression
9. Alzheimer's disease and dementia
10. Chronic obstructive pulmonary disease

Older adults today have more education and financial resources than ever before in U.S. history. Because they initiated the fitness movement, they are more likely to have regular exercise programs. They also have fewer children to assist in their care.

Fewer than 5% of older adults live in nursing homes, assisted living centers, and other institutions. That leaves 95% living in homes either alone or with their aging spouses or family members.

NURSING PHILOSOPHY

I love working with older adults because doing so allows me to practice within the framework of my nursing philosophy. My first job was at a Catholic hospital, and I was taught to "Serve the Sick as Though They Were Christ in Person." I embraced that philosophy and still practice it today. When I care for elderly individuals in all settings, I am able to give them excellent physical and emotional care, and I am able to be caring. When I add holism to my caring approach, I have a successful format for delivering quality nursing care within the framework of my nursing philosophy. This book is based on the two concepts of holism and

caring, and the purpose of this chapter is to share these critical concepts with you.

CRITICALLY EXAMINE THE FOLLOWING

Think about the elderly people (older than age 65) in your family or among your other acquaintances. Identify three people and think about them. Use their name for the heading and list the characteristics of older people, just discussed, that apply to them. What are their race, sex, age, living conditions, general health, source of income, and other factors that contribute to their quality or lack of quality of life? The purpose of this exercise is to assist you in really seeing older adults. If you do not know the answers, go visit the people you chose and ask them just what it is like to be 65+ in the 21st century.

Understanding the diversity and uniqueness of older adults is important to giving them excellent health care. One professional aspect of yourself that will assist you in meeting the objective of excellence is a nursing philosophy.

Have you considered what your nursing philosophy might be? As a beginning nurse, you may not know what a nursing philosophy is, let alone have one defined for yourself. This is a personal concept that has to come from within you. At this point in your career, you may find a philosophical statement that you like, and as you obtain more education and clinical experience, you may change it.

I have shared my philosophy with you. It is (1) simple and (2) specific and (3) has great meaning for me. These are three characteristics of a valuable nursing philosophy. Let me repeat my nursing philosophy: "To serve the sick as though they were Christ in person." Obviously, I am a Christian; this philosophy would not work for someone of a different religion. I suggest you develop your own nursing philosophy to use as a guide and measurement for the work you do in nursing.

Holistic Nursing

Holism is based on a belief that individuals function as a complete unit and cannot be reduced to a sum of their parts. Its very definition makes the word and its concepts important to the profession of nursing.

Holistic care refers to care of the body, mind, social-ization, and spirit of the person for whom you are re-sponsible. Holistic care occurs when you, the caregiver, make healing the whole person (all of the person's "parts") your priority. It goes beyond healing a surgical incision and includes all aspects of the individual that need attention so there is a wholeness of the person.

When you examine the career of Florence Nightin-gale, it will be apparent to you that she was able to in-tegrate holistic concepts into her personal nursing practice. If she were not holistic, she would have con-sidered just the soldier's wound and nothing else. You will learn that Nightingale is known as the "Lady with the Lamp." After the other nurses had gone to bed, she would walk through the wards at Scutari with her lamp to check on the wounded; she wrote letters for them; and she spent her own money to buy them fruit and vegetables so they would have better nutrition. These are examples of holistic care.

Holistic nursing is something Nightingale prac-ticed without a textbook or a teacher to explain it to her. How did she, the Mother of Modern Nursing, capture the essence of holism with her patients in Scutari? More importantly, how do we, as modern nurses, accomplish that vision today?

Basic Concepts of Holistic Care

Understanding the concepts of holistic nursing is im-portant for the practice of 21st century nursing. It is a philosophy that weaves the demanding technical skills of nursing with the social science skills that en-hance the humanity of the nurse and the person re-ceiving care.

CRITICALLY EXAMINE THE FOLLOWING

Ponder the idea of having a nursing philosophy to guide your clinical practice. Remember that it will change as you learn and grow in the profession. It could simply be:

• Be kind and thorough in the care I give.
• Always practice high-level physical and emotional care.

I am hopeful that by the end of this book or even this chapter, you will be able to say some-thing like the following:

• Practice holistic nursing based on the philosophy of caring.

Write a one- or two-sentence personal nursing philosophy and put it somewhere where you will find it again. It will be interesting to read it at the end of this class or at the end of your LPN educa-tion. Your instructor may want to have you share your philosophy in class.

The philosophy of holism, which was first for-mulated in the 1930s, emphasizes the importance of understanding a person's whole being rather than treating only specific parts. When a patient is recov-ering from a total hip replacement, the patient defi-nitely wants the hip fixed and fixed properly! There may be other needs, however, such as loneliness, fear about being able to live alone again, or a mis-understanding about medications. The person needs more than treatment for the hip.

The philosophy of holistic care should put an end to comments such as "the gallbladder down the hall," which ignores the person and focuses on the illness alone. A holistic identification of the "gallbladder down the hall" should be the person's name or some-thing pleasantly descriptive, such as "the grand-mother who knits all of the time."

If you are a holistic nurse, you will take an active role in developing a healing relationship with the patient. This relationship focuses on the multiple needs of people who are ill and how they can best be resolved. The critical activity to promote holistic care is listening. This approach encourages people who are sick to be more involved in their care. The nurse should listen to what has worked in the past for patients and discuss their ideas as to what would be best for them in the current situation. The nurse needs to provide an environment in which the pa-tient is able to make decisions that are honored by the health-care team.

Holistic nursing practice can be implemented in many ways. Following are four basic concepts:

Rule #1: Always follow the physician's orders. If the patient refuses the treatment or medication ordered, call the physician. That is an excellent way to validate that you are listening to the patient. Be sure to share the patient's concerns with the physician.

Rule #2: You will develop clinical expertise; use it.

Rule #3: Draw on the personal intuition and cre-ativity patients have to resolve their own health problems. You will need to consider the patients'

Focused Learning Chart: Components of Holistic Nursing

Holistic nursing is based on the importance of understanding the whole person rather than treating parts of the person

Develop a Healing Relationship	Work With a Team	Excellent Clinical Skills
Unrushed time	Family, friends, and pets	Holistic communication
Truly listen	Interdisciplinary team	Medication administration
Determine what has worked in the past and discuss options.	Other specialists	Assessment
		Bedside skills
		Management skills

---

values and life experiences when devising treatments. Remember, all of the older adults you will be giving care to are the survivors; they are the people who did not die, and they are strong and smart and have lived with their body long enough to know what it needs.

Rule #4: Take every opportunity to develop a closer relationship with family members or significant others. This is your true entry into getting support and assistance for the older person who is ill. You also will learn many things about the patient in your care.

Holistic Care Is Based on Teamwork

The holistic approach to nursing is effective when dealing with most populations, and it is an excellent way to deliver care to older adults. One of the principles of holistic care is that neither you nor the older person is alone. There is always a team of people working for the best outcome for the person needing care.

These teams look very different for each person. Most holistic teams have family members, although that is not always true. Some have a treasured family pet—a very valuable member. Others have an entire health-care team, such as an older adult in a nursing home who has the advantage of an interdisciplinary team. This is a team of professionals, such as a dietitian, physical therapist, nurse, pharmacist, social worker, and others, who work toward the best condition for the resident. They meet at least monthly to discuss each resident, and the resident and family members are invited to attend this meeting.

The premise is that you, the nurse, will work closely with the team members who are most important to the older adult. The focus of the teamwork should be to provide care, health promotion, and, if possible, cure. This means that you will advocate for the 15-year companion, Suzie the dog, to make regular visits to the nursing home. If you have a home health patient who needs assistance with getting into bed at night, you need to work to make arrangements with family, neighbors, or friends for the necessary assistance. If the person to whom you give care has six adult children and you get calls from each one each week, you need to recognize that there are children who are willing to be involved.

A holistic nurse does not wait for the various team members to come to the nurse. Instead, a holistic nurse looks for any sign or mention of the people who will make a difference in the life of the older person. I remember a blind woman who was brought to the hospital for terminal care. She was brought in an ambulance, and consequently none of her personal things accompanied her. She had no children, and her spouse was deceased, but she did have a dear older friend and neighbor. One morning I entered this woman's room and found her crying. With a bit of encouragement, she told me that she missed having her pictures with her. She had several treasured photos of herself and her husband, and she liked to hold them and think about the wonderful life she and her husband had shared. She was blind, right? But she still wanted those pictures! I located her neighbor, who brought her pictures to the hospital. I know that being able to hold her pictures assisted this woman in having a better quality of life before her death. It simply made her happier.

Some nurses would dismiss the need to be concerned about pictures for a blind woman, and others would not take the time to locate her friend. A holistic nurse would do both things because of the reality of caring about *every* aspect of *every* person in his or her care. Holistic care is a powerful concept and works best when complemented by the nursing theory of human caring.

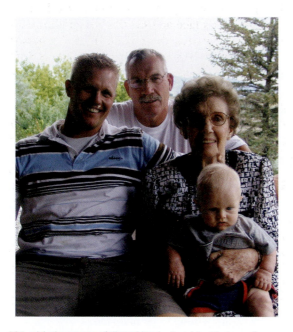

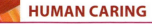
This elderly woman fell and broke her hip 10 days after this picture was taken. Her son and grandson were instrumental in her recovery. Her great-grandson brought her great joy when his parents brought him to see her at the hospital and nursing home.

HUMAN CARING

The Science of Human Caring is a nursing philosophy that was developed by Dr. Jean Watson, founder and director of the Watson Caring Science Institute. Dr. Watson's theory is taught worldwide and serves as the basis of teaching and caregiving for many of the world's nurses. Watson (2018) proclaims that a theory assists us, as nurses, to "see" what it is we do more clearly. It is her hope that the individuals studying and using her theory of nursing will see the world of health care through a "new and different

lens." She wants us to be open to new ideas that are based on caring, and she wants us to put them into practice as nurses.

Watson focuses on looking at the person to whom a nurse gives care as a whole human being, with attention needed for the body, mind, and spirit. This theory calls on you, as a nurse-to-be, to use your imagination and creativity to solve problems in ways that are personal for the people to whom you give care.

There is much more to Dr. Watson's nursing theory, but for the moment, concentrate on these three concepts. In summary, they are:

1. All human beings are valuable, and as a nurse, you have the responsibility to assist, nurture, and provide care for them.
2. It is essential to focus on the human relationship you have with all persons in your care and their relationship with the environment.
3. Developing a human-to-human relationship is critical to being a caring nurse.

Safe, Effective Nursing Care
Human Caring
You are working in a nursing home that takes care of a variety of older adults. After a thorough orientation to the facility, which includes their philosophy of human caring, you are assigned to work on the admissions unit. This is where all new admissions go for the first 3 days to evaluate where they should be placed to receive care specifically suited for their physical and emotional needs. The police bring in a 76-year-old intoxicated man to be admitted. The police tell you he is homeless and an alcoholic. He is dirty, smelly, and uncooperative. His hair is matted, and his beard is overgrown and crusted with food. He has been incontinent, his eyes are bloodshot, and he is drooling. The police remove his handcuffs and quickly leave the area.

Patient-centered care means providing holistic care to *every* patient.

• What is the reaction many people would have about being assigned to admit this man?
• What is your reaction as a nurse who is practicing "The Science of Human Caring"?

• How can you put the relationship you have with this man as the highest priority?
• What can you do to make the environment more conducive to the needs of this person?

Why Study Caring?

Many nurses and other health-care providers tell me they are caring already and ask why they need to study it. I understand the question they are asking. Yet I often see acts of uncaring behavior, as demonstrated by the absence of the human-to-human connection. The following is just one example:

One thing I often see are nurses with lists in their hands as they move quickly from room to room to reassure themselves of the safety of their patients or residents. Many times I have seen a nurse go into a room and say "good morning" without looking at the person and acknowledging him or her personally. Then, with list in hand, the rushed nurse checks the intravenous solution, the bladder catheter, and any dressing or wound, completes the electronic charting, says "goodbye," and leaves the room. Everything the nurse did should have been done, but something very serious was missing. There was no human connection, no transpersonal caring. **Transpersonal caring** is the ability to provide care intentionally focused on caring for the person instead of focusing only on the disease or illness. The nurse was not at all holistic in his or her approach and did not demonstrate transpersonal caring.

How could the same things (checking critical items) be done in a caring manner? First, on the same list with the IV and dressing information should be the person's name. Note it and use it as you go into the room. My personal rule of thumb is to use Mr. or Mrs. the first time I meet an older person. Then, if individuals ask me to use their first names, I do, but only if invited to do so. This is a respectful way to communicate. Look the person in the eye as you say "good morning." Really look at the person's face and see if it has good color, if there are grimaces from pain, or if the person seems sad or depressed. When you get close enough to the person, reach out to touch an arm or a hand if it seems appropriate. This action demonstrates an effort to use transpersonal caring, and it gives you the opportunity to feel if the skin is dry and hot or cold and clammy. Some of these things can be done while you are walking into the room, and none of them take any extra time. After you have connected with the person (human-to-human connection), you can check the IV, the wound, and the catheter. Then lean close so that the older person can see you and hear you, and tell him or her "everything is all right," or "I need to check with the registered nurse (RN)," or whatever is appropriate. Be honest and pleasant in all of your communications. Let the person know approximately when you will return.

Focused Learning Chart: Climate of Caring: Environmental Management

Privacy	Personal Space	Safety	Stimulation/Personalization
Knock on door before entering.	Respect personal items.	No clutter or throw rugs	Multiple opportunities for individual choice
Privacy with family members	Respect personal space.	Proper shoes	Encourage independent function
Respect time to be alone.	Use touch only if it is acceptable to the other person.	Sometimes pets	Cherished furniture and decorations
Pull cubicle curtains.		No frayed cords or broken furniture	Meaningful pictures

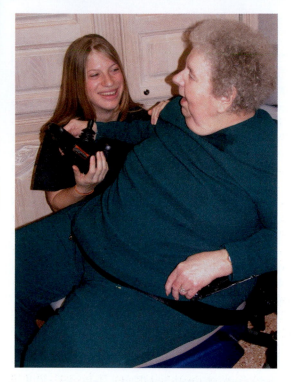

Notice how this LPN is touching the resident and looking directly into her eyes. She is down to the resident's level so the resident can see and hear as the LPN talks to her. What else does the LPN's nonverbal communication tell you?

Cultural Considerations

When providing holistic care to older adults, it is important to assess their individual cultural needs. Promoting the cultural values of any individual assists them in achieving the developmental task of gerotranscendence.

Consider John, the CNA, who is the case study at the beginning of the chapter. After reading the first part of this chapter, do you have a better idea as to how you will help John provide holistic care to the residents assigned to him? What key concepts of Dr. Watson's theory does John need to learn to provide humanistic care to the residents in his care?

Point of Interest

When speaking to older adults, some people address them as "honey," "dearie," or "sweetie." This is an example of the caregiver treating the patient or resident as a child. It is called *paternalism*. Think for whom those comments are generally reserved; it is children. You may hear others use such terms, but you should talk to gerontological patients as the older adults they are rather than as children. It is a matter of respect.

Expanding the Concept of the Science of Human Caring

To truly be a caring person, as defined by Watson, you need to use her principles in all aspects of your life. I do not know your personal or family environment, but I do know that you can choose to behave in any way you wish. I have been screamed at by family members of older adults, but I never scream back. I simply let them "get it out." While they are screaming, I observe them and really listen to their words so I can understand the problem. When the screaming is done, the person generally is crying with sorrow or fear. I keep in mind that there is a reason for every behavior, and I consider it my responsibility to learn the reason for the behavior before I react.

CRITICALLY EXAMINE THE FOLLOWING

Take 5 minutes to think about nothing except how you feel about people with lesser resources for health care. What I mean by that term is people without insurance, people who live at or below the poverty level, people who do not speak English, homeless people, and people with disabilities. These groups of people are often referred to as marginalized people. That means they are on the "margin" of society and not really in it. Can you honestly value each person to whom you give care? Are you willing to use transpersonal caring in your health-care delivery to everyone? Are you willing to make the human-to-human connection with every individual who counts on you for safety and care?

After you have thoughtfully considered how you feel about these questions and any others that come to you, discuss your thoughts with others. They could be classmates, friends, or family. It is an intriguing topic of conversation if you approach it earnestly.

This one application of caring theory in your personal life will improve your ability to relate well to the people you care for the most. Other examples are to listen to people when they are talking and respond thoughtfully. Caring people "get into it" and help others when they need it. This could mean cooking a meal for a sick neighbor, working with the community to make a vacant lot a safe play area, or telling your mom that you love her. (Being a mom, I really like that idea!) I am simply saying that to be a caring nurse, you need to be a caring person, too.

I am confident that you can see how holism and caring complement each other. If you are caring, you look at the body, mind, and spirit of the person. If you are holistic, you also look at the entire person. Both approaches look at how the environment affects the person, and they work with the individual to make the environment more healing.

GEROTRANSCENDENCE

Eric Erickson spent his life studying the psychological developmental tasks of people. His concept was that people would have good psychological health if they fulfilled the developmental tasks associated with each age group. Developmental tasks are the skills and knowledge learned through life experiences that allow us to meet the challenges that occur as we age. Erickson identified eight life stages with specific tasks that need to be accomplished. They are the following:

- Infancy: Trust vs. Mistrust
- Toddler: Autonomy vs. Shame
- Early childhood: Initiative vs. Guilt
- Middle childhood: Industry vs. Inferiority
- Adolescence: Identity vs. Identity diffusion
- Adulthood: Intimacy vs. Isolation
- Middle age: Generativity vs. Self-absorption
- Old age: Integrity vs. Despair

Point of Interest

How do elderly people you know work at achieving gerotranscendence? It is very challenging to develop more connections to others when their normal physical changes do not allow for convenient socialization (i.e., diminished vision and hearing, perhaps the inability to drive). Make some observations and discuss what you learn with someone who is older than you are. See what insight you can develop.

If older adults have accomplished integrity, they have likely experienced **gerotranscendence**, which is one of the critical tasks of old age.

Tornstam (2005) identified the concept of gerotranscendence. He states that older adults desire a life with more connections to other people, a life that is significant to self and others. This concept indicates that aging involves a transition to a lesser concern with material possessions, meaningless relationships, and self-interest. With gerotranscendence, older people are satisfied with the lives they have led and look forward to living a full life for the rest of their days; without gerotranscendence, older people are more likely to feel despair with their lives—past, present, and future. These ideas and other insights into gerotranscendence will be integrated throughout this book in an effort to provide you with information that will assist you to help older adults achieve satisfaction with the lives they have lived.

Evidence-Based Practice

Enzman Hines, M. (2017). A view of caring within holistic nursing. *Beginnings*, *37*(5), 6–24.

This article discusses holistic nursing and the concept of caring. Through caring, nurses provide an increased quality of life to patients by supporting wellness and health. Seven themes of caring include the following:

1. Normalizing the environment—routines and actions that demonstrate respect for the patient
2. Creating sacred space—maintaining a physical environment that is conducive to caring
3. Being rooted in compassion—having an emotional connection with the patient
4. The art of being present—focusing your full attention and thoughts on the patient in the moment
5. Establishing trust-caring—develop a trusting relationship with patients and family members
6. Coaching the family as caregiver—empowering family members to participate in the role of caregiver

7. Inspiration for the future—caring moments with patients foster the desire for nurses to continue providing holistic care

Nurses should incorporate aspects of each of these themes into their practice to help patients live life at their highest level.

Question
As a nurse, how will you incorporate the concept of holistic care into your nursing practice? What aspects of the seven themes do you currently use and which themes need more focus?

CASE STUDY SOLUTIONS

• How does the CNA's behavior conflict with your holistic and caring philosophy?

It seems that he has not embraced either concept into his caregiving, even after you have role-modeled and discussed appropriate behaviors for him.

1. He is not respectful. Examples are the "cutesie" names he uses rather than learning the residents' names and his disrespect toward you.
2. He does not listen to family members and recognize they are part of the care team.
3. He does not listen to the residents. An example is the argument he got into with a confused resident. If he would have listened to the resident, he would have understood the "reason behind the man's behavior."
4. He is not caring. An example is his impatience with the slowness of older persons.
5. He does not give good technical care. This CNA not only is *not* caring or at all holistic, but he does not give good physical care. We know this because of the hair not combed and the dentures that were not in place by mid-morning.

• What are you going to do?

You have worked as an LPN on the memory unit for several years and you know how nursing care should be delivered to these residents. You know that John's care is unsafe and can possibly cause harm to the residents.

You decide that you want to help John to provide better care to the residents but realize it will take some time for him to learn caring behaviors.

You start by asking John what experiences he has had with older adults and if they have been positive. He tells you that he did not have a close relationship with his grandparents and has not spent much time with older adults. You recognize that John needs an opportunity to get to know the residents and to learn to value older adults as human beings. You orient John to the facility and the expectations of physical care that should be provided to the residents. You explain that on the day shift all physical care should be completed before breakfast; this includes combing hair and putting in dentures. You then encourage John to start calling the residents by their name as this is a way to value each person as a unique individual. As part of your care, you demonstrate the importance of touch for the residents and encourage John to hold the resident's hands or touch their shoulder when he is talking to them. Over the next several shifts, as you engage with family members you are able to role model for John the best manner to address their concerns. You explain to him that families only have the best interest of their loved one in mind and that their concerns need to be addressed.

It has been 3 weeks and John mentions to you that he is beginning to feel more comfortable with providing care to the residents. You also see that he is more patient with the residents and their families. Overall, he is now providing what you would consider holistic care. You let John know that you have noticed the change in his attitude and approach to caring and welcome him as a team member.

Key Points

- Gerontology refers to the study of the complex world of human beings. It addresses physical, emotional, social, spiritual, and economic considerations.
- Individuals 65 and older make up 14% of the population. It is predicted that by 2030, 19% of the population will be 65 or older. Baby boomers constitute 30% or the population.
- A nursing philosophy provides a framework for providing quality nursing care. You should develop your own nursing philosophy that is simple, specific, and has personal meaning to you. Your nursing philosophy can be used as a guide and measurement for the care you will provide your patients.
- Holistic nursing provides care to the whole person. The focus is on the body, mind, socialization, and spirit of the individual not just the diagnosis. Holistic nursing weaves technical skills with the social science skills to enhance the humanity of the patient.
- Dr, Jean Watson's Science of Human Caring theory focuses on looking at the person to whom a nurse gives care as a whole human being. The theory is based on three concepts: all humans are valuable, it is important to focus on the human relationship with the individuals in your care, and developing a human-human relationship is critical to being a caring nurse.
- To demonstrate the use of Watson's caring theory a nurse should acknowledge a patient by calling them by their name, provide care in an unhurried manner, touch the patient if appropriate, be honest and pleasant in all communications, and keep in mind there is a reason for every behavior.
- Older adults who have accomplished gerotranscendence are satisfied with the lives they have lead and look forward to living a full life for the rest of their days. They have a lesser concern for material possessions, meaningless relationships, and self-interest. They desire a life that is significant to themselves and others.

Review Questions

1. Gerontological nursing refers to the nursing care of:
   1. The "old-old" population.
   2. People who are older and in need of assistance.
   3. People age 65 and older.
   4. A specialized body of knowledge regarding holistic and caring principles of nursing.

2. Older adults constitute:
   1. 14.9% of the U.S. population.
   2. 8.4% of the U.S. population.
   3. 25% of the U.S. population.
   4. 10% of the U.S. population.

3. The underlying concept of holism is:
   1. To include family and pets in the care plan.
   2. To recognize persons as individuals and to see them as an entire or whole person.
   3. To identify team members who will make the nursing care easier.
   4. To look at the patient's face and note how he or she looks.

4. The purpose of a nursing philosophy is to be able to:
   1. Think like a philosopher.
   2. Have something positive to write on a job application.
   3. Talk to other nurses about philosophy.
   4. Have a personal conviction of the type of nursing care you will give to others.

5. "The Science of Human Caring" is (select all that apply):
   1. A nationally accepted philosophy of nursing.
   2. Authored by Jean Watson, former Dean and Distinguished Professor at the University of Colorado.
   3. A philosophy that addresses the body, mind, and physicality of all human beings.
   4. A philosophy of nursing that calls for the practice of individual caring.

6. Gerotranscendence is:
   1. One of the critical tasks of old age.
   2. Based on Dr. Watson's developmental task of integrity vs. despair.
   3. A concept that refers to an elderly person's transition to a more materialistic mindset.
   4. A task that, when accomplished, makes older people despair the lives they have led.

ANSWERS 1. 3, 2. 1, 3. 2, 4. 4, 5. 1, 2, 3, 4, 6. 1

CHAPTER 2
The Aging Experience

Tamara Dahlkemper

KEY TERMS

ageism
function
prejudice
racism
sexism
stereotype

CHAPTER CONCEPTS

Assessment
Health, Wellness, and Illness
Professional Behaviors
Self

LEARNING OUTCOMES

1. Discuss attitudes toward aging and the impact on the care of older adults.
2. Discuss six common theories of aging.
3. Identify age-related changes as they relate to each body system listed in the chapter.

CASE STUDY

Mr. C. is an 80-year-old man who lives with his wife in their home. Overall, he is in good health but recently started taking medications for hypertension. He had his left knee replaced 2 years ago. He gets about 5 hours of sleep each night but usually naps after his physical activity for the day. Usually he wakes up during the night to empty his bladder.

He enjoys being physically active. During the summer, he rides his bike, golfs while walking the golf course, and plays a game of pickleball on occasion. He also maintains a large garden. During the winter months, he walks on his treadmill and plays indoor tennis with some of his friends.

The last couple of years he has noticed that he experiences shortness of breath and minor muscle weakness and soreness during his exercise so he finds he needs to decrease the level of exertion occasionally. He also notices when he plays tennis or pickleball that his balance is not as good as it used to be. Although these issues slow him down, he understands the concept of "use it or lose it."

Over the years he has developed dark spots on his arms and head. He uses sunscreen when he is outside and wears a hat to cover his head, which is covered with thin graying hair.

Continued

CASE STUDY—cont'd

Mr. C. no longer drives at night, so he relies on his wife to drive after dark. He states that his eyesight is not as good as it used to be and finds that reading in brighter light seems to help.

Mr. C. and his wife have a very active social life and like to travel. Their social activities include going to movies and eating out. He finds that he and his wife cannot eat large meals anymore so they usually share a meal. Although his body is aging, he feels like he is still able to live an active and productive life.

Discussion

1. What age-related changes has Mr. C. experienced?
2. Would you consider Mr. C. to be a healthy older adult? Explain.

INTRODUCTION

The aging experience is a significant part of personal and societal living. Sometimes called "the graying of America," this dramatic change in our population has many ramifications in politics, economics, health care, recreation, and entertainment. All facets of life, not just health care, are affected by the fact that many more older adults are living today than lived in the past.

People 65 years old and older constitute almost 15% of the population in the United States.

Here are two important pieces of demographic information that will impact your practice as a licensed practical nurse (LPN):

1. The older white non-Hispanic population has decreased over the last several years and will continue to decline compared with Hispanic and other ethnic minority groups (National Center for Health Statistics, 2017).
2. The fastest-growing segment of the population in the United States is people who are older than 85 years of age. Projections indicate that the size of this age group will almost triple by 2060 (U.S. Census Bureau, 2018).

IMPACT OF AGING ON NURSING

This significant increase in the number of older people means that nursing practice must be different from what it has been in the past. Current national statistics state that 65% of all patients in acute care hospitals are age 65 or older, as are 83% of people in home care and 92% of residents in nursing homes. As a nurse you will be taking care of older adults in all care settings. The graying of America calls for gerontologically qualified nurses who can work in diverse health-care settings. The purpose of this book is to assist you in meeting that objective.

Health care has changed in various ways because of the number of people who are aging. As a group, older citizens are a very powerful political force; they have influenced the actions of Congress and the president on health-related issues and will continue to do so.

Older adults want and expect to have a say in the kind of health care they receive, where they receive it, and from whom. They are better educated than any other generation of older adults and have the knowledge to make more sophisticated demands on the health-care system. For instance, demand is growing for home care services from older people who need assistance and nursing care but prefer to be cared for at home. This population of new clients in the health-care system requires you, the nurse, to consider them in a new way.

CRITICALLY EXAMINE THE FOLLOWING

Before reading the next section, take the time necessary to complete this critical thinking exercise. Critical thinking is an essential component of nursing. These exercises are a positive way to begin to develop that all-important skill.

How Will It Impact Your Nursing Practice to Have:

1. Increasing numbers of old-old people as your patients?
2. Increasing numbers of older adults from ethnic minority groups as your patients?

ATTITUDES TOWARD AGING

The study of aging is a very important part of nursing. Many myths, **stereotypes** (an assumption that all people of one culture or race have the same personal characteristics), and **prejudices** (a preconceived judgment or opinion formed without factual knowledge) about old age exist in our culture, and nurses need to be able to separate myths and prejudices from fact. Modern researchers are intently studying the aging experience (another indication of the importance of this topic in today's world). This chapter draws from their findings to represent a realistic picture of the processes and effects of aging.

Myths and prejudices about old age are pervasive in our society. Browsing through a greeting card display reveals some very good examples of the stereotypes and fables of aging:

"I won't say you're old," reads one greeting card, "but in horse years, you'd be glue on this envelope."

"Happy birthday, Hot Stuff! Who says people our age can't still live in the fast lane?" reads another. The inside message: "Voila! Adult diapers with racing stripes."

Cultural Considerations

Some cultures value the aged while other cultures view aging as undesirable.

As the contents of many of the cards imply, old age conjures up images of rocking chairs, dentures, memory loss, and incontinence. People laugh at the humor in the birthday cards, but a serious societal danger lurks in such negative and prejudicial images. Stereotypes, myths, and distortions concerning aging and old people lead to actions that discriminate against the aged. American culture glorifies youth. Print and television advertising, clothing fashions, and other expressions of the desirable norm all push the image of zestful youth. Because today's adults have grown up in this culture, they pick up its values and prejudices without realizing it. Fortunately, in recent years, the media has started depicting older adults in a more positive manner as healthy and active.

Although the media do play a role in how older adults are perceived, research shows there are other influences that play a part in our perceptions of older adults. Individuals with limited interactions and lack of knowledge of older adults in general have more negative perceptions. Individuals who have numerous interactions with older adults, either with family members or other acquaintances, and whose interactions are mostly positive tend to have a more positive perception of older adults. Negative perceptions are also decreased if some biographical information is known about the older adult, such as their life history or simply the individual's prior occupation (Hoogland & Hoogland, 2018).

Studies show that health-care providers' negative attitudes toward aging can have an impact on the physical and psychological well-being of patients. Older adults are less likely to receive appropriate preventive care and screening tests that can lead to accurate diagnosis. These factors can all impact patient outcomes. Health-care providers with more positive attitudes toward older adults will provide a higher quality of care overall (Smith et al., 2017).

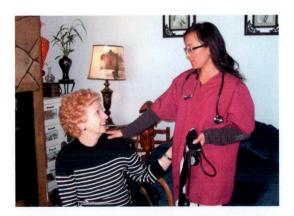

Home health care is one of the health-care changes that elderly people have demanded as part of their health-care options. People want to stay at home and be near family, friends, and the things that are familiar to them.

Point of Interest

The word *geriatrics* is the term that describes the medical study of older adults, and the word *gerontology* describes the nursing study of older adults. You need to know the definitions of both words to discuss gerontological issues knowledgeably.

Evidence-Based Practice

Jackson, J., Clark, A., Pearse, L., Miller, E. A., Stanfield, H., & Cunningham, C.J.L. (2017). Explaining student interest and confidence in providing care for older adults. *Journal of Gerontological Nursing, 43*(3), 13–18.

There is a need for health-care professionals trained and interested in providing care to the aging population in the United States. This study evaluated how students' attitudes toward aging might be associated with their confidence and interest in providing care to older adults once they graduate and start their professional careers. The study included students enrolled in pre-professional programs; nursing, social work, physical therapy, athletic training, and nutrition/dietetics at a U.S. university.

The results showed student confidence and interest in caring for older adults was influenced by their attitude toward older adults based on societal views, positive views towards their own aging, positive attitudes toward older adults in general, frequency of contact with older adults and if the contact was positive, and the age of the respondent. Confidence and interest in working with older adults was highest in nursing and physical therapy students.

The study provided a deeper understanding of how societal views on aging and a person's views regarding their own aging affects choices students make about planning to engage in gerontological care as a career path.

Questions
1. What factors influence your confidence in working with older adults?
2. Does your new knowledge about older adults impact your confidence?
3. What are your thoughts about focusing your career on the care of older adults?

AGEISM

The term **ageism** was coined in 1968 by Robert Butler (1969) to describe negative attitudes and practices that were directed toward old people. He defined ageism as a systematic stereotyping of and discrimination against people simply because they are old. Ageism is very similar to **racism** (prejudice against someone of a different race) and **sexism** (actions and attitudes that relegate individuals of either sex to an inferior status in society), which discriminate against people because of skin color and sex. We as a society are outraged by acts of racism and sexism, but we seem to accept ageism as a norm for behavior. Old people are categorized as confused, rigid in thought and manner, and old-fashioned in morality and skills.

Yet older adults are as individual and unique as people of all other age groups. Ageism allows the younger generation to see older people as different; they subtly cease to identify with their elders as human beings.

In the decades since Dr. Butler first wrote about ageism, a steady improvement in attitudes toward the aged has been seen. This change has partly resulted from general public education, increased attention in the media, and broadening of education about gerontology in colleges and universities. Negative attitudes toward the aged still exist. They appear subtly, covertly, and even unconsciously. Similar to racism and sexism, ageism is still persistent.

Priority Setting

The priority you need to take from this chapter is that of recognizing and combating ageism. Why is that the priority I chose? Ageism is a powerful, negative form of discrimination.

Because you will be giving care to older adults, you need to be their champion and assist them in combating this negative influence in their lives.

How can you meet this priority of recognizing and fighting ageism?

- Start by becoming acutely aware of what ageist behavior is. It could be something as simple as not laughing at the discriminatory cards that mock older people and the aging process. They simply are not funny. Look for age-based discrimination. Once you can recognize it, you can begin to change within yourself if that is needed.
- Look at older adults as "wise and wonderful." They really do have the wisdom of the ages. Just think of all the problems they have solved by living in a tumultuous world (world wars, the Great Depression). They deserve to be heard, so listen!
- Be patient with older people. Their bodies are wearing out because of the *normal* process of aging. Don't hold that against them.
- Along with patience, speak up, move in close so you can be seen, touch if it seems appropriate, smile, and learn to enjoy your time with someone older. You may need to start with enjoying your grandparents or older aunts and uncles. Both generations have so much to offer each other. Don't be too busy to take advantage of this opportunity.

- Be brave! Speak up when someone says or suggests doing something that is ageist. You don't need to be aggressive, but you should state your opinion. You don't need to defend what you say because the statement should speak for itself.
- Read about ageism, ponder what you read, talk to others about it, and consider how you would like to be thought about and treated when you are older. If you don't like what you foresee, how can you change it?

An example is the cosmetic industry, which thrives on the sale of products that eliminate age spots, smooth away wrinkles, conceal gray hairs, and make one look younger than one's actual age. Growing old is represented as a calamity, and being old as having a dreaded disease. The last years of life are pictured as time spent in death's waiting room.

In reality, elderly people do not offer a panorama of doom and death. Many senior citizens live well into their 80s and 90s with "youthful vigor," in relative physical comfort and safety, and in good health. Many others do have chronic health problems, but because the problems are well managed and well controlled, such people consider themselves healthy and lead active, fulfilling lives. Still others have significant limitations that affect their independence and activity, but they are able to enjoy a rich and varied existence because they live with family members or in other protected environments.

Negative images of nursing homes envisioned by some people are in part an expression of ageism. Most nursing homes give excellent care to a frail and vulnerable population that cannot be cared for elsewhere. Another point of information, unknown by many people, is that only 5% of people older than 65 years are in nursing homes at any one time (Larsen, 2019). Today's nursing home is characterized by a concept of *rehabilitative,* not *custodial,* care, a perspective that calls for nursing interventions intended to support the highest possible level of independence despite physical and cognitive limitations.

It is easy for society to judge, criticize, and ignore an older person. Do an internal examination to determine if you are ageist. Do you get impatient when an older person is in front of you driving on the freeway? I tell my gerontology students that they will not pass the class until they have conquered that type of impatience. I give them assignments to sit down and unhurriedly talk to a well elderly person.

I suggest they go with the older adult to lunch or shopping, even to the grocery store. The students are encouraged to ask questions about the older adult's life and how it has been impacted by aging. To change attitudes regarding ageism, individuals who hold ageist views must change their beliefs and behaviors (Teater, 2018).

An important concept to remember is the uniqueness of the individual. Just as every child and every middle-aged adult is unique in some way, so is every older adult. The mistaken belief that one old person is just like another is an expression of ageism, and this perception can lead to potentially harmful treatment. Physicians and nurses sometimes treat older patients as they might treat a child, calling them by their first names without asking how they wish to be addressed or, worse yet, calling them "honey" or "dearie." Caregivers often are guilty of "infantilizing" the elderly. It is easy to see how such treatment increases dependence and frailty, rather than fostering independence, even for a person with limitations. Not all old people are cranky and gloomy, although a man or woman who was cranky and gloomy at age 40 is probably more so at age 80. People tend to become more like themselves as they age. All individuals who work in the health-care field need to examine their own attitudes and biases about older adults in general and about frail or ill older adults in particular to battle ageism successfully.

THEORIES OF AGING

Theories of aging are a scientific effort to assist people to understand what contributes to aging in a positive or negative manner. As a nurse, you need to understand the basic theories to assist and support your older adult patients and residents to live healthier lives. There are physiological and psychological theories to assist you in understanding aging. There are many theories available for study; the following are three from each category that will assist you in giving effective nursing care.

Physiological Theories of Aging
Genetic Factors
The theory of genetic factors is easy to understand if you critically examine yourself and your family members. You already know that you may have inherited your hair and eye color, height, and body size from your ancestors. There are many other things you also may have inherited, such as musical or

athletic ability. Have you considered that the aging of your body also is inherited? This theory says that it is. Interview your grandparents or older aunts and uncles. Are their siblings still alive? How long did their parents and grandparents live? I know of a family in which all of the men died before the age of 50 with heart disease, but the women lived to be in their 70s. I know a family of six sisters who all went through menopause at age 52. I have a friend whose mother had 11 brothers and sisters; they all lived to be in their 80s. Consider Mr. C. in the chapter case study. Can any of his aging issues be related to genetics?

Safe, Effective Nursing Care

Attitudes Toward Older Adults

If you were to ask other students where they plan to work when they graduate, very few will say they plan to work in assisted living or a nursing home. Yet, most nurses working in acute care facilities will work with older adults as their primary patient population. It is important for all nurses to have the necessary knowledge to provide quality care for their older patients.

Because of earlier experiences with older adults, some nurses may have a negative attitude toward their elderly patients. Beyond the ability to know how to provide needed care, a nurse must also value the individual for whom they are providing care.

• What is your attitude toward older adults?
• Do you have any biases toward taking care of older adults?
• What are some things you can do to overcome your personal ageism?

Spend time pondering the issue of ageism. Really grasp what it means for you personally. This can be done by talking to your colleagues and peers and, more importantly, by talking to older people.

This genetic theory of aging claims that animals and humans are born with genes that predetermine their life span. This may seem discouraging to people who are working hard to obtain or maintain optimum health. However, a healthy diet, exercise, and stress control, among other things, will certainly support a higher quality of life, if not add to one's longevity.

Just as nurses interview people about their family history regarding diseases, it would be appropriate use

of this theory to ask about their parents and siblings and their aging process. This information may assist you in working with the patient or resident. The most important aspect of this theory is for you to recognize that it is one way to accept aging as the inevitable process it is. With that acceptance, you should develop an additional acceptance of the normal and abnormal aspects of aging and the eventual death of each of us. According to this theory, it is predetermined and inevitable.

Wear and Tear

If you were to go to a senior citizen center or a nursing home dayroom, you would easily identify the basis for the wear and tear theory. As people age, their body parts show the effects of the complex and sophisticated work the body does through the years. People will be walking with canes or walkers; some will be on oxygen; others will simply moan when they get up from a chair. Similar to any type of fine-tuned machinery, body parts wear out or become less effective. Knees need to be replaced because of the lack of cartilage that comes with aging, joints develop arthritis, and hips break because of decreased bone mass or lack of balance leading to a fall.

Think of all the running and jumping you did as a child. Perhaps you were an athlete during high school. Maybe you are a mountain biker or ride motorcycles or participate in other physical activities. The body is well used and sometimes abused, and its parts simply wear out. Could any of Mr. C.'s physical issues be related to this theory?

Understanding this theory should assist you in accepting that older adults walk slower, hear less effectively, need to stop and rest, and overall do things at a slower and safer pace. If you understand and accept this theory, you will accept the changes that require your attention in giving care to specialized, older people.

CRITICALLY EXAMINE THE FOLLOWING

Spend time with your parents or older relatives and discuss the genetic factor theory with them. Ask questions about your ancestors and identify traits that you may have inherited from them. Inquire about the longevity of your ancestors as well as their major diseases. When you have enough information, predict how long you will live and the predominate diseases you will have. Justify what you predict from your family history. Prepare the information into one paragraph that could be read in class.

Nutrients

Chapter 8 in this book is devoted to nutrition for older persons. When considering the nutrient theory, however, you should focus on your own nutritional intake. This theory states that aging and the quality of aging depend on a person's nutritional intake over the span of his or her life. This is easy to understand because, as a health-care worker, you recognize the negative effects of obesity, lack of exercise, and high cholesterol, all of which may be attributed to food consumption. The quart of chocolate ice cream, mountain of french fries, and large steak are not ways to promote a successful aging process. The nutrient theory states that good nutritional intake at any age assists in improved health as one ages. The longer you eat healthy foods, the longer you will live with a better quality of life. Now is a good time to start.

Whenever you are giving care to an older person, you should examine the individual's eating habits and determine if you can teach him or her something new that will improve health. Suggest having a dietitian visit the person or arrange for fresh fruits to be available for snacks if that would help. You need to take care of yourself and share your knowledge with those you love. Teach them the things you will learn in the nutrition chapter and apply the principles to yourself as well. There is little in life that is better than a healthy old age!

Psychological Theories

Developmental Tasks

Eric Erikson (1963) is known for his eight stages of personal development of individuals. He begins with infancy and progresses through old age. His focus is on ego development, which gives people the strength to manage their lives. The task for old age, according to Erikson, is Integrity vs Despair. If older people can find meaning in the life lived, then they will have the ego integrity to adjust and manage the process of aging. If they do not have integrity, they will be angry, depressed, and feel inadequate; in other words, they will feel despair.

You may encounter older persons who are feeling despair. They complain constantly and keep saying they wish "this" or "that" had happened in their life. Also frequently heard is the phrase "if only ...." Such people need your time and acceptance of them and their lives. Ask them to talk about their life experiences and reinforce the valuable things they have done. Help them to see what they have contributed to the world. Your efforts should focus on identifying the actions in their life that will assist in building the feeling of ego integrity. Similarly, you may also find older adults who are happy in their lives and have been able to adjust to the process of aging. An example is Mr. C. Although he is dealing with issues related to the normal aging process, Mr. C. states that he is "happy with his life and looks forward to the next 10 years." I would say Mr. C. has reached Erickson's eighth stage and has developed ego integrity.

Subculture Theory

This theory defines older people as a subculture, which in anthropological terms means that older people have their own cultural norms and standards. This includes attitudes that are common to multiple members of the group and beliefs, expectations, and behaviors that make them different from others.

You will study cultural and ethnic differences in people throughout your education. It is important to understand people's differences and needs. The subculture theory suggests that elderly people are another group worthy of your study and that they share many similarities. However, it is important to remember that although older people as a subculture exhibit many similarities, they, like all people, are also strongly individualized.

Continuity Theory

In simple terms, the continuity theory states that as people change, their basic personality and behavioral patterns do not change. If you are an angry person at age 20, then you will be even better at being angry at age 70. The same is true of a teacher, who will find a way to keep teaching as he or she ages. A loving mother will find a way to continue to mother people (perhaps her grandchildren or children in the neighborhood), musicians will keep playing, and athletes will still keep trying to win.

The continuity theory recognizes the unique and individualized characteristics of people and their ways of adapting to aging. This theory is easy to apply to your practice. You simply need to talk to the older person and the family members about what type of person your patient was in his or her youth or adulthood. Then you will know what type of behavior to expect now that he or she is an older adult. Don't try to change older people; rather, respect them for who they are.

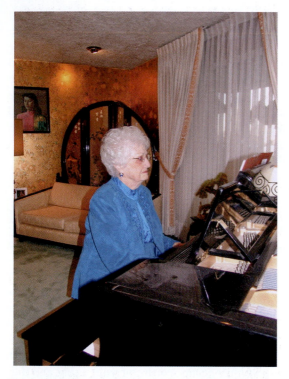

This 82-year-old woman has always played the piano. Now that she is older, she is better at it than ever before in her life. Which psychological theory does this demonstrate?

NORMAL AGING PROCESS

Since the early 1950s, much research has been done in Europe and the United States on identifying and classifying common physiological and psychosocial changes that occur as people grow older. In this context, aging is seen as a natural process, and the changes associated with it are considered to be expected and continuous. If you are curious about your potential normal aging changes, you need to look at your grandparents. What acute and chronic diseases do they have? At what age do people in your family die? Do the men go bald; do the women develop osteoporosis? We all will age until we die.

Focused Learning Chart: Theories of Aging

Physiological Theories	*Psychological Theories*
Genetic Factors *Born with a genetic program that predetermines life span*	**Developmental Tasks** *Eric Erickson defined eight developmental tasks from infancy to old age. The task for old age is Integrity vs Despair.*
Wear and Tear *All life is a fine-tuned machine. Body parts wear out as they age.*	**Subculture Theory** *Defines old people as their own subculture with cultural norms and standards*
Nutrients *Aging and the quality of life depend on the person's nutritional intake over his or her life span.*	**Continuity Theory** *People change physiologically as they age, but their basic personality and behavioral patterns do not change.*

To me, that comment makes aging the desirable choice between the two. I would sooner grow old than die young.

To understand the normal aging process fully, nurses must realize that aging is a normal developmental event and that patterns of aging vary dramatically among older adults. Although the profession studies normal age changes that are universal, every person ages in a particular, individualized way. No two individuals are alike; the number of ways in which people age may be seen as equal to the number of people who have lived into old age. As individuals age, they become more diverse, not more alike. The range of "normal" aging characteristics is wide, and each individual exhibits a unique interplay of physical, social, and environmental influences that define the personal aging experience.

Older adults often have a chronic or acute illness superimposed on age-related changes, but development of disease is not a normal part of aging. It is essential for you, the LPN, to understand this perspective and develop a positive approach to normal aging. It also is important to remember that most older adults live actively and independently in the community and cope successfully with age-related changes and chronic illnesses (remember that only 5% of them are in nursing homes). Health for older adults might be defined as the ability to function at an individual's highest potential despite the presence of age-related changes and risk factors (Box 2.1).

NORMAL PHYSIOLOGICAL CHANGES ACCORDING TO BODY SYSTEMS

Specific age-related changes are described in terms of the body systems with which they are associated. Common functional changes experienced by older adults as a result of physiological alterations also are discussed. The term **function** refers to an older adult's ability to perform activities of daily living (ADLs) and independent activities of daily living (IADLs) and takes into consideration the quality of life of the individual. As the older adult experiences an increase in the number and intensity of age-related changes, functional independence is often jeopardized. Nursing approaches to prevent losses and promote self-care in light of age-related changes also are considered in this section.

Cardiovascular System

The cardiovascular system loses its efficiency with age, but because older adults require less oxygen at rest and during exercise, many people effectively compensate for changes in circulatory function. The high incidence of cardiovascular disease in the older population often makes it difficult, however, to distinguish normal age-related changes from changes related to illness. Older adults now know more about

Box 2.1
Essential Facts About the Normal Aging Process
- As individuals age, they become more diverse, not more alike.
- Age-related changes develop in each individual in a unique way.
- Normal aging and disease are separate entities.
- Normal aging includes gains and losses and does not indicate decline.
- Successful adaptation to the aging process is accomplished by most older adults.

taking care of themselves, which improves the function of their cardiovascular system.

Age-Related Changes
HEART
- Cardiac muscle strength is diminished.
- Heart valves become thickened and more rigid.
- The sinoatrial node, which is responsible for conduction, is less efficient, and impulses are slowed.
- Heart contractions may be weaker, blood volume decreases, and cardiac output declines.

BLOOD VESSELS
- Arteries become less elastic.
- Capillary walls thicken and slow the exchange of nutrients and waste products between blood and tissues.
- The greater rigidity of the vascular walls increases systolic and diastolic pressures.

BLOOD
- Blood volume is reduced due to an age-related decline in total body water.
- Bone marrow activity is reduced, which leads to a slight decrease in levels of red blood cells, hematocrit, and hemoglobin.

Point of Interest
In addition to the ability to take care of one's ADLs—basic personal needs, such as eating, dressing, washing, toileting, and moving—function also refers to the ability to live independently in one's community, performing IADLs including cooking, shopping, taking medications properly, cleaning, traveling locally, and managing finances. This information will be addressed in more detail in Chapter 15.

Functional Changes
With normal aging, some atherosclerosis ("hardening" of the arteries) is expected as well as decreased cardiac output, but cardiovascular response remains adequate if cardiac disease is not present. Older adults usually adjust to cardiac changes but find they may need to pace their physical activity.

Respiratory System
Respiratory functioning shows minimal age-related decline in healthy older adults. The age-related changes that affect the respiratory system are so

gradual that most older adults compensate well for these changes.

Age-Related Changes

SKELETAL CHANGES
- The rib cage becomes rigid as cartilage calcifies.
- The thoracic spine may shorten, and osteoporosis may cause a stooped posture, decreasing active lung space, and limiting thoracic movement.

ACCESSORY MUSCLES
- Abdominal muscles weaken, decreasing inspiratory and expiratory effort.
- The diaphragm does not seem to lose mass.

Intrapulmonary Changes
- Lung elastic recoil is progressively lost with advancing age.
- Alveoli enlarge and become thin, and although their number remains constant, the number of functioning alveoli decreases overall.
- The alveolus-capillary membrane thickens, reducing the surface area for gas exchange.

Functional Changes
Structural changes in the respiratory system affect the rate of airflow into and out of the lungs as well as the rate of gas exchange at the alveolar level. Because of limited elastic recoil, residual volume increases; less ventilation occurs at the bases of the lungs, and more air and secretions remain in the lungs. In addition, the shallow breathing patterns of older adults—secondary to postural changes—contribute to this reduced airflow. Decreased chest muscle strength contributes to a less effective cough response and places an older adult at greater risk of pulmonary infection. The shallow breathing pattern also affects gas exchange. Oxygen saturation is diminished. For example, the partial pressure of oxygen (PaO_2) in alveoli is about 90 mm Hg for a healthy young adult, whereas a value of 75 mm Hg at age 70 years would be acceptable. This decline may result in a decreased tolerance for exercise and the need for short rest periods during activity.

Musculoskeletal System
Most older adults experience alterations in posture, changes in range of motion, and slowed movement. These changes account for many of the characteristics normally associated with old age.

Age-Related Changes

BONE STRUCTURE
- Loss of bone mass results in brittle, weak bones and increases the risk for fracture.
- The vertebral column may compress, leading to reduction in height.

MUSCLE STRENGTH
- Muscle wasting occurs, and regeneration of muscle tissue slows.
- Muscles of the arms and legs become thin and flabby.
- Muscles lose flexibility and endurance with inactivity.

JOINTS
- Range of motion may be limited.
- Cartilage thins, so that joints may be painful, inflamed, or stiff.

Functional Changes
Loss of muscle mass is a gradual process, and most older adults compensate for it well. Regular exercise has been shown to reduce bone loss, promote increased muscle strength, and improve flexibility and muscle coordination. Conversely, immobility and sedentary lifestyles lead to loss of muscle size and strength.

Loss of bone mass and bone density results in osteoporosis and porous, brittle bones that are at greater risk of fracture. In women, loss of bone mass may be due to the estrogen deficiency caused by menopause as well as low serum calcium levels. Treatment may include calcium supplementation, bisphosphonates, and other types of medications that enhance bone mass. Estrogen therapy is no longer recommended for the treatment of osteoporosis in women.

In summary, changes caused by osteoporosis, lack of joint motion, and decreased muscle strength and endurance may affect the functional ability of the older adult. An effective exercise program, together with adequate diet and a healthy outlook that includes independence and an active lifestyle, can reverse or slow down musculoskeletal changes. The phrase "Use it or lose it!" directly applies to an older adult's musculoskeletal functional ability.

Integumentary System
Changes involving the skin and hair probably are symbolic of the aging process more than those of any other system. The formation of wrinkles, the development of "age spots," graying of the hair, and baldness are constant reminders of growing old. In addition, no

other system is so highly influenced by previous life patterns and environmental conditions, particularly sun exposure.

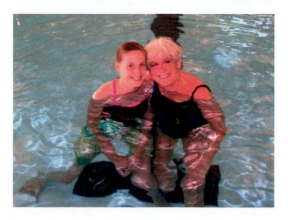

This grandmother and granddaughter team go swimming together twice a week. It provides a special time for them to be together and a great opportunity for meaningful exercise.

Age-Related Changes

SKIN
- The skin loses elasticity, leading to wrinkles, folds, and dryness.
- The skin thins, giving less protection to underlying blood vessels.
- Subcutaneous fat diminishes.
- Melanocytes cluster, producing the skin pigmentation known as age spots.

HAIR
- Decreased activity of hair follicles results in thinning of the hair on all areas of the body.
- Decreased rate of melanin production results in loss of original color and graying.
- Women may develop hair on the chin and upper lip.
- Men may develop an increase in ear, nose, and eyebrow hair.

NAILS
- Decreased blood flow to the nailbed may cause nails to become thick, dull, hard, and brittle, with longitudinal lines.

SWEAT GLANDS
- Decreases in size and number occur.

Functional Changes

Intact skin is the first line of defense against bacterial invasion and minor physical trauma. Age-related skin dryness and decreased elasticity increase the risk of skin breakdown and skin tears, leading to increased potential for injury and infection. Body temperature regulation is impaired by decreased sweat production. Because of this, older adults may not exhibit diaphoresis with elevated body temperatures.

Conversely, the loss of insulation in the form of a fat layer may make older adults feel cold. They often ask for extra sweaters when younger adults are comfortable with the ambient temperature. Nurses need to be aware of temperature discomforts when bathing, dressing, or examining an older adult and respond appropriately to the older adult's concern.

Age-related changes in the integumentary system affect the essential mechanisms of body protection and temperature regulation and greatly influence one's perception of aging. Earlier health practices related to nutrition, grooming, bathing, and physical activity as well as genetic, biochemical, and environmental factors are powerful determinants of integumentary status.

Gastrointestinal System

Changes in the gastrointestinal (GI) system, although not life-threatening, often cause the greatest concern to the older adult. Indigestion, constipation, and anorexia are common GI problems that greatly affect functional status.

Age-Related Changes

ORAL CAVITY
- Reabsorption of bone in the jaw may loosen teeth or cause a loss of teeth, reducing the ability to chew.
- Saliva production decreases.

ESOPHAGUS
- The gag reflex weakens, causing an increased risk of food aspiration.
- Smooth muscle weakness delays emptying time.

STOMACH
- Decreased gastric acid secretions may impair absorption of iron, vitamin B_{12}, and protein.

INTESTINES
- Peristalsis decreases.
- Weakening of the sphincter muscles leads to incompetent emptying of the bowel.

Functional Changes

The slowing of peristalsis and the loss of smooth muscle tone delay gastric emptying so that a feeling of "fullness" is present after eating only small amounts of food. In addition, delayed gastric emptying time and reduced gastric acid secretions may lead to indigestion, discomfort, and reduced appetite. Frequent small meals, rather than three large ones, may be better tolerated. Decreased peristalsis also contributes to slower transit time in the large intestine and allows more time for water reabsorption and hardening of the stool. Because of this factor, the nurse should recommend a diet adequate in fiber and fluids.

Fatigue, discomfort, activity intolerance, and sensory losses may make food preparation difficult for an older adult living at home. This problem could result in a nutritionally inadequate diet. In summary, effective GI functioning creates peace of mind for the older adult and greatly influences well-being.

Urinary System

Changes in the genitourinary system affect the basic bodily functions of voiding. This issue is often difficult for an older adult to discuss. A commonly held belief is that having genitourinary problems such as incontinence is a normal result of aging. It is not, but the belief that it is often causes an older adult to delay seeking treatment. Helping the older adult to maintain optimal genitourinary function is often a challenge for the nurse.

Age-Related Functions
RENAL FUNCTION
• Renal blood flow decreases because of decreased cardiac output and reduced glomerular filtration rate.
• Ability to concentrate urine may be impaired.

BLADDER
• Loss of muscle tone and incomplete emptying may occur.
• Capacity decreases.

MICTURITION
• In men, increased frequency owing to enlargement of the prostate is possible.
• In women, increased frequency may be caused by relaxation of the pelvic floor muscles.

Functional Changes
Despite decreased renal blood flow and the loss of kidney mass, the genitourinary system continues to function normally in the absence of disease. Functional impairments result from decreased bladder capacity and include urinary frequency, nocturia, and retention of urine. These changes may eventually cause dysfunction, leading to infection, urgency, and incontinence. Although urinary incontinence is not a normal outcome of the aging process, cumulative damage to the pelvic floor muscles, often due to pregnancy and childbirth, may contribute to one of the most common forms of incontinence in women—stress incontinence. This condition involves leakage of urine that occurs with coughing, sneezing, laughing, or lifting. Pelvic floor exercises are an effective strategy to strengthen muscle tone and prevent involuntary leakage.

Enlargement of the prostate, which occurs in most elderly men, is most often benign. It can cause, however, urinary retention, frequency, overflow incontinence, and, eventually, renal damage. Older men should have regular examinations of the prostate.

Changes in voiding, particularly incontinence, may contribute to embarrassment and general discomfort for an older adult. By showing sensitivity and acceptance, the nurse can intervene effectively to improve genitourinary functional response.

Reproductive System
Age-Related Functions
FEMALE REPRODUCTION
• The vulva may atrophy.
• Pubic hair may fall out.
• Vaginal secretions diminish, and vaginal walls thin and become less elastic.
• Breast tissue atrophies.

MALE REPRODUCTION
• Testes atrophy.
• The prostate may enlarge.

Functional Changes
Because of the aging process, female genitalia exhibit many changes. As a result of a decrease in vaginal secretions and changes to the tissue, women may experience painful sexual intercourse. Many new treatments, including local estrogen therapy, estrogen-like medications called selective estrogen receptor modulators, and vaginal moisturizers, are available for this condition.

The structural changes in male genitalia can cause a reduction in sperm count, but these changes do not affect the physical ability of men to achieve erection or ejaculation.

Despite the changes in the male and female reproductive system, many older adults are still able to enjoy intercourse and other forms of sexual pleasure (Box 2.2). For many older adults, discussing reproductive issues can be embarrassing, but these issues need to be assessed by the nurse.

Nervous System

Age-related changes in the nervous system affect all body systems and involve vascular response, mobility, coordination, visual activity, and cognitive ability. Most misconceptions about normal age-related changes involve the nervous system. For example, there is a misconception that mental decline or "senility" is inevitable with aging or that intellectual capacity diminishes with age. The nurse needs to teach older adults that general decline of neurological function is not an automatic response to aging and that, in the absence of disease, the older adult's neurological system functions adequately.

Age-Related Changes
NEURONS
- Neurons are steadily lost in the brain and spinal cord.
- Synthesis and metabolism of neurotransmitters are diminished.
- Brain mass is lost progressively.

MOVEMENT
- The kinesthetic sense is less efficient.
- Balance may be impaired.
- Reaction time decreases.

SLEEP
- Insomnia and increased night wakening may occur.
- Deep sleep (stage IV) and rapid eye movement sleep decrease.

Functional Changes
As motor neurons work less efficiently, reaction time slows, and the ability to respond quickly to stimuli decreases. Research studies indicate that although response time may be prolonged, older adults are willing to give up speed for accuracy and tend to respond more slowly but with greater precision. There seems to be little correlation between brain atrophy and cognitive loss. Older adults are generally well oriented to time, place, and person, with minimal changes in memory performance despite decreased synthesis of neurotransmitters and diminished brain size.

Older people are particularly at risk for falls, owing to a slower reaction time in maintaining balance and the potential for hypotensive reactions secondary to decreased blood volume. Resulting symptoms of dizziness, lightheadedness, and vertigo contribute to impaired balance. Nurses should allow older adults adequate time for position change; dangling the legs at the bedside and standing briefly before ambulation may be indicated.

Older adults generally sleep less at night but take naps during the day, so that cumulative sleep time is usually adequate. The frequent awakenings may cause restless sleep and abrupt wakefulness that are often troubling to an older adult. Thorough sleep assessment is necessary to determine actual sleep time. Additionally, the nurse may suggest afternoon exercise and a decrease in stimulants at bedtime. Environmental changes, such as noise control and regulation of room temperature, may be helpful.

Common age-related changes of the nervous system, particularly slowed reaction time, affect movement, sleep, and cognition, the functions of which are vital to optimal performance of ADLs.

Special Sense Organs
The sensory organs of sight, hearing, taste, touch, and smell facilitate communication with the environment. Loss of sensory function, particularly vision and hearing, severely alters an older adult's self-care abilities and quality of life. Age-related changes that result in loss of sensory function may be the most difficult for a person of any age to accept and cope with effectively. The nurse must be extremely sensitive to sensory changes and their impact on each person.

Age-Related Changes
VISION
- Ability to focus on close objects is diminished.
- Increased density of the lens occurs, and lipids accumulate around the iris, causing a grayish yellow ring.
- The production of tears decreases.
- The pupils decrease in size and become less responsive to light.
- Night vision decreases, and the iris loses pigment so that eye color usually becomes light blue or gray.

HEARING

- The ability to hear high-frequency tones decreases.
- The cerumen contains a greater amount of keratin so that it hardens and becomes more likely to become impacted.

TASTE

- Ability to perceive bitter, salt, and sour tastes diminishes.

TOUCH

- Ability to feel light touch, pain, or different temperatures may decrease.

Functional Changes

Despite normal age-related changes in vision, most older adults have adequate visual function using corrective lenses for self-care activities. Because dark and light adaptation takes longer, simple activities, such as entering or leaving a theater or going to the bathroom at night, put older people at risk for falls and injury. Yellowing of the lens makes vision for low-tone colors (violet, blue, green) difficult; use of yellow, orange, or red colors on signs or on bedroom walls increases the older adult's ability to read. Decreased production of tears by the eye may contribute to irritation and infection; artificial tears are often prescribed.

Functional hearing changes result initially in an inability to hear high-pitched tones. The nurse should speak in a normal tone of voice without shouting and without increasing pitch.

Because it takes more sensory stimulation to trigger the taste experience, older adults may use more salt to produce a salt taste on their food. All of these sensory changes have a profound impact on the functional ability of older adults. The nurse must always determine whether the patient uses corrective lenses or a hearing aid and ensure that the older person has these assistive devices available at all times.

Later in this book, the reader will be able to compare abnormal physiological changes of older adults with the normal changes explained here. As a future gerontological nurse, you should have a thorough understanding of both aspects of physiological aging.

CASE STUDY SOLUTIONS

1. Mr. C. has experienced age-related changes in the following areas:
   Cardiovascular
   - Decreased activity tolerance
   - Fatigue with increased activity
   Musculoskeletal
   - Loss of muscle strength
   Integumentary
   - Thinning hair
   - Melanocyte clusters, age spots
   Gastrointestinal
   - Delayed gastric emptying leading to fullness
   - Reduced GI motility

   Genitourinary
   - Decreased bladder capacity
   - Increased frequency
   Nervous
   - Impaired balance
   - Increased night awakening
   Special Senses
   - Decreased night vision
   - Poor vision in reduced light
2. Mr. C. is a healthy older adult because he functions at an optimal level despite the presence of age-related changes. He feels good about his life and looks forward to the next 10 years.

Key Points

- People aged 65 and older constitute almost 15% of the U.S. population. The "graying of America" has many ramifications in politics, economics, health care, recreation, and entertainment.
- It is important to explore the myths, stereotypes, and prejudices about old age to begin the process of seeing older adults as unique individuals who have special histories and life experiences.

- Understanding the various theories of aging can promote a more positive attitude toward the process of aging. Three physiological theories of aging include genetic factors, wear and tear, and nutritional factors. The three psychological theories are developmental task theory, subculture theory, and continuity theory.

- Normal aging changes each person in a unique way. Nurses should embrace the attitude that all older adults are unique and should be encouraged to function at their full potential. Outcomes should be adjusted as appropriate for each individual.
- The cardiovascular system loses its efficiency with age; however, most older adults are able to effectively compensate. Due to the changes in the respiratory system, older adults are more prone to respiratory infections.
- Because of changes in the musculoskeletal system, older adults experience changes in range of motion and slowed movement. Age-related changes to the integumentary system lead to thinning of hair, age spots, loss of skin elasticity, and a decrease in subcutaneous fat.
- Changes in the GI system lead to weakened gag reflex, decrease in emptying time, and a decrease in peristalsis. Aging changes the urinary system by causing loss of muscle tone in the bladder, increased frequency of urination, and decreased renal blood flow.
- The reproductive system is also affected by the aging process. For women, vaginal secretions decrease and breast tissue atrophies. For men, testes atrophy and the prostate can enlarge.
- Age-related changes to the nervous system include decrease in reaction time, increased night wakening, and progressive loss of brain mass. The special sense organs such as the eyes and ears are also affected by aging. Older adults lose their ability to focus on close objects and night vision decreases. The ability to hear high-frequency tones decreases.

Review Questions

1. Your client is 84 years old. What normal change in vital signs would you expect to assess?
   1. A higher than normal temperature
   2. A slower pulse
   3. A shallower breathing pattern
   4. A lower blood pressure

2. Immobility or sedentary lifestyles have what effect on the older adult?
   1. Loss of muscle size and strength
   2. Decreased serum sodium levels
   3. Loss of skin elasticity
   4. Thinning of cartilage in joints

3. Mrs. Jones, aged 86 years, complains of fullness after eating only small amounts of food. This is primarily due to which GI change?
   1. Delayed gastric emptying time
   2. Increased gastric acid secretions
   3. Hypertonicity of gastric muscles
   4. Loss of ability to chew

4. Mrs. Smith, aged 79 years, is admitted to the hospital. Based on your understanding of normal age changes in the nervous system, what behavior might you expect Mrs. Smith to exhibit?
   1. Decreased intellectual function
   2. Forgetfulness and confusion
   3. Lack of orientation to time and place
   4. Longer response time to questions

5. Which of the following statements most accurately describes normal aging changes in an older adult?
   1. As individuals age, they become more diverse.
   2. Most older adults experience chronic illness and functional impairment.
   3. Age-related changes are similar in each older adult.
   4. Normal age changes most commonly describe decline and loss of function.

ANSWERS 1. 2, 2. 1, 3. 1, 4. 4, 5. 1

CHAPTER 3
Supporting Life Transitions and Spirituality

Diane Leggett-Fife

KEY TERMS

progressively lowered stress threshold
   model
religion
self-transcendence
spirituality
stressor
stressors
transition

CHAPTER CONCEPTS

Collaboration
Communication
Culture
Ethics
Grief and Loss
Health Promotion
Patient-Centered Care
Spirituality
Stress

LEARNING OUTCOMES

1. Discuss the significance of transitions and spirituality in the lives of older individuals.
2. Describe what a transition is and its impact on people.
3. List four to six activities the nurse can perform that will facilitate a successful transitional outcome.
4. Define how the "progressively lowered stress threshold" concept can assist in the management of negative behaviors in older adults.
5. Recommend three transitions common to older adults.
6. Compare and contrast spirituality and religion.

CASE STUDY

Akbar Tahan is a 79-year-old male who came from the Middle East with his wife 50 years ago. He is an actively practicing Muslim and has been living at home since the death of his wife from breast cancer 6 months ago. He has a son who lives in another state and a daughter who lives an 8-hour drive from her father. The children call their father at least once a week to check on him and have tried to find a neighbor to also check on him. Since the death of his wife, he has become less social and has begun refusing visitors. His daughter became concerned when a neighbor called telling her he had seen her father wandering in the backyard, looking confused.

She immediately drove to his house and on arrival found her father disoriented, feverish, and unable to clearly answer questions. She quickly took him to an emergency room where he was diagnosed with dehydration and a urinary tract infection. He was admitted and started on antibiotics. His daughter requested to stay with him.

CASE STUDY—cont'd

During the late evening hours, the daughter informed the staff she was taking a walk. Shortly after that, a noise was heard from the room, and the staff entered to find Mr. Tahan on the floor by his bed, crying in pain and attempting to say prayers. He had some minor abrasions on his arm, but an x-ray revealed a fractured right hip.

Following the surgical repair, Mr. Tahan was placed on a soft diet. When the first tray of food arrived, the certified nursing assistant (CNA) held the tray in her left hand while clearing the overbed table with her right hand. She then placed the tray on the table with her left hand. The daughter looked at the tray and told the CNA that the chopped ham sandwich is unacceptable, and her father will not eat anything served with the left hand.

That evening a female nurse entered the room and told Mr. Tahan she was there to get him out of bed. He refused until his daughter was called into the room.

The next day you are assigned to his care. He is slightly agitated and wants to know what is happening and where his things have been taken. He is taken to physical therapy by a male assistant but refuses any treatment because the only therapist there is female and he does not have a family member with him. You are able to locate the daughter and request that she bring some personal items such as pictures and his book of scriptures to help him feel more comfortable. You also talk to the physical therapy department and set up a time when the daughter can be with him.

1. Why was Mr. Tahan attempting to get on the floor to pray? How will you assist in meeting his needs at this time?
2. Why did the daughter refuse to let her father have the foods brought to the room? What information will be necessary to address the nutritional needs of this patient?
3. Why did Mr. Tahan refuse to participate in getting out of bed and physical therapy? How can you assist in addressing this problem?
4. Consider all three problems and determine what you, as the nurse, could do to help Mr. Tahan in his recovery.

INTRODUCTION

With today's harried workloads in health-care environments, you, the licensed practical nurse (LPN), may think that there is not enough time to deal with the issues of transition and **spirituality** (the belief in something more powerful than oneself). There are too many medications, too many treatments, and definitely too much paperwork! In addition, there are not enough licensed nurses and too many budget cuts. It is challenging and difficult for this generation of nurses to be able to deliver humanistic (vs mechanistic) care. Transitions are a consistent part of life, however. Think of Mr. Tahan, who had faced several transitions and was demonstrating frustration from not having personal needs met. Even the choice to be a more humanistic, holistic nurse requires a transitional period, during which time the nurse needs to work out the details of how to treat older individuals in a more caring and holistic manner, while still fulfilling all of his or her responsibilities on time. This chapter will assist you in understanding transitions and spirituality so that you can learn to incorporate holistic care into your daily practice.

SIGNIFICANCE OF TRANSITIONS AND SPIRITUALITY

Whatever your age, you have experienced a lifetime of **transitions**, which are the moments between what was old and what is new. Think of the times you have been driving and enter an area with heavy fog. You find yourself searching for something to help guide you when little can be seen ahead. Your mind races to remember familiar landmarks, and you find yourself slowing down from a feeling of uncertainty. This change creates stress and moments of transition.

You experienced transitions after you chose to attend school. The need to pay for school, arrange child care, complete housework and/or schoolwork, and maintain a part-time job are some possible challenges that you faced during the transition. Do you remember the stressful feelings you had until you worked out the details successfully? That period of stress and the unknown was the transitional period. You eventually resolved the stress of the changes and became a successful student.

Youth is a period of constant growth and learning. A child learns to ambulate by first crawling, then standing up, and then walking; the child may then learn to ride a tricycle and then a bicycle. All of these instances involve periods of uncertainty as the child learns the new skill. Adults, too, experience transitions as they commit to an education and career, a spouse, and possibly children.

As people reach older adulthood, there is still much to learn and many new skills to master; however, it is also a time when more of life's changes include loss. Children leave their parents' home for work, school, or adventure, among other choices. One's parents may die, and siblings or friends may move or succumb to accident or disease. Retirement is a big change for most people, resulting in a loss of work friends, income, and often social position. As people age, some develop the chronic diseases of normal aging and other diseases, such as heart disease, diabetes mellitus, or a debilitating stroke that results in physical and emotional losses.

Many of the life occurrences that accompany aging are challenging experiences, and all of them require older adults to make a life transition. No one experiences only one transition in a lifetime, and sometimes there is more than one transition at a time. Each loss or change requires transitional effort from the person experiencing it. Think of Mr. Tahan and the transitions he has faced: the loss of his wife, living alone, and now the loss of independence and some mobility. All of these required transitional effort on his part.

Another example is a young-old friend who lives out of state, who called me recently. She had fallen while attempting to do yardwork. Although she lives alone, a neighbor noticed that she was lying in her front yard crying with pain. She was found to have a broken wrist and a sprained rotator cuff (shoulder). Her wrist was put into a brace, her arm was placed in a sling, and she was instructed to see an orthopedic surgeon that upcoming Monday. On Sunday, she had so much pain in one of her teeth that she had an emergency root canal (I am not making this up!). She is a strong woman who has lived her life well. When I talked to her this morning, however, she was feeling despair. The changes she was dealing with were major and painful, and she was managing them alone. She needed assistance to move through the changes: someone kind who would keep her informed, provide honest hope regarding her situation, and care for her as the total person she is rather than the crying older woman she appeared to be. Humanistic health-care providers can assist her and people like her through this transition.

Now let us consider how spirituality fits into the concept of transition. *Spirituality* is often part of the process of transition for older people. Most people have a belief in God, the Divine, or a greater power. With this belief, there is a connection with something more powerful than oneself. When individuals have this connection, it links them to others with a similar belief. It also can be a link to nature or to familiar rituals and behaviors. Spirituality is comforting for many people and can provide a method for understanding the losses that they are experiencing.

Spirituality can also provide the purpose for moving forward, for accepting and adapting to the losses that are occurring, and for finding the strength to deal with one's life changes. This ability to "move on" results in an improved quality of life and death. Returning to my friend who had fallen in her yard, she is a very religious person. I know that she would want to see a clergyman and would appreciate someone to pray with her. I realize that you may not believe in God and may not pray. If that is the case, as her nurse you could offer to sit with her while she prays, and you could offer to call the clergyman. Because her religious beliefs have helped her through previous transitions in her life, she will benefit from them again. Accepting and accommodating a person's spirituality to the best of one's ability is one of the many ways a holistic nurse can help a person through a transition. Think of Mr. Tahan and the solutions offered for his care relating to his spirituality. The nurse recognized that he was in a hospital trying to practice his religion. With this information, the nurse asked the family how to help him meet his prayer needs, how the food should be prepared and served, and took time to listen to the patient and the daughter as a caring nurse.

THINK LIKE A NURSE

You have been assigned care of a 70-year-old patient recently admitted for repair of a fractured ulna on the right side. She was given pain medication in the emergency department before being transferred to your care. She does not have family with her at this time and reports that all her family lives out of state. She has been working from home typing reports for a company. She has voiced concern about being able to care for herself and continuing her part-time work for income because she is right-handed. What would be some physical and transitional priorities for this patient?

Responses

- The developmental stage for this patient is to maintain integrity (see Eric Erickson's stages of development in Chapter 2). Communication with and for the patient is key to identifying and meeting the patient's needs. This will be especially important since she does not have family members with her.
- Physical priorities should include pain management to prevent feelings of hopelessness, physical therapy consultation to address changes in mobility and use of the right arm, and occupational therapy consultation to assist in the transition to home from the facility.
- Transitional care priorities would include communication with all health-care providers involved in the care and any family members or significant others (neighbors or friends) who will be assisting in the care. This communication should address available services to be accessed, should provide consistent information to those involved in the care across the continuum, and should be leveled according to the educational level of the patient. The patient needs to feel that needs are and will be met throughout the time of recovery. Remember to include the patient in deciding who should receive this communication.

UNDERSTANDING TRANSITIONS

Ralph Waldo Emerson, a poet, essayist, and philosopher who is described as belonging to the tradition of "wisdom literature," commented, "Not in all his goals but in his transitions, man is great" (Emerson, 1860). Emerson understood change and its powerful impact on the life quest for individuals. Transitions are significant, universal human experiences. Because transitions are interconnected with the growth of the person and, consequently, the world, understanding transitions has rich significance for your personal and professional life and your practice of human caring.

As a holistic nurse, your objective is to assist the older person in your care to be successful in making the transition and managing the stress. Doing so alleviates despair and promotes integrity for the individual,

and it achieves your objective of excellent caregiving. Most people have experienced a critical transition; if you assist people in remembering the behaviors that were helpful to them in the past, they can use those behaviors again to help them through the transition that they are currently facing.

Common Transitions

High school graduation, sudden loss of a job, marriage, significant illness, death of a loved one, pregnancy, divorce, and relocation to a new home are some of the life events you may have experienced. These events are marked by beginnings and endings and a new phase of life change (the time driving in the fog). Joy and celebration at a transition are common, although some transitional events result in a deep sense of loss and sadness. Whether pleasant, painful, anticipated, unexpected, temporary, or permanent, all transitions, by their nature, evoke some degree of stress.

Patients often face health-illness transitions, which occur when changes in health status result in a change in role relations, expectations, and abilities. Multiple transitions occurring simultaneously are common and particularly challenging. For example, a health-illness transition precipitated by a severe stroke can require a person to relocate to a hospital, which could be followed by a second or even third relocation to a nursing home or rehabilitation center. In addition, there are the physical losses from the stroke: perhaps the loss of one's job and social role as the breadwinner. Dependence on others often is a difficult transition for most people to make.

The time span of a complex transition, such as having a stroke, extends from the first anticipation of transition until a sense of stability in the new situation has been achieved. A transitional period can last weeks or months, which indicates the critical need for nursing staff to know and understand the concept of transition. Only by understanding can the nurse be therapeutic.

Priority Setting

The priority for this chapter is to help you understand your own personal transitions. It is only through personal experience that a person can successfully and sincerely apply what is learned to assist others in transition. Examine your own life and critically consider what has happened to you in terms of transitions, and then learn to identify your personal strengths. How did you manage your last three transitions? Were they effective coping skills? What would assist you in the future? When you understand this concept on a personal level, you will be able to apply it to older individuals. Remember, you also want to achieve the highest level described by Maslow, which is self-transcendence so now is a good time to begin working toward it (Personality & Spirituality, n.d.).

Four Common Features of Transitions

Transitions are significant, life-altering experiences. They are processes of change that are lasting in their effects; they force one to give up how they view the world, and they necessitate the development of new thinking and skills. Transitions generally cause great emotion and require the person experiencing the transition to work hard to survive the change. Transitions warrant the attention of health-care professionals.

CRITICALLY EXAMINE THE FOLLOWING

Think back to your most difficult transition. How did you feel? What assisted you to manage the transition? Take the time to make a list of the people, activities, or thoughts that assisted you to persevere while driving in the fog.

According to researchers (Davies, 2005; Jungers, 2010), there are four common features to transition:

1. A phase of turmoil
2. Disturbances in bodily function
3. Mood and cognition changes
4. An altered time perspective

These four characteristics are commonly seen in older adults in health-care facilities. Have you ever encountered an older person who was in a state of turmoil, unable to control bowel or bladder, seemed confused, and did not know the time or date? Disorientation could indicate that a person has a mental illness or dementia; a loss in bodily function is expected when someone has a stroke; and time confusion is something that happens to people who are no longer tied to work schedules or routines.

So are these characteristics being exhibited because of illness or because of transition? All of these behaviors demonstrate a change for the person experiencing them, and so they are due to transitions. As a nurse, you can play a strong role in assisting a person to make sense of the change and to manage it with minimal symptoms. The objective is integrity vs despair. With your thoughtful application of transition theory, you can assist the older people in your care to achieve integrity and improve their quality of life and death.

HOW TO INFLUENCE A TRANSITIONAL OUTCOME

You can influence the outcome of transitions for elderly people. The following factors influence transitional outcomes:

1. Degree of choice in the transitional process
2. Extent or degree of change
3. Preparation for the change
4. Characteristics of the individual experiencing the transition
5. The individual's perception of the change
6. The characteristics of the prechange and postchange environment, including support systems (American Psychological Association, 2018; Jungers, 2010; Ryan & Deci, 2000).

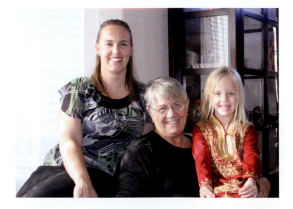

The moments of our lives combine to make a lifetime of transitions. This picture of a grandmother, mother, and daughter is symbolic of that concept.

Let's examine these influences and see how nurses can use these influences to help ease older people into necessary transitions.

Give People a Degree of Choice and Respect Their Decisions

People who think they have freely chosen the transition are more likely to embrace it or own it. Think of the differences between your decision to come to LPN school and the fact that you "had" to go to high school. Choice is an essential part of being human, and it should be honored and respected.

I spent some time as a consultant at a large (700-bed) nursing home on the East Coast. While I was there, I learned some valuable lessons. The most profound lesson that I learned occurred on the very large Alzheimer's unit. Everyone, and I mean *everyone*, included the residents in the decision making. For example, a resident refused his medication, and the polite and caring nurse agreed with the decision and came back within 10 minutes and tried again (successfully). She understood that the resident had the right to refuse any treatment, had the need to have some control over his life, and that—within just a few minutes—may forget that he refused the medication and might be amenable to taking it later. When the housekeeper asked to clean a resident's room and was told no, the decision-making authority to the resident was respected and the housekeeper did not go in, but returned when the resident was not in the room. The housekeeper accepted the negative answer, but did not neglect professional responsibility. Everything was done, just at a slightly later time.

Evidence-Based Practice

Jeffs, L., Kuluski, K., Law, M., Saragosa, M., Espin, S., Ferris, E., … Bell, C. M. (2017). Identifying effective nurse-led care transition interventions for older adults with complex needs using a structured expert panel. *Worldviews on Evidence-Based Nursing, 14*(2), 136–144.

This study used a consensus-focus research design to identify the most effective nurse-led care transition interventions for the complex older adult population. Twenty-three experts in care transitions and patient care were chosen for the panel. Five high-ranking interventions were identified as the most effective at decreasing readmissions, emergency room visits, medication errors, delays in care, and an increase in the cost of care for this population. These interventions included education for all involved in care of the patient, making sure all instructions were understood, using comprehensive communication with standard tools for documentation, fully using nurses' scope of practice for the transitions, and having organizations with strong leadership and accountability for transitions. Older adult care transitions are complex and have poorer outcomes than other care transitions. The use of the identified nurse-led transitions can lead to improved outcomes, but there may be difficulty incorporating them into all organizations.

Questions

Which of the following inferences can you make? State whether the study summary provides extensive, limited, or no evidence to support each inference.

1. Older adults with complex care needs complicate care transitions.
2. Older adults transitioning to other care facilities will benefit from nurses using their full scope of practice.
3. Nurse-led care transition interventions improve patient outcomes.
4. Individuals involved in the care of the older adult should receive education regarding present care and continuation of care.
5. Organizational leadership needs to take responsibility for transition of care with the older adult population.

Mr. Tahan was unable to participate in many of the decisions regarding his care because of the situation. As a nurse, if you realize the importance of the desire to have some degree of choice in decisions, you would have been able to offer him something as simple as choosing the foods for the meal. If he and the daughter had been included in the physical therapy participation appointment decision, the staff would have understood his cultural needs and he may have been willing to negotiate.

Make the Extent or Degree of Change More Manageable

Transitions can be made smoother if the apparent obstacles are removed and the changes are manageable. A family asking their aging mother to relocate from a rural farmhouse to a city apartment to be closer to health-care services would require their mother to make a huge change, which would be very disruptive for the older woman. To ease their mother into the transition, a family member who lives in the city could invite her to stay for either a long weekend or a 2-week period so that she could get a feel for city life. Additionally, when the family members find an apartment that meets the physical requirements necessary for their mother, they could verify that there are people near their mother's age who live in or around the complex. Is there a senior citizen center nearby where she can participate in activities with newly made friends? Is there a grocery store that is within walking distance? These are thoughtful considerations of a loving family that would make their mother's transition easier. They represent humanistic caring rather than mechanistic caring. The mechanistic solution would be to find an apartment that meets the location and safety needs of the mother, while doing nothing to make the transition less stressful. Which approach would you like someone to use with you?

Another example of humanistic caring would be the nurse's willingness to negotiate care with Mr. Tahan. Asking the daughter to bring some personal items to the facility to help in the adjustment of the change may also help Mr. Tahan in his transition.

Help Prepare People for the Transition

Although preparation for a transition is something logical to do, reflect on how often people fail to prepare for a transition even though it is expected. Consider a person who receives a diagnosis of a chronic disease like diabetes. This individual needs to know what to expect and how this disease will impact his or her life to start the transition process. Death is something we all will experience, and yet it seems difficult for people in our society to discuss it and plan for it. Psychologists often say that the closer a family is, the easier it is to discuss the topic. When transitions are identified as part of one's future, preparation is a key factor in being able to manage them.

Talk to your patients and residents about changes that are anticipated. Give them all of the appropriate information and be willing to repeat it as often as necessary. You should involve the family members as well. Use your creative thinking and do all you can for each individual to prepare him or her for changes that are coming.

Consider the Characteristics of the Individual

Transitions can be threatening to persons who are cognitively impaired or who require a high degree of structure and predictability in their environments. Research has shown that relocating people who are mentally ill or confused is associated with higher death rates compared with people with similar impairments who are not moved. Some people who are cognitively intact don't deal well with change, either. It is common for people to fear or avoid change.

A person's personality, past experiences, and coping skills are important factors to consider when helping that person through a transition. Generally, being in good health increases resiliency during stressful times (American Psychological Association, 2018; Sapolsky, 2004). Adequate sleep, nutrition, exercise, and satisfying social relationships are also important to transitional outcomes.

When considering past experiences and coping skills, think back to Mr. Tahan. He had lost his wife only 6 months earlier, had been alone at home, and now was facing another major transition. The nurse took the time to talk to both him and his daughter to discover what coping skills he had used previously.

Learn How the Person Perceives the Transition

All of us create meaning and give our experiences labels. Different individuals can view the same transition as an opportunity, blessing, crisis, challenge, or disaster. Use your communication skills to listen to how a person perceives a transition and gain insight into the unique meanings that are attached to it for the person. It is dangerous to assume that you know what someone is thinking. It is better to invite personal reflection on the transition and accept that there are differences in the way people think.

CRITICALLY EXAMINE THE FOLLOWING

Think back to your decision to go to school. What fears did you experience? Were there changes that you tried to avoid? Now think of an older adult in your life, either someone to whom you have given care or someone who is a friend or family member who has recently experienced a transition. Did you recognize their fears or resistance at the time? Do you see them now? They are there even if you did not recognize them.

Remember the example of the woman who needed to move to the city from her farm? It is possible that she would love to be closer to her grandchildren, that she is excited about being near a wider variety of stores for shopping, and that she recognizes that she needs to be closer to health-care services.

Taking time to talk to individuals, as the nurse did with Mr. Tahan and his daughter, provides valuable information to assist both you as the nurse and the individual with the transition. It is important to listen and, as mentioned, not assume you know what is going to be said. Listening is how you will learn about the individual.

Help Improve Environmental Characteristics

We all live in an environment with its variable aspects. When you walk onto a unit in a hospital or nursing home, can you sense what the environment really is like? I am not talking about cleanliness or colorful or drab decoration schemes, although they are important for a healing environment. I am referring to aspects of the environment such as cheerfulness, relaxation, nurturance, and respectfulness. These environmental components are the opposite of harsh, demanding, restrictive, and joyless environments. In caregiving situations, nurses have the power to co-create, with the older adults, healing environments that are loving, empowering, and respectful. Remember the personal items the nurse requested the daughter to bring to the hospital for Mr. Tahan? Seeing the familiar pictures of friends and family will provide renewed hope to work on recovery.

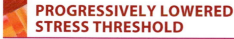

PROGRESSIVELY LOWERED STRESS THRESHOLD

The **progressively lowered stress threshold (PLST)** is a care concept (Hall & Buckwalter, 1987) designed to be used when planning personalized, holistic care for older individuals. The concept of PLST originates from the importance of personal freedom and control. According to the PLST theory, dysfunctional or negative behaviors in humans often occur because of increased anxiety. If people perceive that they have lost their personal freedom or their control

over a situation because of an increasing amount of outside **stressors** (anything causing stress), they can become anxious and stressed, which leads to frustration and anger.

A classic example with which most people are familiar is getting children to eat their vegetables. Imagine a scene at the family dinner table when parents tell their children to eat their vegetables. By telling the children to do something, the children's personal freedom and control are taken away. Generally, this situation results in a power struggle (note: *no one* wins in a power struggle) and in the end, the children not eating their vegetables.

An older person's freedom is restricted during the time he or she resides in a health-care facility. In hospitals and nursing homes, meals are generally served at set times, and baths are given at the convenience of the staff rather than of the patient or resident. No one is encouraged to stay up late and watch or read a good mystery! There are rules in health-care facilities, and they usually are enforced.

When people have limited control over their life, there is a higher likelihood that stress will occur. With unresolved stress comes frustration, and unresolved frustration leads to anger (Lease, Ingram, & Brown, 2017; Sapolsky, 2004). That is a normal human reaction. What does anger look like? It is different for every person because of individual personality traits, but it can include raising one's voice, screaming, hitting, or a high level of criticism of the environment and the people in it. If you perceive that the reason behind the anger is stress because of lack of control, you can apply your understanding of PLST to your practice and work at giving the people in your care as much personal control over their lives as is safe for them.

CRITICALLY EXAMINE THE FOLLOWING

Take some time and think back to any recent experience when you were told what to do. How did you feel? Did it make you feel like a child? That is the feeling that comes to me. I like suggestions, interesting information, even metaphors, but I do not like being told what to do. I have learned over the years how to handle this feeling so that a situation does not degenerate into a power struggle, but I still have to take time to consider my reaction.

Write a brief paragraph regarding how you feel when someone imposes on your personal freedom. Note how you handle being told what to do and what your thought processes are regarding it. Then consider how your feelings compare with those of any older person with whom you have had experience. Does the older adult like being told what to do? How does he or she handle the situation? Be prepared to share your ideas in class either verbally or by handing in the paragraph.

Common Stressors

Five common stressors that tend to result in the highest levels of stress for older persons are:

1. Fatigue
2. Change in environment, routine, or caregiver
3. Misleading or inappropriate stimuli (sounds or noise are examples)
4. Internal or external demands to achieve that exceed one's functional ability
5. Physical stressors such as pain, discomfort, infection, acute illness, or depression (Hall & Buckwalter, 1987)

I am sure that you can immediately see the relationship between transition and these five stressors. It is like the "perfect storm." Changing living environments is tiring (stressor 1), and it is a dramatic change in environment, routine, and caregiver (stressor 2). The person going through the transition may have great expectations from self to "do well" so as not to worry "my daughter/son" or to assure a return to one's home (stressor 4). Deteriorating health or a new illness (stressor 5) may be the very reason the older person was moved.

With this basic information on PLST, do you see how transitions and most other stressors will, in all likelihood, result in the older person showing signs of stress? Even under ideal circumstances, most of us would feel the effects of stress; thus this is something that needs to be recognized as a reality in giving care to susceptible older people.

Application of Progressively Lowered Stress Threshold

Your objective, each day you go to work, is to decrease the stress of the persons in your care. This often includes the CNAs and other people in your work environment. Settle disputes among the staff, keep noise levels low, provide places of rest for older people in the facility to avoid fatigue, and expect stress-related behavior to occur.

When such behavior does occur, don't be upset and get involved in the problem. Instead, use your knowledge, and work to eliminate the stress. Perhaps taking an older gentleman who is angry and combative off the unit for a "special walk" with you will remove him from what is upsetting him. Try to find out what is the **stressor** for any person who is acting stressed, and involve the other members of the health-care team in correcting the problem.

Remember the initial premise of the PLST model. It is to give as much control as possible to the individuals in your care. After all, they are adults who are accustomed to making their own decisions, and, in most situations, they should be allowed to continue. This premise requires the entire health-care team to understand and agree to provide such an environment.

Transition is challenging, and being older can be difficult. The role of the LPN is to do everything possible to make these realities less stressful and enhance the quality of daily life for older adults.

Read the poem on the next page. It is charming and meaningful. Read the poem to enjoy it, and then read it again to look for the impact of transition and PLST on human life.

Point of Interest

I remember a cold and snowy winter afternoon in Utah. My daughter, one of her friends, and I were traveling in the car. The girls were laughing and playing noisy games in the backseat, the radio was blaring something I didn't recognize, and, unbeknownst to me, the temperature was falling. I recognized the fall in temperature the moment my tires started to slide on the newly formed ice into a monstrous snowdrift on the side of the road. If I corrected the slide, I would head into the oncoming traffic. I was stressed!

Within a brief second my entire personality changed. I turned off both the heater and the radio, I literally yelled at the girls to be quiet, and then miraculously (or so it seemed to me) I was able to stop the car with minor damage caused by the snowdrift. When the initial stress was over, I spoke with great concern and tenderness to the girls, turned the heater back on, and got out my cell phone to get the help I needed.

Why did my behavior change so abruptly? It was because of the stress. Without thinking, I turned off the radio and heater because they were stressors to me. Much to my chagrin, I yelled at the girls because their noise was a stressor as well. Then, with less external stress, I could handle the immediate situation.

Have you seen exasperated mothers of young children raise their voice at them in a store? A man swearing out loud because of a flat tire? Two children or two adults hitting each other? I observe that they usually are exhibiting such behavior because they are stressed. Relate the concept of stress and the resulting behavior to yourself. Once you understand how it affects you, you will have a better understanding of how and why it makes a big impact on older people, who often have fewer physiological resources.

Sunshine Acres Living Center
Marilyn Krysl, RN

The first thing you see up ahead is
Mr. Polanski,
wedged in the arched doorway,
like he means absolutely
to stay there; he shouldn't
be there in the first place, put here
by mistake, courtesy of that grandson
who thinks he's a hotshot, and too busy
raking in the dough to take time
for an old man.
If he had any place to go, you know he'd
be out instantly, if he had any money.
So he intends to stay in that doorway,
not missing a thing, and waiting for trouble.
Which of course will come.
And that could be you—you're handy, you look
likely, you have the authority. And you're
new here, another young whippersnapper,
doesn't know ankle from elbow, but has
been given the keys.
Well, he's ready, Mr. Polanski. So you go right
to him. "Mr. Polanski, good morning." You

say it in Polish, which you learned a little of
when you were little, and your grandmother
taught you a little song about lambs, frisking
in a pen, and you danced a silly dance with
your grandmother while the two of you sang.
So you sing it for him in the dim, institutional
light of the hallway, light which even you find
insupportable, because at that moment
it reminds you of the light in the hallway
in the rest home where, when your
grandmother died, you weren't there.
So you're also singing to console yourself.
And at the moment you pay her this silly
little tribute.
Mr. Polanski steps out of the doorway. He
who had set himself to resist you, he who
made himself a first, Mr. Polanski,
contentious
often combative
and always inconsolable
hears that you know the song. And he
steps out
from the fortress of the doorway, begins to
shuffle
and sing along.

This poem captures many aspects of human relationships and struggles. You may want to discuss your insights about the poem's message with fellow students or family members. As an LPN, you will have many opportunities to meet people like Mr. Polanski.

Understanding the mediating factors of control and decision-making, preparation, support, meaning and perception, and maintaining optimal health will assist you in your own transitions as well as in supporting and caring for older people.

COMMON TRANSITIONS FOR OLDER ADULTS

Transitions occur at every stage of life. It is important to examine the transitions that commonly occur in the lives of older adults to anticipate them and develop the knowledge base to be supportive when they occur. As you know, not all transitions happen for everyone, but some can be anticipated because of their frequency in the aging process. Job changes and retirement, family role changes, and health changes are common impetuses for transitions that occur with individuals as they age.

Job Changes and Retirement

Job changes and retirement can have a dramatic impact on the aging population. Common changes include the following:

1. *Role change.* When an older person retires, the role change can be a very difficult transition. The person retiring has to adjust to the loss of what was their purpose and position for 8 or more hours a day.
2. *Lower income.* A retiree's income often is decreased. This can be the cause of several other changes. Health care can be reduced because of the financial need to maintain the house or replace a furnace. Good nutrition may be impacted because of the expense of essential medication. Plans of traveling or other leisure activities may have to be cancelled.
3. *Dissatisfaction with employment status.* Older adults generally were raised with a strong work ethic and believe that unemployment is an unacceptable situation whatever the cause.
4. *Unpreparedness for the future.* Many people do not prepare for their eventual retirement. They have not developed interests outside of work, prepared financially for a decreased income, or nurtured their dreams. Without preparation, retirement can be fraught with profound losses for the individual.
5. *Loss of identity.* For some people, the loss of their job, with retirement or other factors, threatens their identity. Most people derive their identity from the work they have done throughout their lifetime. Be it mother, physician, teacher, or nurse, part of who we are rests solidly on what we do. When that crucial role is gone, it is a struggle to redefine one's personal identity, and that struggle is not always successful.
6. *Lack of social interaction.* Someone who has been focused on their work setting often has many friends there. With retirement comes a separation from those people. This can be a serious transition unless the retiree has maintained relationships outside of work. Without friends to join in social activities, life can be very lonely.

Family Role Changes

Family roles and relationships change as each of us age. Common changes in old age are the following:

1. *Grandparenting.* Because of the aging of America, more people experience grandparenting, and many are able to enjoy this phase of life longer than ever before in U.S. history. There can be serious transitional concerns, however, with the various roles grandparenting can take.
2. *Distant family members.* Adult children move out of the house, and many are scattered throughout the United States or the world. Older people of today frequently were raised with the responsibility to build their adult lives in a location near their parents to promote family closeness and to care for their aging parents. Today's grandparents often have to adjust to not seeing children and grandchildren as frequently as they would like, and they may not be able to count on adult children to assist them to remain in their homes as they age.
3. *Parenting for parents.* Some grandparents are assisting single parents by providing child care or are tending children while both parents work, while others may be grandparenting full time. For many older adults, this can be too much responsibility in the day-to-day activities of their children and grandchildren.
4. *Role crisis.* Parents eventually die. In some situations, the illness and death are lingering, which requires the caregiver to be part of what is known as the "sandwich generation." This role often goes to women. The sandwich generation caregiver is a person who is raising children while caring for aging parents. As this person ages, the children leave the home, and the parents die. This can cause a role crisis because there is no one left who needs the "sandwiched" person.
5. *Death of spouse.* The death of a spouse is more common as people age. It is an event that has a dramatic impact on all aspects of life for the surviving partner. When an older spouse dies, the survivor has lost the person with whom he or she has spent most of his or her life. The intimacy that was shared is gone as is the help, understanding, and often part of the income. Their experiences together can be the most significant happenings that have occurred during their lifetime. With the deceased person go dreams, plans for the future, and a lifelong companion. The loss can be intolerable.
6. *Insufficient income.* More women than men experience the death of a spouse. Because of their age, many older women may not have worked outside of the home or left their profession to raise a

family and are poorly prepared to supplement their income. Their life role generally has been focused on their spouse and children. These women end up alone, without the income they need, and with fewer friends because most of their previous friends were couples. If their children and grandchildren are living in other states, the situation is even more difficult because they are truly alone.

Health Changes

Health changes are complex concerns for older adults. They can affect every system in the body and cause a change in one's health that has a life-altering impact. Some common health changes are as follows:

1. *Illness and disability.* These health changes are major reasons why older adults need assistance and support. It is estimated that 60% to 70% of the population in the United States over the age of 60 is living with at least two chronic diseases. These chronic diseases lead to disabilities that limit doing yard work or housework (National Council on Aging, 2018; Office of Disease Prevention and Health Promotion, 2018). This may extend to cooking as well. Along with the disappointment over what they are unable to do, older adults with disabilities often worry about being placed in an institution such as a nursing home or assisted living facility. The overall fear is the loss of independence.
2. *Acute diseases.* It could be the flu or pneumonia, a heart attack, or some type of infection. Regardless, older adults often do not have the strength to fight acute illnesses as they did when they were younger. The immune system commonly is weaker because of aging (Merck Manual, 2018). Each winter, numerous older people die of complications from influenza because their bodies are no longer strong enough to mount an adequate defense against the disease.
3. *Body image.* Adjusting to a new body image is another challenge of growing older. There may be disability and pain from arthritis that interfere with routine activities such as cooking or walking. The older body gains weight and becomes shorter, hair color changes, and vision and hearing diminish. There are also changes related to acute and chronic diseases. All of these conditions can cause an altered body image or lower one's self-esteem.
4. *Longer physiologic response time.* The aging body does not work as efficiently as it once did. Fatigue is often a daily occurrence along with decreased memory function and slower response time (Delves, 2018; Mauk, 2014).

It is important for you to keep these transitional situations in mind as you care for older people. For example, even if you have seen numerous people put into wheelchairs because of the pain and danger of arthritis, remember that it is each person's first time doing so. During the transition, there is fear and concern on the part of the older adult and the need for support and understanding from you. Preparing yourself to assist people through the transition is a critical aspect of giving holistic nursing care.

SIGNIFICANCE OF SPIRITUALITY

In the lifelong search for integrity versus despair, spirituality has a significant role. Most people feel they are part of something very important when a spiritual bond connects them to others. There is a commonality in belief and understanding of the universe. The belief system often provides a social system as well. These aspects of spirituality are supportive to someone going through one or several transitions.

Religion and Spirituality

There is a difference between religion and spirituality. **Religion** is the organized practice of one's belief regarding God or a higher power. Most religions have a formal building for worship and prescribed actions (prayer) or practices (partaking of sacraments or communion). Some religions worship personages other than a God or simply believe in a divine power. Religion is an organized practice whereas *spirituality* is the feeling within that communicates to individuals there is a higher power at work in the universe. Many spiritual people do not belong to a religion but practice beliefs they feel strongly about regarding a higher power (Fontaine, 2011; Taylor, 2002).

Humans, by their nature, are spiritual. It is the part of being human that seeks meaning through some type of connection such as with nature or with other humans (Gallardo-Peralta, 2017; Taylor, 2002). This makes awareness of and concern for another's spiritual and religious needs a significant aspect of nursing care. Being supportive while sharing and participating in a person's spiritual beliefs is an important aspect of holistic care.

Realizing their connection to something greater than themselves assists all people to rise above their challenges. For older adults, this sense of connection to a greater being is very important because of the numerous losses and transitions they make as they age. Spirituality and the practice of formal religion can assist people to overcome their problems, manage their despair, and find the peace that will help them to accept the change that is occurring (Fontaine, 2011; Gallardo-Peralta, 2017). Spirituality and religion help provide the essential step toward integrity and **self-transcendence** (Personality & Spirituality, n.d.).

Cultural Considerations

It is important to understand that a religion practiced by a group of individuals can also be considered a culture. Many people have immigrated to the United States with groups from their country that practice the same religion. As a health-care provider, you will need to have a basic knowledge of those who have different beliefs or practices than the majority in a facility. If you do not have a basic knowledge, you will need to know where to find the information necessary to treat each person with respect for their beliefs and practices. This will also help you to provide any assistance, equipment, tools, or special items for a patient that can help alleviate stress and improve recovery.

Assessing Spiritual Needs

Assessing people for their spiritual needs and identifying how you can assist in meeting them may be a new skill for you. Most health-care facilities list the religious preference of the person on the chart. That is the place to start. Use your observation skills to identify religious jewelry or other artifacts in the person's personal belongings. Are there religious books in the room such as the Koran, Book of Mormon, or Bible?

The facility where you work may have a spiritual assessment. If not, think about what it is you need to know to be helpful. The information you need should include the following:

1. Does the person belong to a formal religious group? If so, does he or she want the leader of the group or other members to be contacted? Are there special rituals the person would like to have performed, such as a blessing for health, a prayer circle, or something else?
2. You need to know the person's specific spiritual beliefs, so ask. Then inquire if there are any specific practices the person would like to see performed. This may include a Shaman from the Navajo Indian culture, being allowed out of bed to pray on the floor facing east for a Muslim, incense burning, or specific foods. You cannot meet an individual's spiritual needs unless you know what that person believes.
3. When a person in your care is found crying, exhibits depression, or simply does not seem interested in what is going on in the environment, these could be symptoms of spiritual distress. A person may continuously question, "Why is God doing this to me?" or, "What have I done to deserve all of these problems?" Comments of this type often are expressions of an unmet spiritual need.
4. Some people exhibit anger at God or the Divine power because of the severity of the transition that must be made. Loss of basic physical ability because of a severe stroke or unmanageable pain from cancer could be examples. An older adult may feel betrayed by God and express unusual anger. This symptom of unmet spiritual needs should be addressed with understanding and empathy.

Safe, Effective Nursing Care

Respect for Patient Differences, Values, Preferences, and Expressed Needs

Channa Arenson, a 72-year-old woman who practices the Jewish faith, has been admitted to the hospital for pneumonia. She requires oxygen by nasal cannula and has been encouraged to increase her intake of fluids by mouth. She has brought a book that she calls the Hebrew Bible and informed the admitting personnel that it was Passover. You are the nurse assigned to her care for the evening.

At approximately 6 p.m. in the evening, you hear a commotion coming from her room. You enter to find her attempting to climb out of bed, tangled in her oxygen tubing, and mumbling about her head and a shawl. As you try to assist her back to bed, she begins crying and pushing you away. You also notice that her evening meal tray remains untouched, and she refuses to eat anything that is not kosher.

You request assistance to help her back to bed. The individual who comes in to assist has spoken with a family member and informs you of the need for the patient to have her head covered. There is also a desire expressed to allow her to have Passover foods and say prayers with her shawl. With this information, you and the assistant locate her head cover and shawl, then assist her to position herself to pray while making sure the oxygen is still in place. As you help her back to bed after prayers, you notify the primary health-care provider and the dietitian of the patient's desire to follow Passover rituals. You then make a note in the chart of the patient's requests.

- Should the nurse have allowed and/or assisted the patient out of bed? Why or why not?
- How did the nurse and assistant show respect for the preferences of this patient?
- How would you describe the values and needs of this patient?

Resolving Spiritual Needs

Research indicates that a meaningful spiritual or religious practice promotes health and healing in many people (Gallardo-Peralta, 2017; Haber, 2003). Because of this fact alone, you need to strive to identify unmet spiritual needs. When you have identified such needs, determine interventions that will help the older adult in your care. You should do all you can to assist the person to meet the unmet needs. This may require quiet listening, meaningful discussions, and the involvement of outside people from the religious or spiritual groups of the person. Remember the nurse caring for Mr. Tahan and the time she took to work with him to resolve issues of attending physical therapy because of the conflict with religious beliefs. Lack of physical therapy could have impacted his recovery.

To learn what you need to be helpful, you need to *listen attentively*. Ask questions if you do not understand what has been said. Plan time so that you can stay with the person until he or she is through with what he or she wants to say. Then take this new understanding to your nurse manager and, together, identify a way to resolve the spiritual need.

It is essential that you *accept the beliefs* of the person in your care, even if you do not agree with them. Your support of another's belief system is as important as your support when you assist someone to walk. Work with the family and spiritual leaders to provide the spirituality that will assist with comfort and healing.

Provide the people in your care with time alone so that they can participate in religious activities. This time could be spent praying, reading religious or other meaningful books, or meditating in solitude. Solitude is a valuable asset for most spiritual people. Do all you can to provide it for your patients while still caring for their physical needs.

Remember the spiritual need that is expressed with anger toward God or a divine power? It generally is based on the need to make sense of the transition that has occurred. *Do **not** be judgmental* when you hear this anger. Be empathetic, and do all you can to understand the person's point of view. Look at the situation as if you were the person so that you can more readily understand the frustration being expressed. Let's be honest: Some things are not fair, but nevertheless they do happen. Do not join in the anger and do not criticize the anger; rather, listen and make nonjudgmental comments designed to be comforting.

Prayer is a common tool for spiritual people. I realize you may or may not pray; however, if a person in your care requests someone to pray with, please do what you can to assist the person. You might hold a hand or sit near and be reverent during the prayer. If you are uncomfortable with prayer, find a coworker who can assist the person. The objective is to support the person with unmet spiritual needs so that he or she can achieve management of the illness or problems being faced. You play a crucial role in that goal achievement.

Focused Learning Chart: Common Transitions for Elderly Persons

| *Job Changes and Retirement* | *Changes in Family Role* | *Health Changes* | *Spiritual Distress* |

RESOLVING TRANSITIONAL PROBLEMS

At this point, you understand the basics of transitional and spiritual care. I hope that you also understand the importance of meeting the needs that arise based on those concepts. Meeting such needs contributes greatly to improved health, the ability to manage distress, and the all-important objective of achieving integrity and eventually self-transcendence. Self-transcendence allows an older person to live life without regret and to die well, which is something we all would like to achieve. That makes finding a way to implement the resolutions to transitional situations a quality-of-life as well as a quality-of-health issue.

I realize that your workloads are heavy and that fulfilling the medical orders and personal care needs of the individuals to whom you give care is essential for you to do. If you believe in holistic care, however, assisting an older adult who is under the stress of seemingly insurmountable transitions is also essential and needs to be addressed. You may need to talk to your nurse manager and determine if family members or volunteers could be thoroughly oriented to the skills needed to take over that responsibility. If volunteers are used, ensure that there is an effective way for them to communicate with you regarding what they learned. Perhaps the patient or resident mentioned a spiritual person or ritual he or she would like to be with or experience, or perhaps there is a person the patient or resident wronged and wishes to apologize to before death. It is important you learn of the unmet needs so that these can be resolved, if possible.

Life Review

One way to help older people resolve transitional problems and move toward integrity and self-transcendence is life review. Staff members who value the lives of older people are also key to providing holistic care and guidance to aging residents and patients.

The objective of this activity and the activities described subsequently is to assist older people to review their lives and appreciate them. If there are items the older adults feel need to be resolved, life review also gives them that opportunity.

I often hear families complain about having to listen to the same stories over and over again from their aging parent or grandparent. This storytelling is not unhealthy behavior. Instead, it is exactly what the older adult should be doing to achieve integrity.

When health declines and the older person's social system gets smaller, it is healthy to reflect on the accomplishments of one's life. In that reflection, the older person can identify strengths that will assist with current transitions as well as feel the satisfaction of good deeds and good times.

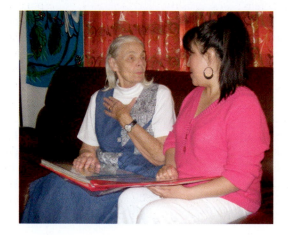

This home health nurse is assisting her patient with reminiscence therapy. Notice how involved the older woman is in telling her story or memory after seeing pictures in her scrapbook.

This crucial behavior requires time from you or others assigned to do life reviews. Volunteers with maturity and a deep sense of responsibility can be taught to do effective reviews.

Sometimes there is an event in life about which the person feels shame and remorse. It may be difficult for you or the volunteer to listen to older persons reveal their mistakes and talk about the people they have hurt. Yet, this information should be shared. Talking about life errors to a kind and attentive listener is therapeutic and should be encouraged. Sometimes referrals to a counselor or therapist should be made. This is a strong reason for you to keep in close contact with volunteers who may do life reviews on the unit. In addition to verbal life reviews, written and visual life reviews can be created by the older adult and their caregivers and loved ones.

Writing One's Life Story

When writing a life story, many adults do not feel as if it is something they can do. It is especially difficult if they hand-write rather than use a computer. This is where a volunteer would be very effective. Initially, the volunteer needs to develop a relationship with the older person. It can be determined if a recording device or simply talking would be the best way to share the person's life story. The volunteer would need to be able to type on a computer while the older person is talking or, if using a recording device, interview the older person and then type the information that was recorded on a computer. There is a great satisfaction in recording one's life events. It is even better when there is a willing listener and facilitator for the project.

Imagine the satisfaction of having your life recorded or documented, even if it is just you who reads it. That is seldom the case, however. This type of life review meets the same needs as previously discussed. Perhaps the family could be involved and copies made for the children and grandchildren. A copy of a life story could be put on each chart or in a specific file so that staff members could read it and know the person better. Keep in mind that you would need permission from the person, whose story it is, to share it with the staff. You will also need to be aware of Health Insurance Portability and Accountability Act regulations regarding the sharing of information.

Collecting and Organizing Photos

Many people I know have boxes of photos that are unlabeled and disorganized. When those boxes exist for an older adult, it could represent the disorganization they are feeling in their life. Suggesting to a family member or recruiting an effective volunteer to assist in the organization and labeling of, quite literally, one's life is a significant thing to do. This is another way to do a life review. It provides the opportunity for the older person to relive precious moments, note the voids in pictures because of a family argument, or simply enjoy the grandchildren's pictures when they were babies.

The final product, the photo album, often becomes a treasured item to be shared with others. The significance of one's life is then visually apparent. The scrapbook provides the opportunity to reassess one's life and experience a sense of accomplishment.

Staff Who Value the Lives of Older People

If you are working on a unit that has a large percentage of older adults, or if you work in a nursing home, I hope that people who value the lives of older people surround you. As you go through your daily workload, take the time to ask older adults about their lives as children or young adults. Hopefully you know about the person and his or her culture and can ask questions that have significance for the person. When you ask a question, take the time to listen. Be especially alert for coping mechanisms that worked in the past for that individual. Listen for accomplishments and success stories that can be shared with the staff, and hopefully someone will ask to have the story told again.

Think of your own transitional stress and what helped you, then provide the same support for your patient. Consciously strive to be a truly holistic nurse by embracing the body, mind, and spirit of the person to whom you give care. You do this by following the medical plan of care (body), addressing transitional stress needs and all that accompanies those needs (mind), and meeting spiritual needs (spirit).

CASE STUDY SOLUTIONS

1. Quietly approach Mr. Tahan after calling for assistance to get him back in bed. Make arrangements with the daughter to provide a method for him to say his prayers to help ease his distress. Let both Mr. Tahan and the daughter know you are there to provide support for the needs that will assist in his recovery. Talk to the daughter in Mr. Tahan's presence about expectations of her father during his stay at the facility.

2. You were thinking about Mr. Tahan and how to help him transition to an acute hospital following the surgery when the CNA comes out into the hallway looking confused. She announces that Mr. Tahan and the daughter said the food and the service were unacceptable. You go to the room and calmly ask what is wrong with the food. The daughter explains that pork is forbidden and the left hand is considered unclean, so it was offensive to her father to have the food served with the left hand. You confer with the CNA regarding food preferences and the importance of using the right hand to serve food for this patient.

The CNA obtains another tray for Mr. Tahan and is careful to serve everything with the right hand. You apologize to Mr. Tahan and the daughter for not recognizing his dietary needs. You reassure them that information regarding pork products and serving food will be given to other

Continued

CASE STUDY SOLUTIONS—cont'd

individuals involved in his care. Take time to listen to the patient and the daughter regarding changes that have occurred over the last year. Listen for clues to what may have assisted him in the time since his wife's death, and determine if any of these strategies would be helpful in the current situation. If it is possible, stay in the room until the CNA completes serving the food, and make sure it is satisfactory.

3. You are back on duty the next morning and Mr. Tahan refuses to go to physical therapy (PT). By this time, you have investigated Muslim practices and were anticipating difficulty if a female assistant were to help him. You realize the importance of following protocol for this patient. You go in and talk to him about PT. You discuss the significance of having PT the day after surgery, and you ask if he would be willing to participate in therapy with a male attendant.

You then locate a male assistant to help get Mr. Tahan out of bed and discuss options for therapy with the PT department. When you are told there will only be a female therapist the following day, you request information regarding exercises the male assistant would be able to perform.

4. When you enter the room later in the day, Mr. Tahan is sitting up in bed with his daughter at his side. He is smiling and excited to show you the pictures and his book of scriptures his daughter brought him from home. You gather information regarding needs for male caregivers and arrange times with the daughter to be present if a male caregiver is not available. Mr. Tahan's recovery will be challenging because of his age, but you have been able to make this transition easier for him by listening and responding appropriately.

Key Points

• Transitions occur throughout the lifecycle. Despite a lifetime of learning and transitions, changes occurring in an older adult's life can create confusion and frustration. Spirituality can assist these individuals as they move through the aging process.

• Transition is associated with growth of an individual. This growth comes from change that can be difficult. It is important to recognize, understand, and help those going through transitions to enhance the quality of life for each person.

• Transitions can have a positive or negative outcome on an individual. As a nurse, you can provide support of a positive outcome with those in your care. Providing a choice, respecting the decisions made by the individual, preparing the person for a transition if possible, and having an understanding of the person and his or her environment will assist in making the transition a better experience.

• The PLST can be used to plan care for older individuals. Understanding common stressors

allows you to lower the stress of the individual by allowing as much control as possible for the individual rather than the health-care team.

• Understanding common transitions for people as they age will help you provide appropriate support for the transitions. This will alleviate some of the fear and concern faced with the changes.

• Spirituality provides a sense of connection for many people. Assessing spiritual needs of those in your care will provide information that you can use to help with resolving spiritual issues or needs.

• There may be individuals who are having difficulty resolving transitional difficulties. You can offer to help with life reviews, organizing photos, and valuing each person enough to take time to listen with caring. These skills will assist an older individual achieve self-transcendence as they approach the last stages of their life.

Review Questions

1. The overall objective of recognizing and assisting clients with transitions is to:
   1. Resolve shame vs doubt.
   2. Decrease complaints filed on your unit.
   3. Achieve Maslow's esteem level of need.
   4. Deliver humanistic and holistic care.

2. The importance of understanding PLST is to:
   1. Give firm directions to older adults so they will not feel insecure.
   2. Provide health-care environments where older people have complete freedom to make decisions.
   3. Lower the stress threshold of the environment where older adults are given care.
   4. Assist older adults in making the decision to make a transition or to perform PLST.

3. The difference between spirituality and religion is:
   1. One is done in a formal building; the other can't be.
   2. One is a feeling that comes from within.
   3. The age of the person determines the difference.
   4. Spirituality is a category of highly functioning religious people.

4. Research with spirituality and religion indicates that:
   1. It does not impact people who believe in a divine power only.
   2. It does promote health and healing.
   3. It should not be considered when planning nursing care.
   4. It is too personal to discuss with patients and residents.

5. The value of life review is to:
   1. Provide useful activities for volunteers and patients.
   2. Keep older people busy while they are hospitalized.
   3. Publish a book of older adults' lives and sell it as a fundraiser project.
   4. Gain understanding into one's successes and mistakes.

6. When discharging (or transitioning) a patient from the hospital to a long-term care facility, it would be important for the nurse to include:
   1. A detailed description of the medications for the patient to review.
   2. Contact cards for the patient of various therapies involved in the care.
   3. All communication, contacts, medications, and therapies for the facility.
   4. Detailed information regarding family involvement in the patient's care.

ANSWERS 1. 4, 2. 3, 3. 2, 4. 2, 5. 4, 6. 3

CHAPTER 4
The Use of the Nursing Process and Nursing Diagnosis

Holli Sowerby

KEY TERMS

activities of daily living (ADLs)
care area assessment (CAA)
care area trigger (CAT)
environments of care model
interdisciplinary health-care team (IDT)
minimum data set (MDS)
North American Nursing Diagnosis Association (NANDA)
resident assessment instrument (RAI)

CHAPTER CONCEPTS

Collaboration
Communication
Evidence-Based Practice
Patient-Centered Care

LEARNING OUTCOMES

1. Describe the nursing process as a problem-solving technique in the context of assessment of the older adult, plan of care, nursing interventions, and nursing documentation.
2. Identify the use of the nursing process minimum data set (MDS) and Care Area Assessments (CAAs) in developing nursing care plans for residents in nursing facilities.
3. Use the nursing process to develop a care plan for the presented case study.

CASE STUDY
Resident Admission

December 1, 2017, 1 p.m.: Mrs. H., 69 year-old, white, widowed, female, is admitted to Room 169 of Peach Valley Assisted Living. She arrived via privately owned vehicle with her two daughters. She was discharged this morning from Mercy Hospital following a 3-day stay. The reason for her hospital stay was sepsis related to a urinary tract infection. She has Parkinson's, diabetes mellitus, and atrial fibrillation. Dietary was notified of no concentrated sweets, and minimal dark leafy greens diet. The following medication orders were faxed to the pharmacy:

- Furosemide (Lasix) 40 mg PO once a day for peripheral edema
- Levodopa-carbidopa (Sinemet) 25/100 mg 2 tablets PO three times a day for Parkinson's
- Atenolol 50 mg PO once a day for atrial fibrillation
- Plavix 75 mg PO once a day for atrial fibrillation
- Potassium chloride (K-tabs) 1 tab PO once a day related to diuretic use

CASE STUDY—cont'd

- Metformin 800 mg PO once a day before noon for diabetes
- Oxazepam (Serax) 20 mg PO nightly at bedtime for insomnia
- Docusate (Dulcolax) sodium suppository prn constipation
- Acetaminophen (Tylenol) 1,000 mg PO every six hours prn pain
- Bactrim 800/160 mg twice a day for 14 days following discharge from hospital on 12/01/2017

The daughter has durable power of attorney for financial and health-care decisions but has not yet signed the advance directive form for "Do Not Resuscitate." Resident has a living will, and her wishes are known to her family.

Daughter reports that she is allergic to penicillin, wears glasses, and used to read often but no longer reads at all, has all her own teeth in good repair, does not use a hearing aid, and uses a walker to ambulate. Her height is 5 feet, 5 inches; her weight is 124 pounds.

Mrs. H. is alert and oriented to self and daughter. She is oriented to time but is unsure of where she is and is unable to respond to location questions; she just shakes her head no. For the past 3 years, she has been living with one of her two daughters for 6 months at a time. Caring for Mrs. H. has been quite stressful at times. She has become increasingly paranoid and sometimes believes that her family is trying to steal from her or hurt her. She has become quite frail and has lost 50 pounds over the past year. Her gait is unsteady and she uses a walker to ambulate. She occasionally leaves the house unattended and has been returned home by neighbors several times. One of her daughters is a school teacher but has had to take a leave of absence to care for her mother, and the other daughter has four children still living at home and has difficulty managing the increasing demands of caring for her mother at home.

Mrs. H. was admitted to Mercy Hospital after her daughter took her to the emergency room because her mother was more unsteady on her feet and slurring her words. Mrs. H. was determined to have a severe urinary tract infection. She was admitted and intravenous antibiotics were started. After several days of discussion between Mrs. H., her primary care doctor, and her daughters, it was decided that Mrs. H. should go to an assisted living center that could provide some rehabilitation and that she could potentially stay there if she likes it. The daughters are expressing much guilt over the decision to place Mrs. H. in an extended care facility, but they admit that she would be safer there.

Mrs. H. is able to walk with her walker but is very unsteady. She forgets where she is and wanders trying to find her way "home." She is able to dress herself but requires help with her socks and shoes. When confused or agitated she will change her clothes several times a day, sometimes putting clothes over top of what she is already wearing. Mrs. H. is able to feed herself but has not been eating well and has lost a significant amount of weight in the past year. Mrs. H. has been generally continent of bladder and bowel except while in the hospital, where she was incontinent of both. She does wear a pad for occasional stress incontinence.

Mrs. H. was a homemaker and enjoyed gardening, reading, and was quite an accomplished pianist. She has no interest in gardening and no longer reads but will sit down at the piano and play for 1 to 2 hours if left undisturbed.

Physical Assessment

General Appearance: Thin white woman.

Head and Neck: White hair. Scalp dry with multiple areas of white dry flaking. Face symmetrical. Skin also is dry. Eyes are clear with no drainage, conjunctiva pink, pupils are equal at 5 mm and react briskly to light, consensual, and accommodative. No drainage from nose; patient is able to breathe through both nostrils. No drainage from ears. Did appropriately respond when asked in a whisper to raise her arm. Oral mucous membranes are pink and dry. No saliva pooling noted between gum and cheek. Tongue pink with no coating; remains at midline when extended from mouth. Throat dry with no pharyngeal drainage or redness noted; no cervical lymph nodes palpable; no thyroid nodules or enlargement palpated.

Chest: Symmetrical chest movements. Breath sounds clear throughout though diminished. Apical pulse: 78 and regular. No extra heart sounds noted. Back has multiple waxy, light brown to medium brown, 2- to 3-cm, flat, raised lesions. Moderate kyphosis of spine.

Continued

CASE STUDY—cont'd

Abdomen and Buttocks: Active bowel sounds in all quadrants. Abdomen soft. No masses palpable.

Genitourinary: Normal female genitalia. Urine amber and foul-smelling.

Extremities: Full range of motion (ROM) of shoulders, elbows, wrist, and fingers. Mild shoulder pain noted when raising arms above head. Radial and brachial pulses strong and equal bilaterally.

Limited ROM of both hips with complaints of pain with movement of left hip. Full ROM of both knees and ankles. Femoral and popliteal pulses strong and equal bilaterally. No complaints of calf tenderness to palpation. Mild edema, nonpitting, on bilateral feet and ankles, toenails are trimmed and polished, patient states she "gets them done every month."

January 10, 23:00 p.m.: Mrs. H. was found in another resident's room, pulling clothes out of the closet. Mrs. H believes she is in her own room and is cleaning out the closet. She does not know the way back to her room. She believes that someone has stolen all her clothes and replaced them with the items she is removing. Mrs. H. reluctantly attends activities when asked to go, but she often leaves the activity early. She naps for 1 to 2 hours in the afternoon and is awake frequently at night, when she wanders the hallway looking for lost items (purse, jewelry, photographs) that she believes have been stolen. Items are always found in her room hidden in drawers or the closet.

Discussion

Use the following nursing diagnoses to organize your assessment data and develop a nursing care plan for Mrs. H. Following each nursing diagnosis, you will find possible problems you can address.

1. Nursing Diagnosis: *Self-Care Deficit* related to confusion manifested by inability to perform **activities of daily living (ADLs)** independently secondary to Parkinson's disease
   ADL Function/Rehabilitation Potential
   Visual Function
2. Nursing Diagnosis: *Injury, high risk* related to altered mobility as manifested by unsteadiness and wandering, secondary to Parkinson's disease.
   Fall Risk
   Behavior Problems
3. Nursing Diagnosis: *Nutrition, altered: less than body requirements* related to lack of appetite as manifested by significant weight loss in last year secondary to Parkinson's disease.
   Nutritional Status
   Dehydration/Fluid Maintenance
4. Nursing Diagnosis: *Urinary Elimination, incontinence* related to confusion mobility as manifested by needing incontinence pad for light bladder leakage
   Urinary Incontinence
5. Nursing Diagnosis: *Confusion* related to inaccurate interpretation of environment as manifested by inability to identify location, and inability to follow commands secondary to Parkinson's disease and possible use of sedative medication.
   Delirium
   Cognitive Loss/Dementia
   Communication
   Mood State
   Behavior Problem
   Psychosocial Well-being
6. Nursing Diagnosis: *Risk for constipation* related to decreased fluid intake as manifested, altered nutrition intake, and dehydration.
   Dehydration and Fluid Maintenance
   Nutritional Status

INTRODUCTION

Licensed practical nurses (LPNs) work in a variety of care settings. Each setting may require the LPN to function in a different capacity, yet each practice area expects the practical nurse to be involved with the assessment, planning, implementation, and evaluation of older adults and the care they receive.

ENVIRONMENTS OF CARE

The **environment of care model** consists of three components: the physical place where care is taking place, the equipment used in providing that care, and the people involved, including the health-care workers, patients, and family members involved. This approach considers the multiple environments in which a patient and nurse interact.

Home Care

LPNs in home care work under the direction of a registered nurse. They provide nursing care such as changing dressings, monitoring blood glucose levels, administering medications, and assessing the status of chronic disease processes in the older adult's home.

Hospice Care

Similar to home care, LPNs who work in the hospice setting do so under the direction of a registered nurse. They provide nursing care in the older adult's home doing the same tasks that the home care LPN does. The goal of hospice care is to provide care that allows the patient to die with dignity and without pain. In addition, hospice care also supports families during the difficult process of having a family member die (National Hospice & Palliative Care Organization, n.d.)

Acute Care

Acute care settings provide care for individuals requiring emergent or unexpected care related to injury or illness. Care is generally provided in a hospital setting that includes inpatient medical and surgery services and emergency care. In the acute care setting, the LPN may be tasked with closely monitoring and reporting vital signs and glucose levels, administering medications, and assessing patients. Often, the LPN is paired with a registered nurse to form a care team in providing nursing care. In an acute care setting, the LPN reports to the RN.

Rehabilitation Facilities

Rehabilitation facilities provide intensive rehabilitation services beyond what can be provided in a skilled nursing facility for individuals who have suffered strokes or spinal cord injuries. LPNs provide similar care to other environments of care but focus is on assisting with mobility and assisting patients with **activities of daily living (ADLs)**.

Extended Care Facilities

The LPN may be employed in many types of extended care facilities. *Skilled nursing facilities* and nursing facilities were previously thought of as nursing homes. These facilities generally provide a high level of nursing intervention. *Assisted-living facilities* provide care to older persons who may need assistance with ADLs but who do not require complex, skilled intervention (Eliopolous, 2018). *Continuing care retirement communities* have several levels of care, including skilled nursing, assisted living, and independent living apartments. Wellness clinics are frequently provided for residents living in independent apartments. LPNs could be employed in any one of these extended care settings.

Priority Setting

There is a great deal of information in this chapter, and all of it points you toward the behaviors and thought processes of a licensed nurse. One of the unwritten objectives for you in attending school is to learn to think like an LPN, and this chapter provides the foundation for that type of thinking. Your priority for this chapter is to learn and put into practice the nursing process.

Using the nursing process in your everyday life will assist you in learning to think like a nurse. Remember the five stages of the process:

- Assessment
- Nursing Diagnosis
- Planning
- Implementation
- Evaluation

I suggest that you purposefully think in those five stages. It would work in most everyday situations. For example, when fixing dinner, you need to assess the number of people who will be eating and their likes and dislikes as well as the food you have on hand. Your nursing diagnosis would be the selection of food you choose to serve to a specific number of people. Then you plan the actual meal, implement the plan by serving the meal, and then evaluate the meal by obtaining feedback from those who ate it.

I know this seems simplistic, but it is critical to learn to think like a nurse. By going through the steps several times a day, you soon will think that way automatically.

In the extended care environment, the practical nurse works with the registered nurse to collect admission data, provide input to the plan of care, carry out the nursing interventions that are outlined in the plan of care, and assist with the evaluation of the effectiveness of these interventions in meeting the goals of the care plan for the older adult. The registered nurse and LPN confer with the **interdisciplinary health-care team (IDT)** to share observations and clarify the plan of care. The IDT consists of a team of members made up of two or more health-care professions who collaborate to set goals and provide care. The LPN in these settings often is responsible for working with nursing assistants to ensure the plan of care is carried out. Practical nurses often call physicians to clarify orders and to report changes in the resident's health status. The practice of LPNs in nursing facilities is the practice model referred to in this chapter. For additional information on environments of care, see Chapter 11.

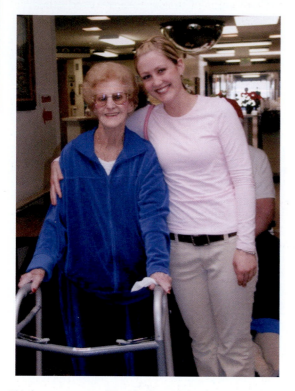

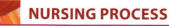

This woman soon will be discharged from a rehabilitation facility where she has been for the past 2 weeks because of a fractured hip. While at home, she will receive nursing and physical therapy as home care. Because of the variety of services available to her, she spent only 3 days in the hospital and will be home much quicker than she would have been a decade ago.

NURSING PROCESS

The nursing process is a problem-solving model that describes what nurses do. It identifies the way nurses approach patient care, and it recognizes the ongoing and changeable nature of the care that nurses provide, care that is based on the individual needs of the patient. Consider the following example.

An LPN in an extended care facility walks into a resident's room and finds the resident with a supper tray in place. The resident is unable to talk and is turning blue. The nurse thinks that the resident is choking. Quickly, the nurse moves the meal tray out of the way and uses a two-handed thrust under the

resident's diaphragm to attempt to dislodge the food that is obstructing the airway. After the nurse does the abdominal thrusts, the resident is assessed for respiratory movements. The nurse decides to do the following based on this assessment: If the person is breathing again, the nurse cuts the resident's food into smaller pieces and observes the resident eating the rest of the meal. If the resident is not breathing, the nurse may attempt another abdominal thrust or reposition the resident so that another abdominal thrust can be done from behind.

This short scenario is an example of the nursing process (Fig. 4.1). When the LPN entered the room and saw the older person with hands clenched on the throat and turning blue, the nurse was collecting data. In a split second, the nurse identified the resident's problem as choking. The nurse's next thought was to set a goal for this resident's care: the resident will expel the food that is causing the choking. With the goal of expelling the lodged food, the nurse designs the plan from nursing knowledge and immediately implements abdominal thrusts. After the nursing intervention, the nurse evaluates the situation to determine whether the resident has expelled the food. If the resident has not, the nurse must rethink and redesign the plan and immediately implement the revised nursing actions.

Nurses are faced with many patient care or resident care problems every day (note that people who have been admitted to extended care facilities are referred to as residents). The nursing process provides

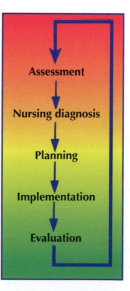

FIGURE 4.1 Nursing process model. The cyclic nature of this model demonstrates that the process is ongoing.

a structure for nurses to plan and give high-quality, individualized care.

Cultural Considerations

The United States is becoming more culturally diverse every year. Experts estimate that by 2080, the non-Hispanic white population will become the minority, with less than 50% of the U.S. population identifying as white. Research has shown that of the factors that influence health beliefs and practices, culture has a major impact. Cultural competence is essential to delivering quality healthcare (Flowers, 2018). As an LPN, you can provide culturally competent care by examining your own biases and educating yourself about the different cultures you encounter in your practice.

Assessment

The first step in the nursing process is to collect all of the information the nurse will need to identify clearly the resident's strengths and current and potential problems. Usually, the assessment starts with the call or written summary from the agency or department that is transferring the resident to your nursing care area. Before the actual transfer takes place, your nursing care area should have the following information regarding the incoming resident:

- Name, age, and insurance identification numbers
- Medical diagnoses, advanced directives, and disease prognosis
- Family support
- Need for equipment (Does the person need special equipment, such as a special bed, oxygen, intravenous [IV] setup, or feeding pump?)
- Functional ability (How does the person transfer, ambulate, move in bed, bathe, toilet, and eat?)
- Medications (Which prescription and over-the-counter medication does the person take?)
- Cognitive ability (Is the person oriented? How is the person's memory?)
- Special needs (Is the person depressed or at risk for skin breakdown or other health risks?)

This information is important for the preparation of the older person's bed and room and makes the transfer to your care as smooth as possible.

After the older person is transferred, the nurse makes a focused assessment that culminates in a comprehensive assessment. The admission assessment includes a nursing history, observations, physical examination, review of laboratory values, and an interview with the older adult and his or her family.

In 1987, the federal government enacted legislation that set minimum standards for the assessment and care planning processes in nursing facilities certified for Medicare reimbursement. This legislation is known as the Omnibus Budget Reconciliation Act of 1987 (OBRA 1987). This legislation was followed by OBRA 1990, which clarified some of the questioned areas of OBRA 1987. The **minimum data set (MDS)** and resident assessment protocols (RAPs) are a part of this legislation that has been implemented across the United States in nursing facilities that accept Medicare and Medicaid funding as reimbursement for the care they provide.

In 2010, the **resident assessment instrument (RAI)** was updated to 3.0, and the RAI 3.0 includes the MDS 3.0. RAPs have been replaced with **care area assessments (CAAs)**.

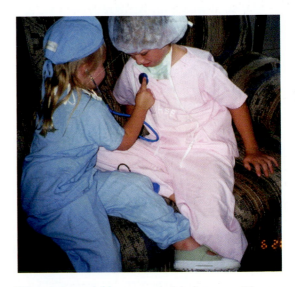

Although these children are only "playing nurse," they are illustrating what each reader of this book needs to do—practice, practice, and practice physical assessment skills until you have confidence in them.

RAI

The RAI for extended care includes the MDS, CAAs, and the RAI Utilization Guidelines. These forms detail a step-by-step process of completing the interdisciplinary assessment and designing a comprehensive plan of care for every resident in an extended care nursing facility (Centers for Medicare & Medicaid Services, 2017).

MDS

The MDS is just that—the absolute smallest amount of information that must be collected on every resident. It is standardized so that the same information is collected on all residents. Nurses in extended care facilities walk around asking each other "… have you done the MDS on Mrs. Hashamoto?" "… on Mr. Nay?" and others. The MDS contains information from all disciplines that work with the resident (i.e., nursing, social work, physical therapy, and dietary). The MDS must be completed within the first 7 days of admission. This allows the interdisciplinary team members some time to get to know the resident as they complete the MDS (Centers for Medicare & Medicaid Services, 2017).

CAA

When the MDS is completed, it provides a comprehensive assessment as well as indicators of risk for the resident. These risk areas are the CAAs. The CAAs are the areas identified with MDS data.

Embedded within the MDS responses are **care area triggers (CATs)**. For example, if a resident has fallen within the last week, a fall risk is triggered. When an area is triggered, the resident needs to be assessed further by using the CAA process to help decide if the area to be addressed is in the resident's plan of care. This is the decision making that is part of the nursing process.

The MDS is the assessment and the CATs trigger the decision-making process. Box 4.1 lists the 20 problem areas that may be identified by the MDS.

Nursing Diagnosis

Developing the nursing diagnosis is a primary responsibility of the registered nurse. It involves the use of diagnostic reasoning to reflect the older person's strengths, problems, and potential problems. The registered nurse considers the assessment data from the MDS and the triggered Care Areas to select the specific nursing diagnosis supported by the data. The **North American Nursing Diagnosis Association (NANDA)** has identified diagnoses that are widely accepted and understood by multiple disciplines and are viewed as the national standards for nursing diagnoses. The NANDA diagnoses are not specific to older people, but they are useful in providing consistent expression of nursing diagnoses for all disciplines and in all settings. An example of a NANDA diagnosis is the following: *Comfort altered, Pain, related to: degenerative joint disease.*

Evidence-Based Practice

Fujita, J., Fukui, S., Ikezaki, S., Otoguro, C., & Tsujimura, M. (2017). Analysis of team types based on collaborative relationships among doctors, home-visiting nurses and care managers for effective support of patients in end-of-life home care. *Geriatrics & Gerontology International, 17*(11), 1943–1950. doi:10.1111/ggi.12998

Researchers surveyed 43 teams that included doctors, nurses, and care managers. The teams were then classifieds into three groups with group A having good collaboration, and group C experiencing poor collaboration, and group B in the middle. Interestingly, the researchers found that in addition to teamwork experience and available communication tools, the patient's condition affected the communication between the team members. The researchers acknowledge some limitations regarding the size of the sample and the fact that the respondents had all previously received training to encourage collaboration. It was found that the home-visiting nurses could help foster teamwork and communication between doctors and care managers.

Questions
1. The minimum data set 3.0 is an interdisciplinary form and process for completing. Do you think there may be disagreements over assessment coding on the form? How do you think these IDT disputes should be resolved?
2. As part of the RAI process, IDT meetings are scheduled with the resident and his or her family. What would you think would be a good agenda for that meeting? What would be the priorities? Who would chair or moderate the meeting?

In the extended care setting, nurses often prefer to use nursing diagnoses that incorporate the MDS language and format. An example of an MDS-related nursing diagnosis is the following: *Potential for joint pain due to degenerative joint disease.* Common nursing diagnoses for older adults include the following:

- Self-care deficit
- Physical mobility, impaired
- Nutrition, altered: less than body requirements
- Injury, high risk for

Box 4.1

Twenty Problem Areas Identified From the MDS

Delirium	Falls
Cognitive loss/dementia	Nutritional status
Visual function	Feeding tubes
Communication	Dehydration/fluid maintenance
ADLs: function/rehabilitation potential	Dental care
Urinary incontinence and indwelling catheter	Pressure ulcers
Psychosocial well-being	Psychotropic drug use
Mood state	Physical restraints
Behavior problem	Pain
Activities	Return to community referral

- Urinary elimination, altered
- Constipation
- Confusion
- Skin integrity, impaired: high risk for

The registered nurse is responsible for ensuring that nursing diagnoses address the comprehensive assessment. The nursing diagnosis is an important part of the nursing process and addresses the potential and actual problems of the older adult.

Nursing Diagnosis and Medical Diagnosis

There are two basic ways to communicate the nature of an older adult's health problems. One way is by medical diagnosis, and the other is by nursing diagnosis. Medical diagnoses are made by a physician and describe a disease or a disease process. Diseases are diagnosed by identifying a specific group of signs and symptoms. For example, diabetes mellitus is diagnosed when a person has elevated fasting blood glucose levels, weight loss, thirst, and a large urine output. A person who has an area of dead brain tissue on magnetic resonance imaging (MRI) and computed tomography (CT) scans, along with speech and swallowing difficulty and left-sided paralysis, would be diagnosed with a cerebrovascular accident. Both of these medical diagnoses are common for older adults and communicate information to the nurse about what physical or psychological processes are happening to the person.

Focused Learning Chart: Resident Assessment Instrument

Federal law requires all facilities that have Medicare or Medicaid residents to have a RAI that has MDSs.

Essential Information That Must Be Collected on Residents	CAAs	Information Is Used for:
Nursing observations	Areas that require further assessments before designing care plans	Meeting federal requirements
Physical assessments	Specialized assessments done by IDT members	Referring IDT members to the list of problems to be addressed
Health history		
Interviews with older adult and family		

Safe, Effective Nursing Care

Support Decision Making Using Available Information

At shift report, the night nurse expressed frustration with Mr. R. because he did not sleep. He paced up and down the hall and in his room all night. She asked if you could call the doctor and get him a "sleeping pill" or something to "knock him out." Because Mr. R. is a new admit, the charge nurse pulled up his chart and his MDS online. She noticed that he had a diagnosis of Alzheimer's disease and that confusion has been triggered as a problem on his care assessment. Going to the plan of care, she saw that one of the written goals in the plan is to decrease agitation, sundowning, and relocation trauma. Suggestions included nonpharmacological approaches such as the following:

1. Keeping the room and hall well lit
2. Having a clock and other visual cues such as a calendar available in the resident's room
3. Having familiar items in the room such as a favorite chair and family pictures
4. Making sure resident is wearing his hearing aid and glasses
5. Giving appropriate care cues to bedtime: helping the resident with brushing his teeth and washing his face along with putting his pajamas on, making sure he empties his bladder and has a glass of water at his bedside, and offering a back rub and a foot or hand massage to help with relaxation
6. Putting on soft music and trying to eliminate bells, alarms, and other irritating noises
7. Introducing yourself with every encounter and reassuring the resident
8. Encouraging family and friends to visit and walk with resident around the facility to help familiarize him to surroundings

The MDS assessment and CATs automatically bring up problems to address in the plan of care. For a new resident, it is important to check the plan of care and to provide appropriate care to the resident.

1. Why didn't the night nurse attempt the approaches identified in the plan of care?
2. How would implementing the items in the plan of care actually save time for the night nurse?

The major problem with planning care based only on medical diagnoses is that they do not describe the individual problems of the older adult or the impact the disease has on the person's day-to-day life. Nursing diagnoses are specific to the individual older person's nursing care needs and frequently relate to the areas in which the older person has difficulty functioning. For example, an obese person who is newly diagnosed with diabetes mellitus may have the following nursing diagnoses:

• *Nutrition, altered: More than body requirements and knowledge deficit related to poor dietary practices*

A patient with long-term diabetes may be experiencing problems with a heel ulcer that will not heal. In this case, the nursing diagnosis would be as follows:

• *Skin integrity, altered*

Both of these people have the same medical diagnoses but different health-care needs, as shown in their nursing diagnoses. When writing your care plan for Mrs. H., you will want to include all of the nursing diagnoses that apply specifically to her.

Planning

After organizing the assessment data and noting the nursing diagnoses identified by the registered nurse, you, the LPN working with the older adult, the family, and the health-care team, begin the planning part of the nursing process. The planning portion of the nursing process includes setting priorities, identifying goals and outcomes of care, and designing and documenting interventions.

Setting Priorities

The nurse reviews the nursing diagnoses and places them in priority order. Remember the example at the beginning of this section? Removing the lodged food so that the resident could breathe would be a higher priority than putting on the resident's shoes!

One of the most popular models used to assist the nurse in setting priorities is Abraham Maslow's hierarchy of needs. This framework gives life-sustaining needs the highest priority. These needs are followed by safety and security needs, love and belonging needs, self-esteem needs, and self-actualization needs.

Because the nursing process is focused on the older person as an individual, it also is necessary to consider the priorities of the resident. Often, a resident will state that the highest priority is to go home. The resident may refuse treatments, medications, and activities that would maintain personal health because no one is assisting in the patient's discharge. Although discharge may not be realistic (at this time), you, as the nurse, will probably be more successful in providing nursing care if the plan of care addresses discharge to home as a high priority.

Following is an example of how the nutrition nursing diagnosis can be considered:

* *Nutrition, altered: less than body requirements*
* Resident refuses to eat and drink.
* Discuss with the resident what is usually eaten at home and how it is prepared.
* Review how the resident's current health status would affect the ability to buy food, prepare it, and eat at home.
* Discuss strategies and plans for ensuring that the resident is able to eat after returning home.
* Include the resident's food preferences in meals.

Goal Setting or Identifying Outcomes

After identifying the priorities for the resident's care, the nurse identifies goals or outcomes for each of the nursing diagnoses. Setting goals is something that most of us do all of the time. Sometimes our personal goal may be to clock out on time or to survive a busy day. The goals that are part of the planning process describe the specific resident outcomes and identify the goals that direct nursing care. To direct care and describe outcomes, goals must be:

* *Measurable*—measurable outcomes need to be identified. "Eating 100% of a meal" can be measured, whereas it is difficult to measure "appetite will improve."

* *Realistic*—the goal must fit in with the resident's abilities. "The resident will recall the correct date and time" is probably an unrealistic goal for a person with Alzheimer's disease.
* *Specific*—the goal should identify certain behaviors or conditions to aid in their attainment and evaluation. "The resident will feel better" is not specific. It could be better worded as, "The resident will state that he has less nausea."
* *Timely*—a time frame needs to be established for the attainment of each goal. "The resident will walk 100 feet" does not specify a time frame for achievement of this goal. Adding "by the end of December" provides a time frame.
* *Attainable*—the goal should be written in such a way as to communicate a motivating factor to the resident and the nursing care staff. For an older adult with left hemiplegia, a goal such as "the resident will be independent in self-care by the end of the year" may be a strong motivator to work harder at the occupational and physical therapy sessions.

In nursing facilities, the documentation regulations under OBRA 1987 and OBRA 1990 require that the status of goal attainment be systematically addressed. These documentation requirements are the monthly summaries (a comprehensive review of outcomes every 30 days) and the quarterly reviews (comprehensive interdisciplinary review of the resident's plan of care every 90 days) (Box 4.2). With new admissions or specific insurance carriers, the nurse may be required to conduct monthly comprehensive assessments of the outcome of care. This provides a 30- or 90-day time frame in which goals can be designed. It also helps the nurse think about what is realistic in that specific time frame. For a resident who is rehabilitating after having a hip replacement, "Ambulate independently" may be a realistic goal in 6 months. "Stand and walk 10 steps with a

---

Point of Interest

Did you notice how many times the term *resident* was used in the previous explanation on outcomes? In the 1987 OBRA Act, the federal government determined that persons living in an extended care facility are to be referred to as residents. The reason is because they live there; they are residents of the facility.

Box 4.2

Assessments Needed for Each Nursing Home Resident

Comprehensive admission assessment including RAI:
1. MDS
2. CATs and CAAs
3. Ongoing nursing assessment
   Annual reassessment including RAI
   Significant change in status assessment
      including RAI
   Quarterly assessment including part of MDS

walker" may be a more realistic goal for 30 days. Following are examples of goals:

- The resident will eat more than 75% of each meal for the next 30 days.
- The resident will toilet independently when reminded to go to the bathroom for the next 90 days.
- The resident will attend one activity daily for the next 90 days.
- The resident will have no signs and symptoms of a urinary tract infection for the next 90 days.
- The resident's supplemental oxygen needs will be decreased to 1 L in the next 30 days.

Look back at these goals. What do you notice about them? Each goal identifies something that the resident will or will not do or will or will not experience. The resident's behavior is the major focus of goals as outcomes. Nursing care is not part of the goal. "Bathe the resident" is a nursing intervention, not an outcome or a goal. Nursing standards also are not part of the goal statements. "Administer all medications within 30 minutes of their ordered time" is a nursing standard, not a resident goal.

Designing and Documenting the Plan of Care

After the goals or outcomes of care are identified, the LPN, along with the other members of the IDT, begins to plan the activities that will help the older person reach the goals. The planning phase involves discussion and pen-and-paper activity. Discussing and documenting the plan of care allows input from all members of the team to be communicated to all staff members who are providing care for that resident. Standards of nursing practice and federal regulations require that each resident have a written, comprehensive, and interdisciplinary plan of care. The plan of care includes the problem or potential problem to be identified, the actions or interventions to be taken to address the problem, the person or discipline responsible for each action, and the goals to be achieved. Because of Mrs. H.'s multiple medical concerns, her care plan may be lengthy, but all of the information pertinent to her must be included for a complete plan of care. An example of interventions in an interdisciplinary plan of care follows:

- Document percentage of food eaten at each meal—*nursing.*
- Feed resident and assess swallowing ability— *speech therapy.*
- Review dietary preferences—*dietary services.*
- Promote feeding of self—*restorative nursing.*

The focus of this chapter is on developing interdisciplinary plans of care using the nursing process. All disciplines caring for the resident need to be represented in an actual plan of care. This is an important criterion for planning interventions: planned interventions must complement the interventions of other therapies. For example, it would be confusing for the resident to be ambulated with a walker by physical therapy and encouraged to walk with two canes by the nursing staff.

It is crucial that members of all disciplines discuss and develop the components of the interdisciplinary plan of care so that confusion among the staff does not occur. Residents who are asked to perform one way in physical therapy and another way on the nursing unit can become confused as to how they should perform. A coordinated approach between physical therapy and nursing helps residents improve quickly and maintain function longer. A coordinated approach among all disciplines enhances the effectiveness of the care given to the resident and minimizes duplication of efforts.

Nursing interventions also must consider the safety of the resident. "Administering a diuretic and a sleeping pill at bedtime" is an unsafe nursing action. The resident may fall while going to the bathroom at night if still groggy from the sleeping pill. Transferring a resident who is able to stand only with the assistance of one staff member may place that resident at risk of falling.

Selected nursing interventions should help to attain the identified goal. If a resident's goal is to "lose 1 pound a week," then giving "dietary supplements between meals and at bedtime" would not assist in achieving this weight loss. When the resident's goal is "will ambulate 100 feet by the end of the month," a nursing intervention must state that the nursing staff will assist the resident to ambulate.

CRITICALLY EXAMINE THE FOLLOWING

Identify the correctly stated resident-based outcomes or goals in the following list. When the outcomes or goals are not properly expressed, explain what is wrong.

1. The resident will walk more in the next 90 days.
2. The nurse will toilet the resident every 2 hours for the next 30 days.

3. The resident will have no areas of skin break-down in the next 90 days.
4. The resident's nutrition will improve.
5. The resident will drink 1,500 mL a day for the next 90 days.

Nursing interventions also must be realistic for the resident, staff, resources, and equipment. A reality in the workplace is that there often is no extra time for staff to talk to the residents. Providing 30 minutes of one-on-one time every shift to discuss pain with the resident is an unrealistic intervention. Stating that each staff member "will ask the resident about hip pain whenever he or she interacts with the resident" is a more realistic intervention.

To be successful and effective, nursing interventions must be developed with input from certified nursing assistants (CNAs). CNAs are important members of the interdisciplinary team. Nursing assistants spend more time with residents in nursing facilities, assisted living facilities, and retirement communities and sometimes in the older adult's home than any other member of the IDT. They can offer important specific information for the assessment of the older adult. Because CNAs are so familiar with the daily routine and functioning of the residents, they can offer pertinent, realistic suggestions for individualized interventions to deal with specific problems. They also are frequently the first people to notice subtle changes in clients' conditions that may indicate onset of a new problem or success or failure of an intervention. A care plan meeting, including representatives of all disciplines, is generally held to discuss assessment information and develop the interdisciplinary plan of care. The CNA who works with the resident to be discussed should be invited to this meeting, and arrangements should be made to facilitate the CNA's attendance. The time away from the unit for the CNA is minimal compared with the value of the CNA's input into the care-planning process.

Successful nursing interventions require the resident's input and should be important to the resident. A resident may not want to "lift weights to strengthen and increase flexibility of his arms" but may be very willing to "comb his hair and wash his face." "Encourage the resident to drink 1,000 mL of water" may not work as well as "encourage the resident to drink 1,000 mL of fruit juice and water."

Nursing interventions also must include continuing assessment and monitoring of disease processes and effects of medications and treatments. If a resident has an IV, the IV site must be "assessed every shift for signs of infiltration, irritation, and infection." If a resident is receiving therapy with digoxin (Lanoxin), the "apical pulse must be taken and recorded before each dose." Residents with heart failure (HF) should be "assessed for edema and dyspnea."

The plan of care is part of the resident's permanent record. It needs to be routinely reviewed and updated as the resident's health status improves or declines. The monthly and quarterly review times provide excellent opportunities to revise the care plan to ensure that the resident is receiving appropriate nursing care.

Implementation

Implementation is the part of the nursing process where a nurse's skills, abilities, and training are used to provide care. Being at the bedside of the resident is one of the most rewarding aspects of being a nurse. Implementation means putting the plan of care into action. Along with providing the nursing care that has been outlined in the resident's nursing care plan, the LPN continues to collect data that can be used to update and revise the plan of care.

> ### THINK LIKE A NURSE
> You are a student nurse working on an acute care unit. You are writing a care plan for your patient. The staff nurse comments that she doesn't write care plans for her patients. How might you respond to this nurse?

Many interventions from the plan of care are assigned to CNAs; this is another strong reason to have CNAs attend the care plan development meeting. If CNAs have an opportunity to provide input into the plan of care and if they are present when it is discussed and developed, they will be more likely to carry out the interventions than if they are merely told what to do or handed a care plan to read.

Because nursing assistants on all shifts cannot attend the care plan meeting, a major challenge for the LPN is communicating the plan of care back to all CNAs. Various communication techniques can be used. Some facilities provide nursing assistants with written assignments that list all of the interventions for each resident. Many facilities place the plan of care in a book and make it available to the staff. Very often, however, the book is not consulted. Meeting regularly with nursing assistants to discuss the plan of care, giving each CNA written assignments with information on the plan of care, and using primary CNAs who care for the same residents each day ensure the implementation of the plan of care. These actions make it a working document rather than a useless piece of paper completed only to comply with regulations.

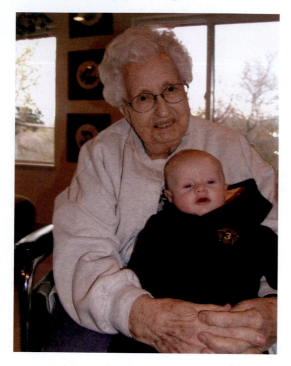

This woman was admitted to a skilled nursing facility with limited mobility, weakness, mild confusion, and heart failure. Her stated goal was to be strong enough to hold her great-grandchildren and to sit up and talk to her grandchildren. The MDS indicated several other goals to implement for her optimum health. As you can see, her priority goal as well as those identified through the MDS were met.

Another aspect of implementation is that it must be documented. Charting is an important part of implementing the plan of care. Documentation of interventions requires recording not only that the intervention was done but also the resident's responses to the intervention. An entry such as the following provides no information about the resident's response to the treatment:

12/16/15 1420 Wet to dry saline packing to coccyx ulcer

A better picture is given in the following chart:

12/16/15 1420 Wet to dry saline packing to coccyx pressure ulcer. Ulcer is 3 × 2 cm and 1.5 cm deep. Ulcer margins are pink, and there is granulation tissue evident. Small amount of yellow serous drainage on old packing. Resident complained of pain when old packing was removed and new packing inserted. Two small (6-mm) scabs on left buttocks from tape irritation. No redness or drainage noted.

Every visit with the resident is an opportunity to reassess nursing diagnoses and their implementation. Following is a simple model that can be used to document the nursing process with nursing interventions and resident responses:

• *Assessment*—What the nurse observed and assessed. Includes:
  • Objective measurements (blood pressure, laboratory values)
  • What the resident did (response to nursing intervention)
  • What the resident said
• *Action*—What the nurse did (nursing interventions): treatments, turning the resident, giving a medication, increasing the oxygen flow rate, hanging a tube feeding, inserting a catheter
• *Plan*—What the nurse plans to do: call the physician, call the family, reassess with the next treatment, refer resident to social services

The assessment-action-plan charting format is simple, yet it sets up a framework for documenting the nursing process in a narrative format.

CNAs also may be involved in documentation and may provide information for the LPN's documentation. For example, nursing assistants can complete flow sheets, which include interventions from the plan of care and activities from the resident's day. Flow sheets can be used to document such interventions as ADLs, walking programs, bowel and bladder training programs, and dietary intake and feeding programs. Results and trends from the flow sheets can be incorporated into the LPN's regular progress charting.

Evaluation

Evaluation is the final step in the nursing process. The main purposes of evaluation are to decide if the resident has met the identified goals and to assess the outcomes of the nursing care provided. Remember how, in the discussion of implementation, the importance of assessing the resident and documenting the resident's responses to care was emphasized? The chart and resident assessments are reviewed as part of evaluation.

When goals have been stated in measurable terms, the LPN should be able to review all of the data and decide whether the goal has been met, has been partially met, or remains unmet. This is a straightforward look at the resident's response to the nursing interventions. The evaluation of goal achievement needs to be documented in a monthly summary, in a quarterly review, or in the nursing notes.

Evaluation also requires that the nurse review the nursing process. This review helps to keep the plan of care up-to-date and reflects changes in the resident's health status. It also is an opportunity to decide which nursing interventions were ineffective (Box 4.3).

The reassessment of the resident and the plan of care in evaluation addresses the dynamic strength of the nursing process. Although the nursing process follows specific, organized steps, no step excludes collecting more data. Data collection is done by assessing the resident, updating goals and interventions, and conducting an ongoing evaluation of the outcome of the care that is provided. Nurses seem to use the nursing process even when they do not identify it as such. Consider the following example.

Mary Jones always was incontinent during the 1:00 a.m. rounds. The nursing staff decided to toilet her at 12:30 a.m.

In this example, the nursing staff assessed incontinence as a problem. Their unstated goal was, "the resident will not be incontinent at 1:00 a.m. rounds." Their intervention was to toilet the resident 30 minutes before she was usually incontinent. After toileting the resident at 12:30 a.m., the resident would be checked for urinary incontinence at 1 a.m. If she was not incontinent, the goal would be achieved, and the staff would continue to toilet the resident at 12:30 a.m. to maintain that outcome. If the resident was toileted at 12:30 a.m. and she still was incontinent at 1:00 a.m., the staff may decide to toilet the resident at midnight. The care plan and charting examples provided in Figure 4.2 demonstrate the use of evaluation.

As this example shows, evaluation is ongoing and occurs daily, not just at the mandatory reassessment intervals. Evaluation does not occur only when the quarterly assessment is due. Would you continue to carry out an intervention that was not working for 3 months until the quarterly review was due? Many people help you evaluate the plan of care each day. Residents give you information through their behavior and by telling you if an intervention is helping or not. Families tell you about changes they notice. Nursing assistants frequently note subtle changes in residents and may alter interventions to accommodate the change in the residents.

Making daily changes in the actual care given is common. Translating these changes into the written plan of care is less common. For the sake of communication and consistency among all staff, it is very important to ensure that the written plan of care is updated to reflect the actual care you want to be given.

COMPUTERS AND THE NURSING PROCESS

Computers and access to documentation supporting and submission networks have dramatically improved the RAI process. Imagine the difficulty interdisciplinary team members have if they all have to access the paper chart for a resident. Having the MDS, CAT, and CAA all available via a computer makes it easier to access the information for the entire team.

If you have never worked within a computerized documentation program before, you may be apprehensive about using it for your assessment and care plans. Completing the MDS and the care plan on the computer has many benefits. One of the most time-consuming portions of the process is computing the CATs—that is, identifying the potential problem areas that need to be assessed further through the CAAs. Most MDS software packages

---

Box 4.3

Significant Change in Resident's Status

Decrease in level of functioning in two or more activities of daily living

Decrease or increase in the ability to walk or to use hands to grasp small objects

Decline in health status that is unresponsive to treatment

Changes in behavior or mood that cause daily problems in assisting the resident to achieve goals

Nursing Diagnosis Problems Addressed	Goals Outcomes of Care	Nursing Interventions	Evaluation
Physical Mobility, impaired related to musculoskeletal impairment as manifested by inability to transfer and ambulate without assistance	Resident will increase ambulation with walker in PT to independent use with minimal supervision in 90 days	■ Assess and document: Orthostatic BPs (lying/sitting/standing) ROM and strength of legs and arms Walking ability with walker and amount of assistance needed ■ Have walker in resident's reach at all times and use for all transfers and walking in room ■ Physical therapy for quad-strengthening exercises and ambulation with walker ■ Put on jogging pants for daily physical therapy	

DOCUMENTATION

October 11, 2015, 1:45 p.m.: Resident is transferred from bed to wheelchair with assistance of one. Uses walker to steady himself when standing. Ambulates with hold-on assistance from physical therapist using a walker. Ambulated two steps without hold-on assistance before becoming unsteady. Orthostatic BPs lying—138/82, sitting—110/80, standing—106/76, complained of being light-headed when he sat up. Dizziness passed in 5 minutes. Instructed to move slowly from lying–sitting–standing positions and not to move to another position until any dizziness or light-headedness passes. Will review medications and fluid intake for possible causes of orthostatic hypotension.

FIGURE 4.2 Sample care plan.

compute the CATs and CAAs in a matter of seconds. Completing the interdisciplinary care plan on the computer saves the nurse from a great deal of handwriting and lends itself to regular updating without further lengthy handwriting. Some software packages print out nursing assistant forms that include all the interventions from the plan of care assigned to the nursing assistant. These forms can be used as assignment sheets that communicate the plan of care to the CNA.

CASE STUDY SOLUTION

There is no specific format in which to write this care plan. Use the format you have been taught by your nursing instructors to develop and document the care plan for Mrs. H.

Key Points

- As an LPN, you have major responsibilities for delivering meaningful nursing care to residents in extended care facilities. Your responsibilities include the management of care given by nursing assistants, working with the IDT, completing documents required by the federal government, and delivering excellent care to the residents.
- The MDS is a valuable tool that helps to identify areas of concern for extended care residents using CAA and CAT to improve resident care.
- As an LPN you have the opportunity to work in several different environments of care including hospitals, home care, hospice and extended-care facilities. A registered nurse supervises LPNs in all these different care areas.

- Learning and applying the nursing process is a key part of learning to think like a nurse. By practicing this skill of assessment, nursing diagnosis, planning, implementation, and evaluation you can become proficient at organizing the care of patients.
- The use of computer charting and documentation in nursing has helped to streamline admissions and make the relevant patient information available to all the team members concerned with a particular patient's care. As the use of paper charting becomes less common, it is important to embrace the new technology and become familiar with the different programs that you will be using to chart nursing care.

Review Questions

1. The nursing process is:
   1. A type of standardized care plan.
   2. A framework for providing nursing care.
   3. A procedure that registered nurses use to make care assignments.
   4. An instinctive method of providing care.

2. The steps in the nursing process are:
   1. Admission, inpatient care, and discharge.
   2. Assessment, intervention, and documentation.
   3. Assessment, nursing diagnosis, planning, intervention, and evaluation.
   4. Admission, physical examination, interview, nursing history, and planning.

3. Nursing diagnoses differ from medical diagnoses because they:
   1. Address the problems of the older person.
   2. Are written in language that nurses understand.
   3. Are standardized for any person who is receiving nursing care
   4. Are designed to address the medical treatment plan.

4. When setting priorities during the planning stage of the nursing process, it is important to consider:
   1. The needs of the physician.
   2. The needs of the family.
   3. The needs of the nursing staff.
   4. The needs of the resident.

5. Evaluation of the nursing care plan is documented by means of:
   1. The nurse's notes.
   2. The resident's care plan.
   3. The physician's orders.
   4. Revising the admission note.

ANSWERS 1. 2, 2. 3, 3. 3, 4. 4, 5. 1

CHAPTER 5
Legal, Ethical, and Financial Considerations

Tamara Dahlkemper

KEY TERMS

advance directive
confidentiality
elder abuse
ethics
informed consent
law
liability
living will
malpractice
Medicaid
Medicare
negligence
omission
restraint

CHAPTER CONCEPTS

Legal Issues
Ethics
Advocacy
Violence

LEARNING OUTCOMES

1. Compare and contrast the terms *legal* and *ethical*.
2. Define the term *liability* and discuss the impact it can have on your career.
3. Define the guiding principles of a restraint-free environment.
4. Outline the role of the licensed practical nurse (LPN) in using advance directives and informed consent.
5. Express an understanding of the ethical responsibility of working with older adults in meeting their sexual needs.
6. Explain the Health Insurance Portability and Accountability Act (HIPAA) law and the significance it has for your nursing practice.
7. Compare and contrast Medicare and Medicaid.

CASE STUDY

As the 7 p.m. to 7 a.m. charge nurse on a 20-bed unit at a skilled nursing facility, you have had concerns about the number of restraints used in the facility. Often, you have found the nursing assistants restraining residents without going through the appropriate process as outlined in the facility policies. You have discussed the problem with the nursing assistants and have taught them about the restraint-free environment at the facility. Despite your efforts, restraints are still being used.

You discussed this problem with your nurse manager, and the two of you reviewed the policy that indicates restraints are not used unless there is a documentable situation that risks the life of the older adult, such as displacement of a nasogastric tube or intravenous needle.

Continued

CASE STUDY—cont'd

Because you are the licensed nurse responsible for what occurs on your shift, you are legally and ethically accountable for the behavior of the nursing assistants who work with you. More importantly, you are concerned about possible injury to the residents due to the use of restraints.

1. What are the ethical and legal ramifications regarding your current dilemma?
2. How will you resolve the problem?

INTRODUCTION

Health-care decisions that are made daily across the United States are based on the legal and ethical definitions of health care. Advances in technology, increased resources, newer drug therapies, and other modalities of treatment continue to bring with them unprecedented ethical and legal problems that require solutions. While the legislators and ethics committees of the United States debate the merits of treatment approaches, health-care providers deliberate every day regarding their own direct care role and often wonder if it is one of help or hindrance.

As a licensed practical nurse (LPN), you will be involved in making ethical and legal decisions that potentially are very complex. This chapter will assist you in understanding ethical and legal issues that relate specifically to the challenges facing older adults and their care.

ETHICS

Ethics is the study of moral actions and values. It is based on the principles of conduct that govern individuals and groups. Many people envision ethics as dealing with principles and moral concepts that determine what is good or bad behavior. The problem with this concept is determining who decides what is good and what is bad. Always ask yourself, "Is this decision one for the older adult, the nurse, the family, or an outside group like an ethics committee?"

A broader definition of ethics considers the value system of a person and the relationship of those values in determining what is good for an individual or group. It is important for LPNs to understand their own value systems and the ethical framework underlying their work performance. As a nurse you need to maintain ethical awareness and skills in decision making that lead to ethical actions, which is considered ethical competence. Ethical competence is developed through personal experience and knowledge and requires administrative support when actions need to be taken. Most health-care agencies have an ethics committee to help nurses and other healthcare providers resolve complex ethical dilemmas related to patient care (Hagedorn Wonder, 2017).

Patient Care Partnership

The Patient's Bill of Rights was a document adopted by the American Hospital Association (AHA) in 1973. This single-page document listed the ethical behavior that was deemed appropriate and proper for care of patients in a hospital. The AHA has updated and added content to the original Patient's Bill of Rights and refers to the document as the Patient Care Partnership. By federal law, each nursing home must have available a similar document that discusses the rights of residents. Other organizations, such as the American Nurses Association, have ethical codes that guide the practice of each professional and are consistent with the Patient Care Partnership. Professional organizations publish standards of care that identify an ethical and legal model of practice. These models are often used in legal cases to determine the acceptable level of care.

CRITICALLY EXAMINE THE FOLLOWING

What do you value in life? Your values create the foundation for your ethical behavior. Make a list of the three things you value most in life in the left column. In the right column, put an example of a nursing situation in which that value would be either tested or proved. Be prepared to discuss your ideas in class. This is an example of how your submission should look.

My Values	Nursing Application
1.	1.
2.	2.
3.	3.

The Patient Care Partnership is based on every individual's right to make decisions regarding health-care treatment. It is designed to serve as a model that defines acceptable behavior toward individuals in your care. All care provided to persons of any age and condition should be based on the principles in the Patient Care Partnership. The document stresses access to health care and coverage. It is clear in not allowing racial or ethnic disparities. It covers billing and collection policies, and it defines the right of every person to be a partner in health-care decisions and delivery. The AHA's vision statement is as follows: "The AHA vision is of a society of healthy communities, where all individuals reach their highest potential for health." (American Hospital Association, n.d.)

Read and review the Patient Care Partnership. The Patient Care Partnership should be the foundation for the work you do with older people. It has special significance when dealing with the older adults who may be struggling with the stress of a new situation, limited short-term memory, or chronic disease.

Point of Interest

You can access the Patient Care Partnership document at http://www.aha.org/advocacy-issues/communicatingpts/pt-care-partnership.shtml. The document is currently available in seven different languages.

Legal Considerations

The legal system is based on **laws**—the rules and regulations that guide society in a formal and binding manner. These regulations are human-made rules capable of being changed by the legislative and judiciary systems of the United States, whose officials are elected and appointed as representatives of the public. The law gives you, as a health-care provider, a general foundation for guiding your work; it may or may not complement your personal value system.

Ideally, the care you give is ethical and legal. It is possible, however, for a legal approach to care to seem unethical to you because it conflicts with your value system. This is when ethical-legal dilemmas occur. For example, the law recognizes the right of a competent person to refuse therapy. All individuals have that right regardless of the agreement or disagreement of the health-care system with the

decision. An older adult has the right to refuse to have a pacemaker replaced. Such replacement is essentially a benign procedure with minimal risk, and not to have it done may cause death. It is the person's right to accept or refuse the therapy, however. The values of the health-care provider do not change the principles of the law.

Another example is provided by Dr. Jean Watson in her theory the "science of human caring" and is explained in detail in her book *Human Caring Science: A Theory of Nursing* (Watson, 2012). In her book, Watson emphasizes the importance of valuing persons as individuals and avoiding objectifying them. She explains that a nurse gives legal care when going into a person's room to perform a complicated dressing change. The nurse assesses the wound site, plans what will be done, removes the old dressing, and replaces it with a new dressing. The dressing is then evaluated for effectiveness. (I hope you recognize the use of the nursing process here.) The law does not indicate that the nurse needs to talk to the person or to explain the procedure or the healing process. For that care to be ethical, the nurse must take the time to talk to the person, however, and treat the person as a human being rather than an object with a wound to dress. Another simple example is

Focused Learning Chart: A Comparison of Ethics and the Law

Ethics	*The Law*
Study of moral actions and values	Rules and regulations that guide society in a formal and binding manner
Principles of conduct that govern individuals and groups; generally complement your personal values	Provides a binding foundation of rules that will guide your work; it may not complement your personal values
Critical to examine and understand your own value system to give ethical care	Must understand and apply the law to every nursing care situation

Note: The highest level of nursing, that of holistic caring, can be given only when both ethical and legal care are administered.

that of bathing persons with dementia. Federal law requires that persons in nursing homes be kept clean. It is possible for a nursing assistant to give a resident a bath that is abusive by allowing no protection of modesty, by not waiting for the water to warm, or by being verbally abusive. This situation could be described as a legal, but unethical, bath.

In the midst of the time pressures of the complex world of health care, one must be careful to define legal and ethical care. Nurses experience legal and ethical issues in their work every day. It is important to be able to distinguish between ethics and the law.

Laws can be developed and passed on national, state, and local levels. Nurses are influenced mostly by national (federal) laws and state laws. Examples of federal laws include the Patient Self-Determination Act of 1990, which requires asking people if they have living wills, durable power of attorney, or advance directives. There also is HIPAA, which includes regulations about patient privacy.

Nurse practice acts are state laws that detail the requirements for licensure and the limits of nursing practice. Every nurse needs to be familiar with the nurse practice act in the state where he or she is practicing. Nurse practice acts differ from state to state, so if you practice in more than one state, you need to know the differences.

Each hospital, home care agency, and nursing home has its own policies and procedures that must be in compliance with the state and federal laws. An employee of each health-care organization is a representative of that agency and is expected to follow all of the rules and regulations. Failure to do so is grounds for being terminated from a job. If an employee believes that laws are being broken by the agency's rules and regulations, there is a citizen's duty to report this to the agency authorities such as a supervisor, or the legal authorities such as the Department of Health, or both. This type of situation can lead to a serious legal and ethical dilemma. It is best to be certain of your facts before you embark on this type of course and to obtain legal counsel.

LEGAL LIABILITY

Most nurses do not commit wrongful acts deliberately, yet they are at risk every day for making a mistake for which they are liable. The term **liability** means that you are legally and morally responsible for an action taken. There are risky behaviors that can increase the possibility of making an error,

increasing your risk of liability. These risks are apparent when the following occur:

1. Working when you are physically or emotionally exhausted
2. Working with inadequate staff
3. Not having the necessary equipment available to meet patient or resident needs
4. Not following the policies and procedures of the institution
5. Practicing beyond the scope of the nurse practice act
6. Allowing an impaired health-care provider to work without reporting him or her

Priority Setting

The priority for this chapter is for you always to identify the nurse practice act for the state where you are practicing nursing as well as the rules and regulations at your place of employment. You are responsible for knowing the law and the policies that determine your practice. No one else can assume that responsibility for you.

The ramifications of the mistakes that can occur during any of the previously listed situations is a serious one and requires your best effort at all times to avoid it. Not only are you liable for your own actions, but you also are liable for any personnel working under your supervision. It is important to delegate only those tasks that an individual has the license or certification and knowledge to perform. For more information on delegation, refer to Chapter 12.

If there is a situation that puts anyone in your work environment at risk, it is your responsibility to do something to improve that situation. You are the licensed person, and not only do you want the situation to be changed, but also you could be liable for the situation itself. If any situation is present that could cause a medical or nursing error—including, but not limited to, the six previously listed risky behaviors and negligence, malpractice, and omission, which are discussed next—you need to work through the chain of command until the problem is solved. Working through the chain of command means going to your charge nurse, your nurse manager, and, if there is no resolution, the administrator. Because you are a new nurse, I understand that the thought of going to a hospital or nursing home administrator might be intimidating. In an ideal situation, you and your charge nurse and nurse manager would notify the administrator together. However, in some cases, this is not possible, and the responsibility for notifying an administrator falls to an individual nurse to prevent potential patient injury.

It is difficult to confront a serious problem, but your ethics will guide you, and I predict you would not be the only nurse troubled by the problem. Gather your resources and, in a patient and professional way, work with your nurse manager, the unlicensed staff, and any others who can support you in making the work environment a safe and risk-free place to practice nursing.

ACTS OF NEGLIGENCE, MALPRACTICE, AND OMISSION

Two legal terms that are important to nurses are *negligence* and *malpractice*. **Negligence** is the failure of any reasonable person to use care and caution to prevent harm to other people in a given situation. **Malpractice** is the negligence on the part of a professional person in providing care to another person. Negligence and malpractice can occur if a medical professional fails to be cautious in doing something or fails to do something that needed to be done; the latter situation is called **omission** (failure to do something).

Every person is ethically and legally responsible and accountable for his or her own actions. Professional people who are licensed to care for others because they have special education, knowledge, and experience are held to a higher standard than other people. For example, as a nurse, you have a duty to protect and advocate for the people in your care as well as provide physical and emotional care for them.

The determination of negligence is based on the level of performance that is expected of an LPN as determined by the state nurse practice act, the policies and procedures for the facility where the LPN works, and what is considered safe and prudent care by other LPNs. For example, if you start an intravenous (IV) procedure, even in an emergency situation, and you are not IV-certified, you have broken the law as outlined in the nurse practice act, and you are liable for your behavior even if there is a good outcome from your actions. Why? Because you broke the law. Even if the outcome is good, you could be sued.

As a licensed nurse, you are liable for any acts of negligence and malpractice that you perform. If you are working on a team with certified nursing assistants (CNAs), you are responsible or liable for their actions as well.

I remember being the charge nurse on a hospital-based nursing home unit when a patient was transferred from the medical/surgical unit. He was an elderly man who had fallen out of bed and had a bruise and gash on his forehead. I asked an experienced and trusted CNA to get him settled into his bed and to let me know when he was settled so that I could come in and do his admission assessment. The unit was full, and I had blood running. Although there were two LPNs working with me, neither of them could legally work with the blood except to observe it. I checked on the blood and the resident receiving the blood. Then I headed to the room with the new admit. Before I got to the room, someone met me and said to come quickly. The new admit was being walked to the restroom, lost consciousness, and fell, hitting his head again. I was horrified that the CNA had not used the wheelchair to move him! Although this case did not go to court, I was liable for the negligence of the CNA. The physician was called, and when he got to the floor, he asked for "... the stupid person who had let his patient fall!" The CNA walked up to him, but I got there in time to say, "I am responsible." It was the truth; I was legally liable for the CNA's actions.

The situation with the CNA was one of negligent care. If a nurse is accused of malpractice and is being investigated and tried in a court of law, how do judges and juries know the difference between good care, malpractice, and negligent care?

The legal system looks at what action is expected from a reasonable and prudent person under the same circumstances. A prudent, responsible nurse is someone who is careful, thoughtful, and wise about his or her actions. This person also is a professional who renews nursing knowledge by reading, attending workshops and conferences, and "keeping up" with the profession. This is something I strongly recommend that you do.

Sometimes there are nurses who cut corners and neglect to follow rules unless someone in authority is watching. Such nurses are not prudent and responsible. A court would not use their behavior as a standard of care. Instead, the court would use expert witnesses, laws, agency rules, and standards of care published by professional organizations to show what a reasonable, prudent nurse would do under the circumstances.

Three conditions are needed to have malpractice:

1. Care inconsistent with standards of care
2. An injury or negative outcome caused by negligence
3. Significant damages suffered by the person due to negligence.

When these three criteria are met, the nurse is legally liable, or responsible, for the action in a court of law (American Board of Professional Liability Attorneys, n.d.).

Many other nursing issues are closely related to meeting the criteria of the law. One additional issue is the concept of omission. Omission occurs when you omit something that is either ordered or expected as a normal part of treatment for a person. Classic examples of omission involve treatment or medication. Omission also could involve failure to notify a supervisor or primary care provider of a situation with a patient. Many lawsuits are based on omissions of care. Although the act is something you did not do rather than something you did do, you are liable for your behavior.

Many issues within the realm of nursing are profoundly affected by ethical and legal concepts. The purpose of the next sections of this chapter is to discuss issues closely associated with nursing care of older adults, such as the use of restraints, advance directives, informed consent, and elder abuse.

USE OF RESTRAINTS

The long-practiced tradition of using **restraints** was an accepted aspect of nursing care of elderly adults until the 1980s. Nursing leaders joined other healthcare professionals in drafting legislation and working with legislators to introduce and pass federal laws for reforming care of elderly adults in the United States. In 1987, the nursing home reform legislation was added to the Omnibus Reconciliation Act (OBRA) and became the law that was instrumental in dramatically changing and improving care of elderly residents in long-term care facilities. Gradually, states wrote and passed their own laws that reinforced the federal law and added improvements for the states. One very dramatic change was the reduction in the use of restraints and the gradual implementation of a restraint-free environment in the care of elderly residents.

THINK LIKE A NURSE
Mrs. Reed has been in bed for about 2 hours but is now awake and very agitated. Your facility is a restraint-free facility. What can you do instead of restraining Mrs. Reed to ensure her safety?

Restraints, pharmacological and physical, are used to prevent an individual from harming themselves or others but should always be used as the last option. Nurses who continue to use restraints often believe they are a means of preventing falls and wandering episodes. Evidence does not support that falls are prevented by restraints. Older adults who are restrained to prevent wandering often are seriously injured because of the restraint. Frequently, their injuries are worse than if they had been wandering and fallen. When restraints are used in large numbers, the injuries and deaths caused by the restraints outnumber the injuries and deaths caused by wandering, even when restraints are applied carefully and correctly. Most restraint deaths are from asphyxiation from crushing the trachea on a side rail or vest restraint or from obstruction of breathing from a resident's head being pressed against the mattress between the bed and the side rail.

Legal Considerations
The legal system considers the use of restraints as well as the threat of using restraints as unlawful imprisonment. Anything that restricts a person's movement is considered a restraint. These items include side rails, protective vests, wheelchairs with trays, safety belts, and geriatric chairs. People fight and strongly resist being restrained, which can cause death, severe injuries, skin excoriation, bruising, and pressure ulcers.

In the remote and rare situation when a restraint seems essential, the decision should be made with the interdisciplinary team (IDT) and by law must include informing the family and obtaining an informed consent from the patient or guardian. In hospitals, it sometimes is necessary to restrain a patient to maintain lifesaving procedures such as a tracheostomy, urinary catheter, or IV tubing. A physician's order for application of a short-term restraint requires the nurse to make careful observation and to perform periodic removal, skin care, and range-of-motion exercises. In an emergency, when it is necessary to protect the older adult or others from danger, a nurse may apply restraints without a physician's order or the IDT assessment and decision making. The circumstances and the observation and care given must be carefully documented. In all instances, the least-confining restraint should be used for the shortest amount of time (U.S. National Library of Medicine, 2017).

Evidence-Based Practice

Shigeko, I. (2017). Advance Care Planning: The Nurse's Role: A consistent, system-wide approach can normalize the process, dispelling fears and misconceptions. *AJN American Journal of Nursing*, *117*(6), 56–61.

This article discusses the importance of what the author refers to as advance care planning (ACP) practice. This entails assisting patients in planning their care in the event they can no longer make health-care decisions for themselves. The author believes that nurses are in a position to take the lead in facilitating ACP practice because they work in all areas of health-care where advanced care planning should be addressed with patients and their families. In most cases, ACP is addressed for end-of-life situations when final decisions need to be made. The author suggests that ACP should be addressed for all adults whatever their age or health status. The discussions need to start at home between the person and the possible decision maker as well as the individual's primary healthcare provider, prior to the person becoming ill.

Some health-care providers, including nurses, do not believe ACP practice is within the scope of practice for nurses. Assisting patients and families by promoting ACP conversations is supported by the American Nurses Association Code of Ethics and is within the nursing scope of practice. Other healthcare providers may need education to this fact. Nurses make up the largest body of healthcare professionals and can play an important role in changing attitudes about the importance of ACP.

Questions

1. As an LPN, what can you do to assist patients with advanced care planning?
2. How will advanced care planning be different for each patient?

Other Considerations

The staff in either a hospital or a nursing home should have some common strategies for managing confused older people. There may need to be a policy of placing mattresses on the floor or of lowering the bed near the floor to keep a night wanderer from falling out of bed. If wandering occurs more frequently at night or in the late afternoon, these are the times the staff should be increased so that residents can be closely monitored. However, in most facilities, evening and night shifts are times of minimal staffing. There are numerous devices available to assist with this problem, including alarmed doors, wristband alarms, and bed alarm pads. With these devices, the older adult has freedom of movement, but the staff is immediately alerted when the older person is moving.

Implementing a restraint-free environment requires the education of everyone on staff, including ancillary staff members, to the principles of working there. The education needs to include clear definitions of restraints and restraint-free care. Staff also need to be educated on the various alternatives to restraints that are available to use instead of physical restraints. Along with the education program, it is important to assist staff to focus on their personal values regarding care for the elderly person. This should help in establishing desirable approaches to care. A restraint-free environment is an innovative care strategy that also requires thought by bright and creative people who feel a commitment to the rights of all people, especially older adults.

INFORMED CONSENT AND ADVANCE DIRECTIVES

Informed Consent

Another similar legal and ethical concern is the concept of **informed consent**. The Patient Care Partnership clearly outlines a person's right to information before giving consent to treatment. The law says that there needs to be a signature on the consent form. The ethical aspect of this situation is that the older adult and others have the right to all the information available on the treatment or procedure for which consent is being given.

As the nurse, you will assume the role of patient advocate. The physician is responsible for obtaining the consent by clearly informing the patient of all possible outcomes of the procedure and any alternatives to treatment that are available. A complete explanation of the procedure is also essential. Would you stop a patient from going to surgery if, as you were assisting him or her onto the cart, the patient asked, "Tell me again, what is it the doctor is going to do?" Legal and ethical knowledge says that you should.

> ## THINK LIKE A NURSE
> You are working with a patient who has a terminal illness and is refusing the placement of a feeding tube, but her daughter is insisting that a feeding tube be placed. You know this patient has an advance directive that clearly states a feeding tube is not to be used. How do you handle this situation?

Ideally, this situation can be prevented by ensuring that the patient has the information needed to make decisions about the health and treatment plan. Informed consent can become challenging when the patient is a frail elderly person who is experiencing behavior that ranges from forgetfulness to dementia. Is it enough just to get the signature when you know the person will not remember the instructions? The answer to that is no, it is not enough.

You would need to ask yourself if you value the patient and his or her rights as outlined in the Patient Care Partnership. Do you value the principle behind the informed consent rule? It is hoped that you do. The work may involve reporting the forgetfulness or dementia to the nursing manager. In a nursing home environment, it would be important to share that information at the IDT meeting. Talking to the family may be something you do or that is delegated to the social worker. The priority is to ensure that the elderly person has complete information when asked to make a decision regarding health care.

Some older adults have a medical power of attorney entrusted to a family member or friend. If so, that is the person who should understand the procedure and sign the consent form. The elderly person also should be well informed even though the person may not remember the information. When elderly people do not have family members to assume this responsibility, the court appoints a legal guardian. The guardian is responsible for all legal documents.

Advance Directives

There are several legal and moral concerns with the issue of advance directives. An **advance directive** is a legal document made and signed by a competent adult regarding life-sustaining issues and other concerns related to end-of-life care. Advance directives came into use when legal cases such as those involving Karen Ann Quinlan and Nancy Cruzan surfaced in the judicial system. In both of these legal cases, a young woman was kept alive on life support equipment but had no quality of life at the time and no possibility of improvement in the future. In both cases, the family members decided to remove the life support equipment and allow their daughters to die. In both cases, the health-care facility refused to remove the equipment, and the parents sued.

In 1989, the U.S. Supreme Court ruled that not even the family should make decisions for an incompetent patient without "clear and convincing evidence" that indicated the person's desire was to die if incompetent. In a five-to-four decision by the U.S. Supreme Court, the following rights were listed for states (Cruzan v. Director, 1990):

- The state has a right to assert an unqualified interest in the preservation of human life.
- A choice between life and death is a very personal matter.
- Abuse can occur when incompetent patients do not have loved ones available to serve as surrogate decision makers.

In 1990, Congress passed the Patient Self-Determination Act that requires all health-care institutions that receive federal funding (Medicare and Medicaid) to ask patients, on admission, if they have an advance directive. This could be a **living will** or a durable power of attorney, which gives another person the legal responsibility to make terminal care decisions (Box 5.1). It is the patient's responsibility to provide the health-care facility with a copy of the advance directive. Some facilities have advance directives that can be completed at the time of admission. If there is an advance directive, it is to be noted in the medical record. When the directive is noted, the patient's wishes should be followed. As an LPN, you need to determine what the law is in your state regarding advance directives. If they are required on admission, you need to know where they are and what they say regarding your patient. It is the role of the nurse to be an advocate for the people to whom care is given. Knowledge about the advance directive and the state laws that govern its use is very important. When one is working with advance directives, there is more involved than just knowing the law.

Box 5.1

Advance Directives

Living will: A written document prepared by a competent person describing the type of medical care that he or she wants or does not want in a particular situation. The document needs to be prepared while the person is still able to make his or her own decisions.

Durable power of attorney or health-care proxy: A written document prepared by a competent person giving permission for someone to make health decisions on his or her behalf under certain conditions. This document should include clear instructions about the patient's wishes regarding feeding tubes, medications, resuscitation, and mechanical ventilation.

The law represents legal responsibilities. These are serious responsibilities and should not be ignored; however, as with every issue, there is also an ethical component. It is the ethical responsibility of every nurse to ensure that the person signing the advance directive is not coerced and has full understanding of what is being signed. In most states, the nurse is not allowed to witness this document. It is important that outsiders who would not wield undue influence act as witnesses. Whenever you are giving care to a patient who is in a terminal condition, it is important that you listen as the person talks and provide honest answers to questions. If someone feels concern over what was written in the advance directive, you should bring that to the attention of the nurse manager. The instructions for completing an advance directive are provided in Appendix A of this book. In all situations, it is necessary to keep in mind the primary objective of the advance directive: to follow the wishes of the person who wrote it.

Cultural Considerations

Cultural and religious beliefs play an important part in end-of-life decisions.

States have various laws regarding the use of a living will, and family members may have different ideas as to what the patient's terminal care should be. The best advice you can have for this complicated issue is to know the policies for the facility where you work and the laws of your state. You also may want to discuss this issue with a more experienced nurse before you have to deal with it. Dying is a personal and permanent issue for each person. It is important for you to know what to do and how to manage the multiple situations that can occur by being prepared.

ELDER ABUSE

Occurrences of elder abuse are increasing in the United States. It is estimated that about 500,000 older adults are abused each year, most often by a close family member. **Elder abuse** includes physical, sexual, and emotional abuse, abandonment, maltreatment, neglect, and exploitation. Approximately 1 in 10 older adults in the United States has experienced some form of elder abuse (National Council on Aging, 2018). This number underestimates the amount of abuse because of individuals unwilling or unable to report their abuse to the authorities or family members (CDC, 2016). Abuse exists in family homes, nursing homes, and hospitals. It is done by family members, paid caregivers, and strangers. Into this scenario comes an increasing number of older people who, as a natural consequence of aging, move more slowly and experience mental changes that require patience from caregivers.

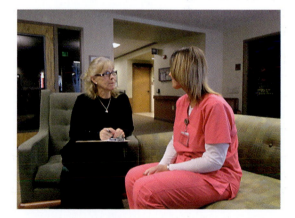

Whenever there is a question about elder abuse, immediately contact the social worker or ombudsman at the facility where you work. This social worker specializes in elder abuse investigation.

Because of a lack of emphasis on understanding and meeting the needs of elderly adults, caregivers tend to experience burnout. Accompanying this phenomenon is the tendency to abuse the elder due to the burnout and frustration they are experiencing (American Psychological Association, n.d.).

Elder abuse is also against the law, and every state in the United States has laws that say that is true. As a licensed nurse, it is your responsibility to determine what the law is in your state and the policies and procedures for handling abuse in the organization where you work. Whatever the particulars of the law are, it will state that you are responsible, under the law, to report all suspected cases of elder abuse. For more information about elder abuse, refer to Chapter 7.

PROVIDING FOR INTIMACY NEEDS

Another ageist concept in our society is that old people are asexual. Biologically, this is simply not true. Sexual needs are as basic as eating and socializing. The aging process does not remove that need from the physiological schema of older adults. The question is, how do you provide for the fulfillment or manage the needs of older adults for whom you are responsible?

Older people need love, too. I recall attending a conference many years ago in which the presenter, a music therapist, made the statement that every person needs 14 hugs a day. I do not believe that she had any scientific data to validate her point, but when she said it, I believed her! She continued to say that most of society finds old people unlovable and unhuggable. I immediately began a lifelong quest to provide as many hugs to older people as I could give in a lifetime. Older people in our society are touch starved; often people do not readily touch or hug them. Does this flash of unscientific insight bring to your awareness that you can do something positive about meeting this need for older adults in your care? It would be very exciting to see a care plan that said: 14 hugs a day evenly distributed over 24 hours.

Safe, Effective Nursing Care

Meeting Your Patients' Individual Needs
You have just admitted Mr. and Mrs. Bennett to your long-term care facility. Although they have a very close relationship, Mrs. Bennett has several health-care needs, so the decision was made by the primary care provider and the family to place them in separate rooms. On several occasions during the day, Mr. Bennett visits his wife in her room. The staff notices that Mr. Bennett sits very close to his wife's bed and rubs her arms and legs. Mrs. Bennett seems very responsive to his touch. On one occasion, one of the nursing assistants suggested that Mr. Bennett crawl into his wife's bed so he could be closer to her. The nursing assistant helped position both of them so they would be comfortable in the bed together. On leaving the room, she placed a "do not disturb" sign on the door.

Patient-centered care means providing for the individual needs of your patients.

• Did the nursing assistant do the right thing?
• Would you have done the same thing?
• Are there any concerns that should be addressed in this situation?

One stereotype that is prevalent in society is that older men have a tendency to inappropriately touch the female body. This stereotyping is generally directed at an older, confused man. Instead of restraining or isolating that individual, you should assess him from a professional level.

An example of an intervention with an older man whose wife recently died could be sitting with him and asking, "You miss your wife, don't you?" to provoke a discussion of his sexual feelings. After your discussion with this man, you may learn strategies that will help him manage his sexual feelings in a more appropriate manner. Perhaps he needs a picture of his deceased wife that he can keep with him at all times, for instance, in the dining room or when he is in the hallway in his wheelchair. It may take something as simple as teaching the nursing assistants to point to the picture of his wife and ask him to tell them about her to ward off his confused attempts at meeting his sexual needs. Perhaps the solution is more complex, and the nursing assistants need to be taught how to stop his inappropriate behavior in a respectful manner that recognizes sexual needs as normal and confusion as a reality. It is your responsibility, in an ethical framework, to determine the approaches and strategies that would provide for effective management of the sexual needs of the older people in your care.

Another problem that occurs sometimes is masturbation. Masturbation is a normal sexual outlet for people. Teenagers generally masturbate as part of their sexual experimentation. Adults often masturbate as part of their sexual relationships with other individuals. It is not abnormal for older people to masturbate. It is something they have either done intermittently or worked hard at suppressing throughout their lives. It is not wrong for an older adult to masturbate; however, because of different levels of cognitive ability, an older person may be participating in this activity in an inappropriate place. Masturbating in the dayroom or in any environment in front of others is inappropriate behavior. If this should occur, it is your responsibility to gently and kindly stop the activity and take the person to his or her room. It is appropriate to leave the person alone there to do as he or she wishes. This approach is an effective one to use if the person is acting out for attention or is forgetful or confused. If you walk into an older adult's room and the person is masturbating, just excuse yourself and close the door.

Often in nursing home settings, there is controversy about allowing married couples to room together or to have time for conjugal visits. Sometimes it is unwise to have couples room together because one may need more care than the other, and the stronger person becomes worn out trying to administer to every need of the ill or degenerating spouse. Abusive behavior brought on because of dementia could be another reason. Only reasons that would jeopardize the health of one or both of the people involved are valid, however, for keeping a married couple separated. It is normal for married people to live together, and it is normal for married people to want to continue intimacy in their relationship.

Another situation that can occur is unmarried, consenting adults having a sexual relationship. You have the ethical and legal responsibility of protecting individuals with dementia and developmentally disabled or mentally ill persons from the sexual advances of others. If that person does not have the ability to make day-to-day decisions, the person does not have the ability to consent to sexual acts. As a licensed nurse, you are responsible for protecting such a person from what could be defined as sexual abuse.

What about elderly residents who are not cognitively impaired? Sexual feelings and expressions are a normal part of living, even if one is old, disabled, or confused. Every dependent human being has the right to expect protection from sexual abuse, but every human being also has the right to express sexual feelings and have their intimacy needs met within the framework of society's norms.

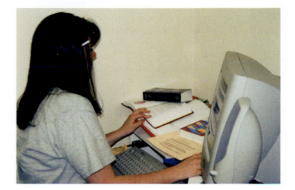

It is your responsibility as a licensed nurse to learn the laws in the state where you practice. The excuse of "I didn't know" is unacceptable in any situation when you have broken the law or violated the nurse practice act.

CONFIDENTIALITY

An underlying rule of professional health care is **confidentiality**. Every individual in the health-care system deserves perfect confidentiality regarding his or her personal information. That includes age, weight, diagnosis, family matters, and any other item of personal living for the individual. No patient has only one caregiver, however. That means information has to be communicated verbally and in written format to others on the health-care team for effective care to be delivered to the person who is ill. This type of professional information sharing is critical and needs to happen in an efficient manner. There is always the possibility, however, of a discussion at lunch or break with a colleague regarding someone or a procedure that is interesting. When you engage in such conversations, you are breaking the law.

The U.S. government developed HIPAA as a strong effort to protect individuals' personal medical information. Confidentiality always has been an aspect of professional nursing; however, the HIPAA law brings the requirement of confidentiality in professional behavior to the forefront of practice. The law allows patients access to their medical records, provides a method for making formal complaints to the government when patients believe their confidentiality has been abused, and gives patients control over how their personal information may be used.

Maintaining confidentiality of information for every patient in your care is an essential moral behavior. It also is a legal responsibility.

FINANCIAL CONSIDERATIONS

In the United States, almost all citizens who have reached the age of 65 have health insurance coverage through the federal Medicare program. Many individuals also qualify for Medicaid if they have few assets and a very low income. Some seniors are still working and may have coverage through a plan offered by their employer.

Medicare

Medicare is a federal program managed by the U.S. government since 1966. It provides health insurance coverage to all people 65 years old and older who have been employed during their lifetime and have become eligible for Social Security benefits. Medicare provides coverage for hospital services, physician and outpatient care, home care, hospice services, and prescription drugs through various parts of the law as described in this section. Coverage is not 100%. There are deductibles that must be met and coinsurance that must be paid by the patient. Some services are not covered at all, most notably long-term care.

Medicare Part A primarily covers hospitalization. It is funded by payroll taxes on all workers that are then matched by their employers. There are no premiums for Part A, and coverage is automatic for anyone 65 years old or older who is eligible for Social Security retirement benefits. Part B primarily covers physicians' fees and outpatient services. Seniors may choose to join part B and must pay monthly premiums to be enrolled. Part D was added in 2006 to cover outpatient prescription drugs. Just as for Part B, those who wish to enroll in Part D must pay monthly premiums. Part C offers seniors a choice. If they wish, they can join a private health maintenance organization (HMO) or other managed care plan (called a Medicare Advantage plan) that replaces the other three parts. Many seniors have chosen to do this because they feel the Advantage plans offer better coverage at lower premiums.

One of the most important things for seniors and their care providers to know is that Medicare does not pay for long-term care. Under specific circumstances, Medicare will pay for some nursing and rehabilitation services but only for a limited period of time. Medicare members who have been hospitalized and on discharge need continuing skilled nursing and rehabilitation services can have those covered for a maximum of 100 days if the need is certified by Medicare and is periodically recertified as care progresses.

Point of Interest

1. Medicare: Federal regulations that provide health care for individuals older than age 65, with end-stage renal failure, and those who are permanently disabled and qualify for benefits
2. Medicaid: Federal and state-supported health care for individuals who are financially disadvantaged
3. Social Security: Federal benefit check paid to retired workers of a specific age, disabled workers of any age, and spouses and minor children of deceased workers
4. Supplemental Social Security (SSI): Federal benefit paid to persons older than age 65 with little or no income or individuals with disabilities that do not allow employment

Medicaid

Medicaid was enacted by the federal government at the same time as Medicare in 1966. Each state is required to set up and manage its own Medicaid program that meets at least the minimum specifications of the federal law and regulations. To qualify for Medicaid coverage, people must have very few financial assets and very low income. Once a person does qualify, however, coverage is very broad, including both acute care and long-term care. There are no premiums to be paid for Medicaid coverage, and copayments are very minimal. Some seniors qualify for both Medicare and Medicaid.

Medicaid is the largest payer for skilled nursing facilities. Even if a resident does not initially qualify for Medicaid, that resident may qualify later after he or she has spent most of his or her assets to pay for care. At that point, Medicaid would take over payment to the skilled nursing facility. If a senior qualifies for Medicaid, it may also pay for portions of acute care, home care, and prescriptions not paid for by Medicare.

Private Health Insurance and Long-Term Care Insurance

A person who continues to work beyond age 65 may be covered through a private insurance plan offered by his or her employer. Such a person is still eligible for Medicare and can enroll if he or she wishes, but by law the employer's plan will be primary. That is, the employer's insurance will pay for services first as covered by that plan, and then Medicare may help fund some of the costs not covered by the private plan.

Neither Medicare nor employer-sponsored health insurance will cover long-term care. Because of this, some people choose to purchase long-term care insurance. These long-term care plans usually pay a fixed amount per day to help cover the cost of care provided in a nursing home, other certified facility, or even home care, as long as the needs can be documented as specified in the policy.

The Patient Protection and Affordable Care Act of 2010

The primary goal of the Patient Protection and Affordable Care Act (ACA) was to increase the number of people who have health insurance, and most of its provisions are aimed in that direction. However, there were some changes affecting seniors, even though nearly all seniors were already covered by Medicare. The reform law made some changes to Medicare Part D that will reduce out-of-pocket costs to members for outpatient prescription drugs. It also expanded Medicare coverage to include more preventive services. States were also allowed to expand Medicaid to include more people, which could make some seniors eligible sooner. Beyond those changes, most seniors will not see direct impacts of the ACA, but there are changes in the way doctors and hospitals are paid for services to Medicare patients that are intended to improve the coordination.

CASE STUDY SOLUTIONS

1. It is unethical and illegal to restrain people without following the criteria discussed in this chapter. When the restraint of older adults occurs, and it breaks the rules and regulations of the facility, your legal accountability is compounded. It is important that you realize that the law is being broken every time the residents are restrained without proper documentation. The ethical problems of restraining residents are as serious as the legal ones.

2. There is more than one approach that could resolve this problem. You may have to use them all before you find an appropriate solution.

   • Clearly state to all the nursing assistants that restraining residents not only violates the facility policies but it is also against the law. Find out if all the nursing assistants know what it means to be a restraint-free facility and if they understand clearly what is considered a restraint. The facility policies need to be reviewed and suggested alternatives to restraints need to be provided. Scheduling a short educational session may be a good approach. Educating the nursing assistants about this information is critical.

   • Use the experience and wisdom of the nursing assistants to process different solutions to the problem of residents wandering or potentially falling at night. The nursing assistants will appreciate being asked to assist in solving the problem rather than being told what to do. Try all ideas that do not go against the policy of the institution, the law, or your ethical standard.

   • Document the unique approaches of care you use on your shift, and share them with the other shifts by means of verbal report and the nursing care plan.

   • Work closely with administration to ensure staffing patterns are appropriate and that staff have the resources needed to provide a restraint-free facility.

Key Points

- Ethics is the study of moral actions and values and is based on the principles of conduct that govern individuals and groups. Ethics considers the value system of a person and the relationship of those values in determining what is good for an individual or group.
- The legal system is based on rules and regulations that guide society in a formal and binding manner. The law gives health-care professionals a general foundation for guiding their work; it may or may not complement their personal value system.
- Ethical-legal dilemmas occur when the legal approach to care seems unethical because it conflicts with a person's value system. The values of the health-care professional do not change the principles of the law.
- Liability means that a nurse is legally and morally responsible for any actions taken. Nurses can also be liable for actions taken by personnel working under their supervision. Risk for liability increases when nurses practice beyond the scope of the nurse practice act, do not follow policies and procedures of their employing institution, or work when they are physically or emotionally impaired.
- Malpractice is the failure on the part of a health-care professional to provide care that meets a reasonable standard and that results in injury to a patient. Negligence is the failure of a reasonable person to provide care to another person in a given situation. Three conditions are needed to have malpractice: care inconsistent with standards of care, an injury or negative outcome caused by negligence, and significant damages suffered by the person due to negligence.
- A restraint-free environment avoids the use of restraints. Implementing a restraint-free environment requires the education of everyone on staff. Facility policies and alternatives to restraints need to be addressed. Staff should review their personal values regarding care of the elderly to help in establishing desirable approaches to restraint-free care.
- Informed consent is the provision of all the available information to a patient regarding a treatment or procedure for which consent is being given. The physician is responsible for obtaining consent by clearly informing the patient of all possible outcomes of the procedures and any alternatives to treatment that are available.

- An advance directive is a legal document made and signed by a competent adult regarding life-sustaining issues and other concerns related to end-of-life care. The advance directive can be a living will or a durable power of attorney. The living will documents the type of care a person wants or does not want in a particular situation. A durable power of attorney is a document the gives permission for someone other than the patient to make health decisions on the patient's behalf under certain conditions.
- Elder abuse exists in family homes, nursing homes, and hospitals. Nurses are required by law to report suspected cases of elder abuse.
- An ageist concept in our society is that old people are asexual. The aging process does not remove the need for affection and intimacy and it is the nurse's ethical responsibility to ensure that an elderly resident's intimacy needs are met.
- Maintaining confidentiality of information for patients is essential. HIPAA was put into place to protect individuals' personal medical information. The law allows patients access to their medical records, provides a method for making formal complaints when patients believe their confidentiality has been violated, and gives patient's control over how their personal information can be used.
- Medicare is a federally funded health insurance program for individuals aged 65 years and older, younger disabled individuals who qualify, and individuals with end-stage renal disease. There are four parts to Medicare. Part A covers primarily hospitalization and does not require a premium. Part B primarily covers physicians' fees and outpatient services. Seniors may choose to join Part B but must pay a monthly premium. Part D is an optional plan that covers prescription medications and also requires a monthly premium. Part C allows patients the opportunity to sign up for a managed care plan that replaces the other three parts. Medicare does not cover long-term care for the elderly.
- Medicaid is a federally funded but state-administered program for providing medical care to qualifying low-income individuals. Coverage is broad, including acute and long-term care. There are no required premiums and copayments are minimal. Medicaid is the largest payer for skilled nursing facilities.

Review Questions

1. Ethics is the study of moral actions and values. One of the dilemmas within ethical thinking is concern over:
   1. Who decides what is right and what is wrong.
   2. Whoever pays the bill deciding what is ethical.
   3. Ethical and legal behavior being the same.
   4. The rules of ethical behavior changing daily.

2. Because of Mrs. E.'s failing health and inability to live on her own, she has been admitted to a long-term care facility. Which method of financing cannot be used to cover her care in the facility?
   1. Medicaid
   2. Medicare
   3. Long-term care insurance
   4. Private pay

3. The legal concept of omission in care applies when:
   1. The physician has missed a diagnosis, and you have omitted treatment for it because nothing was ordered.
   2. You have intentionally or unintentionally missed an antibiotic dose.
   3. Residents are given baths only every other day.
   4. The registered nurse does not work the weekend.

4. A restraint-free environment consists of an environment in which:
   1. Many of the residents fall or wander, but they do not sue the facility because they want to be without restraint.
   2. Mattresses are placed on the floor so that residents will not fall out of bed.
   3. The least-restrictive device is used on each resident.
   4. Restrictive devices are not used for any reason.

5. Elder abuse is a growing concern in modern society. Which of the following statements is correct?
   1. It is against the law to threaten abuse as well as to perform abusive acts.
   2. Elder abuse includes inflicting pain or injury but not confining an older person.
   3. Elder abuse is likely to happen to a male client, older than age 85, who lives with a relative.
   4. It is the legal responsibility of the RN to report all suspected cases of elder abuse; this is not the responsibility of the LPN.

ANSWERS 1. 1, 2. 2, 3. 2, 4. 3, 5. 1

CHAPTER 6
Promoting Wellness

Diane Leggett-Fife

KEY TERMS

holistic wellness
health promotion
chronic disease
self-care

CHAPTER CONCEPTS

Collaboration
Health Promotion
Mobility
Nutrition
Self
Stress

LEARNING OUTCOMES

1. Recognize aging as a normal process of living rather than a disease process.
2. Describe the role nurses play in health promotion and disease prevention activities for older people.
3. Recommend key health promotion and disease prevention activities appropriate for older people.
4. Examine the importance motivation plays in an older person's ability to participate in health-promotion and disease-prevention activities.

CASE STUDY

Mrs. C. is a 70-year-old widow who has lived with her mother since the death of her husband 2 years ago. She retired 2 years ago from her job of 30 years as a marketing director for a large sales firm to care for her mother full time. After retirement, she participated in a health promotion and screening clinic at the senior center. After completing a lifestyle inventory and screening, the following problems were noted in the categories of health promotion:

Nutrition: 10 pounds overweight
Exercise: Does no regular exercise; states she walks around the house plenty to care for her mother
Stress: Cries easily, often unable to sleep at night, complains of fatigue and generally low energy
Relationships: Misses spouse and friends from work; talks about deceased husband; states mother has been confused so she feels isolated without someone for conversation
Substance use or abuse: Drinks one glass of wine before bed and takes an occasional over-the-counter (OTC) sleeping aid. States she worries about being awake for her mother.

CASE STUDY—cont'd

Self-care: Has not seen a physician for regular checks since she had a hysterectomy 15 years ago; has seen a physician for colds or minor discomforts; never had a mammogram and does not perform breast self-examination; has not had a colonoscopy; cannot recall immunization history but is sure she has not had any in the past 10 years; has never had a flu shot or pneumococcal vaccine; recently had blood pressure taken at a drug store machine, which measured 150/92 mm Hg.

Discussion

1. List additional assessment data that should be known in each of the categories of health promotion.
2. How might you determine Mrs. C.'s greatest concern?
3. What part does Mrs. C.'s motivation play in developing a wellness plan?
4. What conditions or disease states might develop if Mrs. C. continues with no changes in her life?
5. What might be the first priority for Mrs. C.?

INTRODUCTION

One of the positive aspects of being a gerontological nurse is the variety of ways you are able to work with older people. The role of the licensed practical nurse (LPN) is crucial in the care of older individuals. You are the person who gives direct care to most older people who seek out health-care services. Many nurses think only of care given in a nursing home when they consider gerontological nursing, yet less than 10% of people older than age 65 are nursing home residents (Institute on Aging, 2018). Where do the others live, and what type of nursing care do they need?

Many older adults need your knowledge and support to stay healthy. To help these individuals, you need skills and knowledge in holistic **health promotion** and wellness. Health has many definitions, one of which is the absence of disease. However, most elderly persons have one or more **chronic diseases** that require ongoing management. Can they ever be considered well? Yes, if you consider the concept of **holistic wellness**. When considered holistically,

health implies "… a wholeness and harmony of body, mind and spirit" (Eliopolous, 2017). Achieving this balance will be the focus of wellness used in this chapter.

The search for eternal youth has a long history. The legends surrounding the "forever young" concept are taking on a new reality and meaning for the aging society in the United States because people are living longer than ever. (Remember the older-than-85-years age group and the elite-old?) The modern version of the legend of the Fountain of Youth is embodied in the concept of health promotion. The focus is on living longer and healthier, an opportunity offered to today's society that has not existed previously.

The older people of the United States are generally healthier than those of previous generations. This change is due to improved nutrition, sanitation, immunizations, and overall safety in work environments and everyday life. Today's older people have benefited from improved health care as well. People older than age 65 are expected to comprise 30% of the population by 2030 (Institute on Aging, 2018), yet they use more than one-third of U.S. expenditures for health care (Johnson, 2016). The remarkable advances in surgery, pharmacology, and the technology available for diagnosis and treatment have made tremendous contributions to the prolonging of life for older people.

Some elderly people complain about getting old. It is important to acknowledge that normal processes of aging include some decrease in vision, hearing, and joint mobility from arthritis. There may also be some weight gain. Aging is associated with losses of friends and family because of death or nursing home placement; the loss of income is also a problem for some older people, as are the acute and chronic diseases that tend to accompany the aging process. Yet, the objective of wellness defined by harmony between the body, mind, and spirit can occur if individuals strive for gerotranscendence as they age. When aging individuals achieve this developmental stage, they are able to accept the naturally occurring losses of the aging experience. They also have plans for their future and have strong relationships with supportive and caring people.

Can you see how important these characteristics are to health and wellness? It can make the difference between good to excellent or poor quality of life. *Remember:* the objective is not to run a marathon or never to experience illness. Rather, the objective is to achieve harmony in the body, mind, and spirit.

Our society views age-related changes and common health problems as diseases experienced by older people, when actually they are normal consequences of aging. Not enough attention has been given to the positive side of aging and the beneficial effects of health promotion activities to prevent disease and to slow the effects of chronic disease. Do you think that this lack of attention is another form of ageism? If so, what can you do about it as a nurse?

Current health-care concepts emphasize vitality and independence for older people as a primary concern. Regardless of age, as people laugh more, walk more, eat better, relax more, and think better of themselves and their relationships, they move beyond the neutral point of good health. Many of the complaints associated with the aging process, such as joint stiffness, weight gain, fatigue, loss of bone mass, and loneliness, can be prevented or managed by basic health promotion activities. One does not have to be free of disease to experience the benefits of health and wellness.

Priority Setting

Do you remember Chapter 2, where your priority was to combat ageism? This chapter is a continuation of that idea.

Most older adults do not have the availability of health promotion facilities, personnel, or financial support that other age groups have. Yet, if the health of older persons could be maintained, the medical bills in the United States would decrease immensely. That is secondary to the improvement in life quality that can happen for the wellness-focused older person.

Your priority for this chapter is to become well informed about wellness facilities and organizations that are specific for older adults. This information will be valuable for you as you render care to older people. You could visit the local center for senior citizens and become familiar with the activities they offer. The center can refer you to other organizations that assist aging people to be healthy. Gather as much information as you can. As a licensed nurse, you need to have a broad spectrum of information available for use as you pursue your daily work of caring for others. Assist

older adults in recognizing the importance of holistic wellness. Encourage them to be involved in the organizations and activities you find. Teach them about the concepts in this chapter that will assist them in their personal wellness program. Become knowledgeable regarding wellness for older persons, and you will enhance the lives of those in your care and become a valuable resource to the health-care team.

Most health-promotion activities focus on exercise, stress management, nutrition, and dealing with substance abuse. In addition, it is important that wellness activities for older adults include relationships and **self-care**.

ILLNESS AND WELLNESS AS A CONTINUUM

If you think of health as a continuum with illness on one end and health on the other, you can understand better the importance of health promotion. By using a holistic approach to examine the continuum, you focus your attention on the person's previous experience with life, existing support systems (for example, family, church), and personal strengths. The point is that everyone wants health, and holistic health promotion activities are one way to achieve that goal.

Primary care providers and nurses traditionally focus on working with patients who are on the illness end of the continuum or who have symptoms of disease or disability. As a person's health improves, traditional medicine becomes less involved in helping the person reach optimal well-being. In contrast, health promotion efforts primarily are focused on wellness, the other side of the continuum. Think of Mrs. C. and how she participated in a health promotion and screening clinic following her retirement. The information obtained at the clinic will assist her on the wellness path.

In more recent years, nurses have begun to use health promotion efforts even when dealing with people on the illness side of the continuum. Special exercise and nutrition programs have been designed for cardiac rehabilitation, exercise and weightlifting programs for chair-bound persons, and weight management programs for older persons. The remainder of this chapter focuses on health promotion activities on the illness and wellness sides of the health continuum.

Motivation

If you, as a nurse, want to be successful in promoting healthy choices in older people, you need to understand the importance of individual motivation. Desire must be present on the part of an older adult to make a change. It is critical to explore what motivates an older person to eat right, exercise, and avoid unhealthy behaviors on an individual basis. This is true for all people, even yourself.

CRITICALLY EXAMINE THE FOLLOWING

Motivation is an important concept to understand. You will understand it best if you comprehend what motivates you. Answer the following questions and be prepared to share your answers in class or submit them to your faculty person.

1. What are you wearing today? There is a reason for wearing it; do you know what that reason is? Whatever the reason, it is your motivation to wear it. It could be as simple as the outfit being your favorite color or being the last clean outfit in the closet.
2. What foods have you eaten today? Why did you choose those foods? Your choice of foods could be healthy or unhealthy, but you were motivated to choose them. What were your reasons for those choices?
3. Why are you in a nursing program? What is your motivation for being here? Spend time pondering this question. Understanding your personal motivation for such an all-important decision is critical.

As a part of human behavior, motivation is the incentive or drive that causes a person to act. Incentive to take action is based on needs and desires that are internal and external to the person. An older person may have an incentive to exercise three times a week if it helps the individual experience less discomfort or immobility from arthritis. For some people, the incentive may need to be more than physical wellness. A need also may exist for a mental wellness experience, such as that derived from socialization with others while exercising, such as in a water aerobics class, playing tennis, or with a group doing mall walking.

The nursing challenge is to assist older adults in identifying their own incentives for participation in health promotion and disease prevention activities. This information allows the nurse to have greater insight into ways to promote health and lessens the frustration experienced from what are often incorrectly referred to as *noncompliant patients*. Compliance occurs only if the individual can personally identify a need or desire to exercise, eat correctly, reduce stress, or make other changes necessary for improved wellness. This is motivation experienced by people individually. Often, assisting to identify the motivation is one way that you, the LPN, can help an older adult. Think about Mrs. C's motivation to participate in the health promotion and screening clinic. Will this same motivation keep her interested in addressing some of the issues listed? What could you do to increase her motivation?

Incentives

Studies have disclosed some of the reasons (incentives) for older people to participate in health promotion behaviors, such as the following:

- A belief that activities improve fitness and health
- The enjoyment of socialization
- A belief that activities help maintain independence
- Influence of significant others (Cassidy, Richards, & Eakman, 2017; Dedeyne et al., 2018)

Knowledge about why a person participates in health promotion (or the incentives for doing so) can be determined through a caring and focused interview. After personal incentives have been identified, you can reinforce them in health promotion activities. In addition to understanding individual motivation, you need to help individuals plan their short- and long-term goals for making health changes. The secret to success in health behavior is to help the older adult choose personal goals with care and then learn to enjoy achieving them. Following an interview with Mrs. C., you may discover several areas that would increase her interest in obtaining the goals. Review her statements regarding missing people at work and her husband. Could socialization with group activities be a stimulus to keep her active? Would she find motivation in improving her fitness if it could help her to continue caring for her mother in her home?

Health Promotion Activities

When older adults have identified an area of health promotion that is desirable, they have an incentive to maintain or improve their health. The challenge is to locate a properly designed activity. Many current health promotion activities can be geared toward younger age groups and may exclude older adults by design. Four reasons underscore why the current focus on health promotion activities is often inappropriate for older people:

1. The focus frequently is on life extension or on reducing the risks of premature death. If a person stops smoking, reduces fat intake, and exercises, the risk of a heart attack at an early age is reduced. For elderly people who have already lived beyond the average life expectancy, life extension may not be as important as quality of life. Stopping smoking, reducing fat intake, and exercising are important at any age, but for different reasons. The focus must be on health promotion benefits specific to an older person.

2. Emphasis is often placed on advancing "youthfulness" and preventing aging. Older people recognize that they do not fit the image of youth and have already experienced some consequences of aging. This does not mean self-image and appearance are not important to older people, but that the image needs to match the older person's self-perception.

3. Health promotion programs focus on preventing chronic disease. It is important to note that three out of four of those aged 65 or older already have two or more chronic diseases (U.S. Department of Health and Human Services, 2018). When these programs focus on management of the symptoms of the disease rather than on its prevention, more older adults have a reason to participate.

4. A focus on self-responsibility for health fails to consider the limitations imposed by personal circumstances. An individual who has a need and desire to walk daily for exercise may live in an unsafe neighborhood. An older adult may desire to eat a healthy diet but because of limited income may be unable to afford the proper food. The external environment may pose barriers to older people that are difficult to overcome. These problems need careful attention.

As you, the LPN, evaluate the key areas of health promotion for older people, your goals must be to design, plan, and provide activities that fit individual needs for the desired results.

Properly designed health promotion activities should be:

• Accessible (transportation, time of day, location)
• Enjoyable and social (mental and physical wellness)
• Reasonable (focus on the right activity for the right reason)
• Sensitive to needs of older people (hearing, vision, functional level)

Health promotion strategies must be based on the belief that the individual is the only one who can choose a path to a healthy life. Consequently, you, the nurse, must be sure that health promotion activities are individually designed so that the pathways exist.

REGULAR EXAMINATIONS

Before appropriate health promotion activities can be designed for an individual, a physical examination of most body systems needs to be completed. An annual physical examination is important for maintaining health and promoting wellness. Many older adults need to be seen more often for the management of the chronic diseases that may accompany aging. Some older people avoid making such appointments because they have limited funds to pay the co-pay; they lack convenient transportation; or they do not recognize that their symptoms can be treated. Some people think that being ill is part of being old, so they accept their condition and do not seek treatment. Some people may be like Mrs. C., who has no health complaints and therefore does not feel that she needs to have regular examinations.

Regular visits to the physician can help prevent acute conditions and are an asset for managing chronic diseases. An acute condition is one in which the symptoms come on rapidly and can be severe but usually have a short course. An example would be the flu, which can be prevented by yearly immunizations. Regular bloodwork as an indicator of overall health is critical, as are screening tests for colon, breast, cervical, and prostate cancers. The physician's visit is the time to obtain immunizations such as annual flu shots and immunizations for tetanus (every 10 years), shingles, and pneumonia ("Recommended Adult … ," 2018).

Medications should be monitored for effectiveness and drug interactions. Encourage your elderly patients to bring a list of all medications, including OTC drugs and supplements, when visiting the physician. The physician needs to know every medication, herb, or supplement taken to prevent problems.

Foot problems are common in the elderly, and regular visits to a podiatrist may be needed to manage care of aging thickened toenails, bunions, corns, and calluses. Vision should be checked annually to monitor for glaucoma, cataracts, and other eye problems. Dental visits ideally should be twice a year and annually for people who wear dentures. Denture wearers still need to see a dentist because everyone should have an annual oral examination to check for denture fit, mouth soreness, or mouth cancer. Audiology examinations do not need to be done unless there is a hearing problem. The benefits of regular examinations of the body are to prevent, treat, and monitor physical conditions. Yet problems do occur even with careful attention to health-promoting activities. Chronic diseases are a common problem.

CHRONIC DISEASE

As an LPN giving care to older adults, you need to understand the promotion of wellness in the holistic sense. This concept needs to go beyond the vision of physically well, older people living in their own homes independently. Remember that greater than 60% of individuals over the age of 60 are living with two or more chronic diseases (U.S. Department of Health and Human Services, 2018). People older than 85 years experience increased difficulty with home management activities and are more likely to depend on assistance in their living situations. Regardless of age, living arrangement, or health condition, the goal for health promotion should be to assist older adults in reaching a state of optimal health.

The most common health problems of older adults are associated with chronic diseases. The most frequent chronic conditions include arthritis, hypertension, heart conditions, hearing impairments, and dementia. Because of these conditions, older people visit physicians more often, are hospitalized more frequently, take more prescription and OTC drugs, and experience more functional problems than younger people. The focus of many medical treatment interventions in the United States is on *curing* acute conditions. Chronic illnesses, which are the predominate illnesses of older adults, cannot be cured, but instead require management with a focus on caring.

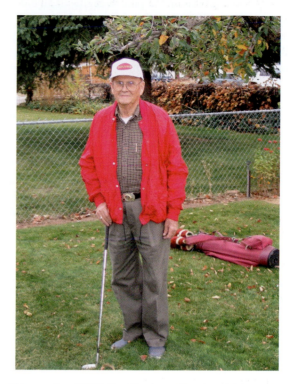

This man has COPD. He still goes golfing but rides a cart and sometimes elects to skip a difficult hole. This man has adapted to his chronic disease.

CRITICALLY EXAMINE THE FOLLOWING

Reread the last paragraph of the introduction. Your health would improve if you paid more attention to the management of your personal exercise, stress, nutrition, substance use, relationships, and self-care. As a student in a very demanding program, you may need to examine your own health promotion critically. Make comments regarding how you can improve your health in the following areas. Be prepared to discuss them in class and relate how what you do for yourself may also assist an older adult.

1. Exercise
2. Stress management
3. Nutrition
4. Substance use and or abuse
5. Relationships
6. Self-care

Treatment Strategies

Management of chronic conditions involves treating symptoms and maximizing the strengths of an older person. You need to understand the aging process and older adults in general and advocate and lobby for what they need. For an older adult who has arthritis and who is in severe pain, it is important to treat the symptom of pain. If pain is minimized, the person is better able to stay active and prevent the further disabling effects of immobility. Nurses are the key people to recognize the symptom (pain) and administer the prescribed treatment (medication). As a gerontological nurse, you must go one step further and consider the impact of the disease and its treatment on the older person's ability to perform activities of daily living (ADLs), which include personal care, dressing, and eating. In addition, instrumental activities of daily living (IADLs), which are often more difficult, need to be considered. IADLs are activities such as shopping, doing the laundry, and cleaning the house. So consider:

- What could be done to prevent the onset of pain?
- What would be the side effects of the pain medication?
- How has the older person coped with pain in the past? Would the same approach be effective now?

An LPN must recognize the importance of good health and its correlation with functional independence among older people. Understanding does not always make it clear, however, what kind of activities would promote health and prevent development of further secondary conditions that result in dependency.

Point of Interest

To meet the needs of older adults, nurses often seek interventions that come from external sources rather than empowering older people to use their inner sources. Most older people have lived a lifetime of taking care of themselves and their families; they have given service to the community; and many have managed devastating challenges. Be sure to use them as a resource by involving them in the planning stage of the nursing process. They will have greater motivation performing activities if they have been part of the planning.

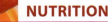

NUTRITION

With advancing age, a person's general health is determined to a great extent by the effects of dietary patterns over the years. Staying physically and mentally active is important to all older adults, but it can be affected by dietary intake. They need to understand the role proper nutrition plays in their lives, even in later years.

As bodies age, four changes occur that affect a person's nutritional status:

1. The body's rate of metabolism slows and no longer needs the same amount of energy and food to do the same amount of work. Older adults often comment that they have not changed how they are eating and exercising, but they are now gaining weight. As people age, lean body mass decreases, and body fat increases. This may result in weight gain and can lead to obesity.
2. The senses of taste and smell may be less keen. Some or all of an elderly person's teeth may need to be replaced by dental appliances. As a result, older people may find themselves eating different foods and drinking less fluid. To enhance the taste of foods, they may use more salt or sugar.
3. Social aspects of eating are important. As people age, they retire, their families grow up and move, and their spouses and friends move away or die. This results in changes in the socialization of eating. One of the most difficult adjustments is cooking for one and eating alone.
4. Environmental factors greatly influence nutritional habits of older adults. Lack of transportation to food stores and restaurants, inability to manage reading labels and shopping, and insufficient money to buy healthy food can be major barriers to eating properly.

Poor dietary habits contribute to many diseases that occur in older persons. Chronic diseases, such as heart disease and cancer, can be slowed—and for some people, prevented—by avoiding obesity and decreasing the amount of fat in one's diet. Studies from the Mayo Clinic (2018b) indicate that high cholesterol levels increase the risk for atherosclerosis, which increases the risk of stroke or heart attack. The American Cancer

Society (2018) found marked increases in the incidence of cancer of the uterus, gallbladder, kidney, stomach, colon, and breast associated with obesity.

It is estimated that osteoporosis, or low bone mass, affects 55% of men and women over the age of 50 in the United States (International Osteoporosis Foundation, 2017). The loss of bone mass and bone strength as a result of this disease leads to broken hips, arms, and legs and to back injuries. Osteoporosis is often referred to as a "silent" disease. Few signs or symptoms appear until a bone breaks. Adding calcium to the diet, participating in a regular exercise regimen (which should include weight-bearing and balance activities), and avoiding alcohol and smoking are key prevention strategies.

Other chronic problems that are frequent complaints of older people include constipation, urinary incontinence, and arthritis. Nutrition plays a role in each of these conditions. More information on nutrition is provided in Chapter 8.

Although one-on-one teaching may be easier, group learning that incorporates an opportunity for socialization and fun is much more likely to result in positive outcomes. You, as the LPN, may want to organize a group of elderly people in the community to participate in learning nutrition principles. One of the principles that should be taught is Choose MyPlate, which replaced the food pyramid in 2011 (U.S. Department of Agriculture, n.d.). (See Chapter 8 for more information.) This information, which may be new to some people, replaces the food pyramid or the basic four concepts that many older people were taught.

Health promotion activities aimed at altering a lifetime of eating habits must be reasonable, and the benefits need to be made apparent. Nurses should clearly understand what motivates the individual. In addition, nurses must be aware of the unique nutritional needs and problems that accompany later years.

Although there is no information regarding nutrition for Mrs. C., she may benefit from some nutrition guidance. Living with and caring for her mother could have disrupted her routine and schedule that was in place when she was working. This and the dietary needs of her mother could affect her food choices. It was stated that she was 10 pounds overweight so planning optimal nutrition could help her reach a healthy weight.

Evidence-Based Practice

Ory, M. G., Lee, S., Han, G., Towne Jr., S. D., Quinn, C., Neher, T., … Smith, M. L. (2018). Effectiveness of a lifestyle intervention on social support, self-efficacy, and physical activity among older adults: Evaluation of Texercise Select. *International Journal of Environmental Research and Public Health, 15*(234), 1–19. doi:10.3390/ijerph15020234

This quantitative study examined the effects on physical activity, a belief in an ability to exercise, and social support for adults age 60 and older. Physical activity has been encouraged as a way to reduce limitations that can occur as an individual ages, but aging brings age-related changes that can affect physical activity. This study demonstrated the ability to decrease sedentary behaviors and increase physical activity with planned, instructor-led, group exercise and education regarding physical activity, even in adults with chronic conditions. The participants showed improvements in feelings of being able to exercise, amount of activity each week, and feelings of social support at 3 and 6 months.

Question
Which of the following inferences can you make? State whether the study summary provides extensive, limited, or no evidence to support each inference.

1. Older adults can participate in physical activity, even with chronic conditions.
2. Group-led exercise and education helped the older adults increase physical activity.
3. Socialization during physical activity for the older adult will detract them from participating fully.
4. Athletic abilities should not keep the older adult from participating in activities.
5. As a health-care professional, encouraging and assisting older adults to participate in physical activity will help them to adjust to age-related changes.

EXERCISE AND FITNESS

The fitness movement in the United States began in the 1970s. By the late 1970s and early 1980s, society began to stress the importance of fitness for older adults. Studies today continue to emphasize the benefits of exercise and its importance to total health for all ages. The body's responses to exercise are fundamentally the same throughout life. Exercise stimulates the mind, maintains fitness, prevents or slows progression of some diseases, helps to establish social contacts, and generally improves quality of life.

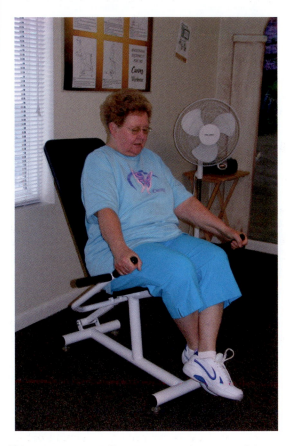

This woman goes to Curves, a women's exercise club, three times a week to maintain her strength. This type of program has assisted her in losing weight as well as increasing her strength. Besides, she says, it is fun to socialize with the people there.

Fatigue and lack of energy, poor sleeping habits, and poor circulation are common reports of older adults. These problems often result in inactivity. Inactivity leads to muscle wasting and weakening of the bones. This vicious circle results in disabling conditions and functional dependency. If exercise could be packed into a pill, it would be the most widely prescribed and beneficial medicine in the world. Chronic conditions such as heart disease, diabetes, osteoporosis, arthritis, obesity, and depression all have been shown to improve or experience a slowing of progression with regular physical activity.

Physiologically, a regular exercise program can build and maintain muscle strength and endurance and can improve the capacity of the heart, circulatory system, and lungs. The commonly heard phrase "use it or lose it" is the overall theme for exercise and fitness in a person's later years. Exercise programs for people older than 60 should emphasize a regular routine of exercise to expand and increase strength, flexibility, and endurance. Such exercise programs can be developed for individuals with a wide range of conditions, from wheelchair-bound or bed-bound frail elderly people to physically active individuals. If an individual 65 years or older is in generally good health and generally fit, the American Heart Association (2018) and Mayo Clinic (2018) recommend 150 minutes of moderate intensity exercise per week with 2 days of muscle-strengthening activities for maximum health benefits. Additional benefits of a good fitness program include increased energy, buildup of lean body mass, and increased self-esteem.

Regular, scheduled exercise for Mrs. C. would bring some routine back into her life, provide for some socialization outside her home, and assist her in reaching her ideal weight. In addition, the increased activity may help to decrease her complaints of fatigue and low energy while improving her sleep.

Strengthening

Strengthening exercises help build and maintain muscle condition by moving muscles against resistance. Simple strengthening exercises are needed to promote activity without tiring a person too easily. Muscle strength is also crucial to the support of joints and can help prevent problems related to arthritis. Improving muscle strength is a primary objective in slowing the progression of osteoporosis. Patients confined to bed lose muscle mass very quickly. It can be restored, however, when exercise is resumed. Something as simple as doing range-of-motion exercises while holding a soup can make a difference in strength for most older adults.

Focused Learning Chart: Significance of Strengthening Exercises

Effects of Exercise	Exercise Plan Considerations
Builds and maintains muscle strength	Should be designed for the individual
Decreases arthritic pain over time	Should not be too tiring
Strengthens joints	Should promote activity
Slow process of osteoporosis	
The greater the muscle mass, the greater glycogen reserves, which means more energy	
Weak muscles lead to falls and possible fractures	

Healthy People 2020

Goal

Increase the proportion of adults who meet current federal physical activity guidelines for aerobic physical activity and for muscle-strengthening activity (Healthy People 2020, 2018).

Point of Interest

If an older person is able to meet life demands, it is unnecessary for the nurse to intervene. The only intervention necessary in this situation is to support the individual in what he or she is able to do and monitor for any changes.

As a nurse, you must be aware of the impact a short-term illness can have on an older person. Something as common as the flu can cause significant weakness and inactivity. Weak muscles lead to falls, which can result in hip fractures and other injuries. If older adults are unaware of the importance of strengthening exercises, no incentive can return them to the normal level of function.

Strength-building exercises are also important for a person with diabetes because the exercises help regulate glucose metabolism by increasing muscle mass. The greater the muscle mass, the greater the glycogen level in the muscles, and the more energy will be available in reserve for periods of exertion.

Flexibility

Flexibility exercises involve slow stretching motions. Medical and fitness experts agree that stretching is the most important part of an exercise program designed to prevent injuries, reduce muscle tension, and maintain range of motion. As a result of the normal aging process, muscles tend to lose elasticity, and tissues around the joints thicken. Flexibility exercises can delay or reverse this process by preventing muscles from becoming short and tight.

All stretching motions should be done gradually and slowly, without any sudden force or jerking motion. You should encourage a variety of stretching exercises for different parts of the body, including arms, shoulders, back, chest, stomach, buttocks, thighs, and calves. All exercise routines should include a warm-up and cool-down with 5 to 15 minutes of stretching exercises. As the older person's range of motion increases, the individual will be able to reach, turn, and move in all directions with more grace and less pain.

Endurance

Endurance-building or aerobic exercises improve the function of the heart, lungs, and blood vessels. A frequent report from older people is "feeling tired." Endurance-building exercises help strengthen the heart to pump blood and the lungs to exchange oxygen and increase the elasticity of blood vessels. These functions are a vital part of fitness and feeling good. Walking, cycling, and swimming or water aerobics are excellent all-around exercises.

As stated earlier, the basic components of an exercise routine for older people include strengthening, flexibility, and endurance. In addition, attention must be given to breathing during exercising. Breathing is a vital part of an exercise program. As a person concentrates on the exercise, it is easy to forget to breathe. Respiratory changes with aging make it even more important to use the correct breathing technique. The correct breathing technique is to breathe out during vigorous effort or exertion and breathe in as the muscles relax.

A last comment on exercise is a caution for older adults who have not been exercising on a regular basis, who are frail, or who have cardiovascular problems. Anyone with heart problems or high blood pressure, who is overweight, or who has been told to be cautious in personal activity level should have an exercise program prescribed by a physician. It is important for anyone, regardless of health condition, to have a check-up prior to beginning an exercise program and to maintain contact with the health-care provider.

Physical fitness is one component of life that enables people to live it to its fullest. As a nurse, you have a responsibility to understand and teach the importance of exercise and fitness to elderly patients. Remember to think holistically. What environment is best for the older person, who is there to be a support person, what is the incentive to make change? If you know these things and assist in making a plan that uses them, the program will be more successful.

Mrs. C. could possibly benefit from the inclusion of exercise, but she has told you she does not participate in regular exercise. Helping her to understand and believe in the benefits of may be the first step to persuade her to include exercise as part of her routine.

Cultural Considerations

Wellness can have different meanings for a variety of groups. When working with an older adult you will need to understand the meaning of health and wellness from a cultural perspective. Asian cultures have a great respect for elders. Family members may be hesitant to urge the older adult to exercise or change eating habits, viewing this tactic as disrespectful. Working with individuals from the Muslim or Hindu faith, you will need to be aware of dietary restrictions and make adjustments to guarantee a balanced diet. Another consideration from these groups is clothing and modesty. Make sure you understand the needs regarding coverings, attendance of family members, or even the need for care from someone of the same gender. Discovering the needs from a cultural perspective will help the older adult to accept modifications in diet or lifestyle, which can improve individual health.

Stress

Stress motivates people to act, forces them to think under pressure, and challenges them to be creative and resourceful human beings. The key is to be able to strike a balance between too much stress and not enough, between positive stress (*eustress*) and stress that is harmful (*distress*). As with all areas of health promotion, it is never too late to improve a technique. Failure to take a healthy approach to dealing with stress can greatly increase the risk of developing or worsening heart disease, cancer, and other chronic diseases (WebMD, 2017).

For most older people, stress is related to three basic areas: environment, body, and mind. Environmental stressors are weather, crime, crowds, time pressures, and the demands of others. The human body can experience stress because of illness, accidents, drugs, lack of sleep, and normal changes related to aging. The mind can create stress for people because of negative attitudes and perceptions, boredom, despair, and hopelessness.

Regularly occurring events such as trips to the grocery store, pain from arthritis, and fear of the unknown conditions of retirement all may create stress for older people. Stress-related problems and symptoms include ulcers (stomach pain), high blood pressure (no symptoms), arthritis (joint pain and muscle tension), heart disease (chest pain and difficulty breathing), cancer (increased susceptibility), headaches (constant worry), circulatory problems (cold hands and feet), and backaches (muscle spasm and chronic pain) (WebMD, 2017).

One of the most important strategies for health promotion is to help older people recognize their personal reactions to stress and their bodies' physiological responses. Tools used to recognize stress include a stress log or journal of daily stressful situations, life change inventory, and stress control inventory.

After an individual has recognized personal stress and his or her response to it, several interventions are available to help relieve it. As a nurse, you should understand and be able to recommend appropriate stress-reducing activities. These activities may be divided into two categories: quick relaxers and long-term stress management skills.

A quick relaxer is something a person can do in 2 or 3 minutes to relax and counteract symptoms of distress. One of the most important, yet difficult, skills for some older people is learning simply to relax. Learning how to relax helps older people sleep better, control blood pressure, lower cholesterol, reduce headaches, relieve depression, reduce or eliminate use of drugs and alcohol, and smile more. Examples of quick relaxers include roll breathing, progressive muscle relaxation, imagining a pleasant place or situation, eye relaxation, and exercise. The importance of exercise was discussed earlier in this chapter; however, it is worth emphasizing that exercise is the most natural way to relax. For the greatest calming effect, an elderly individual can combine fitness activities with breathing and other mental relaxation techniques.

For some older people, dealing with stress requires more than a few "stress-buster" quickie techniques. If stress causes continuous physical and mental discomfort that results in illness, learning how to deal with the source of stress needs to be a major goal. This assumes that the individual understands what is causing the stress.

Using the four stress management options listed here as a teaching tool is very helpful for many people. The four basic options are:

1. Attempt symptom relief (quick techniques).
2. Accept the stressor (change perception or attitude). *Example:* Your children frequently call you at the last minute to babysit your grandchildren. You may accept the stress and decide you really do not need much time to prepare, so say yes and enjoy! Another choice is to lovingly say no!
3. Alter the stressor (change or alter the source of stress so it is no longer there). *Example:* Make the decision that you will not be able to babysit unless they let you know 1 day ahead of time.
4. Avoid the stressor (remove yourself from the stressor). *Example:* Decide you will not be a babysitter for your grandchildren. After the source of stress has been pinpointed, the older person often can decide whether to accept, alter, or avoid it.

Stress management techniques may be unfamiliar to many older individuals, even though stress and recognition of stress have been in the spotlight for some time. Teaching older people stress management can be done very successfully through either group or individual activities.

Think of some symptoms recorded for Mrs. C. Could it be possible she is experiencing stress in her life from the loss of her husband and retirement? Stress management techniques may be another avenue to explore to assist her in being able to sleep at night.

LIFESTYLES

Maintaining a healthy lifestyle at any age involves more than getting fit, eating right, and coping with stress. Other challenging issues that people of all ages encounter are relationships, possible alcohol and drug abuse, and lack of self-care.

Relationships

Human life is constantly defined and redefined by our ties to others. The term *relationship* means any significant bonding in which a person feels a strong sense of responsibility toward the physical and emotional welfare of others.

As people grow older, the reality is that all relationships eventually end. Whether through divorce from a spouse or death of a spouse, child, family member, friend, or pet, the loss redefines one's life. An individual's ability to deal with the process of grief over the losses can result in significant personal and health changes and changes in dealing with others. How strongly these changes affect the rest of one's life depends on how well the individual and those involved in the personal life of the individual cope with the loss. How people have coped with change and crisis in younger years predicts how they will deal with these same stressors later.

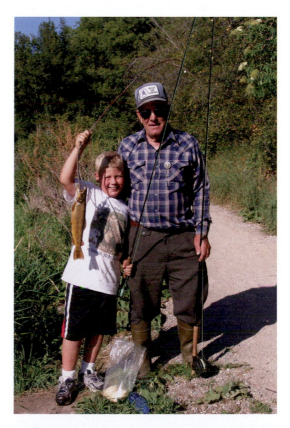

This 65-year-old man goes fishing with his youngest grandson two or three times a week. Fishing always has been part of this man's lifestyle, but now he has the added close relationship with his grandson.

As years pass, life changes can become increasingly complex. Older adults must deal with changes caused by retirement, which can have major impacts on home life, health, finances, and role changes. In addition, the loss of relationships may be frequent and numerous. Mrs. C. has faced multiple losses in the last 2 years. Talking with her about these losses and discovering her previous coping skills may help her at this time.

As a nurse, you have an opportunity to help older adults gain insight into loss and life change. Chapter 11 contains a section on the stages of grief that may be helpful to you in understanding reactions of older adults to loss. You need to assess the effect that loss has on a person's ability to function with day-to-day activities. As an LPN, you must ask questions and allow the older person to share concerns. Health promotion activities that focus on mental wellness can provide an excellent opportunity for older adults to express the concerns they face. The American Association of Retired Persons (AARP) offers resources to help lead discussions about the myths, fears, and reality of change as one grows older.

Alcohol, Drugs, and Aging

Abuse of alcohol and drugs among older men and women may be a more serious problem than most people realize. Until the 1990s, research on drinking and the health effects focused more on the younger generation (Holahan et al., 2014). Since that time more studies have focused on the effects in those 55 years and older. The inattention to this information occurred for the following reasons:

- The elderly population in the United States was small, and few older individuals were identified as alcoholics.
- Chronic problem drinkers (individuals who had abused alcohol off and on for most of their lives) often died before old age.
- Older people frequently have been able to hide drinking problems because they often are retired or have few social contacts.

Some families may unknowingly accept or encourage drinking in older family members. They may have the attitude that drinking should be tolerated because older people have only a limited time left to live and should be allowed to enjoy themselves. Sometimes the alcohol consumption seems to be an insignificant amount to the family, and they blame the resulting impairment on aging (National Institute on Aging, 2018)

The amount, time, and place of alcohol consumption have little significance. The critical issue that needs to be addressed is what alcohol does to an individual's quality of life and functional ability. The substance use of wine before bedtime and the occasional use of a sleeping pill for Mrs. C. would warrant further investigation regarding her quality of life and functional ability. Despite studies indicating that older people consume fewer alcoholic beverages and have less alcohol-related problems than younger age groups, it can lead to a greater risk for health problems. It is important to screen for alcohol use because excessive drinking late in life, often in response to situational factors such as retirement, reduced income, declining health, or the deaths of friends and loved ones, may be a pattern of managing the stress. In these cases, alcohol is first used for temporary relief but later becomes a problem (National Council on Alcoholism and Drug Dependence, 2015; National Institute on Aging, 2018).

The physical effects of alcohol are significant for older people. Alcohol impairs mental alertness, judgment, physical coordination, and reaction time. These problems mimic and exacerbate the deleterious effects of other chronic conditions (dementia, depression, and arthritis) and increase the risks of falls and other accidents.

As people age, they seem to become less tolerant of even small amounts of alcohol, and the effect of alcohol on the body may be unusual. For example, the effects of alcohol on the cardiovascular system may mask the pain of an oncoming heart attack. Older people are the greatest consumers of prescription and OTC drugs. The combined use of alcohol and drugs increases the likelihood of a toxic or lethal effect.

Increased alcohol use in the older adult population is expected to increase with the rising age of the baby boomers. Identifying and acknowledging increased alcohol use as a problem in this age group may be difficult due to fear of stigma and denial (DiBartolo & Jarosinski, 2017). It is easy to overlook or accept problem drinking because the drinking seems to offer enjoyment or comfort. It is much harder to create social alternatives to the life events that lie behind the increased use of alcohol or alcoholism.

As a health professional, you may be tempted to rush over or omit assessment questions referring to alcohol intake. Because nurses often play a key role in recognizing alcohol and drug problems, you cannot afford to avoid such questions. You always should ask what the impact of this problem may be on the older person's ability to function. It becomes easy to see that the physical, mental, and social impact of drinking could contribute to alcohol dependency.

Safe, Effective Nursing Care

Work in Interprofessional Teams; Provide Safe, Quality Client Care

Mr. Smith, an 85-year-old widower of 8 months, has been on the unit for management of his diabetes. He has been taking an oral hypoglycemic, but since the death of his wife 8 months ago, his blood sugars have steadily risen. He states that his wife did most of the cooking and he has not had to plan meals. He has spent the last few days as your patient and has been learning how to balance insulin, diet, and physical activity. He is preparing for discharge but is concerned about his care when he returns home.

During his time on the unit, he has had visits from a daughter, and tells you that he has a son living in another state who contacts him by phone at least once a week. His chart indicates that a social worker has been in to visit with him, and he has agreed to have an assessment by a physical therapist before going home.

You have been assigned to prepare him for discharge.

1. Before discharge, it is advised that you have a meeting with those who will possibly be involved in his care at home. Recommend those individuals who should be in attendance at this meeting, and describe why they should be included.
2. Will it be important to include Mr. Smith in any of the planning meetings? Why or why not?
3. Mr. Smith lives alone and has had little physical activity since the death of his spouse. How would you encourage him to become more active?
4. What recommendations would you have for his safety in his home and his activities?
5. Would you give him any other education regarding activity, diet, and insulin?

The primary health promotion goal is helping older adults and their families recognize when alcohol is a problem. Second, straightforward information must be given to elderly adults regarding the effects of alcohol, especially in combination with drugs. The nurse needs to understand the older person's reason for drinking. Health promotion activities that create alternatives should be made available to an older person with an alcohol problem.

Because of their critical importance, drug issues are discussed in Chapter 20; however, emphasis on the problem of drug dependency and abuse is important. Drug abuse is defined by the relationship of the individual to the drug in question. Regardless of the reason, if an older person misuses a drug or becomes dependent on it, the effects are similar to those of problem drinking. Physical and mental impairments resulting from prescribed or OTC drugs mimic disease states and increase the risk of falls, accidents, and dependency.

One role of health promotion is to offer education and screening regarding drug use. Promoting self-responsibility is the key component. Nurses must assess the impact of drug treatment on an older person's ability to complete ADLs. If a patient cannot afford a prescribed drug, he or she probably will not take the medication as ordered. If the older adult does not understand what outcomes are expected from the drug treatment, misuse of a drug may ensue by taking it for too long or taking too much of it.

SELF-CARE—TAKING CHARGE

Older adults are best qualified to keep themselves healthy and to know when they are ill. As a nurse, you need to respect and explore what the older person reports as the problem. Do not take charge and deny an older adult responsibility for personal health and health management.

Self-care, self-help, and *self-maintenance* are terms often used interchangeably to describe various aspects of an individual's efforts to maintain optimal health and functionality. When an individual cannot assume responsibility for self, the patient has the nursing diagnosis, Self-Care Deficit. Most individuals with this diagnosis need medical or nursing intervention.

From a nursing perspective, the focus is frequently on ADLs, which are the most basic self-care activities engaged in by older adults. It is common to see dependence in at least some basic ADLs for older people. Surveys show that people older than 65 years who live in the community are dependent in at least one ADL. In nursing homes, the prevalence is higher. In addition to ADLs, an older person needs to manage IADLs, such as food preparation, managing medications, and managing personal finances.

Regardless of whether an older adult is attempting to overcome a functional deficit in ADLs or IADLs, the same self-care skills are needed. Self-care involves the following:

1. Accepting personal responsibility for one's own health
2. Adopting healthy lifestyle habits with regard to fitness, relaxation, and nutrition
3. Learning how to make the changes you choose to accomplish the things you want to do

Contributing to personal health and a healthy lifestyle contributes to feelings of positive self-worth. These characteristics complement the concept of self-transcendence by meeting needs of the individual so that person can focus on the needs of others.

Accepting personal responsibility for health behaviors applies to the "why" of the decision more than the "what." *Self-responsibility* means that the older adult does not rely solely on spouse, children, physician, or nurse to determine "what to do to be healthy." The person must be allowed to think through the options and make each decision. This does not mean that a person should not seek the assistance of others, but rather that a need exists to work in partnership with the physician, nurse, or family (separately or together) to make the best decision.

The self-care concept emphasizes the need for encouraging individuals to take a more active role in maintaining or improving their health. Often, the patient does not understand this process, and it is not easy for older people to accomplish. Health promotion strategies related to self-care must include helping the older adult understand how to be in charge of personal health decisions. Your efforts should be focused on enabling an older person to be a wise medical consumer and to know how and when to work and communicate as a partner with the health-care team.

> ### THINK LIKE A NURSE
> You are taking care of a 75-year-old woman who was recently discharged from a rehabilitation facility after a total knee replacement. She is unwilling to get up and walk, cries or shouts at people who try to get her up or move her, and she states it hurts too much to move. How will you handle this situation? How will you apply your new knowledge of self-care?

Your role as a health professional is twofold. First, you must offer activities to develop self-care skills, such as one-on-one or group activities that teach how to be an informed medical consumer, and you must provide information on prevention and screening guidelines, such as for a mammogram or a prostate examination. Second, you must ensure that the environment enables the older adult to use these skills to make choices and assume self-responsibility. If an older adult wants to be a partner with the health-care provider in a health decision, the provider should take the time to answer questions and ultimately let the treatment decision be made by the older adult. This same situation applies to nursing. If the older adult is expected to be involved in a self-care activity program, you, as a nurse, must be prepared to explain the benefits, procedures, and risks and be willing to let the older adult make the decision.

CASE STUDY SOLUTIONS

1. Additional information in each category might include:

Nutrition
What are her daily eating habits? What type and amount of food and fluids does she consume? Does she eat alone or with her mother?

Exercise
What is her normal daily activity level? How does this differ from her daily activity level before retirement and taking on the care of her mother? What activities does she consider exercise in the care of her mother?

Stress
What is her perception of coping with changes such as death and retirement? Has she stated any other physical complaints, such as weakness, headaches? Does she feel caring for her mother is causing her stress?

Relationships
What family or friends are important to her? In what social activities is she involved? Does she have any hobbies? Does she have other family members who could assist her in caring for her mother?

Substance Use or Abuse
When did she begin drinking wine every evening? When did her sleeping problems begin? Has she always taken sleeping pills?

Self-Care
Does she have a primary care provider? Does she understand the importance of exercise and disease prevention? Does she know the danger of combining drugs and alcohol?

2. Asking Mrs. C., "What is your biggest worry or concern in your life at this time?" would be a good start. Although the nurse may see many areas of concern, Mrs. C.'s own concerns are more critical.

3. If the nurse begins by focusing on what Mrs. C. considers most important, it is easier for Mrs. C. to understand her own motivation.

4. Some potential conditions include:
   - Excess weight, which may lead or contribute to high blood pressure and physical limitation
   - Lack of exercise, which may contribute to weight gain but may also worsen arthritis and its effects on mobility
   - Emotional stress, which may lead to depression
   - Relationship concerns, which also may contribute to depression, isolation, and abuse of drugs and alcohol
   - Combination of alcohol and OTC sleeping pills, which may lead to further sleeping problems, alcohol and drug misuse, depression, injury, and further isolation

5. If Mrs. C. has not seen a health-care provider for 15 years (other than for minor illnesses), she needs at least a baseline physical assessment. She has some significant conditions that need to be addressed, such as borderline high blood pressure, sleep problems, and weight gain. In addition, she should have basic screenings related to disease prevention.

Key Points

- Aging has been associated with declining health. It is important to understand that older adults can have good health despite conditions such as arthritis. Health promotion can help aging individuals achieve balance between body, mind, and spirit for optimal health.
- Illness and wellness are on a continuum that changes on a regular basis. The objective of nurses working with older individuals is to help them achieve the highest level of wellness possible despite any physical, mental, or emotional conditions.
- Health promotion is the prevention of disease or complications from conditions that may already be present. This involves regular exams by a qualified health care worker. As a nurse, you should encourage and help schedule routine examinations.
- Many older adults are living with one or more chronic conditions. Health promotion should include methods and activities that allow these individuals to attain the best possible health status. It is important to include the older adult in the plans so that things such as pain will not interfere.

- Proper nutrition will help the older adult stay active and alert. As individuals' age metabolism slows, the ability to taste changes, sense of smell may not be as acute, and social aspects of eating change. It will be important to discover the needs and desires of each person to help them meet nutritional goals.
- Exercise and fitness provide strengthening, flexibility, and increased endurance in the older adult, but should not cause unnecessary strain or injury. This will require education regarding the various types of exercise. Strengthening exercises include lifting light weights or exercising with stretch bands; flexibility exercises include stretching and flexing (yoga is a good program

for this); and endurance can be accomplished with movements such as walking. Regular exercise will help the older adult to manage chronic conditions and stress.
- A healthy lifestyle includes exercise, eating a nutritionally balanced diet, and managing stress. Changes in an older adult's life may bring increased stress and unhealthy coping in the form of increased alcohol intake or misuse of drugs. Education and screening are important to help this age group manage stress successfully.
- Older adults have spent a lifetime caring for themselves. Helping them to accept responsibility for care will assist them in remaining independent as long as possible.

Review Questions

1. Incentives for older persons to participate in health promotion behaviors include:
   1. The belief that they will be young forever.
   2. The belief that activities will help them die well.
   3. The belief that activities will help keep them independent.
   4. The belief that it will please their physician.

2. Health promotion programs appropriate for older people should focus on:
   1. Maintaining functional abilities.
   2. Advancing youthfulness.
   3. Enhancing chronic illnesses.
   4. Developing dependence on others for care.

3. Basic components of an exercise routine for older people are:
   1. Strengthening, endurance, and flexibility.
   2. Strengthening, dieting, and power walking.
   3. Strengthening, dieting, and aerobics.
   4. Strengthening, aerobics, and Choose MyPlate.

4. Age-related changes that affect nutrition include:
   1. Increase in the ability to taste a wide variety of foods.
   2. Increase in body fat with decrease in muscle.
   3. Increase in lean body mass requiring more protein.
   4. Increased metabolic rate because of aging thyroid.

5. It is important to include an assessment of alcohol use in the older adult because alcohol in the elderly:
   1. Decreases the effectiveness of many OTCs and medications.
   2. Masks symptoms of other serious health conditions.
   3. Increases socialization opportunities but decreases family interactions.
   4. Increases dietary intake, leading to weight gain

ANSWERS 1. 3, 2. 1, 3. 1, 4. 2, 5. 2

CHAPTER 7

Safety

Kathleen Paco Cadman

KEY TERMS

abuse
anxiety disorder
cognition
depression
disaster
emergency
hyperthermia
hypothermia
mental health
post-traumatic stress disorder (PTSD)
sexual orientation
impaired skin integrity
substance use disorder

CHAPTER CONCEPTS

Safety
Sexuality
Thermoregulation
Violence

LEARNING OUTCOMES

1. Identify potential fall risks based on diagnosis, medication, and environment.
2. Give examples of measures that can be taken to promote optimal skin integrity.
3. Compare and contrast the manifestations of hyperthermia and hypothermia in the older adult.
4. Apply knowledge of behavioral patterns to help identify potential mental health concerns.
5. Analyze potential health concerns regarding sexuality for older adults.
6. Compare and contrast possible indications of the various forms of elder abuse.
7. Predict emergencies that may arise and evaluate available resources for each situation.
8. Assess what safety issues are present for older adults in the home environment.

CASE STUDY

Mr. Baxter is an 88-year-old man who, before admission, lived at home with his wife and their pet dog, Ziggy. They enjoy hiking with their dog, doing yoga, and travel. Unfortunately, 4 weeks ago, Mr. Baxter had a ground-level fall while at the farmer's market, in which he fractured his right hip and bruised a few ribs. Repairing the joint went smoothly and after 3 weeks in a rehabilitation center he was discharged home last week. He is progressing well with his ambulation but he is becoming frustrated and restless with his limitations.

Aside from injuries sustained during the fall, he has very few health issues. Each day he takes medications for hypertension, high cholesterol, and chronic

Continued

CASE STUDY—cont'd

shoulder pain from a rock climbing injury 20 years ago. The physician insisted that Mr. Baxter use a walker around his home and a wheelchair when out in crowds until he is steadier on his feet.

When you speak with Mr. Baxter about his medications, he mentions that he occasionally doubles the dose of pain medication so that he is comfortable enough to sleep at night. He also states that some evenings he forgets to take his pills, so he takes them with his other pills the next morning. He also casually mentions that he had a small fall in the home just before you arrived, but that it is "no big deal" because his wife helped him back up. Although he downplayed the fall, you notice some minor scrapes and cuts down the right side of his body.

Before leaving the home after this initial assessment, you ask if he has any other questions or concerns that you can address. He mentions his desire to return to his usually active life and wants to know about two activities in particular. He plans to resume his yoga practice soon and wants to know what precautions he should take to prevent further injury. He also wants to know how much longer he needs to wait before having sex again.

Discussion

1. How would you explain that taking medications in this manner can increase the risk for falls?
2. How can you best modify the environment to decrease future falls or other accidents?
3. How can you help prepare for a disaster? What steps can be taken to ensure that he is as safe as possible in case of a health emergency?
4. What guidelines would you give him in response to the questions about yoga and sex?

INTRODUCTION

Although safety is a key component in patient care for all ages, there are specific concerns that disproportionately affect the older adult population, based on both physiological and psychosocial needs. This chapter addresses key concepts for safety considerations.

FALL RISKS

Each year, approximately one-third of older adults will have a fall. Of these, nearly 20,000 falls will have fatal outcomes, and more than 3 million elders will be taken to the emergency department for non-fatal injuries, resulting in nearly a million hospital admissions (Centers for Disease Control and Prevention [CDC], 2017).

Even if the outcome is nonfatal, falls can result in fractures, breaks, lacerations, sprains, organ damage, traumatic brain injuries (CDC, 2017), and other conditions causing severe disability. Once an older adult is disabled, even temporarily, he or she runs a greater risk for further impairment of overall health outcomes (Healthy People 2020, 2018). Although falls frequently lead to disability or death among older adults, much can be done to prevent them.

Healthy People 2020

Goal

Reduce the number of fall-related emergency department visits among older adults by 10% (Healthy People 2020, 2018).

Contributing Factors

Changes in physiology as the body ages place older adults at a higher risk for both fatal and nonfatal injuries resulting from falls. The primary contributory changes are related to the following (National Institutes of Health [NIH], 2017):

• **Musculoskeletal:** As muscles and bones progressively weaken, the ability to maintain a steady gait decreases. Body weight extremes affect this factor. Among thin patients, muscular atrophy and osteoporosis are more common, which places them at an increased risk for broken bones. For obese patients, who may have stronger bones from weight-bearing activities, there is a greater risk of injury from the impact of their own weight on their bones. For older adults, regardless of weight, discomfort during mobility may further decrease range of motion for mobility, which also increases the likelihood of falls.

- **Neurological:** Neuropathy and other neural changes can lead to poor balance and a shift in proprioception. This is particularly prevalent in persons with diabetes or those who have sustained spinal injuries. Arthritis or chronic back pain may result in increased painful sensations during ambulation. Both types of neurological changes can increase the risk of falls if they result in an abnormal or stuttered gait and impaired reflexes.
- **Sensory loss:** Often vision (macular degeneration, glaucoma, cataracts), hearing, and neurological function decrease as a person ages. This loss may be dangerous to the patient if he or she cannot see obstacles, listen to surroundings, or feel items that may be in the way. Vision and tactile losses are potentially progressive and particularly profound in patients with unmanaged or poorly managed diabetes.
- **Cardiovascular:** Orthostatic hypotension, which can be associated with dehydration (hypovolemia) or various cardiovascular abnormalities such as dysrhythmias, results in dizziness upon standing. Initiation or changes made to administration of cardiovascular medications, such as those for hypertension, may increase the likelihood of orthostatic hypertension.
- **Genitourinary and digestive:** Urinary and bowel urgency or frequency for continent older adults necessitates more frequent trips to the restroom, thus increasing the opportunity for injury. When these urges occur at night, the patient may maneuver to the restroom when thinking is hazy and the environment is darker, increasing the risk for falls.
- **Cognition:** Slowed reaction times, as well as confusion and short-term memory loss involving one's ability to self-ambulate, not only increase the number of falls sustained, but may also decrease reflex reaction times, thereby increasing the severity of an injury.
- **Nutrition and hydration:** Fluctuations in blood sugar, as well as dehydration, can cause feelings of dizziness, which increases the risk for falls.

Fall Prevention Measures

Although it is not possible for the licensed practical nurse (LPN) to eliminate all risk for falls, various measures can be taken to help decrease the likelihood of a fall.

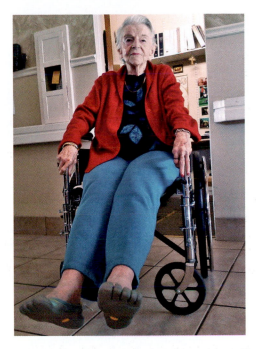

Footwear that fits properly, does not slide or rub, and has good grip or traction is important. Millie, at 99 years old, proudly shows off her favorite shoes. She says that they help her feel safe when she walks, and they have enough grip to let her propel herself in her wheelchair.

- **Clothing:** Ensure that clothing selected for the patient (by the LPN, patient, family, or certified nursing assistant [CNA]) fits properly. Special attention must be directed to the length of pants, robes, or skirts to ensure that the patient will neither trip over them nor get them caught between assistive devices, such as canes and walkers, and the floor. Properly fitting footwear is also crucial; footwear should have thin rubber soles and a method for comfortably yet securely fastening the shoe to the foot so it cannot inadvertently slide out of place. Also, if the patient needs glasses or hearing aids, the LPN must ensure, directly or through delegation, that these are in place and functional as part of the patient's overall wardrobe.
- **Medication:** Administration of all medications must be done according to the physician's orders. The LPN must monitor the potential effects of the medication on ambulation and report any risky changes to the charge nurse or supervisor so that the primary care provider can assess whether the administration times need to be adjusted. Medications that cause drowsiness or dizziness, such as sedatives, blood pressure

medications, and narcotics, are often best given at night, as the patient is going to bed and will not be ambulating as much. Conversely, diuretics and laxatives, which both increase frequency for toileting, are best given during the day, to decrease the risk for injuries that may be sustained by rising too quickly from a lying position or moving through a dark room. It is important to monitor effects of prescription and over-the-counter medications, as well as herbal remedies including cannabis-based products.

- **Nutrition and hydration:** Encouraging ample nutritional intake on a regular basis can help regulate blood sugar levels, decreasing the chance of dizziness. This is particularly important for diabetic patients. Also, encouraging adequate fluid intake can help prevent dehydration, which can contribute to hypotension.
- **Transitional posturing:** Whether caused by dehydration (hypovolemia), medication, or various medical conditions, orthostatic hypotension is common among older adults. The LPN must transition unsteady patients slowly from lying to sitting upright, then pivot them until their feet are on the ground, and then assist them with standing. By allowing ample time between each step, the effects of orthostatic hypotension can be decreased.
- **Durable medical equipment (DME):** Although physical therapists generally assess the need for and order DME for patients, it is within the nurse's responsibility to monitor whether there are new or changed needs for DME, based on a change in condition. If so, the LPN should pass this information on to the supervisor for referral. Although DME such as single-point canes, four-post canes, two-wheel walkers, and four-wheel walkers can help decrease the chance of a fall, improper selection of the DME may inversely increase the chance of a fall. As posturing changes, a patient's DME may need to be reevaluated for proper size as well. Positioning and quality of grips for both comfort and form are also important to note.
- **Physical therapy:** If the LPN in the facility or home setting notices decreases in mobility or increases in contractures, he or she should report this to the supervisor for possible referral to physical therapy. Interventions to prevent falls may include strength training to build muscle mass, increased walks to build endurance, and range-of-motion exercises to promote flexibility. Range-of-motion exercise options include active low-impact exercises such as tai chi or yoga, as well as passive range of motion done by the LPN and other direct care staff.
- **Environmental issues:** Alterations can be made to the environment in which the older adult lives, whether he or she is in a home or a facility setting. This includes indoor issues, such as loose rugs or stairs, as well as outdoor considerations, such as ice, snow, or piles of leaves.
- **Primary living area:** Ensure that the living area for the patient is free of unnecessary obstacles or hazards. Check for adequate lighting, including night lights, to increase visibility. Also, assessing and adjusting tubing (oxygen, nasogastric [NG] tube, and IV lines) and DME location, when possible, decrease the chance of a patient's becoming entangled or tripping while ambulating.

Home health nurses should check the patient's home to be sure that walking areas are free of loose rugs, cords, planters, boxes, newspapers, toys (from pets or grandchildren), and other debris that could cause the patient to trip or lose balance while walking. It is also best practice to ensure that the patient has a telephone and lamp that are user friendly next to his or her bed and primary chair. This decreases risks associated with ambulating to the bed in low-light conditions or getting up in the dark to receive or place a call.

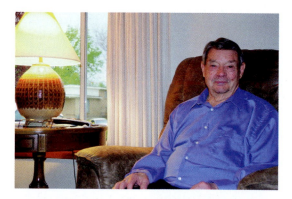

Having commonly used items within easy reach helps reduce the chance for falls that may occur in frequent ambulation and bending to find items. Glen's safety is improved by having a table with good light and his glasses, handkerchief, television remote, and telephone next to his favorite seating area.

- **Bathroom:** Because many falls occur going to, from, or in the bathroom, this area needs particular focus for safety. When applicable, rails should be in place next to the toilet and showering area. Furthermore, ensure that if the patient requires an elevated toilet seat, or a shower stool, this equipment is in place. Nonslip surfaces on the shower floor and a well-anchored shower door or curtain (not on a tension rod) are also imperative in promoting safety. Bath mats must be adhered to the floor to reduce the chance of falls while stepping into or out of the bathing area, and a towel should be easily within reach.

- **Other home setting recommendations:** Walkways to and from the home should be free of leaves, snow, or ice. Lighting outside the home, such as motion sensor or timed lights, can help increase safety not only by reducing falls when going in and out of the home, but also by increasing security. Furthermore, handrails and skid-reduction surfaces should be in place anywhere steps are present, both indoors and outdoors.

Increased safety precautions to prevent falls not only reduce the chance of injury, but also may help improve both the duration and quality of life for older adults. Fall injuries frequently result in broken bones and sometimes a near-paralyzing fear of falling. These factors often contribute to a more sedentary lifestyle, which may lead to further muscle atrophy, progression of osteoporosis, and pneumonia. This combination of outcomes decreases the chance for recovery and often proves fatal for older adults.

Healthy People 2020

Falls

In addition to the initial injury, falls for elderly patients may result in:

- Fear of falling
- Sedentary behavior
- Impaired function
- Lower quality of life

(Healthy People 2020, 2018)

SKIN INTEGRITY

The aging process causes skin to lose elasticity, thus making it more fragile and prone to abrasions and lacerations. Although this is a natural physiological phenomenon, there are measures the LPN can take, both directly and through supervision of the CNAs, to help increase safety by reducing the frequency and magnitude of skin-related injuries. To ensure that breaches in the integumentary system are addressed quickly, the LPN must perform skin checks to assess for abrasions, lacerations, or breakdown, and communicate regularly with CNAs regarding the importance of reporting findings from skin checks performed during bathing.

Injury Prevention

Moving patients while providing activities of daily living (ADLs) must be done gently, to prevent tearing or shearing the skin because of friction. Patients with particularly frail skin should be dressed in comfortably loose, lightweight, soft fabrics that are generally full length, to increase protection of the skin. Clothing should be free from sharp or rough areas, such as elastic bands, and broken zippers, buttons, or bra hooks that could damage the skin. The LPN should also ensure that anyone in close contact with the patient does not have sharp edges, such as long fingernails, jewelry, and lanyards, which could injure patients with **impaired skin integrity**. As the LPN removes adhesive surfaces, such as tape and bandages, he or she must be cautious to remove the surface gently, by pulling skin taut and cautiously lifting the adhesive little by little. Otherwise, adhesive surfaces can tear the skin. A further safety measure to prevent skin tears is assessing edges that are in the patient's environment. This includes looking for particularly rough surfaces, such as a ragged edge to a wooden table, as well as sharp corners or edges. Particularly in the home situation, the LPN must look for heavily worn or broken items that may be hazardous, such as a broken spring protruding through a bed or chair.

Breaches in skin integrity may also occur from hot water burns or scalding. There is increased risk for the older adult if hot- and cold-water faucets are not clearly labeled or if the water heater is set too high. Scalding is of particular concern in this age demographic, due to thinner skin and poor microcirculation (American Burn Association, 2017).

Breakdown Prevention

As skin becomes more fragile, patients are also at increased risk for skin breakdown, including pressure ulcers. Breakdown can lead to infection, which can be detrimental and potentially fatal to the patient if not prevented or treated. The following measures can increase safety by decreasing the chance for breakdown:

- Use of foam pads or pillows to help redistribute weight on bony prominences can help prevent breakdown. This is particularly true for the hip bones, shoulders, and heels.

- Regular repositioning of the patient, as well as any foam pads or pillows, should be done at least once every 2 hours to redistribute areas of pressure and increase circulation.
- Routine application of emollients such as lotion helps maintain skin integrity. Proper levels of moisturizer allow the skin to be less fragile, to not tear as easily, compared with when the skin is either too dry or too moist. Moisturizing includes the application of specialized barrier emollients used for incontinent individuals, to decrease breakdown from excessive moisture. Because older adults often have a decreased immune function, the primary care provider may recommend antimicrobial lotions or creams, particularly in areas where the skin is still largely intact but with some abrasions.

EXTREME TEMPERATURE CONDITIONS

Exposure to extreme temperatures can cause adverse, and sometimes fatal, health reactions for older adults. Both excessive heat and cold, in combination with natural changes in the body's physiological functions, and medication side effects, can cause profound changes in internal temperature regulation, as well as the circulatory and nervous systems.

Heat-Associated Risks

As people age, they often have decreased responses to temperature in their extremities, and they may have less adipose tissue to help insulate them. This combination often leads older adults to feel cold in temperatures that younger individuals may feel are comfortable. As a result, older adults often cover themselves with blankets, even when the temperature is quite warm. This practice, combined with decreased sweat production in older adults and a decreased sense of thirst, may cause internal temperatures to rise to unsafe levels (CDC, 2018).

To help increase safety and decrease risk from extreme heat, the LPN should evaluate the home for an adequate supply of clean water, as well as air conditioning or a fan. If an air conditioning unit is present, the patient should not be seated or lie directly in front of it, to avoid the risk of **hypothermia** from exposure to the cold air.

The LPN should also provide education and demonstration regarding ways to lower body temperature

safely in extreme heat. This includes adequate hydration as well as tepid, not cool or cold, baths for 10 to 15 minutes, or the use of a cool cloth around the patient's neck. When temperatures exceed 90°F, the LPN should be sure the patient is checked twice a day, either personally or by a primary caregiver (PCG), for signs and symptoms that indicate the onset of heat stroke, or **hyperthermia** (CDC, 2018) (Box 7.1).

Cold-Associated Risks

Older adults are often more prone to sedentary lifestyles, which may decrease the body's ability to generate heat. This situation, partnered with decreased insulation from adipose tissue, may lead to excessive heat loss during cold temperatures. For those living in cold environments, even if the patient does not or is unable to verbalize that he or she is cold, the LPN should regularly assess the patients for potential signs and symptoms of hypothermia (CDC, 2017) (Box 7.2).

Box 7.1
Signs of Hyperthermia
- Body temperature higher than 103°F
- Abnormal confusion
- Headache
- Heavy sweating or hot dry skin with no sweat
- Pallor
- Tachycardia
- Fatigue
- Dizziness
- Muscle cramps
- Nausea
- Rapid, shallow breathing

(CDC, 2018).

Box 7.2
Signs of Hypothermia
- Shivering
- Shallow breathing
- Weak pulse
- Memory loss
- Slurred speech
- Decreased responses
  - Mental
  - Physical
- Increased lethargy or fatigue

(CDC, 2017).

To help decrease the chances of hypothermia, the LPN can encourage the patient to wear multiple layers of comfortable clothing and have blankets accessible to further provide warmth. If the older adult is using a fireplace or heating unit, extra precautions should be taken to ensure that blankets or loose clothing are not near enough to ignite and that the patient is not close enough to sustain burns.

Another risk that is particularly dangerous in cold temperatures is the increased chance of heart attack from strenuous activity, such as shoveling snow. This is based on the physiological response of the cardiovascular system to cold. As the ambient temperature drops, the chance of a heart attack increases, particularly among older adults (Malanchini et al., 2017). The nurse may need to help coordinate services for the patient, so that labor-intensive tasks, particularly those that are outdoors, are performed by other organizations or persons.

MENTAL HEALTH AND SAFETY

One of the primary safety concerns for older adults is associated with cognitive difficulties or other **mental health** issues. These alterations in thought process may unintentionally or intentionally place the patient in dangerous situations.

Dementia and Delirium
The cognitive difficulties associated with dementia, including but not limited to Alzheimer's disease, as well as delirium, increase the chances of accidents as well as wandering. If an older adult has a cognitive disorder yet is still physically able, he or she should not be left alone for any duration of time. This includes patients whose baseline cognition is sound but who are having increased cognitive difficulties from delirium, often manifesting as a result of urinary or upper respiratory tract infections.

Those supervising the older adult, including the LPN, and potentially CNAs, family, friends, neighbors, and those affiliated with community services, should pay particular attention to hazardous areas such as the kitchen, where the patient may cook and forget to turn off the oven or stove, and the garage, where sharp, heavy, or toxic items may be stored. Also, precautions should be taken to decrease the chance of wandering or the risk of getting lost as a result of wandering. This may include a silent alarm system or ample scheduling of individuals to be present in the home. Supervision is particularly important in the evening hours because "sundowning" may exacerbate cognitive function impairment.

Furthermore, a "memory-impaired" identification bracelet should be placed on the patient. The bracelet should include the patient's name, a reliable contact number, and a recent photograph of the patient with information such as height, weight, and full name indicated on the back. These bracelets are useful in case it is necessary to contact police for a missing person's report.

Mental Health Disorders
Older adults should be assessed regularly for verbalization or behavior patterns that may indicate a need for proper psychiatric evaluation. If the LPN notes any of the following potential indicators, he or she should promptly report it to the supervisor. Among the major mental health issues affecting older adults are **depression**, anxiety, **post-traumatic stress disorder (PTSD)**, and **substance use disorder** (World Health Organization [WHO], 2017).

- **Depression** may be indicated through verbalization of sadness, decreased socialization, increased sleeping, and verbalization of suicidal ideations, which may include frequent mentioning of wanting to be with loved ones who have passed away.
- **Anxiety disorder** may manifest as increasing insomnia, verbalization of worry, and increasing apprehension about the world around them. Apprehension may be demonstrated by lessening of ambulation based on fear of falling or injury; a frequently stated distrust of others, either of individual persons or society as a whole; or verbalization of fears related to death and the dying process.
- **PTSD**, particularly among veterans of foreign wars, can be amplified by dementia. The memories, or flashbacks, of traumatic situations suddenly becoming more frequent and lifelike, may place the patient at great risk for injury to themselves or others.
- **Substance use disorder** is reported to adversely affect approximately 1% of older adults, and it greatly increases the risk for both unintentional and intentional self-harm, including suicide and overdose.

Social and physical isolation is common among older adults, and it may be cyclical. One common manifestation of decreased cognition or mental health issues, including depression, anxiety, PTSD, and substance abuse, is isolation. This isolation may be based on self-perceptions of shame, embarrassment as memory problems become more obvious, a lack of wanting to connect with others, guilt felt for socializing in the absence of those who have passed away, or an increasing lack of trust of the world around them.

THINK LIKE A NURSE

You have been taking care of a resident in your facility for several months and she has always been in good spirits, but today she is sullen and appears to have been crying. When you ask her what's wrong, she becomes withdrawn and looks away. You know that this past week was the 5-year anniversary of her husband's death. What mental health concern do you suspect, and how can you address this issue?

As patients begin to isolate themselves, it can often cause mental health to decline more rapidly, which may lead to further isolation, and the cycle continues. Any abnormal change in attitude, behavior, or interaction level, including isolation, that varies from the patient's baseline should be noted and continually monitored (WHO, 2017).

Cultural Considerations

The way that mental health and emotions are displayed can vary widely based on cultural influences. Take time to do a thorough mental health screening and communicate regularly with your patient. It may be appropriate to learn more about perceptions of mental health within the patient's culture, but it is also important to not view the patient through stereotypes. Mental health issues present differently for each individual, regardless of cultural norms. Statements made by friends and family about changes or concerns that they notice should be noted and explored, even if the change or concern is not perceived by the nurse.

SEXUAL SAFETY MEASURES

Often, little attention is given to sex and sexuality regarding the older adult population. The LPN, when obtaining the patient's social history, should inquire what the patient's gender identity and **sexual orientation** are, whether the patient is sexually active or not, and if so, whether the patient is using proper protective measures or not. Although these questions may be uncomfortable to ask, the answers should never be assumed. Sex and sexuality are a part of life for people of all ages, and safety should be addressed.

Sexuality

The lesbian, gay, bisexual, and/or transgender (LGBT) population in the United States is estimated to include as many as 2.4 million older adults (American Psychological Association [APA], 2018), but according to the CDC, more than 20% have not disclosed this information to their doctor, often because they have not been directly asked. Of those who have disclosed their sexual orientation or gender identity, many have either been denied health care or believe that they received inferior health care as a result. Many more LGBT older adults, particularly those in same-sex relationships, have been denied housing, in both public and facility settings, based on their sexual orientation ("Movement Advancement Project," 2017).

Point of Interest

Discussions about sex and sexuality with your older adult patients may initially feel a bit awkward or personally invasive. Answers to these questions, however, should never be assumed based on the age of your patient, and addressing these topics may help focus much-needed patient education.

Ask your supervisor whether your place of employment has set protocols for this line of inquiry, and if not, you can help initiate a discussion about the importance of health related to sex and sexuality for patients of all ages.

One possible conversational approach with older adult patients includes the following questions:

"I need to ask you a few questions that may feel very personal in nature, but they are simply part of helping us understand you in a more holistic way so that we can best address your overall health needs. None of the questions are meant as an accusation, and some of the answers may feel very obvious, but asking them is merely standard practice. If there are any that make you are truly uncomfortable, you do not need to answer them."

1. As what gender do you identify yourself (male, female, other)?
2. What is your sexual orientation (lesbian, gay, bisexual, heterosexual)?
3. Are you currently sexually active or have you been within the past year?
4. [If "yes" to question 3] How many sexual partners have you had within the past year?
   a. [If one partner] Is this a mutually monogamous relationship?
   b. [If multiple partners or not in a mutually monogamous relationship] Have you and your sexual partner(s) ever been tested for sexually transmitted infections?
      i. "Yes:" Have you [or they] ever tested positive? [If "yes," then …]
         1. What sexually transmitted infection was diagnosed?
         2. What year was the diagnosis (and month if current year)?
         3. What treatment was given?
      ii. "No:" Educate about the importance of regular testing.
5. Do you and your partner(s) always use condoms or other safety precautions? If "no," educate about the use of protective measures against sexually transmitted infections.

One safety concern specific to this community includes physical and or emotional bullying from peers and staff. LGBT older adults may also have faced bullying or alienation from family members, which could potentially result in lack of a social support system. Aside from the impact on their psychosocial needs, this may also place these individuals in a vulnerable position legally regarding end-of-life decision making and distribution of assets. As a patient advocate, the LPN should provide protection for the older adult in regard to physical safety, psychosocial needs, and enforcement of legal rights, including division of assets and other end-of-life decision making. There are many resources available for the LGBT older adult at a national level and frequently also at state and community levels (MAP & SAGE, 2017) [Box 7.3].

Sexual Activity

The National Poll on Healthy Aging (University of Michigan, 2018) found that 31% of older adult females and 51% of older adult males are sexually active. Although pregnancy is not an issue among older adult women, it may still be a concern for older adult men with younger partners. Also, sexually transmitted infections (STIs) can be transmitted regardless of age, when protective measures are not taken. The National Institute on Aging (NIA) reports that nearly 25% of the HIV and AIDS cases in the United States are in patients older than age 50 (National Institute on Aging [NIA], 2017).

Evidence indicates that many HIV-positive older adults remain sexually active, but that sexually transmitted infection (STI) testing is rarely done on older adults (Karpiak & Lunievicz, 2017). As with patients of any age, sexually active older adults should be educated on the importance of using safety precautions during sexual activity.

Evidence-Based Practice

Karpiak, S. E., & Lunievicz, J. L. (2017). Age is not a condom: HIV and sexual health for older adults. *Current Sexual Health Reports, 9*(3), 109–115. doi: 10.1007/s11930-017-0119-0

Sexually transmitted infections, including HIV, are often associated with younger populations. However, it is estimated that within the United States, 70% of HIV-positive individuals will be age 50 and older by the year 2020.

1. As the nurse providing education to a new patient older than age 50, what information would you provide and what questions would you ask, regarding STIs?
2. What are the anticipated barriers in this patient education? Are those barriers associated with the patient's outlook or your own discomfort?
3. What safety measures could you include in your teaching to help decrease the risk for STIs?
4. What impact do you feel this correlation would have on society? What populations would be most highly affected?
5. What are different possible causes for increasing STI rates among older adults?

Box 7.3

Online Resources for Lesbian, Gay, Bisexual, and Transgender Older Adults

LGBT Aging Center: www.lgbtagingcenter.org
   Services and Advocacy for Gay, Lesbian, Bisexual, and Transgender Elders: www.sageusa.org

THINK LIKE A NURSE

You are taking care of a 74-year-old man who will be discharged the next day. He mentions that he was widowed 8 years ago and has decided to start dating again. His doctor prescribed erectile dysfunction medication for him. What safety issues should you discuss with him?

ELDER ABUSE

Elder **abuse** is an increasing risk facing the older adult population. Recent statistics indicate that 10% of older adults in home and facility settings have been the victim of abuse. However, current statistics are thought to be highly conservative estimates because elder abuse often goes unreported. It is estimated that only around 20% of cases are reported to and substantiated by Adult Protective Services (APS) because many forms of abuse are difficult to confirm if not directly witnessed. Although people often think of physical harm when they hear the term "abuse," there are multiple categories of elder abuse (National Center on Elder Abuse [NCEA], 2018):

- **Physical abuse** involves damage or injury to the older adult's body. This may include broken bones, lacerations, malnutrition, welts, and bruises caused by another individual, and it includes injuries at all levels, not only those warranting medical attention. Injury from abuse may result in exacerbating existing health problems, disability, and premature death.
- **Psychological or emotional abuse** includes yelling or swearing at, belittling, insulting, intimidating, isolating, or manipulating the older adult. It may increase depression, **anxiety,** PTSD, fear, withdrawal from others, and feelings of helplessness.
- **Financial or material abuse** is the taking of money, possessions, or property from older adults without their permission. This also includes the misuse of funds, such as Medicare, Medicaid, and Social Security, which are allocated for care of the older adult.
- **Sexual abuse** includes forced participation of the older adult in any sexual act, whether he or she is giving or receiving the act. This also includes inappropriate touching of a sexual nature while providing care to the older adult. Persons with dementia are particularly vulnerable to sexual assault because perpetrators often believe that there is less chance of being reported.
- **Neglect and abandonment** are purposeful failures of providing the older adult with basic needs, including medical care, psychosocial needs, housing, nutrition, and assistance with necessary ADLs. This can include leaving an older adult alone for extended periods of time when he or she is unable to provide self-care.

Focused Learning Chart: Elder Abuse

Forms of Abuse
- Physical
- Psychological and emotional
- Financial and material
- Sexual
- Neglect and abandonment

What to Look For
- Bodily injuries or malnutrition
- Increased withdrawal or significant change in emotion
- Missing money that cannot be accounted for
- Injury to genitals or mention of sexual aggression from others
- Lack of care provided or marked absence of caretakers

What You Can Do
- Alert an ombudsman
- Depending on level of severity, call:
  - 911 for medical emergencies.
  - local police for urgent issues (excluding medical emergencies).
  - National Domestic Violence Hotline 1-800-799-SAFE (7233) or state APS.

Risk Factors

The risk of elder abuse is increased in situations where the older adult and the PCG have little social support, are highly dependent on others, are unable to care properly for themselves, have drug or alcohol dependency, lack coping skills, are prone to hostility, are under a lot of stress related to other aspects of their life, or have mental health issues (NCEA, 2018).

Prevention Factors

Communication is one of the first steps to preventing elder abuse. The LPN should listen for cues in conversations that may indicate the risk for abuse by others. This includes statements made not only by the older adult, but also by any others involved in their care or living environment. If the older adult is in the home setting with a live-in PCG, it may be necessary for the LPN to assess the PCG's social support infrastructure, ability to physically provide care, knowledge of financial management, and awareness of community resources that can train or aid them in areas where they are still learning (NCEA, 2018).

Reporting Suspected Abuse

Nurses, in most states, are considered "mandated reporters," which means that it is compulsory for them to report evident and suspected mistreatment or abuse. The LPN must report the findings to his or her supervisor and follow through to ensure that it has also been reported to the police, a long-term care facility ombudsman, or APS, depending on the patient's life circumstances and living environment (NCEA, 2018). LPNs caring for older adults should be aware of available resources for the prevention and management of elder abuse within the community (Box 7.4).

Box 7.4

National Center on Elder Abuse: Eldercare Locator

The Eldercare Locator is a public service of the U.S. Administration on Aging that connects users to services for older adults and their families. It can be used by calling 1-800-677-1116 or visiting www .eldercare.gov on the Internet.

SAFETY IN EMERGENCY SITUATIONS

Older adults are at an increased risk for injury or death in an **emergency** situation, often because of physiological or cognitive difficulties as well as multiple health conditions, including the five most common concerns for this age group: hypertension, hyperlipidemia, arthritis, ischemic heart disease, and diabetes (Administration on Aging [AOA], 2018). Although there is no way to prepare an older adult fully for all 21 emergency situations indicated by the Red Cross, and not all emergency situations are applicable to each place, basic measures to decrease the impact of an emergency can be taken (American Red Cross, 2018), and resources such as Ready.gov can be used to see which risks are greatest for each area (Ready.gov, 2018).

Preventable Emergency Situations

Many emergency situations can occur in the home, but it can be possible to prevent, or at least reduce, the risk of occurrence. Among the most prevalent are fire, flooding, carbon monoxide poisoning, and food poisoning (American Red Cross, 2018).

- **Fire** in the home setting is most frequently caused by cooking, but it may also be the result of heating or electrical malfunction, smoking, or an open flame. It is important for the LPN to be aware of fire risks in the older adult's living environment. Heat sources should be surrounded by a clear area, stove and oven knobs should be easy to maneuver, timers on cooking devices should be operational as a reminder, electrical outlets should not be used over their specific parameters for plugs, and the older adult should exercise caution if smoking (National Fire Protection Association [NFPA], 2018). The home or facility should be equipped with functioning smoke detectors, as well as ample fire extinguishers for the living space, and an evacuation strategy should be discussed and demonstrated in case of a fire.
- **Flooding** most often occurs in the home setting as a result of frozen pipes in the winter. This can be decreased by allowing faucets to have a slow drip during subfreezing conditions, particularly for fixtures on an outer perimeter wall.
- **Carbon monoxide poisoning** is most common with fires (NFPA, 2018), but it may also be

present with gas leaks in the living environment. Because carbon monoxide is colorless and odorless, it is often undetected before causing fatalities. A carbon monoxide detector may be used in the environment to alert the older adult or the PCG to the presence of the gas.

- **Food poisoning**, as well as medication toxicity, may occur in the home setting, especially with older adults with dementia. The ingestion of spoiled foods or beverages, as well as improper consumption of medications, may cause illness or potential death. The LPN in the home setting should check the house for rancid or spoiled food and beverages, as well as ensure that medications are properly labeled and appear to be taken in the proper quantity for the time that has passed. If the LPN, older adult, or PCG suspects poisoning from food, beverage, or medication, Poison Control should be called (Box 7.5).

Natural and Human-made Disasters

In the case of a natural **disaster**, many older adults are unable to evacuate themselves. Regardless of the nature of the disaster, many preparation and response actions are similar, such as having a safety bag, knowing whom to contact, and registering the older adult with emergency services (Department of Homeland Security, 2018).

It is recommended to create a safety bag for the older adult, regardless of whether he or she is in a home or a long-term facility setting. This bag should be equipped with the supplies necessary to sustain health for at least 72 hours, in the event that the older adult were to be trapped in the living quarters until help arrived (Box 7.6). The items in the bag may vary

Box 7.6

Items for Safety Bag

- Clothing (including jacket and sturdy shoes)
- Up-to-date list of:
  - Medications
  - Diagnoses
  - Allergies
  - Contacts (physician, power of attorney, family)
  - Necessary equipment
    - Glasses
    - Hearing aid and batteries
    - Dentures and care products
    - Walker/wheelchair/cane
    - Pacemaker serial number
- 10-day medication supply (not expired)
  - Prescription medications
  - Over-the-counter medications
- Flashlight and radio with batteries
- First-aid kit
- Hygiene items
- Cash
- Whistle
- Blanket and/or sleeping bag, and pillow
- Copy of physician orders for life-sustaining treatment, if applicable, and insurance documents
- Nonperishable food and water (for at least 3 days)
  - Not past expiration date
  - Able to be easily opened
  - Include necessary utensils
- Cell phone with charger

(Department of Homeland Security, 2018).

depending on the environment, but the LPN should check to be sure that they are properly stocked with up-to-date items, remove any clothing that may no longer fit, and remove any food or medications that may have expired.

The older adult should have access to an easy-to-operate telephone, when possible, that he or she can use to call emergency services, the LPN, the PCG, or others, as well as receive calls. Having an easily readable list of emergency contact numbers near the phone is helpful, including name, role, and number for each person. This allows responders to know whom else they need to contact. It may also be beneficial for the older adult to wear a life alert system, in case of disaster or personal emergency. Emergency services have registries for older adults, so that responders know which facilities house those who

Box 7.5

American Association of Poison Control Centers

The American Association of Poison Control Centers supports the nation's 55 poison centers in their efforts to prevent and treat poison exposures. Poison centers offer free, confidential medical advice 24 hours a day, 7 days a week through the Poison Help Line at 1-800-222-1222. This service provides a primary resource for poisoning information and helps reduce costly emergency department visits through in-home treatment.

are unable to evacuate themselves. Registration contact information can be found by contacting Eldercare Locator.

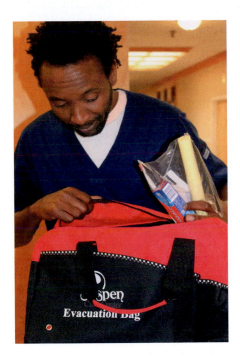

As a nurse, Edwin helps assess the contents of the patients' evacuation bags to be sure that everything is in place, functional, and up to date. This way, in case of emergency, the facility can be sure that each patient has the basic necessities to keep him or her safe and comfortable until more supplies arrive. This facility also has protocols in place for ensuring that the medication carts are part of the evacuation process. For those in a home setting, medications can be included in the bag.

Health Emergencies

Whether because of illness, injury, or other health problems such as heart attack or stroke, older adults in the home setting are at a significant risk for health emergencies. If the older adult is in a facility setting, the LPN must ensure that the call light is within reach and that the patient is able to use it. If the older adult lives alone, or with a PCG who is often away from the home, it may be wise to obtain a life alert system that the patient would wear while alone. This would allow others to be alerted in case of an emergency. Also, having telephones and contact lists in easily accessible places may help the older adult get help in a health emergency.

CRITICALLY EXAMINE THE FOLLOWING

You notice that the facility where you have just been hired does not have any emergency preparedness kits for the residents living there. When you mention to your supervisor that you would like to participate actively in addressing this concern, he schedules a meeting for both of you to pitch the idea to your administrator the following Monday. What resources and information would be good to access before your presentation to her next week?

Safe, Effective Nursing Care

Promoting Safety for the Older Adult

As an LPN, it is your responsibility to provide a safe environment for your patients. Evaluate the CNAs to make sure they are performing tasks correctly; if not, provide the necessary instruction to ensure safe care. Assess the environment and watch for equipment or other items that may cause falls. Also, make sure that a patient's equipment is functioning properly. If not, have it repaired or replaced.

If you notice unsafe care performed by another member of the health-care team or a family member, be sure to communicate your concern to the registered nurse (RN) or nurse manager. If you are aware of errors made, it is your responsibility to report the errors to the RN or nurse manager.

As a member of the health-care team, it is important that you value vigilance and monitoring of care by other members of the health-care team. It is also important to listen to your patients and their families if they voice a concern about the care being provided. By valuing other people's concerns, you will help provide a safer environment for your patients.

SAFETY ISSUES TO CHECK ON DURING HOME VISITS

Many LPNs work in the home health setting and can assess their patient's living environment for safety concerns. First, the most important step to ensure safety is communication. The nurse must listen to what the older adult has to say; use keen observation skills to note potential indicators of safety breaches; and then follow up on any concerns. Second, beyond communication, it is within the LPN's role to survey the environment visually in a way that maintains privacy. Third, the nurse should be aware of community resources that may be able to help in the multidisciplinary efforts to promote safety for the older adult. These steps allow the LPN to implement holistic, safety-focused, care for the patient.

Listening for Safety Concerns

While communicating with the older adult, direct questions can be asked regarding safety, but it is also important to listen for other cues such as the patient's perceptions of their physical environment, as well as the interactions the patient has with others.

- **Fall risks.** Has any change in mental and physical function been mentioned by the older adult? If so, does this affect his or her ability to ambulate safely? Has the patient mentioned feeling more tired, confused, forgetful, or weak lately? Does the patient mention having to get up in the night to use the bathroom more often, or with more difficulty, than before?

- **Skin integrity.** Has the older adult mentioned bumping into things recently? Has he or she recently acquired a new pet? Does the older adult mention itching or dryness? Has the patient mentioned any broken or rough edges in the home? Is the patient more sedentary than before?

- **Extreme temperature.** Does the older adult mention how chilly he or she has been lately, or how warm it seems to be getting? Has he or she mentioned gardening outdoors in the summer, shoveling snow off the walkway in the winter months, or walking his or her dog during either season? Is there any change in speech ability or cognition that may indicate hyperthermia or hypothermia?

- **Mental health and safety.** Has there been a negative change in outlook from normal conversations? Is the older adult more withdrawn than usual? Has the older adult mentioned a change in perception about himself or herself or others? Has the older adult recently lost someone close to them? Is the patient talking much more about those who have already passed away, and how much he or she misses them? Has the older adult stopped talking about the future, even the near future? Is the older adult more fearful than usual?

- **Sexual safety.** Does the patient mention a new relationship? If the patient is sexually active, has he or she mentioned symptoms that could be associated with an STI? Has the older adult mentioned feeling excluded from social situations based on sexual orientation?

- **Elder abuse.** Has the older adult mentioned people who have not been nice lately, or with whom he or she does not get along, who may be a safety threat? Does the patient mention feeling uneasy around someone? Has the older adult mentioned being left alone for long periods of time or being hungry or soiled for extended periods?

- **Emergency situations.** Does the older adult know who to contact in case of emergency? Does he or she know the numbers for those people? Has the older adult mentioned neighbors or family who check on the patient regularly? Has the older adult mentioned any change in physical or mental ability, or has his or her speech changed in a way that may indicate there has been a health emergency?

Visually Inspecting the Environment

It is important to maintain the older adult's privacy when assessing the living environment. It is also imperative to remember that the patient maintains the right to live in a different level of cleanliness than is comfortable for the LPN and to make lifestyle choices different from those that the LPN may prefer. The living environment of the older adult, both in a facility or home setting, may take on many different forms and styles, but if it is unsafe to the point of being physically harmful or fatal to the patient, then the LPN should report this to a supervisor and ensure that it is followed up by any applicable authorities. The following information pertains to individuals living in either a facility or a private home, or both.

- **Fall risks.** Is the older adult wearing any clothing that would put him or her at an increased risk for falls? Does all of the DME appear to be in good repair and properly sized for the patient? Are nonslip surfaces in place where applicable? Are there any broken or missing steps or railings? Is there adequate lighting, including night lights? Are there piles of papers or toys on the floor? Are walkways safe and clear, free from clutter or area rugs? Are there floor-level pets in the home?

- **Skin integrity.** Does the LPN see any rough or sharp edges in the home that may cause abrasions or lacerations? Has a skin check been performed? Is any injury or breakdown present? Has lotion been used regularly? Has the water heater been set to a temperature to prevent scalding? Does water coming from the faucet feel incredibly hot?
- **Extreme temperature.** Is there an operational heating and or cooling system in the home? Does the older adult know how to operate it safely? Is he or she dressed appropriately to be comfortable in the current ambient temperature, or does the patient's skin feel abnormally cool or warm? Is there an ample supply of clean water in the home?
- **Mental health and safety.** Does the home seem to be in more disarray than usual? Is there a pile of newspapers in the driveway? Are any areas of the home filled with soiled dishes or clothing, more so than is the patient's baseline for living conditions? Are there large quantities of empty alcohol or medication bottles? Are any psychotropic medications missing, as if they have run out early? Does the older adult's hygiene seem in accordance with the baseline or has there been a decrease in self-care? Is the patient more tearful, withdrawn, or agitated than normal? Are new obituaries or funeral bulletins visible?
- **Elder abuse.** Are there obvious bruises or injuries? Does the older adult appear more frightened than usual, such as being increasingly jumpy around sudden movements? Does the patient report that he or she cannot find money that had been placed in the home? Are there signs that a PCG may have been absent for quite a while? Does the older adult seem fearful of a family member or a health-care provider?
- **Emergency situations.** Is a safety bag present and up to date? Can the older adult demonstrate ability to contact necessary people in the case of an emergency? If the patient has a life alert system, can he or she demonstrate proper use? Are an easy-to-use telephone, contact list, and light near the areas where the patient resides the most, such as the bed or a chair? Is there a clear path for evacuation in case of disaster? Are smoke and carbon monoxide detectors in place and functional? Are fire extinguishers present? Is there an ashtray near the areas where the patient most commonly resides, and if so, is it overfilled? If the outside temperature is below freezing, are faucets on outer perimeter walls set to drip slowly? Is the kitchen free of expired, rancid, or spoiled food and beverage products? Do counts on medications seem accurate for time that has passed since the medications were refilled, and are the medication properly stored, labeled, and current?

Contacting Resources

Preventing safety hazards can be done in part by constructing a solid support team for the older adult, consisting of friends, family, neighbors, health workers, and those from social circles such as church or other community groups. Communication among the support team members is crucial to help provide a safe situation for the patient.

Resources can be found in most communities to help address safety concerns that may be noted in the older adult's environment, particularly for those in the home setting who may be underserved. If the LPN believes that there is a safety breach present for the patient, he or she must act. If the patient is in immediate danger, then action must be taken, with consideration for the LPN's safety as well, to rectify the situation. This may include the need to call police or other emergency services, including 9-1-1. If no immediate danger is present, then the LPN's next steps would be to report any concerns to a supervisor and educate the older adult in applicable situations.

The supervisor or employing agency will most often have a list of area resources that are available for the older adult. This may include food delivery services; organizations that do home repairs and chores for those in need; lesbian, bisexual, gay, and transgender legal assistance; support groups; and disaster response registries. On discussing safety concerns, the LPN can ensure that interventions are being properly implemented in response. Preventing safety concerns can greatly improve the health and overall quality of life for the older adult.

CASE STUDY SOLUTIONS

1. Mr. Baxter is currently taking several medications that may cause dizziness as a regular side effect. When he takes several doses at the same time, there is an increased chance of dizziness. Instability resulting from learning to ambulate with a walker also places Mr. Baxter at an increased risk for falls. He should be instructed that it is not safe for him to take two doses of medications at the same time. If he misses a dose, you need to notify the RN. You may also want to check with the RN or PCG to see whether any of his medications can be taken earlier in the evening.

2. To decrease the risk of future falls or other injuries, you should make sure that his walker and wheelchair do not have any sharp edges that can scrape his skin and ensure that he is comfortable using both pieces of equipment. You may also want to make sure that his home is free from lose area rugs, cords, and other hazards such as dog toys. Finally, ensure that frequently used items are within arm's reach, so that he is less likely to ambulate without his devices to get items such as the remote, glasses, or to answer the phone.

3. You should discuss with Mr. Baxter the possibility of obtaining an alert system that he can use in the event of a health emergency in case his wife is out of the home. You will also want to make sure he has a telephone that is easy for him to use and is with him at all times. The contact information for friends and family members should be programmed into the phone or listed on a sheet of paper next to his chair. The contact information for the home health agency also should be readily available. In the event of a disaster, he should have a safety bag packed with supplies. It is important to make sure there are 3 to 4 days' worth of supplies for himself, his wife, and his dog in the event they need to leave the home quickly.

4. Although there is no exact guideline for resuming either activity, it is important to discuss with Mr. Baxter the importance of easing his way back into both. You can also recommend exploring position modifications for each as he continues to heal and resume his strength and range of motion. It is important to respond to both questions honestly and respectfully, while not downplaying, dismissing, or discouraging either activity due to his age.

Key Points

- Multiple factors can contribute to falls. It is important to assess the patient's physical and cognitive health as well as their nutrition, medications, and surroundings.
- Maintaining optimal skin integrity can help prevent injuries and infections for older adults. It is important to assess the environment for ways to prevent cuts, scrapes, and tears such as removing, covering, or repositioning sharp or rough edges. Inspecting clothing is also key in decreasing injuries that may come from zippers, hooks, or rough spots from seams or tight elastic bands.
- Older adults are more susceptible to adverse health related to weather extremes because of the normal physiological changes associated with aging. It is important to check for signs of hyperthermia during the summer and hypothermia when the weather turns cold.
- Four major mental health concerns are commonly found among older adults: depression, anxiety disorder, PTSD, and substance use disorder. When engaging with older adults, the nurse should listen for statements and look for visual cues that may indicate a shift in mental health.
- Many older adults remain sexually active, putting them at risk for STIs. It is important to not make assumptions about sexual activity, sexual orientation, or gender identity and instead to have open, honest conversations to learn more about your patient.
- There are various forms of abuse faced by older people: physical, psychological or emotional, financial or material, sexual, and neglect or abandonment. It is possible for a person to be subjected to multiple forms of abuse at the same time. Be aware of statements that are made regarding interactions with others, including loved ones, to ensure that the patient is safe, and no abuse is present.

- Accidents, emergencies, and disasters can occur suddenly. It is important to have plans and provisions in place to prevent emergencies as much as possible or respond to emergencies and disasters as quickly and efficiently as possible.
- A thorough assessment of the older adult's living environment can have a significant influence on their health outcomes. Whether in a home or facility setting, focus must be placed on assessing the environment to decrease risks, listening to safety concerns, and visually inspecting their surroundings. Remember that each individual is entitled to have their surroundings maintained in a manner that is comfortable to them.

Review Questions

1. You recognize that your patient may be an increased risk for falls when she states, "I've felt so dizzy today." You know this dizziness could be directly linked to (select all that apply):
   1. Weather.
   2. Hydration.
   3. Mild dementia.
   4. Nutrition.
   5. Medication.
   6. Infection.
   7. Drug or alcohol misuse.

2. As your patient is brought back indoors, he seems confused, less responsive than normal, is breathing shallowly, has a weak heart rate, and is slightly slurring his speech. In addition to alerting your supervisor, which initial intervention do you perform?
   1. Check to see whether his extremities feel cold to the touch and place a few extra blankets on him.
   2. Remove his light jacket and turn the air conditioning up to high.
   3. Seat him in front of the fan and bring him a glass of ice water.
   4. Instruct the CNA to keep an eye on him and then take his vitals again in 1 hour.

3. All of the following may lead to increased anxiety in older adults, except:
   1. A ground-level fall.
   2. Death of a spouse.
   3. Alcohol consumption.
   4. Beginnings of short-term memory loss.

4. On an initial home visit your new patient, Sheila, frequently speaks about a woman named Elizabeth who lives with her. As you look at the mantle you notice many pictures of the two of them, so you:
   1. Assume that they must be a lifelong friends who moved in together for companionship after their husbands passed away.
   2. Know that Sheila and Elizabeth must be lesbians in a relationship together.
   3. Redirect the conversation back to health-related questions because the ambiguity of the situation makes you feel uneasy.
   4. Ask Sheila to tell you more about Elizabeth's role in her life.

5. Abuse may manifest as all of the following:
   1. Lacerations, bruises on the face, broken bones
   2. Increased tearfulness, withdrawing from others, feelings of worthlessness
   3. Bruising on the genitals, increase in pressure ulcers, weight loss
   4. All of the above
   5. 1 and 3 only

ANSWERS 1. 1,2,4,5,6,7; 2. 1 ; 3. 4; 4. 5. 4

CHAPTER 8
Nutrition

Tamara Dahlkemper

KEY TERMS

complex carbohydrate
complete protein
essential amino acid
fat-soluble vitamin
functional protein
incomplete protein
malnutrition
nonessential amino acid
simple carbohydrate
structural protein
therapeutic diet
water-soluble vitamin

CHAPTER CONCEPTS

Metabolism
Nutrition

LEARNING OUTCOMES

1. Perform a nutritional assessment on an older adult.
2. Develop a nutritional plan using MyPlate as a guide.
3. Identify the influence carbohydrates, proteins, and fats have on maintaining a healthy body.
4. Identify the influence vitamins and minerals have on maintaining a healthy body.
5. Discuss therapeutic diets for older adults with special nutritional needs.
6. List four basic causes of electrolyte imbalance.

CASE STUDY

Mrs. Salvador is a 75-year-old Hispanic resident who enjoyed good health until about 6 weeks ago, when she fell and fractured her left hip and left elbow. A week after her surgical procedure, Mrs. Salvador was transferred to a rehabilitation facility for care. She will need physical therapy before she will be able to care for herself at home. She has a history of hypertension and diabetes. You have been caring for Mrs. Salvador for the past 3 weeks. You notice that Mrs. Salvador has lost 6 pounds since her admission to the unit and the nursing assistants report that she is not eating well at mealtimes. You decide to complete a nutrition assessment on Mrs. Salvador. Any problems identified on the assessment will need to be addressed before Mrs. Salvador goes home. What are your findings?

INTRODUCTION

A nutritious intake of food is essential at any age to achieve optimal health. Good nutrition is a major contributor to feeling well. Healthy eating provides the body with energy to do things, such as work or play. It promotes clear thinking, fights disease, and usually tastes good. Nurses are key to teaching and supporting older persons in their care to understand and use the vast nutritional choices available in the United States. Eating nutritionally is a crucial behavior for positive health in every aspect of living.

The amount and type of food necessary to promote health generally change as people age. Younger people can "get away" with eating donuts or candy, whereas older people generally cannot eat such things without a weight gain or an increase in their blood sugar because of their slower metabolism and other physiological changes that occur with aging. Foods that contain carbohydrates, proteins, fats, vitamins, and minerals in the appropriate amounts must be included in dietary planning for older adults.

Evidence-Based Practice

Astrup, C., & O Connor, M. (2018). Fuel for life: A literature review of nutrition education and assessment among older adults living at home. *Home Health Care Management & Practice, 30*(2), 61–69. https://doi.org/10.1177/1084822318754843

Adequate nutrition is important in managing chronic illness and health in older adults. The risk of complications from chronic illnesses such as diabetes, obesity, osteoporosis, heart failure, and hypertension can be decreased with the provision of good nutrition. Good nutrition also plays a role in wound healing and decreasing physical and cognitive decline. In most cases, the responsibility of providing good nutrition to an older adult in a home setting falls on the family caregiver who may not know the nutritional needs of the person in their care. Older adults living at home are also more prone to nutritional issues due to social isolation, frailty, functional decline, and lack of financial resources.

A literature review was conducted related to nutritional education and assessment of older adults living at home to identify best practices.

The researchers reviewed 317 articles; only eight articles met the two review themes of nutritional interventions and barriers to providing nutritional education and assessment. The literature showed barriers to treatment that included lack of third-party payers to cover nutritional assessments and services and lack of provider referrals for nutrition services. It was also noted that the Outcome and Assessment Information Set (OASIS), a tool used by Centers for Medicare and Medicaid Services to determine reimbursement and quality measures for home health care, does not specifically address nutritional assessment. The literature also showed that many nurses and other health-care professionals felt they did not have the proper education needed to meet nutritional needs of their older patients. The researchers suggest that nutritional education be provided to home health aides and nurses, especially related to chronic conditions impacted by poor nutrition.

Questions
1. What additional information do you need to feel comfortable addressing your patients' nutritional needs?
2. Beyond the information in this textbook, what additional resources are available to you to enhance your nutrition knowledge?

As a licensed practical nurse (LPN), you need to be aware of physical changes related to aging that affect food intake. Examples of these changes are gastric disorders caused by normal gastrointestinal (GI) changes and chronic diseases or illnesses that impact nutritional requirements. In addition, certain foods and medications can cause adverse drug reactions. Older adults may have difficulty chewing or swallowing food because of disease or poor dentition. Sensory changes in seeing, smelling, and tasting foods may influence an older person's appetite. Loss of appetite can occur as psychosocial changes bring on depression, dependency on others for meals, and changes in cognitive skills. Physical changes can also impact an older adult's ability to access or prepare food. As you perform nutritional assessments on older adults, you need to think about reasons why they may have nutritional deficits and ways you can assist them and their family in overcoming the problem (Box 8.1).

Box 8.1

Risk Factors for Malnutrition in Older Adults

Physical immobility
Sensory changes
Poor dentition
Pain
Inability to acquire or prepare food
Depression or loneliness

Unless otherwise stated, *Lutz's Nutrition and Diet Therapy*, 7th edition (Mazur & Litch, 2019) is used as the reference for the nutritional information in this chapter.

NUTRITIONAL ASSESSMENT

Nutritional assessment tools are not always available at every facility. A variety of tools are available and may vary from nursing home to hospital. In many facilities, a dietitian does the nutritional assessment, but that is not always true. You need to be mindful of the basics of a nutritional risk assessment so that you can perform one successfully wherever you are working. A common and easy-to-use nutritional assessment is the Mini-Nutritional Assessment (MNA) (Nestle Nutrition Institute, n.d.). The MNA assesses the following areas that indicate nutritional concerns:

1. Decline in food intake in the last 3 months
2. Weight loss or weight gain during the last 3 months
3. Mobility issues
4. Psychological or acute illness in the last 3 months
5. Taking more than three prescriptions
6. Presence of pressure sores or skin ulcers
7. Living independently
8. Type and quantity of food consumed daily

Concerns in any of the areas listed are nutritional risks that can lead to malnutrition and can compromise health. **Malnutrition** is defined as inadequate or excessive exposure to nutrients. You need to report the nutritional risks you identify to your supervisor. Good nutrition is essential to good health. Reconciliation of the basic problems listed is critical to improved health.

The objective in gerontological nursing is to help the individual attain the best health possible for the best possible quality of life. Good nutrition is a powerful tool in making that happen.

MANAGING WEIGHT

Monitoring weight also is an effective tool in assessing nutritional status. You need to be attentive to any changes in an older adult's weight. If there is weight gain, the person may benefit from becoming more active. It also is important to check for edema because the weight gain could be caused by a more serious underlying problem. If there is weight loss, it should be reported to the registered nurse (RN) to assess for possible causative factors.

Most of the common reasons older adults lose weight are related to physical or socioenvironmental changes. Older adults generally have less mobility and may be unable to prepare meals efficiently or go shopping. Some older people generally do not like to eat alone and may be less likely to eat complete meals. Some elderly people are forgetful and may neglect to prepare meals.

Priority Setting

The priority you need to set, to ensure good nutrition for the older adults in your care, is your commitment to their health. First, learn the information in this chapter. There is quite a bit of detail, but these are only the basics. This information is the minimum you need to learn to be effective in promoting nutritional health. Then:

1. Apply the information to your own life.
2. Work with team members to see that effective nutritional assessments are done on admission for all patients.
3. Support your nurse manager or volunteer to assist in putting the pertinent information from the assessments into the care plans.
4. Put up signs so the staff will know what assistance and encouragement each person needs. Examples are: "Offer fluids or juice every 2 hours and record." "Cut up fresh fruit for Mrs. Jonas." "Stay and visit with Mr. Tanaki while he eats. Encourage him to eat more food." "Mr. Welling has a food journal at the desk. Please record all food consumed."

As a caring professional, you are one member of the health-care team who can work with others to identify and manage nutritional problems that exist with older adults.

Older adults often have a decreased income, so they may not have the money or transportation to obtain adequate food. I remember an elderly woman who attended a gerontological clinic and asked me if it was "OK" for her not to take her antihypertensive medication so she could buy food. This is a serious problem because standard Medicare does not cover medications, so without a supplemental insurance, medications are very expensive for someone on a set income. A thorough and caring interview should reveal many of these problems and others that are age related.

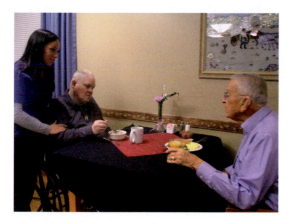

These older adults are enjoying the socialization that comes with dining together.

There are several disease-related reasons why an older adult may lose weight. Are there changes in health that could cause weight loss, such as a prolonged illness? Does the older adult have metabolic changes that affect food absorption, digestion, or elimination? Have you noticed the older adult experiencing chewing or swallowing difficulties or an inability to self-feed or even to see the food? Perhaps the person is depressed, or maybe the food does not taste good. If you are doing home care, there could be reasons the older adult cannot purchase, prepare, or eat the food. Be sure to ask about any problems related to nutrition. Part of a good assessment would be to ask the older adult why, in his or her opinion, the weight loss is happening.

Reasons for weight gain can be related to the process of aging. Weight gain is a problem for people of any age but seems worse for elderly persons who often have health conditions that can decrease their activity level such as arthritis or heart disease. In addition, as the human body ages, it has less lean body mass (muscle), and an increase in fat tissue (adipose tissue), which leads to a decrease in the basal metabolic rate. Unless people compensate for that normal physiological change by eating less, they gain weight. Because adipose tissue metabolizes more slowly than lean body mass, it does not burn calories as quickly.

TRACKING NUTRITIONAL INTAKE

During an illness, nutrition performs a vital role in the body's ability to heal. The critical foods—foods that provide energy and nutrients—are divided into three groups: carbohydrates, proteins, and fats. Each food group is necessary to maintain and repair the body during health and illness. It is important to have the knowledge to assess the inclusion of these food groups in a person's diet. This assessment can be done by evaluating if the person's diet includes a variety of fruits, vegetables, and meats or other protein-rich foods, including grains. The assessment can be done by observing what the older adult is eating during mealtime or by keeping a food journal. If you have observed a patient or resident eating minimal amounts of food or showing signs of listlessness, you should talk to the RN about the problem and suggest a food journal. A food journal is a designated place where the person removing the food tray writes down not only the percentage of the food eaten but also the actual food. Next, a dietitian or other nutrition professional is assigned to determine whether the person is eating enough calories and specific nutrients. The journal needs to be kept for only 3 to 5 days. It is a great way to gather the detailed information needed to assist an older person with obtaining good nutrition. The dietitian is an excellent resource when there is a problem with someone not eating nutritious foods. It may be helpful to complete a food journal for Mrs. Salvador in an effort to see exactly what she is eating at each meal.

A review of the food groups—carbohydrates, proteins, and fats—can help you in your ability to assess and evaluate nutritional needs of older adults. Carbohydrates, proteins, and fats are found in various fruits and vegetables, meats, milk, and breads, and cereal foods. It is important for older adults to eat a variety of foods with these nutrients to ensure that the body can maintain and repair itself.

NUTRITIONAL NEEDS OF OLDER ADULTS

Regardless of the health status of an older adult, he or she needs to have food that provides calories for energy and nutrients to maintain body functions. A person's food needs for optimal health change with age, physical activity, and health status. In 2011, the U.S. Department of Agriculture debuted a new visual depiction of suggested daily food intake called MyPlate. Scientists at Tufts University introduced MyPlate for Older Adults that describes the nutritional needs for individuals as they age. The modified graphic shows a plate divided into four sections: vegetables and fruits; whole grains and breads; protein and fats; and oils and spices. The size of the section represents which types of food should be consumed in what quantity. Each section displays pictures of the types of foods that can be eaten for each category. The graphic also includes a section representing physical activity and liquids that can be consumed as part of a good nutrition plan.

The new MyPlate food guide is important to your knowledge base for teaching and supporting older people in their quest for nutritional health. Frequent use of the food guide will assist you in mastering the information necessary to give meaningful nutrition information to your patients. The food guide will be helpful to you in teaching Mrs. Salvador what she should be eating.

Carbohydrates

There are two types of carbohydrates: complex and simple. **Complex carbohydrates** are those that the body breaks down slowly and that sustain energy over a longer period. **Simple carbohydrates** differ from complex carbohydrates in that they are easier for the body to digest and they provide a source of quick energy.

You need to know which foods provide carbohydrates that promote health. Carbohydrates come from grains, beans, nuts, milk, meat, fruits, and vegetables. Honey, molasses, sugar, and syrups also contain carbohydrates. The more carbohydrate foods are processed, the more the dietary fiber will be broken down, and some of the carbohydrate nutritional value will be lost. Simple carbohydrates come from milk and foods high in sugar content, and they are a source of quick energy. MyPlate provides a visual representation of the sources of carbohydrates that need to be included in a healthy diet.

MyPlate for Older Adults

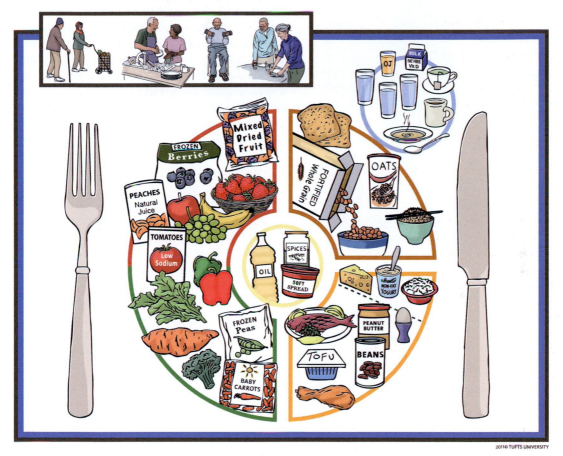

MyPlate for Older Adults. With permission from Tufts University School of Nutrition.

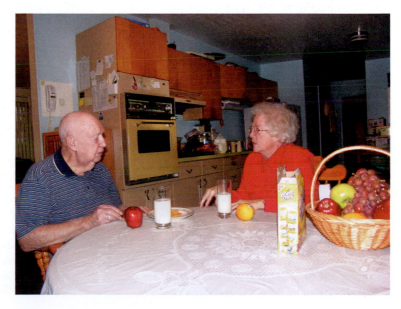

This couple has learned the value of healthy nutritious food. Their meals focus on fresh fruits and vegetables, sodium restriction, calcium intake through dairy products, and low-fat proteins.

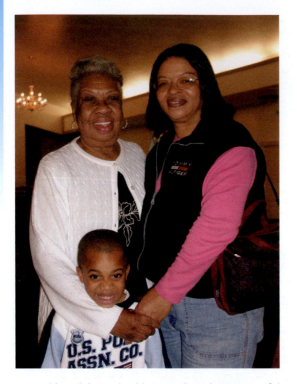

Most older adults eat healthier meals and eat more of the meal if they are eating with family members. This daughter and her son have dinner with grandma three times a week. This assures the grandma of good food and company. She says she really looks forward to these dinners.

Proteins

Proteins are the building blocks of the body and are divided into two categories: structural and functional. **Structural proteins** contain the amino acids that provide support for various body parts. Examples of structural proteins include keratin, collagen, and elastin. These proteins make up the hair, ligaments, tendons, bones, and skin. **Functional proteins** help the body perform the activities that keep the body alive, such as hemoglobin that transports oxygen through the circulatory system and antibodies that fight off bacteria and viruses. The body requires a supply of proteins to repair worn-out or damaged tissues and to build up new tissue. They also play an important part in maintaining the body's metabolic activities and the body's defense system.

When using the term *protein,* you need to remember the term *amino acids.* There are thousands of different proteins, and they all are made of various combinations of amino acids. The two classifications of amino acids are essential and nonessential. You should not confuse the terms *essential* and *nonessential*

amino acids with their value to the body because both kinds of amino acids are important for good health. **Nonessential amino acids** refer to amino acids the body can make in adequate amounts to meet its needs. **Essential amino acids** are the amino acids the body cannot make in sufficient quantities for metabolic needs and usually come from the diet. Essential and nonessential amino acids are necessary for the body to function properly.

The terms *complete* and *incomplete proteins* refer to the foods that supply proteins to the body. A **complete protein** comes from animal sources and contains essential and nonessential amino acids. Milk, cheese, yogurt, beef, fish, and poultry are good sources of complete proteins. **Incomplete proteins** come from plant sources, but plants lack some essential amino acids. Dried beans and dark green, deep yellow, and starchy vegetables are considered good sources of incomplete proteins. (Refer to the MyPlate food guide for a visual representation of the sources of proteins that need to be included in a healthy diet.)

Eating different plant sources during the same meal supplies the body with both complete and incomplete proteins that provide the essential and nonessential amino acids for building, maintaining, and repairing the body. Think of eating beans and rice in the same meal. Each of these foods is an incomplete protein food. When they are eaten in the same meal, however, the body uses them as a complete protein. This way of obtaining protein for the body is used by millions of people who prefer a vegetable-based diet instead of an animal-based diet. Having Mrs. Salvador maintain a good diet, including complete and incomplete proteins, is needed to repair body tissues as she recovers from her accident and subsequent surgery.

Age, sex, chronic diseases, fevers, infections, surgery, and traumatic injury are factors in determining the need for added protein for the body's maintenance and repair. The primary care provider (PCP) may order laboratory tests to determine adequate protein intake. These tests may include serum prealbumin, albumin, and blood urea nitrogen (BUN).

Fats

Fats provide a source of fuel for the body, support internal organs, provide insulation, and help with the absorption of certain vitamins. Excess fat in the diet can increase the risk of diabetes, cardiovascular disease, obesity, and certain cancers.

Fats are found in plants such as beans and nuts and in oils produced from plants. Fats also are found in beef, poultry, fish, shellfish, dairy, and eggs. The food guide MyPlate provides a visual representation of the sources of fats that are heart healthy, are vital for a healthy body, and should be included in the diet.

Vitamins

Vitamins are needed in the body for maintenance of metabolic processes and growth. Vitamins are classified as either water-soluble or fat-soluble. **Water-soluble vitamins** are absorbed in water. **Fat-soluble vitamins** require fats for adequate absorption and include A, D, E, and K. With one exception, which you will see shortly, vitamins are not produced by the body and must be extracted from foods (or nutritional supplements).

Vitamin A is a fat-soluble vitamin that comes from animal and plant sources. Plant sources of vitamin A are dark-green leafy vegetables and deep yellow or orange fruits and vegetables. Vitamin A is necessary for good vision, growth, and immune system function. Vitamin A can be stored in the body's fat; a deficit in vitamin A may not be noted for some time. Taking large doses of vitamin A may cause toxicity in the body. Symptoms of excess vitamin A include ataxia, dry skin, poor appetite, and liver damage. Always ask about the consumption of food supplements and carefully document what is being taken. This is especially important to do with vitamin A intake.

The B vitamins are listed as the B vitamin complex. Vitamin B_1 (thiamine) is necessary for energy metabolism and cell function. Older adults who drink excess alcohol or have poor nutritional intake may need to take thiamine supplements. Foods rich in thiamine come from whole grains or enriched cereals, nuts, organ meats, pork, and legumes.

Vitamin B_2 (riboflavin) is essential in building and maintaining healthy tissue. Foods rich in riboflavin are milk and dairy products, enriched cereals, eggs, and meats.

Vitamin B_3 (niacin) is essential in maintaining healthy nervous and digestive systems and skin. Foods rich in niacin are whole grains and enriched breads, liver, meats, poultry, fish, tea, and coffee. Niacin supplements are often used to increase high-density lipoprotein (HDL) cholesterol. Niacin can interfere with blood glucose control so people with diabetes should take niacin supplements with caution. Symptoms of niacin toxicity are diarrhea, vomiting, gastric ulcers, and liver damage.

Vitamin B_6 (pyridoxine) assists in the metabolism and use of glycogen that has been stored as a fuel. Pyridoxine is required for brain activity and normal functioning of the central nervous and immune systems. Food sources of pyridoxine are eggs, whole-wheat products, nuts, vegetables, and animal sources. Pyridoxine can be lost during processing of frozen foods, luncheon meats, and cereal foods. Toxicity from pyridoxine can occur with the intake of large doses of dietary supplements. The classic symptom of toxicity is lack of muscle coordination, neuropathy, sensitivity to sunlight, heartburn, and nausea.

Vitamin B_{12} (cobalamin) is essential for the production of hemoglobin and for proper nervous system function. Gastrointestinal changes related to normal aging can decrease the absorption of vitamin B_{12}, requiring older adults to take supplements of B_{12}. The best foods containing vitamin B_{12} are meat, fish, poultry, eggs, and milk products. There are no plant food sources for B_{12} so older adults who eat primarily a plant-based diet may require a supplemental source of vitamin B_{12}.

Folate is the most naturally occurring form of folic acid and is essential for healthy cell growth and function and red blood cell formation. Folate can be found in green leafy vegetables, legumes, liver, and fortified grains and cereal. Symptoms of folate deficiency include fatigue and weakness, heart palpitations, bright red tongue, and shortness of breath. High doses of folic acid can cause colorectal cancer.

Focused Learning Chart: Significance of Folate

Benefits of Folate	Folate or Folic Acid Can Be Found in:
Healthy cell growth and function	Leafy green vegetables
Red blood cell formation	Dried peas and beans
	Organic foods
	Liver
	Foods and vitamins enriched with folic acid

Vitamin C is also known as ascorbic acid. Vitamin C is water-soluble and is easily lost in cooking. Vitamin C cannot be stored by the body, so there must be a daily intake of food containing vitamin C. The body needs vitamin C to build and repair body tissues and bones, to keep teeth and gums healthy, and to aid with iron absorption. Lack of vitamin C causes wounds to fail to heal, bones to weaken, and muscles to degenerate, and puts the older adult at risk for infections and falling. Scurvy, an uncommon disease caused by a deficiency in vitamin C, can occur in the elderly and alcoholics. Good sources of vitamin C include citrus fruits, strawberries, kiwi fruit, cantaloupe, broccoli, and Brussels sprouts.

Vitamin D is one of the fat-soluble vitamins. Vitamin D is not actually a vitamin because it is produced naturally by the body. The body can produce its own vitamin D if there is enough exposure to the sun. However, the ability to absorb vitamin D in the intestines decreases with age. Few people have enough sun exposure, however, to produce sufficient vitamin D. Vitamin D is necessary for the absorption of calcium and phosphorus to maintain bone tissue and many other body functions. Older adults are at risk for vitamin D deficiencies if they are not eating enough fortified foods. Older women who have vitamin D deficiency are at risk for bone loss, which increases the risk of fractures due to osteoporosis. Vitamin D occurs naturally in very few foods. The food sources of vitamin D are liver, fish oils, egg yolks, and foods fortified with vitamin D. Excessive amounts of vitamin D can cause loss of appetite, constipation, polyuria, and muscle weakness. Low levels of vitamin D have been associated with cardiovascular disease and sleep apnea.

Vitamin E (alpha-tocopherol) is a fat-soluble vitamin. Vitamin E is a powerful antioxidant that provides protection for many body tissues and slows the aging process. Studies are ongoing to determine the role of vitamin E in preventing cancer and heart disease. Foods rich in vitamin E include peanut butter, nuts, seeds, wheat germ, and vegetable oils. Large doses of vitamin E may interfere with blood clotting so patients taking anticoagulants should only take the recommended amount of vitamin E.

Vitamin K is a fat-soluble vitamin. The main roles of vitamin K are blood-clotting functions, aiding in bone development, and regulating blood calcium. Foods that supply vitamin K are leafy vegetables, cabbage, broccoli, cauliflower, Brussels sprouts, and kale. Vitamin K is extracted by bacteria in the intestine from food sources that contain vitamin K. While vitamin K deficiency is rare, it can occur due to long-term antibiotic therapy. Antibiotics prevent the absorption of vitamin K from the intestinal tract. Vitamin K decreases the effectiveness of anticoagulants so a person taking anticoagulants should limit intake of vitamin K and foods containing vitamin K.

Encouraging older adults to eat a diet full of foods that will provide the required vitamins is important. The nurse should also recommend vitamin supplements with caution and always ask about the supplements patients may be taking. Consider the body's need for vitamins in helping Mrs. Salvador recover from her accident and subsequent surgery. Which vitamins will be the most valuable in her recovery?

Minerals

Along with the necessity of vitamins in the diet, minerals are also required to maintain a healthy body. Minerals are inorganic substances that are found in nature and in the human body and are classified according to the amount needed to maintain a healthy body. Major minerals (macrominerals) are needed in greater amounts than trace minerals (microminerals). Major minerals include calcium, phosphorus, sodium, magnesium, chloride, and potassium. These minerals are known as electrolytes (see the following material).

THINK LIKE A NURSE
Design a daily meal plan for an older adult taking a blood thinner. Which foods will you include? Which foods will you suggest the person does not eat?

Calcium is the most prevalent mineral found in the body. Bones and teeth are composed primarily of calcium. In older adults, additional calcium is necessary for the maintenance of bones and teeth. Calcium also is required for many other body functions, including blood clotting, muscle contraction, and nerve conduction. Calcium is best absorbed with vitamin D. Calcium is found in milk and milk products, leafy vegetables, legumes, salmon, and fortified food products. Osteoporosis can occur if there is a calcium deficiency. Mrs. Salvador's calcium intake should be assessed to ensure she is getting the appropriate amount to aid with bone regeneration.

After calcium, phosphorus is the most common mineral in the body. Phosphorus combines with calcium in the maintenance of bones and teeth. Phosphorus is found throughout the body and is required for metabolism and cell membrane maintenance. Phosphorus helps maintain the body's chemical balance and is necessary for vitamin absorption. It is readily available because it is found in all meat products, whole grain products, fruits, and vegetables. Low phosphorus levels are usually not a concern because it is so available in food. High phosphorus levels may be seen in people age 55 or older, or individuals with kidney disease. Individuals taking over-the-counter sodium phosphate medications used to treat constipation should not exceed the daily recommended dose as this can cause phosphorus toxicity.

Magnesium is necessary for energy, maintaining cell membranes, and insulin regulation. It assists calcium and potassium to cross cell membranes, which is important for muscle and nerve function. Sources of magnesium are whole grains and green leafy vegetables. Magnesium deficiencies occur with malabsorption disorders, alcohol abuse, and diabetes. Older adults are also prone to magnesium deficiencies because of decreased intake of magnesium and poor absorption in the stomach. Older adults are also more likely to have chronic diseases, such as diabetes, cardiac disease, and osteoporosis, which are linked to magnesium deficiency.

Sodium is responsible for maintaining the water balance in the body and contributes to acid-base balance. Sodium is necessary for nerve and muscle functions. Sodium is found naturally in foods such as milk, milk products, and several vegetables. Sodium is also found in processed foods. Table salt is the most common dietary source of sodium. To lower sodium levels, an older adult may be advised to limit salt intake and to reduce processed foods in the diet.

Sodium deficiency is rare unless an older adult has chronic diarrhea, vomiting, excessive sweating, or cardiac, liver, or kidney disease. The body usually excretes excess sodium through the kidneys.

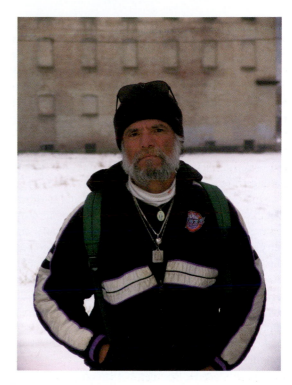

This homeless man has learned where to go for the best meals possible. He goes to the Salvation Army for lunch and the homeless shelter for dinner.

Chloride is found in the body's tissues and fluids. Despite the fact that the body contains only a small amount of chloride, this mineral is important in digestion and in maintaining fluid balance and acid-base balance. The main source of dietary chloride comes from table salt and is also available in vegetables such as seaweed, tomatoes, and celery. Chloride deficiency is rare but can occur with excessive perspiration, vomiting, or diarrhea. Too much chloride can result in fluid retention.

Potassium is responsible for nerve conduction, metabolic activities, contraction of muscles including the heart, and regulation of acid-base balance. The best sources of potassium are unprocessed fruits and vegetables and salt substitutes. Potassium is water-soluble and can be lost when vegetables are cooked in water. An older adult who has a potassium deficiency (hypokalemia) may have muscle weakness or abnormal heart rhythms. Decreased amounts of potassium can be caused by diuretics, excessive use of laxatives causing prolonged diarrhea, and kidney disease. Increased levels of potassium (hyperkalemia) are usually caused by impaired kidney function.

Trace minerals (microminerals) in the human body include iron, zinc, iodine, and fluoride. Iron is important to the formation of hemoglobin, which carries oxygen throughout the body. Good sources of iron include red meat; liver; grains; dark green, leafy cooked vegetables; oysters; and clams. Deficits in iron may be caused by poor absorption by the body or health conditions that cause blood loss such as cancer, gastrointestinal disease, and heart failure. Excess iron may increase risk of infections, organ damage, and joint disease.

Zinc is essential for wound healing and it aids in metabolic and immune functions. Zinc comes from red meat, seafood, poultry, pork, whole grains, and dairy products. Zinc intake is directly related to protein intake; individuals who have low protein intake are at risk for zinc deficiency. These individuals may include the elderly and people living at or below the poverty level. Deficits in zinc may cause hair loss, impaired wound healing, and eye and skin conditions. The effects of zinc on the common cold are still unclear.

Iodine is needed for metabolism and the production of thyroid hormones. Iodine deficiency can cause hypothyroidism or an enlarged thyroid. Excess iodine is rare and may decrease the function of the thyroid gland. Sources of iodine are iodized salt, saltwater fish, shellfish, and seaweed.

Fluoride has a role in bone and dental integrity. Fluoride's main source is fluoridated water. It can also be found in tea and processed food and drinks. The main concern with lack of fluoride as well as excess fluoride in the diet is dental caries.

The quality of foods containing minerals is related to the soil where the foods are grown. Fruits and vegetables that are grown in soils rich in a particular mineral contain more of that mineral.

Water

The need for water is more important than any other nutrient. Tap and bottled water are the most common sources of water. High amounts of water can also be found in vegetables such as iceberg lettuce, celery, and carrots.

Water is the main component of the body and serves as a transport for nutrients and wastes, is a lubricant to body parts, is a solvent for the body's chemical processes, and gives form to the cells and tissues of the body. Water helps maintain the body's temperature. The water lost by sweating during an activity or the increase of environmental temperature serves as a coolant to maintain a normal temperature.

Blood and other body and tissue secretions are transported or circulate through the body. The circulated fluids carry oxygen, nutrients, and other materials to all body cells. Circulating fluids also carry waste materials from the cells.

Point of Interest

It is best to check skin turgor over the forehead or sternum in older adults. You check the skin turgor by softly pinching the skin and then observing how fast the skin returns to normal. If it is slow to return to normal, the person is dehydrated.

Water is essential for the chemical processes in the body. It is vital for the body to maintain a water balance. Older adults are at risk for dehydration because of inadequate fluid intake caused by not feeling thirsty, medications, and chronic diseases. It is important to assess the older adult frequently for oral fluid intake.

Body Electrolytes

The minerals that make up the body's electrolytes are calcium, phosphorus, sodium, magnesium, chloride, and potassium. Each of these minerals carries a chemical charge. Some have a positive charge, and others have a negative charge. You may decide to do a quick review of chemistry to understand better the chemical processes that maintain the body's electrolyte balance. For now, you need to be aware that all of the electrolytes must be maintained in a chemical state of neutrality. An imbalance puts a person at risk for complications such as muscle spasms or weakness, fatigue, or irregular heartbeat. These electrolytes are moved through the body by fluids. Consider fluids and electrolytes lost as a result of vomiting, diarrhea, excessive perspiration, or urination, and then consider the person's potential for electrolyte imbalance.

Plasma proteins consist of protein and globulin and control the water movement in and out of cells. Blood volume is strongly influenced by plasma proteins. Electrolytes and plasma proteins must be kept in balance to maintain healthy body functions.

DIET PLANS

As an LPN, you need to be aware of the various diet plans that can be used to meet the nutritional needs of the people in your care.

A regular diet is prescribed for older adults who are healthy, have no special nutritional needs, and are capable of making nutritious food choices. Amounts of foods depend on the person's appetite, and selections of foods are made by personal likes and dislikes.

A modified diet is prescribed for older adults if they have a prolonged illness and have not eaten or if they have difficulty chewing or swallowing food. Foods in the modified diet range in consistency from clear liquids to soft foods.

Clear-liquid diets are foods that are liquid at room temperature and can be seen through. The PCP or dietitian needs to write directions about what foods are to be included in this diet. Clear or strained juices, teas, carbonated drinks, clear broths, and gelatins are some of the choices. Most clear-liquid diets do not provide adequate nutritional requirements, so they should be used for the shortest period of time possible. Patients receiving clear-liquid diets are moved to a full-liquid diet as soon as their health condition allows.

Full-liquid diets are composed of the foods included in the clear-liquid diet with the addition of foods that are liquid at room temperature but are not necessarily clear. This includes custards, ice cream, milk, some strained cereals, and blended fruits and vegetables. The full-liquid diet meets more of the person's dietary requirements but not all nutritional requirements. The dietitian gives you instructions on the food to include in a full-liquid diet.

Foods in the soft diet include those from a regular diet that have been modified for people who have difficulty chewing foods because of improperly fitting dentures or sore gums. Foods in this diet are mashed, chopped, or ground.

A **therapeutic diet**, a diet designed to control the intake of certain foods, may be ordered for people who need tailored nutritional choices. The person may need more calories or fewer calories in the diet. There may be an order to increase or decrease the amounts of carbohydrates, proteins, or fats in the diet. The person may need dietary restriction on foods containing sodium, potassium, iron, or micronutrients. Examples of therapeutic diets are a diabetic diet or the DASH (Dietary Approaches to Stop Hypertension) diet for a person with hypertension. Fluid restrictions may be necessary for some patients with chronic kidney disease. Older adults may have food allergies or may be unable to tolerate some foods; such foods should not be included in the diet.

There are health conditions in which a person's GI system can digest food but the person may be unable to consume food. Enteral, or tube, feedings are required for these people. Commercial or blended formulas are used to provide nutritional support by using a nasogastric or gastronomy feeding tube (placed directly into the stomach or GI tract through the abdomen). The physician and dietitian determine types and amounts of formulas to be used.

Older adults with chronic illnesses or injuries may require parenteral nutrition (total parenteral nutrition [TPN] or partial [PPN]). An RN is responsible for the maintenance and monitoring of this type of therapy. The RN should instruct the LPN about how to monitor a patient receiving parenteral nutrition.

It is the responsibility of the nurse to assure the older adult is receiving the appropriate meal plan to meet his or her nutritional needs. By working with the PCP and a nutritionist, an appropriate meal plan can be determined.

THINK LIKE A NURSE
You are assigned to care for Mrs. Pearson, an 81-year-old woman who has had abdominal pain, nausea, and vomiting. Which type of diet most likely will be ordered for her? Explain why.

CASE STUDY SOLUTIONS

1. If the weight loss occurred since her admission, you will want to address issues directly related to the care and treatment provided to her. Pain medications and a decrease in physical activity can decrease appetite. If Mrs. Salvador is eating her meals in her private room, you may want to encourage her to eat with the other residents or have family members visit during meal times. You will also need to make sure the food that is served is to Mrs. Salvador's liking.

2. Mrs. Salvador may have foods specific to her culture that are not being served at the facility. Ask her what foods she would like to eat and check with the facility dietitian to see whether these foods can be provided.

3. While trying to meet food preferences for Mrs. Salvador, it is also important to consider a therapeutic diet to address her diabetes and hypertension.

4. Additional areas you will want to address from the assessment are the effects of the current illness on eating patterns and medications affecting diet.

5. Any identified risks should be documented and addressed with the RN.

Key Points

• Nutritional risks can lead to malnutrition and can compromise health in an older adult. Nutritional risk assessments are used to determine poor nutrition in older adults and can be performed by nurses. An easy assessment tool to use is the Mini Nutritional Assessment (MNA).

• Tracking nutritional intake is important to ensure that the critical food groups are incorporated into the diet of an older adult. A food journal is one method to track food intake and is useful in identifying food that is eaten during a specified time period. The journal can be kept by the older adult or used by the nursing staff to monitor intake at meals.

• A person's food needs for optimal health change with age, physical activity, and health status. MyPlate for Older Adults is a visual depiction of suggested daily food intake specific for older adults. The graphic shows a plate divided into four sections that represent the main food groups. The size of each section represents the types of food that should be consumed in that quantity.

• The foods that provide energy and nutrients are divided into three groups: carbohydrates, proteins, and fats. Each food group is necessary to maintain and repair the body during health and illness. Carbohydrates provide energy for the body. Proteins are necessary for building and repairing body tissue. Fats provide a major source of fuel for the body. Fats also support internal organs and provide insulation for the body.

• Vitamins and minerals are needed to maintain healthy tissue and the normal function of the nervous and cardiac systems. They also produce hemoglobin and play key roles in metabolism. Fat-soluble vitamins include A, D, E, and K. Water-soluble vitamins include the B complex vitamins and vitamin C. Minerals are divided into the categories of major or trace minerals. Major minerals include calcium, phosphorus, sodium, magnesium, chloride, and potassium. Trace minerals include iron, zinc, iodine, and fluoride.

• Minerals that make up the body's electrolytes are calcium, phosphorus, sodium, magnesium, chloride, and potassium. For the body to function well, the electrolytes must maintain a chemical state of neutrality. Electrolytes are lost as a result of vomiting, diarrhea, excessive perspiration, and excessive urination.

• Therapeutic diets are ordered for individuals who need tailored nutritional choices. An individual may need dietary restrictions on certain food groups or foods containing sodium, potassium, iron, or other vitamins or minerals. Common therapeutic diets include the diabetic or DASH diet.

Review Questions

1. You are completing a nutritional assessment on an older adult. Which of the following statements should be of concern?
   1. "I eat at least three meals a day."
   2. "I have access to food."
   3. "Because of my arthritis, I find it difficult to prepare my meals."
   4. "My husband and I eat our meals together."

2. Consider an older adult with bone and soft tissue injuries from a fall. Which diet would be the most effective for this type of person?
   1. High-carbohydrate diet, which would assist in giving the person enough energy for physical therapy
   2. 1,000-calorie diet, which would assist in weight reduction and make ambulation easier
   3. High-protein, high-carbohydrate diet, which would assist in cellular rebuilding and energy
   4. TPN, which would provide all nutrients and save energy for the older person

3. Which of the following diets would be appropriate for an older adult who has problems with blood clotting?
   1. Diet low in sodium
   2. Diet low in potassium
   3. Diet high in vitamin A
   4. Diet high in vitamin K

4. All of the following can cause electrolyte imbalances *except:*
   1. Vomiting.
   2. Diuretics.
   3. Diarrhea.
   4. Antibiotics.

5. You admit a man who is very lethargic. Through your admission interview, you identify that he is a chronic alcoholic. He is thin and has poor skin turgor. You are concerned about his overall nutrition. He states that he *never* eats green and leafy vegetables. What nutrient do you recognize he needs and is not receiving?
   1. Magnesium
   2. Chloride
   3. Sodium
   4. Phosphorus

ANSWERS 1. 3, 2. 3, 3. 4, 4. 4, 5. 1

CHAPTER 9

Activity, Rest, and Sleep as Criteria for Health

Tamara Dahlkemper

KEY TERMS

circadian rhythm
insomnia
sleep apnea
stress

CHAPTER CONCEPTS

Comfort
Mobility
Sleep and Rest
Stress

LEARNING OUTCOMES

1. Express an understanding of the importance of activity for all older adults, including those with chronic conditions.
2. Describe normal rest and sleep patterns for older adults.
3. Identify older adults who are most at risk for developing rest and sleep disturbances.
4. Apply nursing interventions to older adults who are experiencing problems with activity, rest, or sleep.

CASE STUDY

Mrs. McDonald is an 86-year-old woman who lives with her eldest son, Sean, and his active family of five children. Mr. McDonald died the previous year of heart disease. Prior to her husband's death, Mrs. McDonald enjoyed working in her yard and taking short walks. She also enjoyed cooking and fixing meals for herself. After her husband's death, Mrs. McDonald started spending more time sitting in her chair and became less able to care for herself. Being concerned about his mother, Sean moved her into his home with his wife and five children.

After living with the family for one month, Mrs. McDonald began complaining that she was unable to sleep at night. Mrs. McDonald has her own room, but all of the bedrooms are on the same floor. Sean has two teenagers who often have friends over to the house. They are noisy and tend to stay up until 9 p.m. or 10 p.m. in the evening on the weekends. There also is a 5-month-old baby who wakes up crying twice a night. Mrs. McDonald is always tired and started napping four to five times a day. Instead

CASE STUDY—cont'd

of getting up and doing things for herself, she has the 5-year-old and the toddler running errands for her frequently during the day.

Sean's wife, Mary, began to complain of having to wait on the children (baby, toddler, 5-year-old, and the teens) and Mrs. McDonald. "She won't get out of her chair or do anything for herself or help around the house," Mary told Sean one day as she was crying. Sean felt caught between the needs of his mother and the needs of his wife and children. He was committed to not putting his mother in a nursing home because she was adamant about not going to live in one. Sean called a local home care agency to see if they could help him with his problem. You are the nurse assigned to Mrs. McDonald. What are you going to do? This is a holistic problem because the entire family is involved, so approach your solution with that in mind.

INTRODUCTION

Activity promotes life physically and psychologically. Even minimal activity has several physical benefits (see Box 9.1). The psychological benefits of activity include the sense of well-being that comes with having the freedom to move from one place to the other and to take care of oneself, even if that care is minimal. Frail health in older adults is associated with inactivity.

Box 9.1

Benefits of Physical Activity for the Older Adult

Decreased risk for obesity; diabetes; and cardiovascular, respiratory, musculoskeletal diseases
Improved quality of sleep
Preservation of muscle strength and endurance
Increased aerobic capacity
Greater bone density
Greater mobility and independence
Better bowel control
Better appetite control
Improved balance
Improved joint function
Decreased risk of falls
Improved memory and learning capabilities
Increased sense of well-being

Rest and sleep are also necessary to an individual's well-being. However, older adults often experience changes in sleep patterns that lead to diminished sleep quality and quantity. Sleep deprivation in older persons can be a very serious consideration when planning nursing care. The importance of managing activity, rest, and sleep is critical in giving care to older people.

Priority Setting

The priority for this chapter is for you to allow all older adults to do as much for themselves as possible. The challenge is that the person may not want to do all he or she can do. Perhaps he or she needs good pain management so that moving is not so painful. Perhaps the older person feels that they do not need to be active. Whatever the challenge, you need to use the information in this chapter to determine what is keeping the person from doing everything possible as independently as possible. Be clever, be smart, be caring, and be holistic.

ACTIVITY

Activity for people in the United States has changed over the years. As society has moved from an agrarian (farming) society to an industrial one, the natural activities that dominated society, such as farming, have changed as well. To accommodate the change in activity, many people now go to gyms or join organized community sports groups to get enough exercise to be healthy. According to the Centers for Disease Control and Prevention (CDC), about 12% of adults 65 years and older get the recommended amount of aerobic and strength training activity (Clarke, Norris, & Schiller, 2017). Studies show that a person's health status plays an important role in activity level. The healthier an individual perceives themselves the more likely they are to participate in physical activity. Likewise, a person experiencing several health issues may be less likely to exercise. There are several barriers to physical activity in older adults. Older adults may not exercise because they are afraid of injury or falling. They may experience lack of self-motivation or are unsure of the appropriate physical activity that is best for them. Other older adults have a concern for safety when exercising in their neighborhood. And some older adults just prefer to participate in more sedentary activities (Bethancourt, Rosenberg, Beatty, & Arterburn, 2014).

Older persons who golf, mow their lawns, or walk their dogs are using the health they have and are working to maintain it. Even those using canes or who need oxygen and who do their grocery shopping in an electric cart are exercising. Although they are not walking, it takes effort to get up, eat, dress, and manage getting to their car and then the store. They are interacting with an environment different from their home and have to stretch and move to get the items they need from the shelves. It is wonderful to see people moving at whatever their physical activity level is.

Advantages and Disadvantages of Exercise

As a nurse giving care to older adults, you have several complex concerns to manage in activity and exercise for older adults. The most important is managing an older person's chronic conditions (Box 9.2). Degenerative arthritis makes it difficult to walk; pulmonary disease makes it challenging to move at all. With the aging of society, many old-old people use canes, walkers, wheelchairs, and oxygen that add to the need for planning when exercising. Nevertheless, elderly people need to exercise.

When people exercise, they are assisting all of their major systems. Exercise improves the functioning of the cardiovascular, respiratory, musculoskeletal, digestive, and excretory systems. Studies also show improvement in cognitive function and general well-being. Setting goals and having meaningful things to do, all of which require some activity, combats depression, insomnia, and boredom.

Box 9.2

Ten Most Common Chronic Conditions in People Older Than Age 65 in the United States

1. Hypertension
2. High cholesterol
3. Arthritis
4. Ischemic heart disease
5. Diabetes
6. Chronic kidney disease
7. Heart failure
8. Depression
9. Alzheimer's disease and dementia
10. Chronic obstructive pulmonary disease

(National Council on Aging, 2017)

Focused Learning Chart: Advantages of Exercise

Assist to Prevent	Assist to Manage	Can Improve
Osteoporosis	Pressure ulcers	Joint immobility
Diabetes mellitus	Arthritis	Most pulmonary conditions
Heart disease	Depression	Insomnia
Boredom	Obesity	Indigestion
	Psychosocial health	Constipation

When older people do not exercise, they are subject to osteoporosis; joint immobility; indigestion; constipation; pneumonia; weakened cardiac and

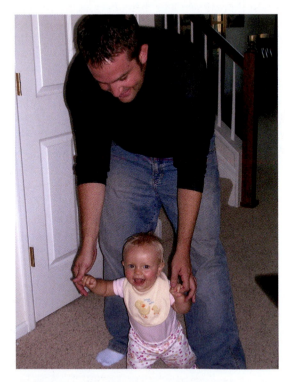

When this child was learning to walk, she needed assistance from her parents. She would walk and walk and walk until she learned to do it independently. Can you draw an analogy from this child to an older adult who has experienced an injury that limits mobility?

other muscles; pressure ulcers; as well as depression, insomnia, and boredom already mentioned. The aging process is a challenge to maintaining a healthy lifestyle. The instrument for avoiding the pitfalls of inactivity in older adults is the care given by you, as a licensed practical nurse (LPN), and the members of the family, who you are responsible to teach.

How to Help Older Adults Stay Active

The first rule when working with older persons and their exercise needs is to allow them to do as much for themselves as possible. This sounds very simple; however, in the real world of your clinical practice, it is not. There is pressure to get everyone to the lunch room in a skilled facility in a timely manner, and walking residents to meals is more time-consuming than putting them in wheelchairs to transport them. Yet, walking residents to the lunch room is an excellent way to give them some exercise. This could become problematic for you as you organize your time. It is critical that you and the people you manage (the nursing assistants) organize yourselves so that everyone can be assisted in walking to their meals, if possible. Once there, the residents can use their time to visit with each other and discuss the day's events. The difference between getting them to lunch at your convenience and ambulating them to lunch with time for socialization is one of quality of care and caring.

In the hospital, you may need to assist an older adult to a chair so that meals can be eaten while sitting upright (better digestion, less acid reflux). Assisting someone to the toileting room, without the use of a wheelchair, promotes bowel elimination, and the walking is important for muscle strengthening (including the heart) and the avoidance of increased osteoporosis.

The "allowing people to do as much for themselves as possible" rule extends to all of the care you render to people in a nursing home, hospital, or home. Allow individuals to brush their own teeth, comb their own hair, and dress themselves as much as possible. These are all activities of daily living (ADLs) that older adults should be encouraged to do on their own in any care setting including at home. All of these actions take time but are excellent for range of motion and self-esteem building. Teaching this principle to family and friends further enhances the quality of life of older adults. Tell them what you are doing and explain the "why." You need to model safe and caring ways for assisting the person in your care. During the time you are assisting older persons, talk to them, listen to what they have to say, and value their wisdom and experience. This valuing behavior helps build self-esteem, and it is a caring and wise way to use the time you are spending in activity with your clients.

While planning exercise for specific older adults in your care, be aware of their physical ability. Consider Mrs. McDonald in the case study. Although she has no physiological reason for why she does not walk on her own, because she has been somewhat immobile for several months, she will need to start slowly with her activity. It is not helpful to put people in a situation that puts major demands on their bodies that could be unsafe. For some people, sitting in a circle and throwing a ball from one to another is good use of their upper body and is fun. For other people, it could be boring and beneath their physical abilities. Begin with a conservative plan and increase it if it does not physically stress the person.

Cultural Considerations

The importance of exercise can vary among different cultures as well as within a culture. Conveying a message about the importance of exercise and activity should be done in a manner that recognizes cultural values and behaviors. Rehabilitation, exercise, and fall prevention programs should be culturally appropriate. Incorporating the positive influence of social support by family members can help encourage individuals to participate in these programs.

Four types of exercise are recommended for older adults (Box 9.3). Endurance or aerobic exercise increases respiratory and cardiac function. This type of exercise might include walking, doing yardwork, or dancing. For a frail individual, endurance exercise may be just walking a certain distance each day

Box 9.3
Types of Exercise for Older Adults

Endurance
Muscle strengthening
Balance training
Flexibility

and increasing that distance as tolerated. Muscle strengthening helps an older adult more easily rise from a chair, climb stairs, and carry groceries. This exercise includes any type of resistance exercise, such as weight lifting or the use of resistance bands, and can be as simple as a person sitting in a chair lifting their arms and legs. Light weights may be added as tolerated. Good balance is important for preventing falls in older adults. Balance training includes standing on one foot or walking heel to toe. A more formal type of balance exercise recommended for older adults is tai chi. Maintaining flexibility improves an older adult's overall movement and helps them stay active. Flexibility exercises include any exercise where the muscles are being stretched. Yoga is recommended for older adults. Doing all four types of exercise regularly will help older adults carry out their daily activities more successfully (National Institute on Aging, 2018).

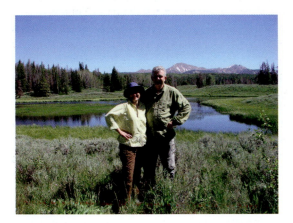

These older adults are getting their physical activity for the day.

 REST

Rest is something most people want to experience more than they generally do. It is common for busy students to want time off to do nothing but rest.

When dealing with older adults, you have a specialized group of people who have specialized rest needs.

Because of the number of chronic conditions older people tend to have, they may be unable to rest due to pain or **stress**. In another scenario, the person may feel that all he or she does is rest. The key to managing the rest needs of older people is to identify what their needs are.

Pain

A common reason people cannot rest is because they have pain that keeps them awake. Pain needs to be identified and managed. It not only interferes with rest and sleep, but it also decreases activity. Chronic pain may leave a person fatigued and unable to participate properly in a restorative care program. In addition, some behavioral problems in institutionalized older adults stem from ineffective pain management. A psychiatric evaluation may be requested for screaming or abusive behavior on the part of a resident of a nursing home who in fact is experiencing physical pain. A failure to identify pain as a factor affecting behavior and function may result in poor medical management. Pain in older people is frequently either overtreated or undertreated simply because it is difficult to assess. Some older adults want every ache treated with a drug, whereas others maintain a stoic attitude: "Why bother? There is nothing that can be done anyway."

Older people often perceive pain differently. Some pain receptors may not be as acute as they were in the past. Medical journals document clinical cases describing "silent" myocardial infarctions or "painless" intraabdominal emergencies. These cases may not be silent or painless but may reflect an older person's normal aging situation. Cognitive impairments, delirium, and dementia are some of the barriers to pain assessment. People who have a dementia process or a stroke and become aphasic may be unable to give an accurate pain history. They may be unable to describe when the pain started or at what point in the day the pain becomes most severe. Most people describe the pain in the here and now. A person in pain is often self-absorbed and inattentive to activities in the environment. A sensitivity to other medications that results in delirium makes pain management difficult for older people. Delirium may also be one manifestation of an attempt to treat a person's pain. An assessment for delirium should be made whenever there is a change in cognitive function after the start of any new pain medication. Refer to Chapter 17 for information on assessing delirium. Multiple chronic disease processes and acute processes compound the difficulty. There may even be an acute exacerbation of a chronic problem. These multiple sources of pain make diagnosis difficult, and pain management becomes a challenge.

There are many myths regarding pain in older adults. One myth is that pain is normal. As body systems begin to wear out, one might expect an increase in pain. At any age, pain is the most common symptom of a disease process and should be investigated and treated. Another myth is that pain and sleep are incompatible. Nurses often disbelieve a patient's complaint of pain when they bring a pain pill and find the person asleep. The wrong conclusion is drawn. It is believed that an individual really in pain could not possibly sleep. The exhaustive feature of pain is seldom considered in the assessment process. The last myth is that narcotic drugs are not safe for older people. Narcotics provide effective pain relief that can improve quality of life for individuals with chronic conditions and terminal illnesses. However, these drugs should be used with caution in older adults. It is best to prescribe a lower than normal dose and increase the dose as needed to provide appropriate pain relief. Longer periods of time between doses are also recommended (Guerriero, 2017).

Although pain is a highly subjective experience, there are two methods for assessing it. Simple observation from a nurse who knows the person well can be very effective. A grimace or clutch of the chest provides a vivid picture of pain. A second method is to use assessment questions following these observations. Clinical practice guidelines for acute pain management identify the quantifiable measures of pain that should be considered in an assessment, including the intensity, duration, and quality of the pain, as well as the personal meaning this pain has to the older adult. The impact on the person's functioning is also included. Assessment tools are available. A good tool addresses the older person's pain history and coping strategies for dealing with pain and medications in the past that have been effective. It is important to ask questions that help to describe or define the pain. Noting the intensity and duration assists in providing an objective measure to a highly subjective experience. Simply asking "How is your pain today?" may prompt the response, "Well, it is there."

The simplest method of pain assessment is the use of a pain intensity scale. The nurse can draw a line indicating that the far left (L) end of the line defines no pain and the right (R) end represents the most pain the person has ever experienced. The person can point to the place on the line that reflects current pain level. Another commonly used method is to ask the older adult to rate the pain on a scale from 1 to 10, with 10 being the worst pain imaginable. Assessing pain in an individual with dementia or cognitive impairment can be more difficult. There are several assessment tools that can be used and the tool used will vary from facility to facility. A commonly used tool is the Pain Assessment in Advanced Dementia Scale (PAINAD) Tool. This tool assesses facial expressions, breathing patterns, body language, and the ability for the person to be consoled (Horgas, 2018). It is your responsibility, as the LPN, to identify the pain and share that information with the registered nurse (RN) or health-care provider. It is the responsibility of the RN or health-care provider to do a comprehensive assessment to determine the causative factors related to the pain. Your responsibility, besides reporting the pain and its impact on the resident or patient, is to check for more common possible causes of the pain. Is the individual positioned properly? Are position changes made often enough to prevent pressure ulcers from starting? Have you checked the medications to see if there is a drug reaction or interaction? Listen to the person experiencing the pain and carefully describe it in the chart. Providing adequate pain relief is part of giving holistic care to your older patients. For more information on pain management, refer to Chapter 20.

Safe, Effective Nursing Care

Individualizing Activity

You have the knowledge to determine a safe and meaningful activity for each individual. Think of the person holistically—for example, what the individual can do and what he or she enjoys—and then plan accordingly. Washing dishes in warm water is a successful way to exercise arthritic hands and fingers with less discomfort. Encourage arm and ankle exercises while watching television or ankle exercises while working at the computer. A walk outside to the sidewalk and back may not seem like much unless you are the person with pain or dyspnea doing the walking. Suggest a pet if it seems appropriate. The value of pet therapy is well published and taking care of a pet requires physical movement.

All exercise plans for older adults in your care need to be ordered or approved by a primary care provider (PCP). In addition, all reputable nursing homes, hospitals, and home care agencies have access to physical therapists. Use the physical therapist to teach you and the family the best approaches and techniques to use with each individual.

1. Consider the older adults in your life. What forms of activity do they incorporate into their daily lives?
2. Discuss what you can do to help them become more active.

Point of Interest

For a healthy older adult, the World Health Organization (WHO) recommends a minimum of 150 hours of moderate aerobic physical activity each week and muscle strengthening activity 2 or more days a week working all major muscle groups (WHO, n.d.). The exercise can be divided into smaller increments of time as long as each session is at least 10 minutes long. Older adults with poor mobility should do physical activity to improve balance three or more times per week. For older adults who are in poor health, just keeping them moving is important. For example, having the older person walk to the kitchen to get a drink of water is better than having someone get it for the person. Having the older person do two or three arm extensions while holding a soup can in each hand is better than not doing any. As you plan your care, think of ways you can involve older adults that make movement necessary

CRITICALLY EXAMINE THE FOLLOWING

Look at your own busy life and holistically plan an exercise program for yourself.

What are you currently doing for exercise?

What do you want to do (lose weight, walk further, play ball better)?

How can you do it?

Do you already have an exercise program that works for you?

Evidence-Based Practice

Whitehead, B. R., & Blaxton, J. M. (2017). Daily well-being of physical activity in older adults: Does time or type matter? *The Gerontologist 56*(6), 1062–1071. doi:10.1093/geront/gnw250.

This study evaluated if daily "purposeful exercise" (exercise) or "non-exercise physical activity" (activity) is sufficient for providing daily health benefits and if the amount of time spent matters. The participants in the study ranged in age from 60 to 95 years old. Participants completed surveys reporting their daily exercise and activity, perceived positive or negative affect, perceived stress, and perceived health and sleep quality.

The results showed that the individuals who regularly exercised experienced less negative affect, lower daily stress, and better perceived health. Individuals who performed some type of daily activity experienced better sleep. Individuals who exercised about 60 minutes a day had a higher positive affect. However any amount of time exercising decreased daily stress. The amount of time spent performing daily activity did not matter and any amount of time lead to a positive affect and better sleep. This finding may be a motivator to older adults to maintain some type of daily activity even if they can only do 10 or 20 minutes per day.

This study supports the common understanding that exercise or activity of any type is beneficial for older adults. However, older adults should be encouraged to participate in more formal exercise to experience positive psychological well-being (positive affect, decreased stress, positive health perceptions).

Questions
1. How can you use this information to increase the level of activity for your patients?
2. List some exercise and activity that could be encouraged for residents in a long-term care facility. What exercise and activity could be encouraged for your home health patients?

Stress

Every person has his or her own personal ability to manage stress. This is very important because stress is a normal part of life. Think of the stress in your own life. Without deadlines, you would not be stressed enough to get your school papers or care plans written and prepare for your tests. Every day people manage the stress of weather changes, worldwide events (war, hurricanes, floods), interactions with others, time constraints, and other physical and emotional stressors. For some people, getting up and getting dressed in the morning are major stress points. Stress is part of everyone's life, and it will not go away. The key to stress is not elimination; it is management.

Life is a series of stressful events. Much of the stress actually enhances our lives (getting up in the morning and getting dressed). Some stress assists us in achieving our goals and other stress simply makes us feel alive and assists us in avoiding boredom. The problem with stress is that there can be too much of it; this is called "distress" and can be damaging to our lives physically and emotionally. The potential for the negative effects of distress is why stress management is crucial to understand. The informative section in the chapter on promoting wellness (Chapter 6) would be valuable for you to reread. The content supports the principles of achieving rest by managing stress. Refer to Chapter 6 and apply the information to the concept of appropriate rest for older adults.

CRITICALLY EXAMINE THE FOLLOWING

Look carefully at your life and identify the three major stressors you currently are experiencing. Then, (1) list the stressor, (2) state whether it is "good" stress or "bad" stress, (3) describe how you are managing it, and (4) indicate whether your management of it seems to be successful. If you feel you are not managing the stressors satisfactorily, indicate a plan that would assist you in more effective management of the stress.

"All I Do Is Rest!"

If you hear this or similar comments from your elderly clients, you need to assist them and their family members to understand the information in the activity section of this chapter. All people need to move to the extent of their ability. The movement works their muscles, and that encourages the body to rest. One of the main considerations when planning activity and rest is to assist the older person to alternate them throughout the day. Many older people have worked for most of their lives and consider daytime

the right time to "do their work" or activities, and they rest in the evening.

As most of us age, we have less stamina for prolonged activities, such as working for 8 consecutive hours. It is important to teach older people and their families to modify the level of activity in a day to what works best for the individual. A combination of activity and then rest, activity and then rest again is generally the best way to stay healthy and happy as an aging person. The older one becomes, the more common this tends to be. It is common for older people to take one or two naps a day. Napping is perfectly natural because of the aging body. Encourage naps that are intermingled with episodes of activity throughout the day. You need to be aware of the possibility of oversleeping because of boredom or depression, however.

Take a moment to consider if the person is bored. If so, find out what interests the person has and then find an avenue to help the person to pursue their interests. Is he or she interested in volunteering for an organization? Or interested in participating in the activities at the senior citizen center? If the person is unable to leave his or her home, are there activities that can be brought into the home? Do the neighbors need to know that their visits are very welcome, or is there an adopt-a-grandparent program at the local high school? Adopt-a-grandparent programs pair a teenage volunteer with one particular older person. Generally, this arrangement results in a very satisfying relationship for both individuals.

Keeping older adults engaged in life is important. Take the time to talk to the older adults to whom you give care and learn about their life interests.

SLEEP

Sleep is the most significant activity people can participate in for quality health. Every person, at whatever age, needs sleep to function normally. During sleep, the body physically repairs body tissues and emotionally resolves the issues of the day. Some people need only 6 hours of sleep, whereas many need the traditional 8 hours. It is recommended that older adults get a minimum of 7 hours of sleep. Generally when people age, they feel less rested, and many need more sleep than they get.

What Is Sleep?

The central nervous system controls sleep-wake patterns. There are two types of sleep: REM (rapid eye movement) and non-REM (NREM). Every individual of every age needs to experience both types of sleep every night. The sleep cycle has four stages of non-REM and one stage of REM sleep. The non-REM stages progress from relaxation to deeper and deeper sleep. The REM stage is the deepest sleep and is essential for a good night's rest. People often go through this sleep cycle four times a night, with each cycle allowing for deeper and more restful REM sleep. If the person's sleep is interrupted, the cycle starts over again from the beginning, and much of the deep sleep needed for optimal health is lost. This deep sleep is the healing sleep. As individuals age, they get less deep sleep and sleep for shorter periods of time (WebMD, 2016). When you wake up from a night's sleep and feel really great, you have, in all probability, had uninterrupted cycles of sleep.

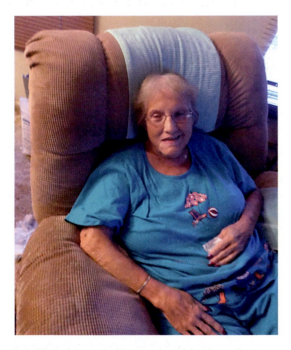

This older adult is taking a nap during her busy day.

Another aspect of individual sleep patterns is the person's **circadian rhythm**. This is the body's ability to synchronize the activity of the body to the 24-hour cycle of the external environment. This cycle is dependent on exposure to sunlight during the day and darkness at night. Within this cycle, people develop personal responses to their sleep needs. It is common for older adults to develop circadian rhythm changes. In most cases these changes go unrecognized unless the individual experiences significant sleep disturbances or the inability to function during

the day. A common problem is that as people age, they wake up earlier. As a result, they get tired during the day and need one or more naps. The daytime fatigue comes from normal physiological changes in the person's circadian rhythm. This normal physiological change causes many older people to want to stay up late so that they do not wake up at 4 a.m. or 5 a.m. Getting up early also reinforces the need for naps throughout the daytime hours. Box 9.4 provides suggestions for helping older adults improve their sleep.

THINK LIKE A NURSE

Now that you know about normal sleep patterns and changes in circadian rhythms, what have you observed that indicates nursing in general does not consistently address this problem when giving care to older adults? Make a list of three nursing care approaches that could be altered to meet the personal sleep needs of older people.

1. In nursing homes, residents often are put to bed between 7 p.m. and 9 p.m. Putting people to bed so early does two things that have negative consequences. The first consequence is that putting adults to bed at the same time as one would put children to bed does not focus on the residents' needs but rather on the needs of the staff and the tasks they must complete by a certain time. All adults with normal mental capacity should be able to determine their bedtime, rather than being put to bed like children. This behavior is demeaning to older persons. In addition, it forces the person to lie in bed awake for lengthy periods during the night and early morning because he or she simply cannot sleep that long at one time. Remember that their circadian rhythm has changed as a normal part of aging. It may be inconvenient for the staff to allow people to go to bed at the time they wish to go to bed, but it provides autonomy for the individual person in a system that does not always allow for individual decisions.

2. In most hospitals, it is noisy at night, and older people, who generally are lighter sleepers, may have difficulty staying asleep once they get to sleep. This constant awakening disrupts their NREM and REM sleep cycle. It is essential that nursing staff make regular rounds, take vital signs, and do other things such as checking

dressings and IV fluids. For most older people, all that movement and noise interfere with sleep. It also is helpful if the activities that need to be done in a patient's room all are done at one time so that there are fewer sleep interruptions. Could the IV or dressing check be done when medication is administered? Staff always should use flashlights rather than turn on the room lights. Noise in the hallways and at the nurses' station should be kept to a whisper level so as not to disturb the patients.

3. If older residents or patients do get up early, is there a place for them to go to read, watch the early morning news, or have a cup of coffee? Because early awakenings are normal physiology, the staff should have a way of managing this occurrence in a positive manner.

Sleep Disorders

There are various sleep disorders diagnosed, but the end result tends to be the same. Older adults often have trouble falling asleep and staying asleep, and they awaken fatigued, which can last throughout the day. People who do not get enough sleep are often irritable, and in older adults, lack of sleep can lead to cognitive impairment (Cabrera & Kornusky, 2018). Sleep disorders in older adults may be an early sign of cognitive decline (Kim & Duffy, 2018). The management of sleep disorders is an important aspect of the care you need to be giving to older adults.

A common sleep disorder is **insomnia** (Richards, Demartini, & Xiong, 2018). Insomnia occurs when people have difficulty getting to sleep or remaining asleep, or they simply feel that they do not get enough sleep. Insomnia is not a normal part of aging. It is more common as people age as a result of medical and psychiatric conditions as well as medications.

Box 9.4
Measures to Assist With Sleep

Balance daytime activity and rest.
Provide activity during the day.
Provide socialization.
Limit number and length of naps during the day.
Maintain bedtime routine.
Provide 2 to 3 hours of uninterrupted sleep during the night.

Another common cause of sleep disorders in older adults is **sleep apnea**. Sleep apnea occurs when a person's airway is partially obstructed during sleep. A common symptom is fatigue on awakening and throughout the day. People with sleep apnea are very tired all of the time. They often snore throughout the night, which can result in disruption of sleep for their sleep partner.

Sleep apnea is treated with continuous positive airway pressure (CPAP) while sleeping. The CPAP machine eliminates the airway obstruction by forcing air into the trachea throughout the sleep period. Complications of sleep apnea include hypertension, heart disease, stroke, diabetes, and depression (Jaffe & Schub, 2018). The typical symptom of sleep apnea is excessive daytime sleepiness. It is important to report such complaints to the RN or physician rather than dismiss the complaint.

Other common reasons for disruption in sleep include frequent nocturnal urination, gastroesophageal reflux disease (GERD), chronic obstructive pulmonary disease (COPD), heart failure (HF), depression and anxiety, and medication side effects. These medical conditions should be treated by the PCP. It is your responsibility, as the LPN, to report symptoms related to these conditions and their management to the RN or PCP and apply nursing interventions where applicable. People with COPD and HF sleep better when the head of the bed is raised. The same is true of someone with GERD. Provide a calming environment for someone with anxiety and monitor medications for possible side effects.

CRITICALLY EXAMINE THE FOLLOWING

Nursing interventions often bring necessary information and comfort to patients and residents experiencing insomnia. Consider the situation of frequent urination as a causative factor for insomnia. There are nursing actions that theoretically can improve this situation. Make a list of things you can do and the reasons why. Focus on nursing knowledge and not medical knowledge, such as medications. One action and rationale is provided as an example; then you need to complete the list. Be prepared to submit your plan to the faculty person.

1. ACTION: If possible, terminate drinking fluids at 6 p.m. This is a challenge for anyone accustomed

to drinking throughout the evening, but a worthwhile behavior. The nurse will need to give sips of fluids with medications at bedtime. Be pleasant and supportive to the person giving up the fluids.

RATIONALE: If the kidneys do not have fluid to process, there is minimal urine. Remember how important it is that any person sleeping has continuous sleep? If not, then refer back to the section on sleep. This action may be all that is necessary to stop nightly urination. You should write three more nursing actions that can assist this type of patient.

Nocturnal movement is another physiological condition that causes insomnia. There are two common types of nocturnal movement. The most common is restless legs syndrome (RLS), which is an irresistible urge to move one's legs. This can happen several times a night, and each episode is capable of awakening the person. RLS can be managed with regular exercise; maintaining a regular sleep pattern; and decreasing or eliminating alcohol, tobacco, and caffeine. Medications may help but are not effective for everyone. For some people, heat application or massage also helps the legs to relax. Be sure to report this disruptive complaint to the RN or PCP so that it can be effectively treated.

Another disruption to sleep is periodic limb movement disorder (PLMD), which is repetitive kicking movements of the lower extremities. Cramping can also occur. This happens without warning and is very disruptive to sleep. PLMD is often linked to RLS. Again, report it rather than ignore it as "just another complaint." PLMD is not a part of normal aging, and medications can assist in managing the disorder. These problems are true concerns when considering sleep patterns and, subsequently, the overall health of the people to whom you give care.

Dementia is a deterrent to effective sleep for the person with dementia and his or her sleep partner. Sleep patterns are altered in someone with dementia, which often results in being awake and wandering at night. This is very disruptive for the caregiver, who most often is the spouse of the individual with dementia. The result is two people who are sleep deprived and having difficulty because of fatigue. This is one reason why many communities have respite programs for caregivers of persons with dementia. The person with dementia is taken to the respite center for constant care, and the caregiver has a few hours or a weekend to rest, visit relatives, or engage in other activities important to a quality of life.

Psychological conditions often are detrimental to effective sleep patterns. People who are depressed often awake early and have hypersomnia, which is sleeping during the time people normally are awake. Anxiety often is related to difficulty falling asleep and frequent awake periods during the night. Psychiatric disorders can be treated with medication and therapy. Several disorders interfere with sleep and other life issues. Be diligent in your awareness of what is going on with the people to whom you give care. Talk to family members to gather information and an accurate past history. Share what you learn with the RN and PCP so that a psychiatric assessment can be made and treatment can be started. The benefits will be much more than a good night's sleep. Box 9.5 provides a list of common risk factors for sleep.

As you evaluate and teach the patient and the family about healthy sleep, refer to the risk factors in Box 9.5 to develop your teaching plan. It is your responsibility to make the environment conducive to sleep, to teach the patient and family members about what disrupts sleep, and to report any medical conditions appropriately so that they can be treated. Carefully examine and talk to any person in your care who seems fatigued. Fatigue is not a normal outcome of aging; it is a problem.

Box 9.5

Risk Factors for Sleep Disorders in Older Adults

Medical conditions
Psychiatric disorders
Sedentary lifestyle
Psychosocial stressors
Medications
Lifestyle changes
Environment changes

CASE STUDY SOLUTIONS

Gathering Information

You ask the admitting RN if you can accompany him on his first visit. He agrees that you should be there. While the RN does the admission, you ask Mary to show you Mrs. McDonald's room and the bathroom. While you are walking down the hallway, you talk to Mary about the problems she is having. It is obvious the entire family needs help if you are going to assist Mrs. McDonald. The following items need your attention.

Depression

Mrs. McDonald's behavior indicates that she could be depressed and has been since the death of her husband. You use the Beck Depression Scale to assess Mrs. McDonald; the results indicate that she is clinically depressed. You talk to her and observe her to see if what you hear and see support the results of the test. Your observations lead you to talk to the case manager, who contacts the physician. After talking to Sean, the physician orders a mild antidepressant for Mrs. McDonald. You will observe her closely for the next 3 weeks to determine if there has been a change. If the medication does not relieve the depression symptoms, you may need to suggest psychological therapy to assist her in managing her feelings regarding the death of her husband. You know that if the depression is managed, Mrs. McDonald will sleep better and be better able to care for herself during the day.

Strengthening

Mrs. McDonald needs more activity to become stronger. You arrange your first visit to be when the entire family is at home. Mrs. McDonald also is present at this family meeting. You explain the "first rule" of activity for older adults: It is for the person to do all activities possible for himself or herself.

Mrs. McDonald likes the idea of being more independent, so she agrees to listen to your plan, which follows. You also explain to everyone that the more activity Mrs. McDonald has during the day, the better she will sleep at night. You also explain that some physical activity during the day will help with her depression.

1. She will come to the dining room for all meals. (Mary has been feeding her in her room, which contributes to Mrs. McDonald's depression.) Mary agrees to walk her to the dining room for breakfast and lunch in time to enjoy eating with the family. The teens agree to take turns walking their grandma to the dining room for dinner.

2. The 5-year-old volunteers to "work out" with grandma while she does arm exercises with a soup can in each hand twice a day. You need to evaluate how many lifts she can do with her current muscle strength. You will reevaluate this frequently.

3. The teenagers agree to take turns taking grandma for a walk each day. You emphasize that "a walk" initially will be a short trip in the hallway. You will monitor Mrs. McDonald's strength and add to the distance traveled as is appropriate. The length of each walk will be increased as tolerated. The goal is to get Mrs. McDonald outside taking long walks around the neighborhood.

4. As part of the family discussion, Mrs. McDonald states she is also interested in taking on a few responsibilities around the house. Mary suggests that maybe Mrs. McDonald could dust the house each week and help her prepare dinner on the days Mrs. McDonald feels up to it.

5. Her son also suggested that they plant a small elevated vegetable garden that he and his mother could maintain. This will give Mrs. McDonald a chance to do something she enjoys that will also provide some additional exercise for her.

Sleep and Rest

Mrs. McDonald naps four to five times a day and still feels exhausted. You should ask her to keep a log (with Sean's help, if necessary) about her sleep. What time does she go to bed? What time does she wake up? How many times a night does she get up or become fully awake? What causes her to awaken? This information should be shared with the RN or the PCP so that decisions can be made about medical and nonmedical interventions for Mrs. McDonald's fatigue.

In the meantime, you can get to work on basic nursing interventions. Is the room quiet at night without disruptive lighting? Does Mrs. McDonald avoid alcohol, smoking, and caffeine, as they are things that can disrupt her sleep? Is the room warm

Continued

CASE STUDY SOLUTIONS—cont'd

enough, and is the bed comfortable for her? Does she need a new nighttime ritual, such as reading or taking a bath prior to going to bed? Would she like the family to come into her room and have family prayer at bedtime? There are several interventions you can investigate.

It would be an effective idea for Mrs. McDonald to try to take only two naps a day. She needs to be tired when she goes to bed. Staying awake, if it is reasonable, along with her new strengthening exercises and the increase in her daily activity will help her sleep.

There are other plans you could work out for Mrs. McDonald and her family. Consider at least two more and write them as part of this case study solution.

Key Points

- To have maximum health, all people need activity that fits their physiology, rest that accommodates their lifestyle, and sleep that allows them the ability to function without fatigue.
- Exercise improves the functioning of the following systems: cardiovascular, respiratory, musculoskeletal, digestive, and excretory. Studies have also shown improvement in cognitive function and general well-being.
- The four types of exercise older adults should participate in are endurance, muscle strengthening, balance training, and flexibility. A combination of these types of exercise can increase cardiac and respiratory function, improve movement, prevent falls, and provide the older adult the ability to more successfully carry out daily activities.
- Encouraging older adults to move is an important role for the nurse. Assisting a resident to walk to the dining room and encouraging patients to perform their own activities of daily living are ways to encourage daily movement.
- Due to the number of chronic conditions older adults tend to have, they may be unable to get the amount of rest their bodies need. Unmanaged pain can hinder a person's ability to rest. It is the nurse's responsibility to assess for pain and provide proper measures to relieve the pain.
- There are two types of sleep: REM and NREM. Every individual needs to experience both types of sleep each night.
- A person's circadian rhythm also has an impact on how a person sleeps. Within this cycle, people develop a personal response to their sleep needs. It is common for older adults to develop circadian rhythm changes. In most cases, these changes go unrecognized unless the individual experiences significant sleep disturbances or the inability to function during the day.
- Older adults should get 7 to 8 hours of sleep each night. When sleep is disturbed at night, they will usually nap during the day. Nurses can assist older adults get better sleep by helping establish a bedtime routine, encourage daytime activity and socialization, and limit the number and lengths of naps during the day.
- Sleep is the most significant activity people can participate in for quality health. Sleep disorders are common for older adults and include insomnia and sleep apnea. Common reasons for insomnia include GERD, heart disease, depression, and medication side effects.

Review Questions

1. When considering activity for older adults, the greatest challenge is:
   1. Getting them up and about without hurting your back.
   2. Keeping their weight within normal limits so that it is easier to move them.
   3. Managing their chronic conditions.
   4. Doing as much for them as possible as a pain management intervention.

2. The normal sleep cycle for older adults:
   1. Has four non-REM cycles and an extra REM cycle. This occurs approximately four times a night.
   2. Is not affected by the interruption of the non-REM/REM cycles.
   3. Has a built-in mechanism, which develops as people age, that makes awakening more difficult.
   4. Does not change or adapt as people age.

3. Measures to assist with sleep include all but the following:
   1. Maintain a bedtime routine.
   2. Limit number of naps during the day.
   3. Balance daytime activity and rest.
   4. Encourage light exercise before bed.

4. Older adults who are most at risk for rest/sleep disturbances include all but the following:
   1. Older adults with sleep apnea and obesity.
   2. Older adults with depression or dementia.
   3. Older adults with RLS or PLMD.
   4. Older adults who are underweight.

5. Many sleep/rest problems can be managed with effective nursing interventions. Choose from the following list the activity that is not a nursing intervention:
   1. Sleep apnea testing
   2. Limiting fluids before bedtime
   3. Provide daytime activity.
   4. Promote a bedtime routine.

ANSWERS 1. 3, 2. 4, 3. 4, 4. 4, 5. 1

CHAPTER 10
End-of-Life Issues

Jamie Wankier

KEY TERMS

advance directive
cultural sensitivity
end-of-life issues
grief
hospice care
palliative care

CHAPTER CONCEPTS

Communication
Culture
Grief and Loss
Spirituality
Stress and Coping

LEARNING OUTCOMES

1. Define palliative and hospice care and the patient benefits.
2. Identify the stages and symptoms of grief that patients and families can experience.
3. List the qualities necessary for a nurse to give end-of-life care.
4. List the eight signs of imminent death.
5. Describe advance directives and how they relate to your patients.

CASE STUDY

Mr. Reed is an 80-year-old patient with terminal pancreatic cancer. His wife died 10 years earlier from lung cancer. Mr. Reed lives alone but does have numerous friends and an active social life. He was initially treated with chemotherapy but when the disease progressed, his physician decided that further treatment would not benefit him. Due to the severity of his prognosis, he was originally referred to palliative care service to provide management of pain and other symptoms as well as psychological and social support. His symptoms have become increasingly difficult to manage on his own and he has no one to care for him at home, so he is being admitted to a long-term care facility. He has two daughters who both live out of state but have come into town to help Mr. Reed with his transfer to the facility. Since his admission, Mr. Reed has been very quiet and has not said much about his current physical condition or shown any emotion. Because he was previously a very active and social man, the change in his

142

CASE STUDY—cont'd

emotional state has his daughters worried. On meeting Mr. Reed's daughters, Liz and Joyce, you find they are concerned about their father's rapidly declining physical and emotional condition. Liz does not understand why the cancer is not being treated and wants to contact the physician to start treatment for the cancer. Joyce is saying that it is time to let their father die and maybe they should now consider hospice. The suggestion of hospice makes the one daughter angry and she states "Dad is not ready to die yet. If you put him in hospice he will just die sooner."

Discussion

1. What methods would you use to communicate the variety of issues with the two daughters?
2. How will you bring Mr. Reed into the discussion regarding his thoughts about his death?

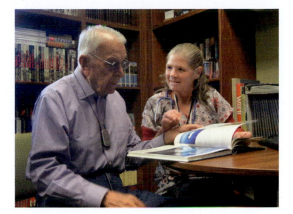

This nursing assistant is helping this man to enjoy the last few months of his life.

THE MYSTERY OF DEATH

As all people know, death is an inevitable and natural human experience. It has, however, been shrouded in mystery and envisioned as an experience of great suffering, generally contemplated with fear. Dying, on the other hand, is an unpredictable event. The exact moment or situation in which someone will die is never known. As people move through the dying process, they and their family members will experience many emotions ranging from acceptance, denial, fear, anger, joy, and confusion. Those emotions are very real to patients and families. As a primary caregiver in this situation you will also experience a variety of emotions as you encounter the dying individual and their family members. Individuals should be allowed to cope with death in their own way, even if it is to deny death's reality until the end. As the caregiver to older adults, you need to be educated about the variety of EOL issues. Some of the skills necessary to provide a "good death" for your patients are the ability to communicate issues, listen and work closely with family members when trying to fulfill patient wishes, work as a team with other caring professionals, maintain a positive and open work environment and apply the guiding principles of gerotranscendence for yourself and your patients. Without skills in these areas, the quality of EOL care for older adults is diminished.

INTRODUCTION

End-of-life (EOL) issues are vital issues in health care throughout the United States. Americans want to experience a "good death" without being burdened by symptoms or technology. Increasing numbers of patients with chronic and advanced disease plus the advances of symptom management have placed EOL care in the focus of health care. Nurses have an essential role in maximizing EOL care by improving symptom management; communication; and education about choices, referrals, and psychosocial treatments. You, as the care provider, have the responsibility to explain to older adults and their family members all of the options, referrals, and resources available. As you review some of the options in this chapter, it is very important that you examine your own attitudes, values, and beliefs regarding death. You need to consider what happens if your personal beliefs conflict with the choices and decisions made by an older adult in your care. The focus of this chapter is to explore how to assist older adults to die well through the excellent care and support you provide them as they approach the end of their lives.

Priority Setting

This chapter describes the role of an EOL nurse. It talks about what you need to learn and explains many things you should work to understand. Caregivers cannot apply information regarding EOL in an effective way unless they have come to an understanding within themselves about death. That is your priority for this chapter. Take the content you read and internalize it. Think about people who have died who were important to you. How did you feel, react, and grieve? If you are confused or uncomfortable with death experiences, where can you go to get more information? Who can you talk to about the death of someone who was close to you? Do you have religious or spiritual beliefs that comfort you or friends who can assist you to accept the death? What are your cultural beliefs and do they assist you in preparing for or understanding death? Do you understand gerotranscendence, through which individuals plan for their own good death and accept it? Do you apply gerotranscendence to your own life?

To give effective EOL care, you need to be at peace with death and its complexities. You should see it as the personal, meaningful, unique experience it is and then be able to share that with the patients, residents, and families with whom you work.

GRIEF

Grief is a reaction to loss. We can experience grief when someone we are attached to dies, but we can also experience it when we lose anything of great significance to us. Understanding and compassion are essential when relating to people experiencing losses.

CRITICALLY EXAMINE THE FOLLOWING

Now that we have discussed various aspects of EOL issues, it is time for you to express some of your thoughts on the topic. Take a few minutes to contemplate and consider what you would call a "good death." The purpose of this exercise is to have you apply the information you have just read. Some of the questions you should answer are listed below. Answer them and then add more

detail. Consider this a "free write," where anything you say will be respected.

1. How old will you be when you die?
2. What will be your general health condition?
3. Who will still be alive and be with you as you die?
4. How will you die?

Add other comments you want to make.

Now consider your ancestors and how and when they died. You have described your perfect death, but few people get to experience such an event. By looking at your parents' and grandparents' health and the death of family members, you will see your genetic predisposition. What do your genes indicate as a possible death?

Do you have any potentially dangerous hobbies such as skydiving or car racing? Do you drive an excessive number of miles in a year? Do you have poor health habits? What do these lifestyle behaviors indicate about your eventual death?

You will die. By trying to understand your own death, you will be able to give better care to people who are at the end of their lives.

Dr. Elisabeth Kübler-Ross, a Swiss psychiatrist, spent much of her life defining the stages of grief. Death, the greatest personal loss a person can experience, was the focus of her grief work. If you understand the five stages of grief, you can recognize them within yourself, the older adults to whom you give care, and their families. Understanding grief is a valuable tool you can use in your care of patients.

Death can be hard. We can experience it many times as a bystander with family and patients, but we only experience it once ourselves. This makes death a unique and powerful experience. The dying person loses friends, family members, home, work, accomplishments, pets, favorite hobbies, and the beauty all around them.

The stages of grief demonstrate the normal human reactions that people can have when facing the loss of a loved one or the loss of something significant to that individual. In addition to death, the stages of grief can be seen with other major losses: divorce, jobs, and extremity through amputation or loss associated with a stroke or other illness.

Kübler-Ross (1969) identified the five stages as follows:

Acceptance
Depression
Bargaining

Anger
Denial

Think of these terms as steps in the process of re-solving grief. The person experiencing the loss can go from one stage (or step) to another and then move back up or down the stages. There is no exact formula or prescription to follow because people are individuals and manage their grief in very personalized ways. Nurses need to allow this type of independent grieving.

Denial

When a significant loss occurs, a person's psyche has difficulty accepting it. Consider a young mother who leaves her aging and confused mom outside for "only a moment" while she goes in the house to get her baby. When the young mother comes out of the house, her mother has wandered out into the street, is hit by a car, and eventually dies in the hospital. Some denial behaviors are shock, praying for it to not be true, walking about, or standing and saying, "No, not Mom" over and over again.

Denial is the psyche's way of protecting itself from the harsh, bitter truth. It is as if the young mother were wrapped up in a soft, protective cocoon. This psychological protection is there until the person's psyche can deal with the loss. You may have heard of or seen people who "were in a daze" during the funeral of a loved one. This person could be experiencing denial. Do not attempt to force someone or talk someone out of denial. The individual will move to the next stage when he or she is able. During this time of grief, people need to be protected from neglect, injury, and financial abuse. Family members need to understand this stage of the grief process and be willing to take care of other children, prepare meals, and support the grieving person.

THINK LIKE A NURSE

You are taking care of a patient who is expressing anger about his impending death. What will you explain to this patient about the anger he is experiencing? Is it important for this person to learn to control his anger at this point in his life?

Anger

When an individual develops the strength to face the specific situation, he or she may exhibit behaviors such as anger or aggression that tend to push others away. This act of anger or aggression is a necessary part of the grieving process. Anger can be defined as strength and can give temporary structure to the emptiness of loss.

Anger demonstrates an awareness of the loss and its consequences. This is one step toward adjusting to the loss. It is also an outlet for the outrage the grieving person feels. Assist the grieving person not to hurt himself or herself or others with the anger. The family needs to understand the advantages of the anger so that they can accept what is happening and support the behaviors that occur. Can you think of some of the advantages of the grieving person showing anger?

Bargaining

When the grieving person recognizes that the "bad thing," or the loss, will not go away, he or she often turns to God or another higher power to question why this loss occurred. This behavior often is demonstrated by bargaining.

Bargaining is seen as something like prayers to a higher power stating that the person will donate a great deal of money to a charitable organization, will never sin again, or will actively do good for others. The thinking is that if one trades something of value, like goodness, with a higher power, then a miracle will be performed. Often, bargaining is expressed as "What if I did this?" or "What if I had done that?" This stage can be very heartbreaking for family and friends. Many say they prefer anger over the wrenching episodes of bargaining. The negotiation process is the final chance to change the situation. If the higher power cannot "fix things," then no one can. This time in the grieving process requires patience and gentleness. People can become exhausted in efforts to support the grieving person. Praise them for staying with the grieving person throughout the entire experience. Try to give them strength and courage to see the experience to its conclusion.

Not everyone believes in God or a higher power. Work with grieving people in whatever way they are bargaining. The principles are the same for all forms of grief bargaining.

Depression

Depression can be a challenging condition in any situation. In the grieving process, it can show that progress is occurring. When a grieving person is depressed, it means that the individual does not accept the loss but accepts the fact that nothing can change it. The denial, anger, and bargaining did not work. It makes sense that the grieving person would be depressed.

As with all forms of depression, actively assess for suicidal thinking. If you identify it, keep someone with the grieving person and contact the registered nurse (RN). Suicide is a preventable outcome, so be alert to its possibility. Depressed people cry, they sleep a great deal, and they have low energy. Teach this to the family members. Ask them to support the grieving person through this last hurdle to acceptance.

Depressed people do not need to be told, "Everything is all right." For them, nothing will ever be all right again. They need love and support while they find a way to continue on with their lives.

Acceptance

When the grieving person reaches acceptance, there is a sense of relief. The individual still is searching for life structure without the loved one who died. It is possible that once acceptance is reached, the grief process may be over. It is important to remember that the stages of grief are fluid and individuals can move

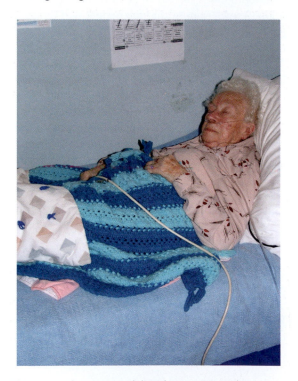

This woman has accepted that she is going to die. As is common with so many people, she does not want to interact with the world anymore. She is done; she has accepted the fact that she is close to death. Notice that she has her call light in hand "just in case." She also must have slowing circulation, as indicated by the afghan, blanket, and oxygen.

forward or backward at any time. Even after reaching acceptance, it would be normal for the grieving person to still call out the name of the deceased person or be found crying after finding a piece of clothing of the loved one, or just sit quietly contemplating the life of the person who died.

The grieving process is difficult for the person experiencing the loss and the family members. The management of the experience can be improved when you, the licensed practical nurse (LPN), know the stages of grief and readily share them with appropriate people. Some of the symptoms to look for in patients or family members experiencing loss are listed in Box 10.1.

After reading this last section, consider the daughter Liz from the case study. What stage do you think she is in currently? As a nurse, what can you do to support Liz during her grieving process?

KNOWLEDGE AND SKILLS NEEDED TO PROVIDE END-OF-LIFE CARE

Many nurses have difficulty talking about EOL matters with patients. You need to learn new skills and acquire new knowledge to improve the care of older adults who require EOL care (Box 10.2). Some new knowledge you may need includes communication skills and knowledge of resources and available services.

As a nurse, you have tremendous potential to change the care of dying older adults and the support given to their families. It is crucial that you understand human nature as you give care to people who are dying. You need to be able to identify the stages and symptoms of grief and discuss these issues with patients and family members. Because grief is unique

Box 10.1

Symptoms of Patients and Families Experiencing Loss

Headaches
Sleeplessness
Exhaustion
Muscle aches/pains
Confusion/dizziness
Loss of appetite
Agitation, anger
Depression
Breathlessness

Box 10.2

Qualities to Develop Before Working With Dying People

- Motivation
- Emotional maturity. Death is serious and individualized and happens only once for each person.
- Tolerance and empathy. Nothing goes according to a formula or procedure. This is true of the dying process and people.
- Communication skills. You need the ability to empathize with all people involved in the death experience.
- Confidentiality. A sense of discretion and respect for patient and family privacy is essential.
- Flexibility. You must be willing to do what patients and their families need, not what you think is best.
- Dependability. Dependability turns into trust.
- Good listening skills. Listening is a wonderful gift you can give to someone who may be feeling frightened and alone.
- Sense of humor. Humor in difficult situations can be a plus. It is OK to laugh with patients and families.

and expressed individually, you need to be able to comprehend the impact on specific individuals and understand the nature of the people involved.

Tolerance and Empathy

Each individual you encounter as a care provider is unique and different. Understanding those you care for requires that you learn to become tolerant and empathetic. Synonyms of tolerance are compassion, endurance, patience, impartiality, and open-mindedness. Synonyms of empathy are understanding, sympathetic, identifying with the patient, and providing insight and feeling in your care. To provide appropriate tolerance and empathy, you must strive to create an environment that meets the physical, emotional, social, and spiritual needs of each dying person. You will also need to show tolerance and empathy for the family members of your dying patients. The two daughters from the case study are both dealing with the reality that their father is going to die and will need care and understanding as they support their father through a difficult time.

Sense of Humor

Having a sense of humor with the dying person is a simple way to assist in relieving, reducing, and soothing the symptoms of a disease. You must know the personality and mood of the older adult in your care before making jokes about the situation. You must

make sure that it is done at the right time and in the right situation. Think about a time and place when you were suffering and laughter helped with the cure.

Communication

Communication is crucial in most situations. When it comes to death and dying, this situation has the possibility of being discussed in a context of hope, meaning, and opportunity. With strong communication skills, uncertainty is replaced with certainty, hopelessness is replaced with faith, and despair is replaced with empowerment. Communicate openly and honestly with what you know related to EOL care. Communicate with the RN and other team members about the specific patient and family issues you are witnessing.

Good Listening Skills

Being a good listener is the greatest skill any nurse can have. Take time to listen to older adults' stories about their children and grandchildren, stories about falling in love, and possibly stories about losing their loved ones. Older people enjoy sharing their life experiences. It is important to remember when talking to an older person that you need to speak in a voice that he or she can hear. Move in close to the person, touch his or her shoulder, smile, and listen to what he or she has to share.

To listen, you must be fully present and attentive to the other person. You are not listening if you:

- Are in a hurry.
- Are thinking about yourself.
- Interrupt.
- Ask the same question twice.
- Do not ask any questions.
- Assume that you know what the other person is going to say.

A good listener is one who does not think about what to say until after the other person has finished speaking. When talking to Mr. Reed about his concerns regarding his death, it is important to listen quietly while he talks and ask questions for clarification.

CULTURAL SENSITIVITY

In addition to the previously mentioned qualities that are needed to care for individuals nearing the end of their lives, it is important to be familiar with the cultural diversities of the older adults in your care. **Cultural sensitivity** is being aware of the different cultures and beliefs of those you care for and being

Focused Learning Chart: Understanding Tolerance and Empathy

A care provider's goal is to understand the needs of people experiencing an end-of-life situation.

Tolerance	Empathy
Compassion	Understanding
Impartiality	Identify with person
Endurance	Sympathetic
Patience	Be insightful
Open-mindedness	Allow self to feel situation

sensitive to how those beliefs may be different from your culture and beliefs. A person's culture influences the decision-making process regarding various treatments. Spirituality and religious beliefs are also important factors when assessing patients' and family's needs as they relate to EOL issues. These can often overlap with cultural beliefs and can be just as influential in the choices that patients and families make.

In many cultures, a family's interdependence, harmony, duty, and obligation to an older family member are obvious. Some cultures believe that it is inappropriate to tell someone that he or she is dying because it would create a sense of hopelessness and sadness. Some cultures believe that a sick individual should not be allowed to make any decisions about EOL care but rather have the family or the eldest son make those decisions. Cultural and spiritual needs should be addressed immediately on admission to any facility. It is very important that the LPN is aware of the family's and the individual's diverse needs and maintain sensitivity to those needs.

Cultural Considerations

Cultural beliefs can have an impact on how a person grieves and the type of care they want to receive at the end of their life. Cultural beliefs can also have an impact on how a nurse will communicate with the patient and their family. It is important for the nurse to be aware of these individual needs so culturally specific care can be given.

END-OF-LIFE DECISIONS

As a care provider for individuals who are nearing the end of their lives, it is crucial that you recognize the importance of being aware of the decisions a person has made about his or her current and future medical care and to honor his or her preferences. Discussing EOL issues can be difficult for many older adults and their families. As a nurse, it is your role to guide the patient through this discussion and make sure the patient's wishes are documented. Having the patient make these decisions provides the health-care team the information they need to provide the best care to the patient. It also helps family members understand the wishes of their loved one so they can provide support to the patient during a difficult and stressful time.

Gaining an understanding of all of the issues surrounding EOL care can be daunting. You may encounter challenges about knowledge and skills in assessing and managing pain in cognitively impaired older adults. You may experience frustration about primary care providers being unwilling to consider a nurse's assessment and recommendations. You may find it difficult to deal with the strong emotional attachments that are formed with older adults at the EOL stage. These are all reasons to learn and study EOL issues.

Palliative Care

Palliative care can be defined as specialized medical care for those individuals with serious or chronic illness. This type of care is focused on managing the variety of symptoms these patients might have.

Palliative care is not limited to a hospital setting because an older adult may receive palliative care in a long-term care or assisted living setting. Palliative care is the art and science of quality EOL care. The goal is to improve quality of life for both patient and family members and it can be provided by a team of doctors and or specialists. You may encounter patients who will be candidates for this type of care. LPNs have an opportunity to take the initiative in offering and providing palliative care that ensures comprehensive, holistic EOL care for all older adults who are experiencing life-threatening, progressive illness. It is an opportunity to be sensitive and respectful to the older person's values, religious beliefs, family traditions, individual cultures, and beliefs.

Hospice

Hospice care can be described as a program through which the palliative type of care intensifies as the patient gets closer to death. Typically patients will transition easily from palliative care to hospice care.

"Hospice" comes from the term "hospitality" and can be traced back to medieval times, when there was a need to find a place of rest for weary and ill travelers. Today, hospice organizations are located all over the United States. Although hospice services are being used more widely, most hospice organizations report being underused. The reasons why hospice is underutilized is complex. Some of this complexity can be attributed to patients with multiple conditions and some of these diagnoses are not typically covered by hospice. Other reasons that add to underutilization is a lack of education and awareness of how hospice works and the benefits provided by hospice. The hospice team provides care to the patient as well as support and education to family members. Hospice care can be provided in a care facility or home setting (Box 10.3).

In the past, referrals to a hospice came "too little, too late" to be most effective. Studies have shown the benefits of improved EOL care for patients enrolled earlier into a hospice program. The number of hospice admissions is improving; currently at least 50% of dying patients are referred to hospice. This percentage will improve with added education and awareness of hospice services (Duggan et al., 2017). An example of providing successful care is that of patients with Alzheimer's disease. Providing them with palliative care may be the primary long-term mode of care. When death is imminent, generally around the last 6 months of life, a hospice team should be called on to provide their specialized knowledge of care for the transition from dying to death. Your role in this transition is to provide education to patients and families about the benefits of palliative and hospice care and how they both can support the patient in their quality of life and death. Providing Mr. Reed's daughters with information about hospice is important. They have many decisions to make regarding the best care for their father, and the palliative team and/or hospice providers can provide assistance in making those decisions.

Box 10.3

Essential Components of Hospice Programs

The following qualities can be found in an excellent hospice program:

- Serves patients, families, and the community with sensitivity to different cultures, values, and beliefs
- Provides interdisciplinary teams of palliative care experts educated to give competent, compassionate, highly skilled, state-of-the-art care to dying people
- Has a low patient-to-worker ratio
- Is responsive 24 hours per day, 7 days per week
- Elicits and responds to patient and family needs and wants and encourages involvement of patient's own physician
- Produces accurate, reliable data about care, outcomes, and costs
- Earns community support

Adapted from St. Christopher's Hospice. (2001). http://www.stchristophers.org.uk/

Safe, Effective Nursing Care

Respecting Patient and Family Needs

John has been taking care of a 75-year-old patient with terminal cancer who is receiving chemotherapy and is on home-care service. The patient's wife, Ann, has provided most of his care while he has been ill. For the last week, she has been voicing to John her concern about her husband's recent decline and increased need for pain medication. Ann is concerned that her husband is not comfortable and worries that the chemotherapy is not helping him and wants to stop all treatment. She states that she is physically and emotionally tired. She also states that she feels guilty about "giving up" on her husband. John spends the next hour listening to Ann while she tells him how she doesn't want her husband to suffer anymore. John then talks to her about hospice care and the services it can provide and suggests she make an appointment to see about getting her husband on a hospice service.

Patient-centered care means providing support to family members and diversity of their needs.

1. Do you feel the patient's wife is "giving up" on her husband?
2. What emotions is Ann struggling with at this time?
3. Do you feel John was inappropriate in suggesting hospice care to Ann? Why or why not?
4. What services can hospice provide Ann?

ADVANCE DIRECTIVES

One of the most difficult situations that health-care professionals face when caring for older people is how to assist patients and families who are trying to make decisions about whether to start, continue, or stop life-sustaining treatments. Elderly people as a group account for 73% of deaths each year, making EOL treatment decisions far more prevalent among them. An **advance directive** is a written statement of a person's wishes regarding medical treatment, often including a living will, made to ensure those wishes are carried out should the person be unable to communicate them to a health-care provider. This process can be defined as advance care planning and might include advanced directives, in which an individual specifies a durable power of attorney for health care (health-care proxy) or another person authorized to make health-care related decisions for them and a living will that specifies the patient's wishes related to life-sustaining treatment,

The health-care proxy has the authority to make health-care decisions if the individual loses the ability to make decisions or communicate personal wishes. The proxy can make decisions as the need arises and is not restricted to a decision that was made previously without knowledge of the current situation. In addition, physicians can complete a "do-not-resuscitate" (DNR) order after a discussion with the patient and family (McDonald, du Manoir, Kevork, Le, & Zimmerman, 2017).

The other type of advance directive is known as a living will. This is a legal document that allows individuals to share their opinions and wishes regarding their death. The living will can list in detail the types of treatments a person wants or does not want to receive, such as mechanical ventilation, cardiopulmonary resuscitation (CPR), or a feeding tube.

Despite the importance of an older adult's completing an advance directive, many aging Americans are reluctant to complete the appropriate forms. Federal law requires health-care providers and institutions to give patients advance directive forms, but most patients do not complete them. Completion rates currently range from 18% to 31%

(Miller, 2017). The legal statutes that govern the use of advance directives vary from state to state. As an LPN, you must clearly understand the advance directive laws where you work. For more information about legal issues related to advance directives, refer to Chapter 5. You can also refer to Appendix A for an example of an advance directive.

Evidence-Based Practice

Miller B. (2017) Nurses in the know: The history and future of advance directives. *Online Journal of Nursing Issues, 22*(3), 2–11.

Nurses play an important role regarding advance directives. This conversation often occurs when the patient and family are in the midst of a crisis, which may not be the most appropriate time to have these conversations. Nursing education related to advance directives is very important because it increases the confidence of the nurse to engage in these critical conversations. Federal legislation supporting the use of advance directives was first introduced in 1990; since then, the Patient Self-Determination Act (to ensure that patients are provided information about advance directives and can accept or refuse treatment) has been revised and updated several times.

Laws are continuing to evolve related to dying with dignity. It is the nurse's responsibility to understand the laws of the state they practice in and understand the policy and procedures about advanced directives in the places they work. Nurses in all fields of practice play a critical role in the completion of advance directives, assurance of quality of care, and in the aim to honor a patient's wishes related to death.

Questions
1. As an LPN, what education can you provide to your patients and family members regarding advanced directives?
2. For a patient without an advanced directive, how can you support the family as they make life and death decisions for their loved one?

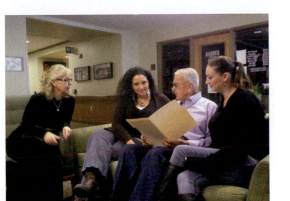

This family is discussing EOL issues with their parent and completing an advanced directive.

IMMINENT SIGNS OF DEATH

As an LPN, it is important for you to know the imminent signs of death. It is easy to assist someone in his or her preparation to die if the person has received a diagnosis of a terminal illness. A terminal diagnosis allows individuals to realign their priorities, mend various relationships, and say goodbye to loved ones. In addition, a terminal diagnosis allows staff the opportunity to prioritize their care and assist persons in meeting their goals and achieving a peaceful life closure.

CRITICALLY EXAMINE THE FOLLOWING

Have you considered what you would like written in your living will? Do you want to be pain-free? What about use of antibiotics? What about use of mechanical ventilation? What about a feeding tube? Use Part 2 of the advance directive in Appendix A to begin writing your living will.

When death is near, body functions slow, and certain signs and symptoms occur, including the following:

- Withdrawal—physical, emotional, and increased sleep
- Reduced food and fluid intake
- Confusion/agitation
- Change in breathing patterns; dyspnea and periods of apnea
- Noisy respiration (pooling of oral secretions in back of throat)
- Incontinence of urine/stool
- Changes in skin temperature and color

Hearing is one of the last senses to be lost. Because dying individuals continue to hear, it is important to talk to the patient. Families members should be encouraged to do so to say good-bye and may even want to encourage their loved one that "it is OK to go" (Ferrell, Coyle, & Paice, 2015).

A common sign of imminent death is terminal restlessness (TR), another term for agitated delirium. This is a common occurrence for individuals nearing the end of their lives. It may appear as involuntary muscle twitching or jerks, thrashing or agitation, tossing and turning, or yelling and moaning. Reports indicate that more than three-fourths of dying patients experience this condition. TR occurs in the last hours of life. It is caused by the diminishing of physiological functions and can be very distressing to the older adult who is dying and to family and staff members. At this time so close to EOL, there is a crucial need for careful and thoughtful intervention to provide the dying person with comfort and to be able to control his or her symptoms.

Your role will involve collaboration with the physician and team, collaboration with the RN, providing reassurance and education, role modeling comfort care, honoring spiritual and culture preferences, and providing physical comfort with the use of medications and other medical interventions.

Medications can be used at the EOL in a variety of ways. Opioids are commonly used to manage pain. Careful pain management assessment is important at the EOL due to changes in consciousness and potential pain medication toxicities. Palliative sedation at EOL may be considered due to excessive pain and/or other final symptoms. Palliative sedation may include the use of benzodiazepines, neuroleptics, barbiturates, and other medications to help manage pain and sedate the dying person into a more comfortable status (Ferrell, Coyle, & Paice, 2015).

Dying is an individualized experience. It is something that has never happened to the dying person before, and the individual may need your assistance in making death easier. One thing you can do is talk to the person to identify individual attitudes and knowledge regarding death, disease, and support systems already in place. Formal assessments are done by the assigned RN; however, you, as the LPN, are giving the bedside care and need to be prepared to respond to questions that are asked after the RN's assessment. The goal of your assessment is to be able to gain a clear understanding of the older person's experiences with his or her illness. In addition, you need to be able to identify distressing symptoms that need management, convey your concern and empathy to the persons involved, and evaluate any risk that may be expressed owing to current distress or feelings. It is important for you to take immediate action when a problem is detected.

The LPN can play an important role with the death process, providing support and education and demonstrating compassion and caring for the dying patient and family. The nursing staff often bear witness to the act of death and with this comes much responsibility. It is important to assess all components of the dying person. You might ask a variety of questions related to pain or distress. For example, "What hurts or distresses you most, and how can I help?" Another good opening question to ask is what the person worries about most when the illness is at its worst and what has been most difficult throughout the process.

The dying person may be experiencing psychosocial changes like introspection, and fear of dying or loss. Your assessment should review the older adult's various abilities to cope with stress and anxiety. For example, "During periods of discouragement, some people wish all this suffering were over. Have you felt this way? Tell me about it." "You seem to feel as if life is not worth living. Are you thinking of doing something to hasten your death? Tell me about it."

The patient's emotional needs are very important during this time and it was demonstrated that patients require the following communication during their final hours:

• Need for information
• Disclosure of feelings
• Maintaining sense of control
• Need for meaning
• Need for a sense of hope
  (Rozalski, Holland, & Neimeier, 2017)

One of the roles of the LPN during this time frame is offering presence, or providing an emotionally safe place for the dying person and their family members to express their thoughts and feelings.

Through the comprehensive assessment process your findings will give you information on how to adequately support the patient and the family through their final hours and after death has occurred. Following death, the bereavement care process begins, including communicating with family, preparing for the next steps, and the technical tasks of preparing the body. Collaboration with the interdisciplinary team and bereavement services during this time frame is important to provide holistic support for the family (Ferrell, Coyle, & Paice, 2015). Bereavement support can occur at any time during the aforementioned processes and for much time after the dying person has gone. Providing families with a list of supportive services is a role that the LPN can play during this time.

Family members will always remember the last days, hours, and moments of their loved one's life. Nurses have a unique opportunity to be invited to experience and witness those last moments with the patient and the family. You also have an important opportunity to make those final hours as positive and fulfilling for the dying person, the family members, and yourself.

CASE STUDY SOLUTIONS

1. As an LPN, you need to assess what Mr. Reed understands about his cancer and the fact that his physician has decided to stop treatment. You also need to identify his attitude toward his own death and any concerns he may have about the dying process. As part of this assessment, you will want to identify any cultural or spiritual needs that may have an impact on Mr. Reed and how the nursing staff could support Mr. Reed and his daughters during the dying process. This discussion needs to be a private conversation between you and Mr. Reed at a time when he is rested and comfortable. During this discussion, you need to be willing to answer all of Mr. Reed's questions honestly. If you are unable to answer specific questions about his cancer, you will need

CASE STUDY SOLUTIONS—cont'd

to make sure there is an opportunity for Mr. Reed to address these questions with his physician. Once you know what Mr. Reed thinks and feels about his cancer and eventual death, then you will be able to advocate for his needs.

2. You will want to encourage Mr. Reed's daughters to discuss with their father what he is thinking and feeling about his death. They need to have an open discussion about their father's wishes regarding his death.

3. As part of this process, you will want to contact a hospice agency to talk to Mr. Reed and his daughters regarding the services hospice can offer. You will want to identify whether Mr. Reed has completed an advance directive. If not, you will want to discuss with Mr. Reed and his daughter the importance of having an advanced directive. You need to provide the appropriate forms for their review and signatures.

Key Points

- Death will occur to everyone with the loss of friends or family and with our own eventual death. As care providers, our job is to support the patient and families as they travel through the many stages towards a "good death." Nurses must exhibit compassion and the ability to communicate openly and honestly during these time periods. Demonstrating ability to listen and be present with our patients will support them through their EOL.

- Knowledge and skills necessary for providing EOL include the ability to communicate issues, listen and work closely with family members when trying to honor patient wishes, work as a team with other caring professionals, maintain a positive and open work environment, and apply the guiding principles of gerotranscendence.

- Grief is the normal and natural emotional reaction to a loss or change of any kind. There are several stages involved with grief including acceptance, depression, bargaining, anger, and denial. It is important to remember that every person handles grief individually and may easily move through the aforementioned stages at different times during the grieving process.

- When dealing with EOL issues it is important to be familiar with the cultural diversities of the older adults in your care. Spirituality and religious belief are also important factors when assessing our patients' and families' needs as they relate to EOL issues. These can often overlap with cultural beliefs and can be just as influential in the choices our patients and families make.

- Palliative care is specialized medical care of people with serious illness. It focuses on providing patients with relief from physical, mental, emotional, and even spiritual symptoms. The goal is to improve quality of life. Hospice care is the next step beyond palliative care for patients with a terminal diagnosis and aims to make the time left for the patient as comfortable as possible.

- Advance directives are written statements of a person's wishes regarding medical treatment, often including a living will. Advanced directives may also include a durable power of attorney for health care.

- When imminent death is near certain signs and symptoms occur: withdrawal, reduced food and fluid intake, confusion and agitation, change in breathing patterns, incontinence, changes in skin temperature and color, and loss of hearing (which often occurs last).

Review Questions

1. When an elderly client experiences terminal restlessness (TR), he or she will display symptoms such as:
   1. Involuntary muscle twitching or jerks.
   2. Extreme fatigue.
   3. A sudden energy for life.
   4. A calm affect causing the body to have no reactions.

2. Palliative care is described as:
   1. The type of care aimed at a cure or active treatment of a certain medical condition.
   2. The type of care that provides comfort and management of symptoms.
   3. The type of care that allows the family to make all of the decisions.
   4. The type of care that provides bereavement support to the family for 1 year after death.

3. The stages of grief in order are:
   1. Denial, anger, bargaining, depression, acceptance.
   2. Denial, communicate, pain, sadness, joy.
   3. Denial, affection, bartering, acceptance.
   4. Denial, anger, acceptance, joy, peace.

4. When speaking to an elderly dying patient, it is important to:
   1. Never talk to the patient, but rather communicate all decisions through family members.
   2. Communicate clearly, possibly with a sense of humor, in a manner that the patient will be able to hear what is being said.
   3. Explain your frustrations with the patient and his or her care in front of the patient and the family.
   4. Be sympathetic rather than empathetic with the patient and the family.

5. Four of the eight signs of imminent death are:
   1. Increased blood pressure, warm extremities, bowel and bladder incontinence, and pallor and mottling of the skin.
   2. Loss of hearing, dyspnea and periods of apnea, and increased bowel and bladder control.
   3. Increased sexual drive, slow pupil response to light, increased awareness of surroundings, and more communicative.
   4. Rapid weak pulse, confusion/agitation, loss of hearing, and noisy respirations.

ANSWERS 1. 1, 2. 2, 3. 1, 4. 2, 5. 4

CHAPTER 11

Environments of Care

Tamara Dahlkemper

LEARNING OUTCOMES

1. Discuss the role of the licensed practical nurse (LPN) as an environmental manager.
2. Describe at least two components of the physical environment that nurses need to consider.
3. Discuss the aspects included in a climate of caring.
4. Identify at least four settings in which nursing care for older adults is provided.
5. Describe how nurses in various care settings meet the needs of older adults.
6. Discuss relocation stress syndrome and ways in which a nurse can help an older person adjust to a new environment.

CASE STUDY

Your neighbor, Sally, asks your advice about finding good care for her 80-year-old grandmother. The grandmother, Mrs. Gilmore, lives at home alone in an isolated section outside the city limits. She recently was discharged from the hospital after injuring her right arm in a fall at home. Her right arm is in a full cast from fingers to upper arm, which makes it difficult for Mrs. Gilmore to cook and perform other self-care activities. Your neighbor is unable to visit her grandmother daily because of work and child care commitments. Sally is worried about her grandmother's ability to remain at home. She invited her grandmother to move in with her for at least a month, but Mrs. Gilmore insists on staying in her own home. Sally asks for your advice. She ends the conversation with the statement, "I just don't know what else we can do to make sure Grandma is safe and taken care of in her home."

Continued

CASE STUDY—cont'd

Discussion

Based on the previously described situation and your reading of this chapter, what advice would you offer Sally?

INTRODUCTION

One of the most important tasks for a nurse is to manage the patient care environment. Florence Nightingale saved the lives of hundreds of soldiers during the Crimean War simply by cleaning the wards, opening the windows, and providing the soldiers with daily hygiene. Nightingale and her nurses also provided direct, caring, "hands-on" nursing to the soldiers under their care. Before Nightingale's interventions, there were more soldiers dying in the hospitals because of the lack of hygienic conditions than there were dying in the battles. Improved health for the men fighting the Crimean War required environmental management and quality nursing care.

The role of a nurse is not that of a housekeeper but that of an environmental manager. To be effective caregivers, nurses must be aware of the influence of environment on the health and functioning of the patient. Nurses are responsible for the manipulation of environmental conditions to improve patient care. In Nightingale's era, environmental management included such tasks as opening windows to clear the patient's room of stale, potentially illness-producing air; managing raw sewage because plumbing was not available; and controlling the population of mice and rats in the hospital. Modern nurses also must understand the effect that the environment can have on enhancing or impeding the progress and functioning of older adults.

SETTINGS OF CARE

Older persons may receive health-care services in various settings. This chapter does not discuss all such settings or services but reviews some of the most commonly used settings of care.

Safe, Effective Nursing Care

Using Teamwork to Provide Patient-Centered Care

Mrs. B. was moving from her home of 40 years to a retirement community. She had some short-term memory problems and walked with a slow gait. To help with the move, Mrs. B.'s son packed for her and sorted through all of her belongings. He identified what items to take and what to give away. Because many of her things were very old and worn, her son decided to purchase all new furniture and decorations for her new apartment. The new apartment looked beautiful. However, after moving, Mrs. B. became extremely disoriented and paranoid, and she accused everyone of stealing her belongings.

Her son was very upset, and the evening certified nursing assistant (CNA) reported that the son was trying to figure out what to do next. The CNA contacted the administrator and registered nurse (RN) to arrange a meeting with Mrs. B. and her son. In the meeting, the son expresses his concerns about the dramatic change in his mother's demeanor and behavior. Mrs. B. talks about the move from her home and her concerns and distress about her new apartment. The administrator acknowledges that although the new furniture and items in Mrs. B.'s apartment are very nice, the lack of unfamiliar things may be contributing to her confusion and paranoid behavior. She suggests that the son bring some old family pictures, the anniversary clock, and some of Mrs. B.'s handiwork to give the apartment some familiar touches.

In some care areas, you will have to enlist the help of different individuals assigned to the care of a resident. In this situation, the administrator and RN may not have direct patient care responsibilities, but the well-being of the resident is their job. They have the resources and connections to ensure the best outcome for this resident and her son.

1. As the nurse in the retirement community, what would you have suggested to Mrs. B.'s son about preparing his mother for relocation?
2. What suggestions would you have to avoid this problem with future residents?

Adult Day Services

Adult day services (ADS) are available in many communities to provide supervised activities for older adults. Day treatment centers for older people with psychiatric problems and day hospitals for older persons with considerable physical disability are available in many localities. Day treatment centers and day hospitals focus on a particular type of older person and provide specific services to meet their physical and psychiatric needs. Many ADS provide transportation for the older person to and from the center. Fees for daycare may be charged on a sliding scale, according to the ability of the older adult to pay. Some ADS are private pay while others may participate in a Medicaid waiver program. As a general rule, Medicare does not pay for ADS. Generally, the older person or the family must pay for these services personally.

A typical day in this care setting includes planned activities such as group discussion, current events, exercise, snacks, and lunch. Volunteers may visit a center to speak on community affairs or health promotion topics or to present entertainment programs that encourage group participation. Many centers have activity directors who plan and schedule events that are appealing, offer a variety of choices for the older adult, and promote group interaction.

Nurses working in ADS provide numerous services, according to the needs of the individual. Assessment of the older person's physical, psychological, and emotional functioning is a critical component of the nurse's role in the daycare center. Health teaching to older persons and their families also may be included in the nurse's role.

Some older people may need assistance with mobility, toileting, or eating. Other older adults may need help in taking medications. Still others simply need encouragement to participate in center activities. Nurses in adult daycare centers need a solid foundation in gerontological nursing to help them in their daily interactions with older people. This foundation ensures that subtle physical or emotional changes are not disregarded or blamed simply on "old age."

Acute illnesses in older adults can manifest in atypical fashion. A nurse who knows and appreciates normal aging is better prepared to assess subtle changes in older persons and to be alert to the possible implications of these changes. Because so many older adults have chronic illnesses, medication administration often becomes a major responsibility for the nurse in an ADS. The nurse needs to be skillful at administering medications and needs to know their expected effects and possible side effects. The nurse also can use knowledge of medications to teach the older person and family members the importance of safe and accurate medication use. Do the older adult and family members know which medications are being taken and why they are prescribed? Are the older adult and family members aware of possible side effects, potential drug interactions, and the necessary steps to take if problems are suspected? The nurse, as teacher, has an important role in this setting.

Ongoing assessments of ADS participants are especially important. Frequent contact with the older person allows nurses to see subtle changes in function that may signal serious underlying physiological problems. The nurse's powers of observation and knowledge of the aging process are crucial in detecting actual or impending illness. Is an older person experiencing mobility changes? Are you seeing decreased participation in formerly active participants? Has an older person had changes in weight or affect? If you note these changes, the next question to ask is why they are occurring. Good communication skills may uncover a change in family living conditions, changes in medication, or exacerbation of the effects of a chronic illness.

ADS provide opportunities for socializing and staying involved in the world. Many families use daycare to give respite to the main caregiver for the older adult. The stresses of caregiving can have a strong effect on the older person, caregiver, and family. Respite allows caregivers some time to attend to their own needs. Grocery shopping, housekeeping, socializing with friends, and participating in enjoyable activities for the caregivers can often mean the difference between continued home care versus institutionalization for an older adult. Nurses in ADS are able to use their assessment skills to identify the older person's strengths and weaknesses, help elders to continue to participate in daily living activities and provide information for older persons and their families about community resources.

THINK LIKE A NURSE

You are the licensed nurse at an adult day service. Mrs. Y. attends the center every Monday, Tuesday, and Wednesday until after lunch, when her husband picks her up. This Tuesday you notice, for the second day in a row, that Mrs. Y. has been unsteady when she walks. She stops to rest frequently when moving around the center and has been falling asleep during group activities. These behaviors are unusual because Mrs. Y. normally ambulates well, participates enthusiastically in center activities, and often encourages others to "join the fun." What further assessment do you now want to make? What types of questions would you ask her husband?

Although ADS nurses may perform few technical nursing procedures, they use a variety of different nursing skills. ADS nurses must have particularly strong physical and psychological assessment skills. They also must be adept in communication and teaching. An ADS nurse also must have a thorough knowledge of community resources and be able to refer older persons and their families to appropriate services in the area.

With the increasing awareness and concern about care for people with dementia, some programs are now available to provide ADS specifically for older persons with cognitive impairments. These ADS are designed to give care that takes into account the abilities and safety needs of patients with Alzheimer's disease or other types of dementia.

Home Care

Home health-care agencies provide numerous services for older adults in the home. These agencies provide nursing services, given by licensed nurses and nursing assistants, and therapy services, such as physical, occupational, and speech therapy. Many agencies also provide medical supplies and equipment. Most agencies are licensed and eligible for state or federal reimbursement for services. Medicare, Medicaid, and community funding may pay for limited home health-care services if the older person qualifies for such reimbursement.

Home care may be provided on a daily basis or intermittently, according to the needs of the patient. Nursing care provided in the home has become more complex in the past two decades. It is not unusual for people who need help during their recovery to be discharged from the hospital "quicker and sicker." Older adults with a chronic illness may be receiving home care to avoid frequent hospitalizations.

The LPN in home care works under the supervision of the RN case manager. In the home health role, the LPN is assigned basic nursing care, medication administration and teaching, and dressings and wound care. The LPN often is assigned to work with a CNA in coordinating care for the patient.

Evidence-Based Practice

King, D. K., Faulkner, S. A., & Hanson, B. L. (2018). The feasibility of adopting an evidence-informed tailored exercise program within adult day services: The Enhance Mobility Program. *Activities, Adaptation & Aging*, 42(2), 104–123. https://doi.org/10.1080/01924788.2017.1391030

Providing regular exercise for individuals with dementia improves mood as well as functional mobility such as improved gait, strength, and balance. The improvement of strength and balance help to decrease the risk of falls. Studies show that just 60 minutes per week of exercise is all that is needed to provide the benefits listed.

The purpose of this study was to identify the feasibility of implementing an exercise program for older adults with dementia into an adult day services program. The chosen exercise program, Enhanced Mobility (EM), is a group exercise and walking program. The group exercise component of EM consists of 20 exercises repeated three times during a 30-minute period. The walking component is of a 20-minute duration. The 20 minutes can be divided into shorter increments of time as needed. Twenty-two participants began the study and 20 completed the final assessments.

After 8 months, the participants were reevaluated. The results showed no significant improvement in the participant's ability to complete a chair stand. However, participants were able to balance for a longer period of time and their gait speed was improved. Staff also noticed the individuals were more likely to have improved general mobility and better able to get up and walk on their own. The staff also noted that participants showed some psychological improvements such as better mood, increased self-confidence, and better focus.

Concerns for implementing the program included need for dedicated space and equipment, trained staff to teach the exercises, and adequate staff to assist the participants with their exercise. The staff were able to overcome these challenges and a year later the EM program continues to be used with good results.

Questions

1. What exercise programs have you noted when doing clinical rotations at various facilities?
2. If a formal exercise program is not available for your patients/residents with dementia, what are some ways you can increase their physical activity?

A certain amount of creativity is needed in home care nursing because of limitations in the type of equipment and supplies that are available. As in other settings, it is helpful for the nurse to be aware of resources available to the older adult and of ways to gain use of those resources. Nurses who choose home care nursing can expect a variety of older persons and conditions. Caring for older adults in the home can be very rewarding and challenging. Because a home care nurse generally visits the older person on a less-than-daily basis, patient and family teaching is very important. Teaching may be necessary to help the family ensure a safe environment for the older adult. Education about fall prevention, medication safety, positioning, and transferring techniques for older persons and families also should be addressed. A family also may need to learn more complex procedures, such as how to change dressings or give injected medications.

THINK LIKE A NURSE

As an LPN for a home care agency, you are assigned to Mrs. E. Mrs. E. is 75 years old and lives with her husband in their home. Mrs. E. was just discharged from the hospital after surgery to pin her broken right hip. She is not capable of weight-bearing, and the physical therapist is scheduled to visit her at home twice a week. Mrs. E. has mild dementia and frequently forgets that she is not permitted to walk. Her husband, Mr. E., wants to keep her in bed to remind her not to walk. What care do you need to teach Mr. E.?

The amount of time spent with older persons is often limited by the nurse's workload and the reimbursement for care given. The nurse is responsible for assessing and documenting care needs and providing prescribed treatments. Good communication skills are important to ensure that all members of the health-care team are aware of the older person's needs and progress.

Community-Based Care

Nursing opportunities are available in various settings not linked to formal institutions, such as hospitals or nursing homes. **Community-based care** settings are noninstitutional settings that include community clinics, dialysis centers, or physician's offices. In these settings, the nurse may practice under the direct supervision of a physician rather than RN. Practice in these settings often includes assisting with physical examinations and treatments, and nurses in these settings are frequently an important source of information and clarification for patients. The nurse uses assessment skills and provides information on resources available in the community to meet the older person's needs. Contact with older adults in these settings may be more infrequent than in other care settings.

Hospice

Hospice care is designed to provide care for a dying person and the family. A team approach is central to the hospice concept. Team members include physicians, nurses, social workers, and nursing assistants as well as other ancillary workers. The goal of hospice care is to help dying persons remain at home, if possible, with all the support needed to ensure a "good death." In this case, "good" means that the older person is kept comfortable and able to receive the support of family and loved ones in a familiar setting.

Hospice work allows nurses to give direct patient care and develop a close relationship with the patient and family. As in the care settings previously discussed, the nurse's role as a teacher is especially helpful. Most families are not prepared to meet the needs of a dying family member. The hospice nurse can teach family members how to provide for the comfort of their loved one. The nurse also can identify hospice resources available to help families and older persons cope during this extremely demanding time. Nurses who have not worked in a hospice setting may be reluctant to try this type of nursing because all of the clients are terminally ill. Talking with nurses who work in a hospice often shows, however, that the team support and the closeness to patients and families provide a high degree of job satisfaction.

Assisted Living Environments

As people age, there is a tendency to simplify lifestyles and living space. The size of the home needed to provide adequate living space for a family can become more of a burden than an asset to older adults. **Assisted living environments** are an increasingly popular way for the elderly person to have a home without homeowner responsibilities. Not having yard work and other maintenance tasks associated with a large home relieves numerous burdens. Assisted living communities generally offer apartments with community dining and activity areas. They have a nurse, an activity director, CNAs, and housekeepers. The goal for these retirement communities is to appeal to a broad range of older adults by offering security and various conveniences and services. Although communities for retirees have been popular for quite a while, assisted living facilities that also provide services for older adults with physical care needs are now increasingly common. Many assisted living complexes have a satellite branch of a home health agency on site.

The goal of assisted living units is to provide older persons with help in performing ADLs. Frail older persons who do not require continuous care are able to have help in such activities as meal preparation, grooming and bathing, laundry, and housekeeping. Most assisted living programs require that the older person be ambulatory and fairly independent. Much of the care provided is done by nursing assistants rather than LPNs. The LPN in an assisted living program often provides supervision for nursing assistants, medication administration, basic documentation of care given, and assessment of the older person's ability to function.

The nurse in an assisted living community also must use creative talents to ensure that the environment is as homelike as possible. The nurse must be flexible in tailoring care to the individual needs of each older adult. The nursing assistant in assisted living care may be called a resident assistant and perform many functions that do not relate directly to ADLs. Nurses and nursing assistants working in assisted living care often are very involved in activities and social planning for residents.

Some assisted living facilities provide a continuum of care for older adults. Elderly adults can be admitted to their own apartments, but if their health changes, they can also be admitted to the skilled nursing section for care.

For many older adults, the appeal of a continuing care retirement community lies in the fact that adults are able to stay in a familiar environment regardless of their health status. Nursing in a continuing care retirement community offers many opportunities. Home visits, health promotion or screening activities (for example, blood pressure monitoring clinics), health teaching, and direct bedside care to nursing home residents are a few of the opportunities available to nurses in continuing care communities. As in assisted living situations, supervisory ability is a valuable asset for the LPN. Retirement community nursing allows nurses to work with older adults who have various needs and abilities. The ability to apply your knowledge of the aging process in this setting helps you enhance the quality of life for the older persons there.

Long-Term Care Facilities

Generally referred to as nursing homes, **long-term care facilities** provide an area of practice that has been available to practical nurses for many years. With the growing number of frail elderly adults and old-old (85 and older) adults, the need for nursing home care is great. Some nursing home residents need a full range of nursing care; others may be independent physically but have cognitive changes that require a high degree of supervision to maintain their personal safety. Two categories of long-term care are defined by federal regulation. The first category is the skilled nursing facility (SNF) and the second is the nursing facility.

All nursing homes must be licensed by the state in which they operate. If they wish to receive reimbursement from Medicare or Medicaid for the services provided to residents, they also must meet additional federal requirements and be certified by the federal government. A nursing home may choose not to accept Medicare and Medicaid funding and admit only private-pay residents.

In an SNF, licensed nurses provide care around the clock, and an RN is present at least 8 hours a day, 7 days a week. A SNF also offers the services of allied health professionals, such as speech, physical, or occupational therapists, at least 5 days a week. A nursing facility generally does not have the same level of staffing by RNs or therapists as an SNF.

Regardless of category, long-term care facilities offer a team approach to meeting the older person's needs over time. Facilities that receive federal funds are required to offer the services of a social worker and an activity director and dietetic consultant. Licensed nurses can gain input from various sources in planning and delivering care by being actively involved with the interdisciplinary health-care team.

In long-term care, the LPN has traditionally been responsible for supervising the nursing assistants who give hands-on care to residents; the LPN also gives medications and performs treatments.

A nurse interested in long-term care has the opportunity to get to know residents well over a long time. Because of the changing needs and physical condition of residents, the long-term care nurse needs very good assessment skills. Long-term care nurses use skills such as monitoring resident responses to treatments, observing for signs of decreasing function, and assessing subtle changes in condition on a daily basis. Accurate documentation; skillful use of the nursing process; and good interpersonal skills in working with residents, staff members, and family members are valuable tools in long-term care.

Patient Education

As an older adult anticipates transitioning from an acute care setting or an assisted living facility to a long-term care facility, he or she will have questions about how to choose a facility. Nurses can be instrumental in helping patients and families in the selection of a nursing home. The following is a list of some key elements that should be addressed when visiting a facility.

- The environment is clean, well maintained, odor free, and secure.
- There is a provision for private areas and the ability to personalize rooms.
- The overall atmosphere is calm and welcoming.
- Residents are well groomed, and personal equipment such as wheelchairs and walkers is clean.
- Staff are professional in appearance and are attentive to the residents.
- The schedule for daily care is flexible to allow for individual needs.
- The facility provides restorative programs and resident and family councils.

- Meal schedules are flexible and provide a variety of options.
- There is an adequate number of staff members with low turnover.
- Safety equipment is used appropriately.

The person and family should visit several nursing homes for comparison. The visits should be done at different times of the day to ensure that patterns of care are consistent from shift to shift. If it is allowed, the person should ask questions of the staff, residents, and family members about the care that is provided. The Centers for Medicare and Medicaid Services has developed a checklist that can be used when visiting a nursing home. The checklist and other information can be accessed at https://www.medicare.gov/Nursing-HomeCompare/checklist.pdf

Centers for Medicare and Medicaid Services [n.d.]. Your guide to choosing a nursing home or other long-term care. Retrieved from: https://www.medicare.gov/Pubs/pdf/02174-Nursing-Home-Other-Long-Term-Services.pdf

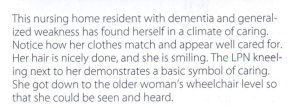

This nursing home resident with dementia and generalized weakness has found herself in a climate of caring. Notice how her clothes match and appear well cared for. Her hair is nicely done, and she is smiling. The LPN kneeling next to her demonstrates a basic symbol of caring. She got down to the older woman's wheelchair level so that she could be seen and heard.

Care in a long-term care facility differs from hospital care in many ways. The skills required of the nursing home nurse are no less challenging and the tasks no less difficult than those of the hospital nurse. The goal for a hospital patient is to cure illness in a brief time. For a long-term care resident with multiple chronic conditions, cure is often not possible. Instead, the primary focus is on providing care rather than a cure. When you make the care given to residents transpersonal caring, the quality of that care improves remarkably.

Acute Care

Acute care settings include hospitals and clinics. Most hospital admissions are patients 65 years and older. Depending on the source used, it is estimated that 40% to 65% of hospital admissions include older adults. Nursing practice in a hospital setting presents many opportunities and challenges. Usually, LPNs are responsible for a set number of patients, and, depending on policy, they may perform various procedures. Most patients are hospitalized only briefly. The emphasis on cost containment and federal mandates means that reimbursement for care is often limited to a set period. Hospital-based practice requires all of the basic skills an LPN possesses. Acute care also involves brief contact with a large number of patients.

There are several challenges in giving nursing care to older adults in the hospital setting. These challenges include establishing a trusting relationship over a short period, dealing with problems secondary to relocation stress or medications, and resisting the tendency to stereotype patients because of their age. In addition, a major challenge for a nurse working with older people in the hospital setting is to create a safe and caring environment that facilitates independence; this must be done while the tasks required for the cure and treatment of the person are accomplished. Environmental management, as discussed earlier in this chapter, is the most difficult task to accomplish in the hospital setting. The short time frame and the urgency for treatment in many situations do not readily accommodate the slowed responses and abilities of older persons. It is your challenge to slow things down so that the older adult can manage them.

THINK LIKE A NURSE

Mr. W. is a 90-year-old resident of a nursing home who was admitted to your floor at Hoover Medical Center for treatment of heart failure. He has significant dementia, is incontinent of bowel and bladder, and is very unsteady on his feet. As his primary nurse, what can you do to make his hospital environment more like home? What steps will you take to ensure that Mr. W. is receiving continuity of care between the nursing home and hospital? Who will you communicate with to assure Mr. W. is receiving continuity of care between the nursing home and the hospital?

Priority Setting

As with the other chapters, everything mentioned in this chapter is important. The question is: What is the priority?

As a novice nurse, you need to know about the different environments of care so that you can:

1. Recognize the best place for you to be employed. It is important to have a satisfying job that allows you to be the most effective caregiver possible.
2. Function most effectively as a member of the health-care team. By knowing about different environments of care, you have more information to share with the team where you are working. This is an important aspect of being a valuable member of the health-care team.

One of the positive things about being a nurse is the fact that there are so many opportunities for different types of work.

As a gerontological nurse, it is important to understand the special needs of older adults. They have difficulty seeing and hearing. They move much slower, and they need clear explanations as to what is happening. When you recognize these needs of older adults, you have a responsibility to meet the needs and assist others involved in the care of the older adults to slow down and focus on those needs as well.

ENVIRONMENTAL MANAGEMENT

Providing care to older adults must include environmental management. Assessment of the environment is the first step. As an LPN, you need to examine the total environment starting with where the older person is living. There are multiple environments of care in which an older adult might live. If the person lives at home, you might ask the following questions: What is the neighborhood like? Is it a safe neighborhood for an older person? Is there a security system in the home or building?

If an older adult lives in a long-term care facility or is receiving care in a hospital or rehabilitation center, you might ask the following questions: What is the staffing ratio? Is the environment clean and free of odor? Is there a place where the older adult can socialize with family and friends?

If an older adult lives in an assisted living environment, you might ask: How far is it to the dining room? Are there activities that interest the person? Is there a nurse available 24 hours a day?

Assessment of the physical environment includes all aspects of the older adult's living situation that can be seen, heard, touched, or smelled. Each of the physical items in the environment can either contribute to

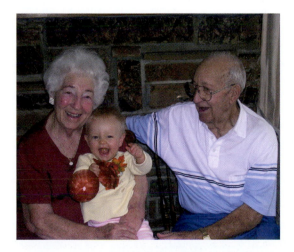

This couple are both past 80 years of age and have lived in their current home since they were a young married couple. They have made it clear to their children that they do not want to leave their home if they become ill. Many older people have a strong aversion to leaving their homes, which is why home care is such a valuable resource to older adults.

or detract from the optimal functioning of the older person. A room that is too hot may make the older person tired, lethargic, and unwilling to participate in personal care activities. A room that is too cold may likewise result in lack of activity because the older person is unwilling to get out of bed or to come out from under the cover of an afghan.

A crucial question to ask throughout the assessment of the physical environment is how well the older person functions in the living areas. Is the environment as barrier-free as possible? Can the older person walk unencumbered or wheel a wheelchair through the entire setting? Are there features in the environment to promote physical function? These may include grab bars in the bathroom by the commode, shower, or bathtub seat and handrails by stairs. When assessing how the older person carries out ADLs, be aware of possible alterations that may improve function. Lowering a mirror or moving a storage area below shoulder level may improve safety and convenience. The risk of falling can be decreased with adequate room lighting and the use of night lights. The room where the older person reads should have high-intensity illumination. When assessing Mrs. Gilmore's home you will want to keep the safety of her current environment in mind.

THINK LIKE A NURSE

People do better when they are in a caring environment. Remember Dr. Jean Watson's theory of human caring? She has spent her career researching and documenting the significance of caring in our lives. When a nurse and a patient connect in a caring way, Dr. Watson refers to it as "transpersonal caring." This happens when you, the nurse, relate to the older adult in a holistic manner that is based on caring, or, in other words, you care about every aspect of the person's life, including his or her environment.

Climate of Caring

Another important part of the environmental assessment is evaluating the climate of caring. The **climate of caring** involves the people in the environment and the environmental tone and atmosphere. The people in an older person's living environment may include family members, neighbors, friends, and paid caregivers.

The people in an environment are extremely important to the older adult's potential for improvement and optimal function. Families, staff members, and visitors can be encouraging and uplifting or depressing and discouraging. A climate of caring includes persons who present a positive but realistic outlook. An older adult's personal space is respected in a caring climate. Such an atmosphere also affords opportunities for privacy, encourages activity and involvement, and facilitates independence.

Safety

In any setting, safety for the older person is a primary concern. Are there any environmental hazards, such as frayed extension cords, malfunctioning equipment, or broken furniture? Falls among elderly people are common. Although not all falls can be avoided, what can be done is to keep the environment free of fall risks. Such risks include clutter, throw rugs, wheelchair leg rests, and poorly fitting shoes or slippers. A pet sometimes can be a fall risk as well. Refer to Chapter 7 for other safety issues.

Stimulation and Personalization

Opinions vary on whether environments for older adults with cognitive impairment should be very stark and nonstimulating or should contain eye-catching and stimulating components. What is more important is a personalized environment for the older person. Personalized items help older adults relate to the environment and maintain a sense of identity. A special picture can be displayed in a hospital room or nursing home. In some settings, such as nursing homes and retirement communities, the entire bedroom or apartment can be personalized with cherished furniture and decorations.

A climate of caring facilitates optimal independence and autonomy for each older person living in the setting. Sometimes the routines and regulations necessary to operate a large health-care facility such as a hospital or nursing home cannot accommodate the individual needs or desires of older adults. Although a nursing home may need to serve meals at particular times because of regulations and staffing, the rule that all residents must be dressed for breakfast may be unnecessary. This rule does not allow for each resident to take the time personally to do as much of the dressing as possible. Such a rule can force a resident to be dependent on staff for dressing. A climate of caring provides multiple opportunities for individual choice in the environment and encourages the older person to function as independently as possible.

Personal Space and Territoriality

Personal space and territory are important to every human being. **Personal space** is the area around a person. Some individuals define their personal space very close to their bodies, whereas others define it as a broader area. It is viewed as an intrusion for someone to invade another individual's personal space. In providing nursing care, nurses must frequently invade the personal space of the patient. Nurses must be conscious, however, that they do not do so unnecessarily.

Territory is the space used by a person and seen as owned by the person. People tend to be territorial because it meets the need for privacy, security, and autonomy. These needs cannot be met unless individuals can defend their space (Giger, 2017). Think about a current class. Do the students tend to sit in the same seats during each class session? Technically, you and your classmates do not own the seats, but the tendency exists to define a territory and return to it habitually. The seating arrangement in a dining room in a nursing home or retirement community is frequently consistent for each meal. This consistency tends to occur whether or not seats are assigned. Individuals defend their territory if an unwanted person intrudes. An older person who has a favorite chair at home or in the nursing home may fiercely defend it from others.

Privacy

All human beings need time to be alone. People need to have opportunities for privacy and for human contact. It is difficult sometimes for an older person living in a health-care setting to find opportunities for privacy. Many hospitals and nursing homes have multiple-occupancy rooms so that the patient may never have a chance to be truly alone. As a nurse working with older persons in a congregate setting, you must be aware of the older person's needs for privacy. You should respect that right to privacy by knocking on the door before entering, pulling cubicle curtains during care, and arranging private time for the older adult.

Cultural Considerations

In cultures where privacy is valued, nurses should allow and provide opportunities for patients to have their privacy. This can be difficult if the patient is in a shared room. In cultures where priority is given to group needs and not individual needs, nurses need to adjust their care to include family members and other group members as identified by the patient (Giger, 2017). In any care setting, the patient should be asked about their privacy needs. Some considerations may be difficult to address depending on the care setting, but nurses should do what they can to meet individual privacy needs.

Activity and Involvement

As a person ages, the number of social roles fulfilled tends to diminish. An older woman who was once a daughter, a wife, a mother, a neighbor, an accountant, a scout leader, and a bridge player may hold none of these social roles at 90 years of age. Because of aging and disability, these roles may no longer be possible. Involvement with others is still a need, however. A climate of caring affords each individual multiple and diverse opportunities for activity and involvement with others.

As a nurse working with older people in multiple health-care settings, you can help to provide important opportunities for active involvement. It is important to find out the older person's prior social roles, particularly the ones he or she most enjoyed. Activities that include tasks associated with these roles should be encouraged. It also is important to create opportunities for social interaction. By introducing the older person to others in the setting who may share similar interests and by arranging seating for natural conversation rather than against walls, the nurse can be instrumental in encouraging social exchanges.

CRITICALLY EXAMINE THE FOLLOWING

You are taking care of a resident with dementia on a memory care unit. You understand the importance of managing the environment of this individual and know aspects of the living situation that can be seen, heard, touched, and smelled should be evaluated. For an older adult with dementia, what will you consider for the following components of the environment?

Climate of Caring
Safety
Stimulation and Personalization
Personal Space
Privacy
Activity and Involvement

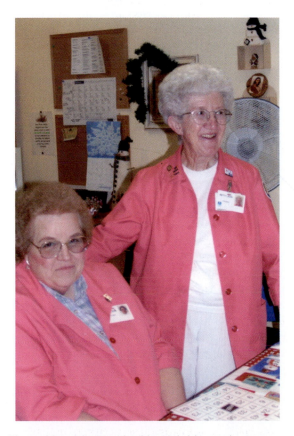

These older women are healthy and able to volunteer at their community's local nursing home. They assist others with making the transition to a new environment and provide many services that otherwise would be unavailable.

RELOCATION STRESS SYNDROME

Moving from one environment to another is stressful. Anyone who has ever moved from one house to another or from one city to another can appreciate the stress of relocation. It takes time to adjust to and become familiar with a new setting. During times of crisis or illness, one has less energy available to deal constructively with stress. Older adults are particularly susceptible to being overcome with the stress of relocation.

Older people use a considerable amount of energy coping with chronic illness and disabilities. The onset of an acute illness or some other major crisis requires additional coping. If the crisis or illness results in the need to move to another living situation, the older person's coping abilities may be exhausted. A crisis, superimposed on the day-to-day stresses of living with disability and dysfunction, frequently leaves the older person with little coping reserve to deal with the stress of relocation and transition. When the stress is overwhelming, and the older person is unable to cope with the situation, signs of decompensation appear. These may include disorientation, agitation, acting out, and hallucinations. It is common for an older adult newly admitted to any of the health-care settings described in this chapter to exhibit some of these signs. The movement from one environment to another can be extremely disruptive to the older adult; this disruption has been termed **relocation stress syndrome**. You will want to consider the possible impact of relocation stress syndrome on Mrs. Gilmore when assessing her situation. Will moving her to a care facility even for a temporary period of time cause more health issues for her?

In addition to identifying and understanding relocation stress syndrome, the nurse can help to relieve relocation stress. Relocation stress syndrome is temporary, and the behavioral signs of decompensation should diminish as the older person becomes familiar with the new environment. You can accelerate the process of adjustment, however.

Limit stimulation and the introduction of new activities and people on the older person's first day in the setting. Orient the older person to the environment slowly so that he or she can incorporate new areas and routines gradually. On the first day, introduce only people and places that are absolutely necessary. For example, placing an older person in the dining room of a nursing home with 20 other residents shortly after admission may be overwhelming.

Focused Learning Chart: Relocation Stress Syndrome

Symptom of Decompensation	Nursing Care
Disorientation	Temporary condition
Hallucinations	Familiar items such as furniture and photos
Agitation	Involve family and friends.
Acting out	Caring attitude
	Limit stimulation (people, places, and activities) for the first few days.

Look for ways to provide links between the old environment and the new one. The more familiar the new environment is to the older person, the easier the transition is for the person. Bringing favorite furniture and objects, such as pictures, to the new setting increases its familiarity to the older person. Including the older person in planning for the move is ideal. This is not always possible, however, if the move occurs because of an acute illness. If it can be arranged, involve the older person in selecting the items to take to the new location.

CASE STUDY SOLUTION

When a nurse assesses her friend Sally's grandmother, Mrs. Gilmore, she finds that Mrs. Gilmore's home is all one level and has been remodeled to consider the needs of an aging homeowner. Grab bars have been installed throughout the bathroom. The shower is a simple step-in model with a seat allowing Mrs. Gilmore to sit and operate the shower water controls. The toilet is a tall model and the sink is raised. Mrs. Gilmore has a wide-step aerobics step next to her bed that she uses to get in and out of the bed. She also has an emergency alert system that is part of her home security system. Her neighbors have a key to her home if there is an emergency.

This is a relatively safe environment and moving Mrs. Gilmore to a care facility for even a temporary period of time may cause relocation stress syndrome. The main concerns are personal cares and meal preparation. Home care or private duty home health aides could be enlisted to help Mrs. Gilmore with personal cares and meals.

Key Points

- There are multiple care settings where an LPN can provide care to older adults. They include daycare services, home care, community-based care, assisted living, hospice, long-term care, and acute care. Each setting provides different opportunities for LPNs. LPNs should determine the best setting in which to work based on their interests and skills.
- The care provided by the LPN in each setting is different. In settings such as long-term care, assisted living, acute care, home care, and hospice, the LPN will provide more direct patient care. In some of these settings, the LPN may also function as a supervisor for nonlicensed personnel. In a community-based care setting, the LPN assists with physical examinations and treatments and provides resources available in the community to meet the older adult's needs. Depending on the setting the LPN is supervised by a registered nurse or physician.
- Managing the environment of patients is an important role of a nurse. Assessing the environment includes all aspects of the older adult's living situation that can be seen, heard, touched, and smelled. A crucial question to ask throughout the assessment is how well the older person functions in their living areas.
- There are several components to consider when assessing the environment:
  - Is it a caring climate?
  - Are safety concerns addressed?
  - Is personalized space provided that is stimulating?
  - Do residents have an area they can call their own (territory)?
  - Is privacy provided?
  - Do residents have the opportunity for activity and involvement with others?
- The climate of caring includes the people in the environment and the environmental tone and atmosphere. The people in the environment may include family members, friends, and paid caregivers or facility staff that respect the older adult's personal space. A caring environment also provides privacy, encourages activity, and facilitates independence.
- Relocation stress syndrome is the stress experienced when moving from one environment to another. It takes time to adjust to and become familiar with a new setting. During times of crisis or illness, one has less energy available to deal constructively with stress. Older adults are particularly susceptible to being overcome with the stress of relocation.

Review Questions

1. Mr. D., 75 years old, is discharged from the hospital after a right-sided cerebrovascular accident. He requires at least 6 weeks of further nursing care and physical therapy. The facility most likely to meet these needs is:
   1. A continuing care retirement center.
   2. Hospice care.
   3. An intermediate care facility.
   4. A skilled nursing facility.

2. Hospice care provides a multidisciplinary approach to caring for people with:
   1. A chronic illness.
   2. An acute exacerbation of a chronic illness.
   3. A terminal illness.
   4. A contagious illness.

3. The major benefit of living in a continuing-care retirement community is:
   1. Low household maintenance requirements.
   2. Services available for a continuum of health-care needs.
   3. A safe environment for older adults.
   4. The presence of a hospital in the complex.

4. Mr. J., 83 years old, has Alzheimer's disease and has wandered from home on several occasions. Mrs. J. is concerned for her husband's safety and desires some respite services. You recommend that she investigate:
   1. A local nursing home.
   2. The local senior center.
   3. A home health-care agency.
   4. An adult daycare center.

5. In the home health-care setting, the LPN can expect:
   1. A limited amount of equipment and supplies to be available.
   2. Intermittent contact with clients.
   3. To care for clients discharged from the hospital with many physical care needs.
   4. All of the above.

6. When discharging (or transitioning) a patient from the hospital to a long-term care facility, it would be important for the nurse to include:
   1. A detailed description of the medications for the patient to review.
   2. Contact cards for the patient of various therapies involved in the care.
   3. All communication, contacts, medications, and therapies for the facility.
   4. Detailed information regarding family involvement in the patient's care.

ANSWERS 1. 4, 2. 3, 3. 3, 2, 4. 4, 5. 4, 6. 3

CHAPTER 12

Management and Leadership Role of the Licensed Practical/ Vocational Nurse

Ann Rocha

KEY TERMS

bullying
delegation
evaluation
incivility
leader
manager
transformational leadership

CHAPTER CONCEPTS

Caring Interventions
Clinical Decision Making
Collaboration
Communication
Managing Care
Professional Behaviors

LEARNING OUTCOMES

1. Identify the five management styles and determine when each would be effectively used in the gerontological setting.
2. Identify communication skills and techniques that can be effectively incorporated into your role as a charge nurse.
3. Identify delegation skills required for the licensed practical nurse (LPN) charge nurse in the gerontological setting.
4. Integrate decision-making skills into safe patient care scenarios.
5. Recognize the use of the planning hoop in setting priorities.
6. Define and give examples of bullying and incivility in nursing.
7. Identify three common errors made in doing employee evaluations.

CASE STUDY

Nurse White graduated as a licensed practical nurse (LPN) 6 months ago and has been steadily employed at a skilled nursing facility (SNF) for 5 months. For the past 3 months Nurse White has functioned effectively in the role of charge nurse of a 25-bed unit on the 0600 to 1800 shift. This 25-bed unit is full and has one certified nursing assistant (CNA), in addition to the LPN charge nurse, on the day shift.

As Nurse White arrives for his shift:

- He is greeted by 10 students, their instructor, and the newly hired LPN, all eager to get their assignments.

Continued

CASE STUDY—cont'd

- The charge nurse who works the 1800 to 0600 shift is not at the front desk and Nurse White is anxious to receive his report before delegating assignments.
- Passing of medications is to begin at 0630.
- Patient assessments are to be reported at the 1000 interdisciplinary meeting. The interdisciplinary care-planning session begins at 1000, which includes a report of this morning's assessments.
- As he goes to find the night nurse, he sees the CNA coming out of a patient's room in tears. The CNA rushes by Nurse White and loudly exclaims "I cannot work with that family. They continually treat their mother like she is an idiot, and now they are treating me the same way. I'm done!" Nurse White goes into the room to find the patient crying and the patient's daughter insisting the medications have not been given correctly for the past 2 days. She wants to review her mother's medications immediately.
- The instructor of the students rushes down the hall to find Nurse White and tells him that Dr. Jackson just called and was in her usual uproar over her new admit in room 222. Evidently, the new admit was incoherent on admission last evening, and the night nurse had called to report a fall and a possible fracture to the right lower extremity; the night nurse left a message for Dr. Jackson that this did not appear to be an emergency and the patient was complaining only of mild pain. Dr. Jackson is just returning the call and would like him to call her as soon as possible.
- A student nurse greets Nurse White and the instructor as they are exiting the patient's room and tells them that the night nurse is in the bathroom and is very ill.

Discussion

Imagine you are Nurse White. Review the situation and, using critical thinking, begin to develop a list of priorities. Create a plan of action with explanations on how you arrived at your decisions. You will have opportunity to reflect on your initial plan at the end of this chapter.

INTRODUCTION

Management and leadership, as they apply to the LPN in the geriatric setting, are constantly changing to keep pace with changes in the health-care delivery system. Up to this point you have been educated through a directed program of study that incorporates the process of nursing with an emphasis placed on physical sciences and research. The basics of physiology, pathophysiology, pharmacology, and the basic medical and surgical procedures and skills have been your primary concerns. Somewhere along the line, leadership and ethics may have been touched on, but only briefly, and certainly not in the context of the LPN's role in management and leadership.

Entering into the position of a novice nurse, as an LPN, and being expected to understand your role as a manager and leader can be somewhat daunting. You may readily understand the role of a patient caregiver at the LPN level, and all of the accompanying requirements of being a safe patient caregiver but may lack the full understanding and experience with the management and leadership skills associated with this position. Education to enhance what may or may not come naturally to you can help you become a good manager or leader.

An important attribute to identify, as you read through this chapter, is how to motivate yourself to be a good manager and how to lead, inspire, and empower others whom you manage.

MANAGEMENT AND LEADERSHIP ROLES

Recognizing that the work of an LPN will always require management and leadership skills and accepting that the scope of practice and responsibility may frequently change is a first step in helping you recognize what your management responsibilities are in any setting. It is challenging enough to be an LPN prepared to assume the responsibility of management, but when it is done with skill it can add to the outcome of safe patient care in a multidisciplinary work environment.

In some nursing homes, LPNs are directors of nursing, whereas in some hospitals, they are not allowed to administer medications. This diversity in scope of responsibility is important to understand. If a registered nurse (RN) is on the health-care team, the LPN is responsible to the RN. This is always true because of the dictates of licensure. It is possible for an RN and an LPN to have the same job description in an organization, just as it is possible for an LPN to be the director of nursing or shift supervisor. Even if you and an RN have the same job description, you have different licensure; the licensure and its scope of practice are critical for you to follow. The LPN must know and follow the appropriate scope of practice.

At the time of employment, the LPN should clarify the scope of responsibility and role expectations to be fulfilled. Determining that the duties assigned are not in conflict with the state nurse practice act also is important. As licensed nurses, all LPNs are responsible for knowing the law governing practice. This responsibility should not be delegated to a supervisor or another nurse.

MANAGEMENT AND LEADERSHIP STYLES

In this chapter, the terms "management" and "leadership" are presented synonymously. However, it is important for you to understand that you can be a **leader** without being a **manager**. Each of us has the potential to be a leader even if we are not in an authority role. According to Grossman and Valiga (2017), leadership skills include vision, communication skills, being a change agent, stewardship, and ongoing development and renewal of followers. In other words, leaders see a different world and inspire others to work toward this vision. Leaders possess communication skills and are not discouraged when change is required. Stewardship is the desire to serve others and not just focus on personal wants and needs. Finally, leaders continue to motivate and keep followers committed to the vision. Gaining an understanding of the different leadership styles will help you function as a leader or a manager. As you read through this portion of the chapter, compare the traits associated with each of the management and leadership styles as they relate to the type of manager you would like to become. Most of you have worked with people you consider good managers. As you look at the different traits of each of the following leadership styles, make sure you identify those traits in people you have worked with or know well. Also, decide what method you would like to use, in specific situations, as you develop your own leadership

and management skills. The type of leadership style you display may have a significant impact on recruitment and retention of staff, staff turnover, and quality of care (Saleh, O'Connor, Al-Subhi, Alkattan, Al-Harbi, & Patton, 2018).

In this chapter, five basic styles of leadership will be discussed:

- Authoritative (autocratic)
- Permissive (laissez faire)
- Democratic (participative)
- Multicratic (eclectic)
- Transformational

Other leadership styles exist, and many leadership theories have been proposed. The LPN nurse manager should understand the basic styles and be flexible enough to incorporate other information into the clinical decision-making process as it becomes pertinent. The overall objective for defining and comparing the basic styles of leadership is for the LPN to determine an effective but flexible leadership style for professional use.

Authoritarian

In the strictest sense, authoritarianism functions with a high concern for tasks done and low concern for the people who perform those tasks (Dahlkemper, 2018). The authoritarian style demonstrates control and overall direction from a boss or a manager. It is certainly not the preferred style in our society as many of us do not respond well to dictators. This style can be oppressive and decrease motivation among workers when the majority of the decisions are made by the manager and when the employees are allowed little feedback or recognition.

An authoritarian manager does not allow for creative thinking or new ideas. No opportunities are presented to try new concepts on a patient or resident care plan unless the idea is the manager's own. This type of manager is more interested in seeing that the work is done rather than that the patients are being lovingly cared for and their individual needs are being met. As an example of this type of management, the workload plan would require baths to be completed by 11 a.m. instead of treating the patients as individuals and allowing them autonomy in planning their morning care.

However, the authoritarian management style has a purpose and a place. There are times when this type of management can and does work; it is usually situational. It is very effective in a code situation when one person needs to take charge to save a life. It can also be effective if there are time factors dictating a massive amount of work needing to be accomplished in a short period of time or if your level of knowledge is such that direction is required. Although you may not want to adopt this management style permanently, it could be used effectively as situations demand.

Situations exist in which this type of management style is crucial for success, such as during an emergency. If a visitor or older adult falls to the floor in cardiac arrest, this type of manager would take over, give orders, and, in all likelihood, save the life of the person. The problem with this management style is that life is not a constant series of emergencies. This style does not allow for the creative and caring approaches that are necessary for effective gerontological nursing. Often, older persons miss out on the best possible care, and the employees miss out on opportunities to learn and grow as they implement new care practices.

Permissive or Laissez Faire

The permissive style can be either very effective or completely chaotic. There is no real direction displayed in this type of management as there is often more delegation rather than guidance. In general, with this management style, the employee must be able to function on his or her own. This can be very advantageous if your employees are able to function at higher levels and take responsibility for the outcome. The basic strategy is to allow the employees to make the decisions, do the planning, set the goals, and essentially manage the organization. This management style views employees as ambitious, responsible, intelligent, and creative.

It is important to examine this type of management style in relationship to organizations involved in gerontological health care. For many people, especially those who need guidance, the permissive style can result in a feeling of no direction. It is not motivational or empowering for those who need direction and can actually create a sense of havoc. In some instances, it can set up a situation detrimental to patient safety.

It is difficult to envision the federal guidelines for safety (Occupational Safety and Health Administration [OSHA]) or for nursing home licensure carried out in a permissive or laissez faire manner. The same is true for quality-assurance programs in health-care environments. Most facilities providing care to older adults require specific attention to the documentation that keeps an organization in operation. It also is necessary to have layers of responsibility that ensure that every person in the facility receives the best possible care with attention to detail.

In other environments, permissive management is very successful. An example is a group of highly motivated, professional people, such as a group of researchers, for whom independent thinking is rewarded. Conversely, it is difficult to imagine an effective nursing home or hospital unit being managed with this style of leadership.

Democratic or Participative

The democratic style is thought to be the preferred style in most situations. Allowing decisions and input from others and encouraging participation can help to create a high-functioning team. When we discuss communication later in this chapter, you will see that a democratic team approach is effective, and the synergism created allows for more to be accomplished.

The democratic management style places strong emphasis and value on the people on the team. The manager gathers information from the other team members and presents it to the group. All suggestions from the group are considered before decisions are made by the group (Dahlkemper, 2018). This is a very open system of management, yet it identifies the individuals who are responsible for the various projects being managed.

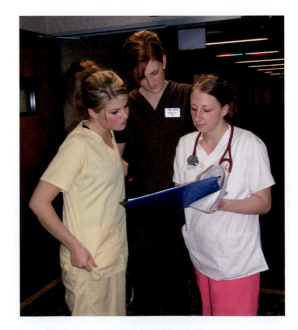

A democratic management style involves others in decision making.

The advantage of this type of management is that a majority of the employees will accept decisions because they have been part of the decision-making process. The disadvantage is that it often takes longer for decisions to be made, and it may not be the best management style when quick action is necessary. Generally, however, the results are positive, and employees tend to be very satisfied. This is a style that works well in gerontological environments because it is focused on people and includes the employee, the older adult, and the older adult's family members. It is a system that considers continuous change and improvement and assigns responsibility for such ventures.

Multicratic or Eclectic

Multicratic or eclectic allows the use of all styles of management discussed already. Different styles are needed for individual situations. This style of management allows for maximum participation and optimal outcome in most situations. The disadvantage of using a multicratic style is that managers must be highly skilled. They need to know and understand the different management styles and be able to assess what each person and/or situation needs to achieve optimal outcomes. The disadvantage is that it also allows for misjudgment of situation, an employee or peer, or a patient or patient situation.

Transformational

In a **transformational leadership** style, leaders work to meet the needs of employees and patients, allow and encourage participative decision making, strive to bring out the best in everyone, provide ongoing support for staff and patients, and strive to remove barriers to practice and empowerment (Grossman & Valiga, 2017).

The main concepts associated with transformational leaders include consideration of the individual, intellectual stimulation, and inspiring motivation (Qarani, 2017). Transformational leaders encourage staff to perform at their highest levels and empower them through mentoring and professional development. This type of leader welcomes staff ideas and innovative thinking. Staff are inspired to think outside of the normal routine and create ideas and plans that improve patient care. Transformational leaders encourage others to work toward the common good rather than focus on self-interests. Studies have indicated that transformational leadership inspires employees to exceed patient care standards and may

influence patient outcomes. The advantage of using this style in gerontological settings is it places focus on motivating and supporting staff and their individual needs with the goal of helping them become better care providers, which improves patient care for older adults.

As an LPN nurse manager, you need to evaluate yourself and determine with which general management style you are most comfortable. Then consider whether it is a style that is best used in the care of older people. If it is not, you need to learn more about other management styles and, with that knowledge, consider making changes in yourself. You may need to find a mentor who has a management style you would like to learn more about and ask that person to assist you. This mentor could teach you, become a role model for you, and assist you in applying the management techniques you want in the real-world setting. Being a manager is a challenging facet of your professional life. Take the time to learn the skills and patterns of thought that you need to function at your most effective level.

Evidence-Based Practice

Saleh, U., O'Connor, T., Al-Subhi, H., Alkattan, R., Al-Harbi, S., & Patton, E. (2018). The impact of nurse managers' leadership styles on ward staff. *British Journal of Nursing, 27*(4), 197–203.

These authors studied the leadership styles displayed by nurse managers from the viewpoint of the staff working in the acute environment. This study noted four leadership styles as perceived by their employees:

1. Relational—Collaboration and cooperation between nursing leadership and staff to enhance patient outcomes
2. Preferential—Differential treatment of staff by nurse managers based on nationality or other reason
3. Communication chain—Use of a chain of command for assistance when encountering issues, which may lead to conflict when staff are not given feedback regarding resolution or if the request was forwarded to the next higher level
4. Ineffectual—Lack of awareness on the part of managers about employee satisfaction, fairness, unequal treatment, being proactive, involvement of staff in decisions, and listening

This study found that perceived management styles had a large impact on staff recruitment, retention, turnover, and satisfaction, all of which affect patient care.

Questions

1. Think about the strategies you could implement to improve communication and relations with your colleagues and supervisors/supervisees in a multicultural clinical nursing environment.
2. As a new manager, what can you do to eliminate or minimize staff nurses' perception of preferential leadership style in your clinical setting?

population. Culture is described as behaviors and beliefs of a group of interacting humans. Cultural differences are now common and require the health-care system to be sensitive to what a particular group may think, feel, experience, expect, and believe. Health-care employees are often multicultural and must understand each other to work collaboratively. Nurses and other staff must display cultural sensitivity and competence to work effectively with other staff, patients, and families from different cultures. Look for opportunities to meet and talk with members of another culture to enhance understanding.

COMMUNICATION

The most important skill in any style of management in any situation is communication. Nurses in gerontological care spend 85% of their time communicating with a variety of people who are involved in the care of older adults. Mastering the skills of communication is essential for a successful LPN. Communication involves delivering messages that will be understood; listening to messages that may or may not be confusing; and properly interpreting messages that have been misdirected or are delivered with intense emotion, such as anger.

For the LPN, the art of communication involves various groups of people. The LPN needs to be able to communicate successfully with the older adult, the family, or other members of the person's support group, and the numerous members of the interdisciplinary health-care team. Being part of a team, especially a high-functioning team, is not an easy task; it requires effort on the part of every team member. Your communication skills, along with collaboration, credibility, compassion, and coordination, are important factors in demonstrating competence and respect to all, including the patients in your care. Expertise in communication is demanded every day from individuals who manage, direct, or administer care to older people.

Cultural Considerations

Globalization, the interaction of people, communities, and governments around the world, has led to a diverse workforce as well as a diverse patient

Verbal Communication

Verbal communication is the exchange of ideas and understanding through the use of spoken words and phrases. For the message to be received, the sender must use words and phrases that are appropriate for the listener. The success of all communication is measured by the question: Was the message properly received?

It should be easy to remember sitting in a class and "listening" to a lecture or presentation when you did not "receive" the message. Perhaps you were too tired to concentrate, or the instructor was boring or had inappropriate content to share. For communication to occur, being present is not enough. The critical measure is whether the listener actually understood or "received" the message. The best way to ensure the message was received correctly is to ask for feedback. What did the recipient hear you say? Obtaining feedback allows you to clarify any misunderstandings while emphasizing key points.

Nonverbal Communication

Nonverbal communication is the ability to share messages without using words. It refers, among other things, to a person's body posture (is the person tired and slouched over, or excited and alert), the tone and speed of the voice, the kind of clothes a person wears, and hand and facial movements. Nonverbal communication is considered to be the most honest communication a person can receive. Someone may say, "I'm having a great day. How are things for you?" in a cheerful-sounding way, but an examination of his appearance may indicate something different. The face is not smiling, and the posture is one of fatigue. The person's hands may be clenching and unclenching as a symptom of stress. Another classic example is a resident in a nursing home who is asked each morning, "How are you?" and each day responds verbally, "I'm fine." The person asking the question is busy with the breakfast tray or the linen change and does not look at the sad and worried face of the resident who answers with the reply that is expected, rather than with the truth.

The ability to recognize honest communication and respond to it is crucial for a successful nurse manager. The nurse manager must learn to develop the refined skill of understanding nonverbal communication because it conveys valuable information about patients and employees. Nonverbal communication is an honest method of communication and allows the LPN to follow up on problems and concerns that otherwise might not have been recognized.

Communicating With Patients and Residents

The decision to work with elderly adults is a commitment to accept the normal physiological changes that accompany the aging process. That commitment requires knowledge of the normal changes that occur in elderly people (see chapter 2) and the skill to work with them successfully as they move through the change process. A tendency exists in our ageist society to judge older people negatively because of the normal aging processes they exhibit. Normal aging changes that might affect communication are slower speech, presbycusis (difficulty in discriminating sounds), presbyopia (difficulty seeing near objects), and overall slower movements or responses to what is being communicated. The knowledgeable LPN recognizes these as normal occurrences and responds to them with skill and compassion.

Some people are impatient and negative about the aging process. This is ageist behavior and is unacceptable in any setting. The skills necessary for successful communication with older adults must be firmly based on respect for them as individuals. If that ingredient is missing, communication is unsuccessful. Consider the following strategies (not every older adult would need every strategy):

- Do not approach the person from the side because you may not be seen, and the person could be startled by your sudden appearance. Approach only from the front. This factor is important because of the gradual loss of peripheral vision that often accompanies aging.
- Place yourself on eye level with the older person so that a comfortable presence occurs during the communication process.

- Reach out and touch the person if it seems appropriate; this is often the bridge to a trusting relationship.
- Speak at a normal rate and do not shout, even if the older person is having trouble hearing. Shouting does not overcome the problems of presbycusis. Speak in a normal tone and speak slower than usual, but not so slow as to insult the person.
- If the patient is having trouble hearing you, move closer and speak in a normal tone. Moving closer often allows for lip reading or the reading of facial expressions.
- Pleasantly repeat what is being said, if necessary.
- Do not be impatient or judgmental.
- Place yourself and the older adult in a setting where there is a bright but not glaring light.
- Use a setting without disturbing or distracting noises.
- If the older adult gets confused while speaking or responding to a question, give the person time to collect personal thoughts. Do not rush the person.
- Repeat questions or comments in a different sentence structure if the older person is having trouble understanding what is said. Do not keep repeating the same information in the same way.
- Reflect on what the older person has said by repeating it back in a different way; for example, "Do you mean that you are lonely because your wife is in the hospital and not able to visit you here in the nursing home?"
- Listen carefully to the words used and verify what they mean.
- "Listen" carefully to the body language and other nonverbal communication and verify what they mean.

Your goal is to have the message successfully received. The use of these basic, caring strategies enhances your achievement of that goal and your relationships with the older adults in your care.

Communicating With the Families of Older Adults

Often, the family members of older patients or residents are worried, exhausted (if there has been extensive care given at home), and experiencing feelings of guilt over the condition of their family member or the necessity of admitting their loved one to a healthcare facility. Successful communication with this varied group is challenging because of the emotions involved. The issues involved often go beyond concern over an admission to a hospital or nursing home

Focused Learning Chart: Understanding Nonverbal Communication

Critical to Learn, to Recognize, and to Respond to as a Nurse Manager	The Most Honest Form of Communication	Examples
		Posture
		Facial expressions
		Tone and speed of voice
		Personal hygiene
		Type of clothing being worn
		Hand and facial movements
		Symptoms of stress

to such highly charged questions as the right to die, the decision whether to do an amputation, or dealing with a diagnosis such as Alzheimer's disease.

Point of Interest

Most of you have either played sports or watched sports being played, by your children or professionals. In each sporting activity there is a certain etiquette that is followed if the game is played well. The etiquette, or the rules, are not the same for each sport, but the rules for each sport are equally important. For instance, in basketball, body contact denotes a foul. Depending on how many fouls or what kind of foul, the opposing team may be awarded an extra shot or two, which can culminate in a loss to the offending team. Soccer penalizes teams when players are "off sides." Baseball has a set of rules that readily change depending on your age, your gender, and your league. The rules for each type of sporting activity are somewhat different, and the penalties for each variation of the game rules also differ. The primary concept is that if you are playing the game and you violate the rules—even if you do not know the rules—you will receive a penalty. Ignorance is no excuse when you are playing the game. The better you are, the more you play, and the more skilled you become, the more you will understand the subtleties of the game rules or etiquette. The same is true for understanding the

scope of practice or the appropriate etiquette for leadership and management for the LPN. Remember these words: "Ignorance is no excuse." Knowing there is a protocol and that the protocol changes for each place of employment, or each unit or floor, at your place of employment is important. Know the rules and use them to your advantage as you maintain the highest level of safe patient care.

It is crucial for the LPN to recognize the emotional environment of the family members before communicating with them. The goal is still the same: You want the message to be received by the listener. Some communication strategies for families are as follows:

- Listen before you attempt to impart information. It is essential that you evaluate the emotional environment to determine if they are able to listen to you. Often, just listening allows for you to learn critical information that you otherwise would not learn.
- Plan to spend time with the family members. They have questions and concerns, and they deserve to have them addressed.
- Family members often feel guilty over some issue with their loved one and need to discuss these issues and have them clarified. Families need not feel guilty unless evidence of elder abuse is found.
- Find a quiet place to speak to the family. It should be a place where they can sit comfortably and be

together as a group. The nurses' station is never an appropriate place for meaningful communication other than the simple sharing of facts.

- As nurse manager, the LPN needs to facilitate the sharing of information with the family. This could mean arranging an appointment with the social worker or assisting a family member to reach the physician.
- The older adult's family is as important as the older person. Generally, strong personal relationships that are interdependent exist. Always treat the family members with the same high level of respect and concern that you use with the older adult.

Interdisciplinary Team Communication

As an LPN you will interact, possibly on a daily basis, with an interdisciplinary team (IDT) that can provide services and knowledge to enhance the well-being of your individual patient, as well as provide a greater benefit to your organization as a whole (Lancaster, Kolakowsky-Hayner, Kovacich, & Greer-Williams, 2015). Working with a dietitian to help determine the best diet for your diabetic patient when the patient is discharged from your facility may help your patient understand better why it is necessary to check blood sugar three times a day and adjust diet and insulin accordingly. Involving a medical social worker to provide follow-up care for this same patient has the potential to increase your patient's compliance and safety once in the home environment. Including family members who can give encouragement as the patient with newly diagnosed diabetes learns to make life changes will provide the support the patient needs to maintain compliance with this required change of lifestyle. The combined knowledge and skills of these team members provides a much better outcome than if any one of these team members were to try to go it alone. This type of collaboration in patient care is an active form of synergism that can significantly benefit safe patient outcomes and reflect positively on your organization. Generally, the care given to older people in all settings is based on the interdisciplinary approach. It is critical that the nurse manager be an active and contributing part of this team. Generally, nurses are with the patients 24 hours a day, or if the older person is a home patient, the nurse generally sees the individual more frequently than other members of the team. This constant attention provided by the nurse to the patient provides a vast amount of personal and

pertinent information. It is essential that the nurse manager be active in contributing to the knowledge base and planning of the IDT.

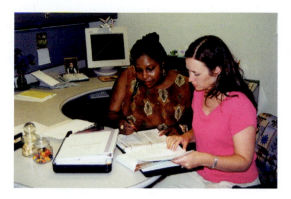

When working with a colleague on patient or resident care or other projects, be sure that your message is received. It pays to check and double check.

Concern arises over how to share information the nurse has gathered about the older person. It needs to be shared with skill so that the message is received. This process is different in a group setting than it is with an individual patient or family members. The group consists of professionals who have specialized knowledge regarding the older person. There is rarely sufficient time to discuss the patients in a thorough, relaxed manner. A time crunch often exists in IDT planning that establishes a unique atmosphere for communication. Following are strategies for communicating with an IDT:

- Come prepared! There is no time to waste in these meetings, whether in groups or one on one.
- Plan ahead and have priority concerns in your mind or on a piece of paper.
- This is not just a team of nurses, and members of an IDT may not understand a nursing concept that is very familiar to you. Because nursing is its own specialty, you may be asked to justify your requests or concerns or to teach the team about a nursing concept.

In most situations, the nurse has the role of patient or resident advocate. This occurs naturally because of the amount of time nurses spend with patients compared with other disciplines. This time allows for personal information and concerns to be communicated. It is crucial that the patient advocacy role be accepted by the nurse so that the patient is protected from the system and its potentially depersonalizing effects.

ADDITIONAL COMMUNICATION SKILLS

Specific skills are necessary for successful communication, and each of these skills can be used appropriately in all settings. Such skills are necessary to clarify communication errors, or potential errors, and are commonly necessary in difficult situations. They are important for every LPN to add to their communication skills checklist, and their importance can be compared with that of being expert at cardiopulmonary resuscitation (CPR). You may not use the skills very often, but when they are necessary, you need to know how to use them.

Assertive Communication Skills

The normal physiological reaction to being attacked physically or verbally is "fight or flight." This reaction occurs without thinking about it; it is normal physiology. When a situation occurs in which you are being attacked verbally or feel threatened by what is being said or done, the normal response is to fight back (an argument) or to take flight (avoidance). In the framework of assertive communication, these two normal responses are more formally identified as *aggressive*—fight—or *passive*—flight. The third concept that belongs on a continuum between these two is *assertive*—dealing with the problem.

Ideally, you would use assertive behavior when someone has violated the rights of an individual either verbally or physically. Assertive behavior is the most effective response to that violation. The major rule regarding the concept of assertive communication is simply that the assertive response *must not* violate the rights of the person who just infringed on your rights. What does that look like? An argument is the best example. Someone comes to the nurses' station and criticizes you in an angry, loud manner. There are residents or patients, visitors, and co-workers in the area listening to this *aggressive* communication. It is embarrassing and humiliating to be the victim of a communication delivered in such an inappropriate way. The normal physiological response is either to run away, perhaps crying (*passive*), or to scream back (*aggressive*). Screaming back or starting an argument is a violation of the other person's rights. It does not matter if he or she deserves it; it is still wrong. The *passive* behavior, or running away, does not violate the other person's rights, but it does not resolve the situation or problem.

Assertive communication requires that the person being violated not respond in a normal physiological fashion to the situation. Instead, it is necessary to resist the normal response and use the skills of communication to promote problem-solving. This is done most effectively in a private area. Assertive communication often follows this response format:

- *"I feel"*—Tell the other person how the aggressive attack made you feel. Perhaps you feel frustrated, devalued, angry, or frightened. Many other options are available for you to describe how you feel about what has been said.
- *"When you"*—Describe for the person the behavior that has caused you to feel the way you do. It could be "when you raise your voice at me," "when you talk about private concerns in public," "when you demand things from me that I cannot do," or "when you criticize me in front of others." Many other statements could be used here. The statements used must not be personal statements that attack the other person.
- *"We should"*—Together determine a solution to the problem. Ask what the two of you can do to prevent this from happening again. The aggressive person may respond with more hostility; in that case, restate your words in a calm manner.

Active Listening

Another communication skill that complements assertive behavior is that of *active listening*. Most people respond to aggressive and negative remarks with defensive communication. While the aggressor is making comments, the person being attacked generally is mentally preparing the defense to the aggressor's attack. These are the defensive comments that often provoke an argument. They follow the script of "It is not my fault; now let me tell you why!"

Active listening requires that the person being verbally attacked listens to what is being said. Because of the natural inclination to prepare a defense, listening is challenging. Just listen, and, while listening, try to determine the cause of the problem beyond the apparent anger.

The person who is out of control must be removed to a private setting, such as an office or a place away from other people. This prevents that individual from self-embarrassment in front of others, and it places you in an environment with fewer distractions.

After the angry person has finished saying what they need to say, he or she will take a deep breath and stop talking. This is where the person uneducated in communication skills presents his or her defense. You, the nurse manager, need skills beyond the ordinary person, however. Active listening is one of those skills. The deep breath is the signal to use the information you learned, while listening, to clarify the problem and negotiate a solution.

CRITICALLY EXAMINE THE FOLLOWING

Think back to the last "failed communication" you either observed or took part in. Would it have helped make the conversation successful if the skills of assertive communication had been used? Briefly describe the failed communication and then reword it using the assertive communication pattern.

Assertive Communication Pattern

"I feel . . . "
"When you . . . "
"We should . . . "

Comments such as "You seem so frustrated with … ," "It is unlike you to be so upset," or "How can I help?" are effective ones to use. They are not what the aggressive person expects to hear and generally prevent the person from losing control again. They are helpful comments that show caring and problem-solving skills. These are hallmark behaviors for nurse managers. The next move is for the two people involved to sit down and look at the problem rationally and work on a solution. The whole process begins with the nurse being able to stop "self-defending" and focus on listening.

The format for active listening is as follows:

- Remove the conversation to a private setting.
- Listen.
- Do not prepare a defense.
- Listen for the deep breath that means the person has finished speaking.
- Show support for the other person's feelings.
- Negotiate how to resolve the problem.

Some LPNs reading this text may feel concern over being responsible for assertive communication and active listening skills. They are two of many possible communication skills that may have been discussed in this book. They are listed for a very specific purpose. LPNs, in management roles, have very challenging positions that may place them in

serious situations that must be managed rather than ignored. You might think to yourself, "But I am just an LPN!" and feel that your role does not involve managing and solving problems of this nature. If you are a nurse manager, however, you have an obligation to develop the skills necessary for managing these acute and potentially destructive problems.

CRITICALLY EXAMINE THE FOLLOWING

During the next week, carefully observe yourself or others as they communicate in professional settings. Determine whether you observe the following actions. Record your thoughts and make comments regarding each communication technique.

1. Passive communication:
2. Aggressive communication:
3. Assertive communication:
4. Active listening:
5. Inactive listening:

THE PLANNING HOOP

Decision making is one of the most important skills you will use in nursing. When you consider that nurses are the largest group of caregivers in our health-care delivery system, and that nurses provide the majority of care, then you have a better understanding of why good decision-making skills are so important. Your sound clinical judgment is central to your patient's well-being and optimal outcome. Your ability to assess a patient and identify all pertinent factors surrounding that assessment are of primary significance.

Every day, decisions must be made regarding the workload of the LPN and others that affect the scope of LPN practice. These are decisions that should be made with careful thought and planning, rather than casually and without attention to detail. The decision that may be required of you could be as simple as who will get the first bath as you give morning care, but even this decision may have serious implications for the patients or residents who are recipients of your care. Other decisions that may be required of the LPN nurse manager could include counseling an employee whose behavior is unacceptable, making care assignments, confronting a physician or therapist with an alternate plan of care for a resident, or managing daily staffing. None of these tasks—or the many others that are required of a nurse manager—are easy or simple. They require the highest level of skill and attention to manage the process of making such decisions effectively.

To set priorities and make excellent decisions, the LPN nurse manager must understand the importance of planning, which is an intelligent process of thinking based on facts and information, rather than on emotion and wishes. An example is the holiday schedule. Staff members want Christmas Day off to be with their families. You, the manager, want everyone on your staff to be happy, but you have a clear picture as to what would happen if you granted everyone's wishes for Christmas Day. Instead, you need to make a rotation plan for the holidays, or perhaps draw names out of a hat, assign requests according to seniority, or determine some other way for the Christmas Day shift to be adequately staffed.

Planning is a process that never ends. It can be thought of as a hoop with notches where you stop and enter another phase of the planning process; then you continue going around the hoop over and over again. It is unrealistic to develop a plan and think that it will never change. It may be perfect for the moment, a week, or even an entire year; but the complexity of health care and the individuality of patients or residents and staff members require that your excellent plan be continuously reevaluated. The planning (Fig. 12.1) begins with an assessment.

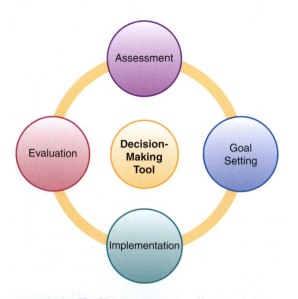

FIGURE 12.1 The Planning Hoop. An effective nurse manager must determine that planning is critical to getting the total workload done effectively.

Assessment

What is the problem or potential problem that concerns you? You know how to do a physical assessment. This is a similar process. Look at the problem from "head to toe" and assess what really is wrong. If it is a staffing problem in a nursing home, look at the mix of licensed and unlicensed personnel. Is it right for the needs of the residents?

Is the problem a lack of knowledge? If it is, you need to assess where the lack is, who needs to know the information, and how to teach it most effectively. Do not be distracted by other issues as you do your assessment. Keep focused on the problem you are trying to resolve and learn all you can about it. Otherwise, it would be similar to trying to assess two residents at the same time. One does not get a clear picture of the problem unless a focused effort is made.

Goal Setting

The next step in the planning hoop is to set goals. Now that you have a complete set of data regarding the problem, you have enough information to set goals. This is very similar to the nursing process. Instead of writing a care plan, you are preparing a plan to resolve a management problem. Make the goals reasonable and achievable. Not everyone can have Christmas Day off. If the problem is an unbalanced mix of licensed and unlicensed personnel, your goal could be to correct the mix through attrition and selective hiring within the next 6 months. If the problem is knowledge, your goal would be to have 100% of your staff attend a class on the information needed by a specific date. The goals should be meaningful and reflect your most careful and organized thinking.

Implementation

Implementation is the test of good planning. Was your assessment done accurately, and are your goals realistic? Perhaps the actual implementation requires you not to hire an RN or LPN when one applies because your staff has too great a proportion of licensed personnel. Or, implementation may mean that you need to find the budget money to pay the staff to attend the education program you determined they needed. In addition, you need a plan for getting everyone to attend. This could involve bonus money or other rewards, and in all likelihood, it would mean presenting the education program several times. Implementation is the actual performance of your plan.

Evaluation

Did your plan work? Was Christmas Day successfully staffed, and did the staff feel that the staffing decisions were made with fairness? Within 6 months, was your staff mix at the level where you needed it to be? How effective was your education program? Did it bring about the change you wanted? Such questions initiate the process of **evaluation**. A nurse manager cannot just do something and consider the problem solved. Instead, a careful evaluation must be performed so that the cycle of the planning hoop can begin again—once you have evaluated your plan, you need to do another assessment and begin the circle again.

Many people do not spend a great deal of time planning solutions to the unit's problems. The profession of nursing is filled with "doing" types of people. One of the critical skills of being a manager is to learn to quit "doing" and begin planning "to do." It is a challenge to take the time necessary to plan because planning does not enter into the conventional description of a "good nurse."

When a person is planning, that person is sitting somewhere quietly thinking. The profession of nursing generally does not see that as productive because beds need to be made, and there are baths and treatments to be given. With those unfinished care issues, how can a real nurse take the time to sit and think? A real nurse manager soon learns that doing the thinking or planning is critical to getting the total workload done effectively. So, fight the urge to be busy when planning is needed. Teach the staff that the time you spend planning is critical to the overall picture of care for patients and job satisfaction for them. Be courageous enough to use the planning hoop to resolve problems and prevent new ones. Because if you do not, the situation may then become a crisis that needs urgent management.

Crisis Management

A crisis manager is a person who does not take the time to plan. This manager waits until the week before Christmas to resolve the problem of the staffing crisis. A great deal of hysteria, excess energy, and distress are involved in solving problems when they occur, rather than foreseeing them and taking the time to plan a solution for the problem. The phrase, "All I do is run around and put out fires!" is indicative of the crisis manager. It is not effective management and can be prevented by the implementation of the planning hoop into your management style. Look

to the future and anticipate problems. Then devise a plan for solving them before a crisis happens.

Some situations still will become a crisis for even the best manager. Accept this, solve the problem, design a plan so it will not be a crisis the next time, and move on to the next situation.

THINK LIKE A NURSE

Prioritizing is actually a highly learned skill that can become a great asset to you, as well as the people in your care. It is an art when it is done correctly. Keep in mind that if you do not learn to prioritize correctly, you could very well put you and your patient at risk. Refer back to the case study at the beginning of this chapter. The ability you demonstrate in prioritizing your tasks and implementation of patient care can make a huge impact on your patient's outcomes. You need to make sure that the order of your prioritization can create an optimal outcome for the patient in a safe and caring environment.

PRIORITY SETTING

Every LPN has learned how to prioritize the work of giving patient or resident care. Traditionally, the sickest patient receives the nurse's attention first, and the least seriously ill person waits until last. This concept assumes that each patient is assessed and observed frequently, rather than being ignored until his or her turn comes to receive care.

Priority setting in management situations has a similar format. The priority of each management problem is determined after the assessment of the situation has been completed. The method for determining priority problems generally is based on determining what is essential for the organization or the person at the time. Staffing for Christmas Day is essential, as is giving pain medications in a timely manner.

The nurse manager needs to think of the entire organization when determining priorities. They often are divided into two categories: (1) concerns that relate to patient or resident care, and (2) concerns that relate to the process of running the business of the institution.

Each category should be considered separately. However, many of the same issues and concerns often arise that apply to both categories when implementing problem solutions. Each concern needs to be listed as a *need* or a *want*. Needs should be met before wants. It is helpful to use this method for categorizing your management concerns before prioritizing them.

Making Care Assignments for Older Adults

One of the day-to-day management skills used by LPNs is that of making care assignments for older adults. The skill of making effective assignments is crucial to any clinical area. The goal of making successful care assignments is to match the appropriate caregiver with the older person in a manner that allows for the best nursing care to be administered and received. As the manager, you also need to focus on an assignment that affords the highest level of employee satisfaction. This requires sensitivity, awareness of the skills and attitudes of others, and the ability to form a plan and to follow through on it. Several aspects of making care assignments should be examined.

When making care assignments, you must consider the personal skills of each person you are managing. You have learned how to assess older adults; now your question might be, "How do I accurately assess a nursing assistant's skills?" Dr. Patricia Benner (2001), who developed her nursing theory in her book, *From Novice to Expert*, describes a specific way to identify clinical skills. Benner's theory focuses on intensive care RNs, and their clinical expertise along the following five skill levels:

- Novice
- Advanced beginner
- Competent
- Proficient
- Expert

As a nurse manager, it is important for you to understand the five levels of clinical expertise and how you can use them to identify skill levels for CNAs and other individuals who work under your direction:

1. *Novice*—CNAs performing at this level have no prior experience with certain situations. They do not understand the detailed information regarding what is happening. They simply do not have the experience to understand what is going on in the situation. For example, a CNA may have several years of employment as a CNA but may not have any experience working on an Alzheimer's unit. As a nurse manager, you should be aware of such a lack of skill and may want to assign a novice CNA to work several shifts with a CNA who is experienced in caring for people with Alzheimer's disease.

2. *Advanced beginner*—CNAs functioning at this level can demonstrate limited acceptable performance. Advanced beginners generally have had multiple clinical experiences, independently or with a mentor, so that they have a general understanding of the clinical situation. Advanced beginners perform tasks using behavior that follows instructions only, rather than appropriate behavior for a specific situation.

   As the nurse manager, you may ask a CNA to assist a resident into the shower. When the CNA enters the room, the resident is found confused and combative. Rather than gauging the situation and deciding that this may not be the best time to give this resident a shower, the CNA does everything possible to complete the task of giving the shower. The focus is on the task, not the aspects of the specific situation or the needs of the older person.

3. *Competent*—A competent CNA has an increased level of skill and ability. The knowledge is based on following the positive role-modeling of other CNAs and dealing with various situations in which clinical skills were learned. A competent CNA still focuses on organizing the assigned tasks, however. A competent CNA makes sure the time is managed well in an effort to complete the tasks on the list, instead of basing work decisions on the older person's needs.

   As a nurse manager, it is critical that you ensure that the resident's needs are actually being met by the CNA in a timely manner. Otherwise, the individuals you manage may give care based on a schedule and a list rather on than the needs of older adults.

4. *Proficient*—A proficient CNA is much more comfortable with clinical skills and has the ability to deal with different situations as they arise. A proficient CNA engages more with the older adult and family members instead of focusing on required tasks. The focus of nursing care of a proficient CNA is on the needs of the older person rather than on a list. An advantage to working with proficient CNAs is their ability to reprioritize the workload based on patient or resident needs. As a nurse manager, you may delegate several tasks to a proficient CNA, who then decides in what order they should be completed.

5. *Expert*—An expert CNA has experienced many different situations and has learned from the experiences. These experiences assist the CNA in making decisions based more on intuition (referred to by Benner as "intuitive knowing") than on timetables and rules. An expert CNA knows the older adult's patterns of behavior and is able to anticipate the unexpected. This complexity of skill and thinking assists the CNA in making decisions based on the "big picture" or the holistic needs of the person receiving care.

An expert CNA walks into a room where an older adult is behaving differently and spends time with the person in an effort to identify the problem. The expert CNA takes vital signs and asks questions so there are data to report to the licensed nurse. The expert CNA knows what to do for this patient.

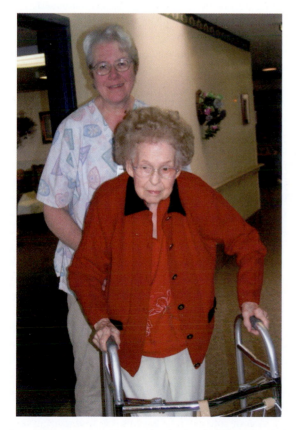

It is worth your time to consider the level of expertise that the CNAs who work with you have achieved. This knowledge influences your scheduling, educational programs, and, most importantly, the quality of care provided to older adults. It is your responsibility to identify and assist CNAs who need more education or experience.

Are you able to identify where your CNAs fit in Benner's five points of clinical expertise?

Do you have a new CNA who is still working at the novice level? If so, that person should be assigned to older adults who require only basic skills that were learned in the CNA class. A novice CNA also should be assigned to an expert CNA who can assist with care when needed and serve as a positive role model. Novice CNAs should not be assigned to give care to challenging patients or residents. They could be assigned to work with another CNA who has the challenging patient or resident and, in that way, have experiences that eventually lead the CNA to the level of expert without hurting an older person in the learning process.

Do you also have a CNA who has worked at the facility for several years, is very familiar with the residents, and has excellent clinical skills? That is the CNA who should be assigned to the most challenging individuals so that these older adults can benefit from the CNA's skills and knowledge. This may not always be the sickest patient on the unit. The assignment could be to the latest admission, in which the older person and the family are having a difficult time adjusting to the transitional stress of the admission.

It is important when developing staffing patterns that a team should not consist of a novice CNA and a novice licensed nurse. A better staffing pattern would be an expert CNA with a novice nurse or expert nurse with a novice CNA. The mix of novice and the levels of expertise that lead to expert are important to acknowledge and use as you manage care.

When you, as the nurse manager, have identified the expertise levels of each nursing assistant, you should praise each one for their special skills and allow them to use those skills. Assist employees to develop skills related to their interests and abilities and recognize them for the skills they develop. Assign staff members to older adults who would benefit from their skills and knowledge. This assignment ensures quality of care and employee self-esteem, which enhance the entire organization.

When working with older adults, it is generally more effective to assign the same employee to an older person for several days in succession. This practice allows the caregiver to learn the personal needs and nuances of the person receiving care and address each successfully. When a "new" person is assigned to an older person each day, it puts a demand on the older adult to explain once again that he or she cannot hear out of the right ear, that the older adult wants two cups of coffee on his or her breakfast tray, or that it is the older adult's right knee that does not work very well. Generally, a comfortable camaraderie and sense of teamwork develop between the caregiver and the care receiver, enhancing the work of healing as they work together over time.

Sometimes a difficult or demanding older person requires more energy and patience than most employees can provide day after day. When this occurs, the nurse manager should rotate the assignment in a direct effort to avoid burnout of the employees.

Another consideration for making assignments is that of physical demands. Often when caring for older adults or chronically ill patients, a heavy physical demand is made in turning, positioning, and assisting the older person to ambulate. When the nurse manager makes the assignment, the physical demands of the care required should be considered so as not to overwork a particular employee. Another consideration is the geographic placement of the rooms. It is unnecessary to make assignments that require an employee to travel to both ends of the hall or in other diverse patterns. Make a strong effort to group the room numbers assigned to avoid unnecessary walking. Most workdays are tiring enough.

Delegation

As the LPN manager, you need to know what is involved in delegating to CNAs or unlicensed assistive personnel (UAP). The goal is to delegate tasks while maintaining quality patient and resident care. Your first step is to familiarize yourself with the nurse practice act for the state where you work. This document defines the roles and responsibilities of a licensed nurse. You need to determine if the nurse practice act allows for **delegation** and, if so, whether there are any limitations as to what tasks or duties you can delegate to a CNA or UAP.

Your next step is to become familiar with the policy and procedures for your facility and the written job descriptions. Any job you assign must be within the employee's job description. After you have identified a task that can be delegated, you need to use sound delegation approaches. Also keep in mind how delegating this task would affect the safety of the older adult. Has the older person been accurately assessed, and are there any safety issues that need to be addressed? The National Council of State Boards of Nursing (NCSBN) has developed guidelines to help nurses ensure safe and proper delegation to

CNAs and UAP. The NCSBN's Five Rights of Delegation provides a checklist that nurses can use when making delegation decisions. The Five Rights of Delegation are:

1. The right task
2. The right circumstances
3. The right person
4. The right direction
5. The right supervision

Additionally, a joint endeavor by the American Nurses Association and the NCSBN produced the delegation decision tree, which is particularly helpful to nurses in a supervisory role (see Web Resources at the end of the chapter).

Generally, CNAs can do tasks that assist older adults with basic needs and activities of daily living. They cannot assess, plan, or evaluate any aspects of patient care. If an older person is taking digoxin (Lanoxin) for his heart, the nurse can delegate to the CNA the task of taking an apical pulse and notifying the nurse what the heart rate is when the pulse is taken. The CNA cannot decide if the older adult can have medication based on the pulse observed by the CNA. In addition, the nurse makes the decision as to when the pulse should be checked again. When working with CNAs, it is very important that the nurse give clear instructions regarding what time the task should be completed and whether the CNA needs to report back to the nurse directly after completing the task. It is a good practice to encourage CNAs to take notes and provide feedback to you as you are giving the information regarding the delegated assignment. When delegating a task to a CNA, you still are responsible for the older adult's care. If you delegate a task to a novice CNA, and the task should have been delegated to an expert CNA, or if you do not give proper supervision, you may be held responsible for the outcome of the care.

As a manager, you should always be willing to delegate certain projects. As organizational needs arise, you may be assigned a project that would not allow you to complete your regular workload. This is a good time to delegate routine work that can be done appropriately by someone else.

In your role as an LPN, you will find it necessary to do effective delegation. Does that mean that you delegate the projects that you do not want to do? Does delegating make you a lazy person? The answer to both of these questions is "no." Delegation of routine tasks to someone else frees the manager to work on more complicated unit needs. Because delegation is crucial to effective management, you want to ensure you are doing it as efficiently as possible. When delegating to anyone, your responsibility as the manager is to identify if they have the basic skills or education necessary to complete the assignment. You also should ensure they have the time to complete the assignment by the deadline without requiring them to put aside their regular job responsibilities. Delegating to someone who is interested in the assignment is a good choice.

When the individual for the assignment is identified, you should give him or her clear, direct instructions on what is to be done, including why the individual is doing the assignment. How the person completes the assignment should be an individual choice. This is often the most difficult part of delegation. When you delegate a responsibility in the manner described earlier and receive feedback, you must now allow the person to do the work. You can "check in," determine whether the person needs something, or just observe so that you can step in if there is a critical situation. Giving the employee the appropriate amount of autonomy in deciding how to complete the assignment is a positive factor for the employee and the key to successful delegation. It also is important that you do not over-supervise the employee. If you are going to watch and participate in every step of the project, you may want to ask yourself why you chose to delegate the task in the first place.

Definite timelines for completion of any delegated project should be discussed, and the manager should check in periodically to ensure that the deadline will be met. Monitoring the assignment periodically allows for questions and discussion regarding the project as the work is being done. Being available for interaction is an important concept. You always should be available to assist the employee if he or she is having difficulty or simply wants reassurance. Taking the delegated project back would be a last-resort behavior because it makes the employee feel like a failure and "demotivates" rather than motivates. When the project is complete, you must evaluate the performance, giving praise and additional information to the employee. This feedback lets the person know what was done well and what may be done differently next time he or she is given a similar assignment. Delegation is an effective way to assist someone to move from novice to expert because of the opportunity to develop new skills and have new experiences.

Wagner (2018) reviewed the process of delegation by nurses to CNAs and UAP. Nurses participating in the study reflected on the difficulty of delegation, including what is appropriate and the tendency to delay delegating due to lack of understanding of role expectations. Wagner noted that following a learning intervention, nurses, CNAs, and UAP had a better understanding of the roles and responsibilities of each. Rather than equate delegation with lack of trust or respect, each role acknowledged the need for delegation and noted an increase in teamwork with enhanced working relationships. It was interesting to note that following the learning intervention, there was a decrease in patient falls as well as an increase in patient satisfaction. The author recommends a brief huddle of staff following report where patient as well as unit needs are discussed, and all staff have an appreciation for the roles of each discipline.

Medication Aide–Certified

The Medication Aide–Certified (MA-C) is a developing role in health care, especially in the long-term health-care setting. The MA-C expands the education and knowledge of the CNA position by attending additional classroom and clinical hours in accordance with state regulations. It is the job of the MA-C to administer specifically selected medications safely under the supervision of a licensed health-care provider. Understanding appropriate delegation is important when working with this new health-care provider.

The MA-C must work at least 1 year, or 2,000 hours, as a CNA before taking a MA-C course. Concepts the MA-C learns and incorporates into patient care include the basic principles and techniques this position needs to know about medication and medication administration. The MA-C does not have the expanded knowledge or education of the licensed caregiver, but he or she does gain an overview of common drugs, including their effects and side effects and common interactions. MA-Cs are taught medication use in a diverse population and how to avoid common medication errors. This knowledge greatly increases patient safety, as long as the licensed personnel understand what can and cannot be delegated to the MA-C.

Drug classifications, basic principles, drug action, drug interactions, and general drug information are concepts covered in the MA-C course. Considerations to gender and age, including distribution, metabolism, excretion, and monitoring, will help the MA-C determine safe administration of medications in diverse health-care settings. Knowledge of how to work with a nurse to determine the correct drug order and ordering methods are among the skills taught in a MA-C course.

State laws and regulations associated with the role of the MA-C in the safe administration of medications in the health-care setting are important knowledge for the MA-C and for the licensed caregiver who delegates medication administration to the MA-C. There are legal and ethical aspects associated with the responsibilities of the MA-C and regulations that are identified for the licensed nurse in the delegation process. It is important for you, the LPN, to know and understand your state practice act as it is associated with this new position. Communication and accountability in giving safe patient care are extremely important skills for the licensed nurse.

The most important factor for the LPN is to always be cognizant of patient safety factors, the progression of delegation in the nursing process, and how the MA-C interacts and functions in this process. The skills discussed in this chapter on leadership will go far in helping you work in collaboration with the health-care team, including the MA-C, for optimal patient outcomes.

Rounding

Becoming a nurse manager is an ever-evolving process in terms of leadership, delegating tasks, making assignments, and ensuring quality care. Another way for the nurse manager to ensure the unit is functioning well is to periodically round on all staff and patients. Individual institutions may have policies as to when and how often rounding is to be done; ensure that you know what your facility requires.

Hugill, Sullivan, and Ezpeleta (2017) note that rounding enhances staff engagement, improves patient perceptions of the care received, reduces the likelihood of hospital created morbidities such as falls, and provides opportunities for staff and management to share goals, reduce confrontations, and promote an environment of respect and trust. The authors discuss the concept of coaching while rounding; nurse managers are able to share knowledge and experience with staff personnel while participating with employees in reflective thinking and critical decision making.

The overall conclusion reached through this study is that a program of rounding and coaching by nurse managers with other staff personnel enhances communication skills, eases the change process, and provides a safe environment for reflective thinking and decision making.

MANAGING PERSONNEL

As a nurse manager, you will be involved in, if not responsible for, the hiring and evaluating of employees. This is a critical aspect of your job and one that requires the highest level of professional skill and performance. This work cannot be done by intuition or "best guess." All personnel decisions directly affect the lives of the employees of the institution. Employees deserve as much care and attention as the patients.

The hiring process is where the employee begins a career with your organization or, if not employed, will leave with an impression that will be taken out to the community. It should be your desire to have that impression be a good one. Many legal issues are involved in the hiring process. Be sure to clarify them with your personnel manager or administrator. Laws exist that involve the advertisement of a job and how the interview is conducted, and federal rules identify questions that cannot be asked in an interview because of concern over discrimination. Be alert to these rules and follow them.

The purpose of interviewing someone for employment is to find someone who fits with the philosophy and vision of your institution. The applicant needs the licensure or certification that the job description demands and the experience to perform the job at a satisfactory level. The interview also allows the nurse manager to determine the shift availability and whether the potential employee is available for part-time or full-time work. An effort should be made to learn the specific interests of the applicant so that plans can be made to use any special skills and knowledge the person possesses. The screening process of the personnel department presumably would eliminate anyone unqualified for the job. Unqualified people do not need to be interviewed.

Interviewing

The purpose of the interview is to exchange information. Be prepared to give positive information about your facility to all applicants whether they are offered a position or not. You want applicants to say favorable things about your organization even if they are not selected for the job. During the interview, the nurse manager is expected to determine the applicant's:

- Dependability
- Skill level
- Willingness to assume the responsibilities of the job
- Willingness and ability to work with others
- Interest in the job
- Adaptability
- Consistency of goals with available opportunities
- Conformity of manner and appearance to job requirements

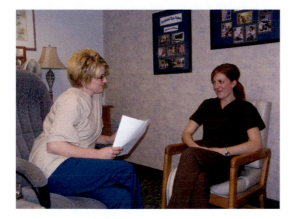

When interviewing someone for a position, establish a friendly and positive atmosphere. Be consistent in the interview process with all applicants and be honest in your assessment of qualifications.

The interview has definite purposes and should be conducted in a professional manner. It is not the place for social chitchat; however, some warm and friendly comments at the beginning of the interview should put the applicant at ease so that the interview can be less stressful.

The greatest predictor of the applicant's future success is past performance. Is this someone who has worked with older adults previously and enjoyed it? Has the applicant sought additional educational experiences that would enhance work in your type of setting? Was this person a desirable employee at the last place of employment or, if a new graduate, a good student? These crucial pieces of information should be noted on the application and verified in the interview.

It is your responsibility as the nurse manager to set the tone for honesty in the interview. Be specific and direct in your comments. It is helpful to have an interview guide available to use for every interview. This guide is a written document that contains questions, directions, and pertinent information to be shared with the applicant. The presence of an interview guide ensures you, the applicant, and the institution that the same process is being used in every interview. It avoids the gathering of prejudicial information and provides consistency in the interview process.

Questions on the interview guide should cover subjects such as which shifts the applicant is willing to work, whether part-time or full-time work is desired, and feelings about working with older people. It also could contain a brief case study or scenario about a gerontologically focused situation that requires a response from the applicant. The presence of two or three such questions gives you additional information about the potential employee. All applicants must be asked the same questions to avoid discrimination or the appearance of discrimination in choosing future employees. You also need to review the Title VII Civil Rights Act carefully before conducting any interviewing. This federal law prohibits discrimination in any personnel decision on the basis of race, color, sex, age, religion, or national origin. A comfortable format for an interview is as follows:

- Use an opening to establish rapport and put the applicant at ease.
- Share the interview procedure with the applicant.
- Discuss the applicant's interests in being employed at your facility.
- Obtain an educational history.
- Discuss future plans of the applicant, such as upward mobility and future education.
- Share case studies and situations and discuss them.
- Inform the applicant about the organization.
- Allow time for the applicant to ask questions and clarify information given and received.
- Close by clarifying how to reach the applicant after the interview, informing the applicant when the decision will be made, and thanking the applicant for considering your organization for employment.

Employee Evaluation

After the nurse manager has made a decision to hire an applicant, a very focused effort must be made to give that person a thorough and extensive orientation to the job, its standards, and its expectations. The quality of personnel hired and retained in the organization determines the success of the organization. The quality of the orientation directly determines the overall success for the organization and the employee.

After the employee has had the opportunity to work with other qualified employees and to establish an effective working routine, the new employee can be allowed to work independently. A resource person should always be available, in some way, to the new employee for the first 3 months of employment. This provision indicates that a sincere effort is being made to ensure success for the organization and the employee.

Each organization has an established process for evaluating employees. The first evaluation may occur at 3, 6, or 12 months. Earlier and more frequent evaluations take more of the manager's time but also provide regular feedback for the employee. Overall, it is generally time well spent. Your organization also should have an established written form for evaluating employees. This process should be consistent for all employees to avoid discrimination.

For all employing organizations, a performance appraisal may be based on the following five basic realistic assumptions:

1. The appraisal is intended to help an employee improve the management of the workload.
2. Employee appraisal is a difficult process, but it is a skill that can be mastered with hard work.
3. Few people like the current form (a perfect one simply does not exist).
4. The employee's supervisor makes the appraisal.
5. Information must be gathered on a day-to-day basis.

THINK LIKE A NURSE

One of the most effective habits you can develop as a manager who does performance evaluations is that of gathering evaluation information on a daily basis. With the use of computers, it is much easier than it used to be to get this information organized. A file or folder can be created on a computer for each employee. When something happens, you simply record it. It could be a compliment from a family member or a display of poor judgment. Making notes on your performance disk is something like doing your patient charting: It needs to be done every day. You won't make a note on every employee every day, but it is important to record the significant things that have happened for the day. This technique for organizing data will make your evaluation process much easier. Remember that this information should be password-protected if you are using a shared computer.

The challenge to the nurse manager is that the performance appraisal must accurately reflect the person's actual job performance. It cannot contain prejudicial information, hearsay, or undocumented information. It is designed to be helpful to the employee, and by assisting the employee to improve, it is helpful to the organization.

Traditionally, potential evaluation problems can contribute to an inaccurate evaluation. The first one is *leniency error*. This occurs when a supervisor wants everyone to be buddies or to be the manager's best friend. It results when the manager "looks the other way" or gives an employee the "benefit of the doubt" rather than finding out what really happened.

A competent nurse manager cannot afford to be "best friends" with employees. The manager needs to be the manager. It is crucial to success for the manager to be an honest and fair person who does not lose the ability to be objective. The leniency error does not help an employee improve, and it does not contribute to the overall functioning of the organization.

The *recency error* is an indication of a manager who has forgotten the basic assumptions of evaluation and who has not kept records of employee performance over the year. Because of the lack of written record, the manager evaluates only on what is remembered most recently. All employees know when their annual review is scheduled and often find it easy to "look good" during the time just before their evaluation. This type of evaluation process enhances neither the performance of the employee nor that of the organization.

The *halo error* is allowing one trait to influence the entire evaluation. It could be either a strongly positive trait or a strongly negative one. Either way, it clouds the objective evaluation of an employee if only the halo behavior is remembered. Evaluations need to be fair and comprehensive regarding the employee's behavior and skills.

The evaluation process is critical to the growth and stability of the organization. Evaluation standards cannot be successful if they are ambiguous. The process of rewarding a strong employee and counseling a poor employee must be valid. This happens only if the manager maintains a professional and consistent attitude toward the evaluation process.

Negative or probationary evaluations are very difficult for all managers to give. Use the same process you would use for a positive evaluation. Make it fair and comprehensive, and share the information you have in a professional manner. For all terminations, the process of counseling the employee must be carefully documented over time. This is an act of fairness toward the employee and a protection against litigation for the institution.

Providing Education for Employees

This chapter has discussed management concepts needed to supervise employees. Now the question is, "What is the nurse manager's role in providing continuing education to the staff?" What can the nurse manager do to move CNAs from novice care providers to expert care providers? Health care changes on a regular basis, and as licensed professionals, we all are trying to keep up with the changes. It is important for unlicensed health-care providers to keep up with health-care changes as well. As a nurse manager, you need to assist with this endeavor.

Several areas of education need to be addressed. The first is the orientation process for new employees. It is suggested that orientation programs for new CNAs should last at least 3 months. An orientation program should match, one on one, a new or novice CNA with a veteran or expert CNA. The program should provide the new CNA with the information needed to function as an effective member of the nursing team at the end of the orientation period. The orientation information should include the policies and procedures for the facility, information about the daily operation and schedules for the facility, and, most important, detailed information about the older adults and the specific skills needed to give excellent nursing care.

The expert CNA who is willing to be a role model and mentor for the new employee should be a valued employee who consistently demonstrates expert clinical skills and care behaviors. This is a CNA who demonstrates willingness to orient the new employees as well. It is appropriate to demonstrate valuing of employees who participate in the orientation program through some type of a reward.

Novice CNAs must have continuity of instruction throughout the orientation. If the facility has five units, the CNA should spend equal amounts of time on each unit. The time spent should be consecutive days so that the CNA can become acquainted with the staff and procedures on one unit before moving to the next. This approach also provides consistency of care for the older adults who are getting to know the new employee.

At the end of the orientation period, the new employee should be evaluated. The nurse manager must decide at this time if the employee is acceptable for the facility. If you are not satisfied with the employee's performance, a plan of action should be developed to assist the employee in meeting the requirements necessary for successful employment. This also may be the time when the nurse manager may make the difficult decision to terminate the employee.

When a nurse manager hires an employee, an effort should be made to increase and maintain the skills of the employee. There are various ways to accomplish this goal. Mentorship programs match individuals together when one person has the required skills and the other person needs to learn them. These programs generally last for a longer time than orientation and in most cases are less formal. A CNA who is interested in becoming an LPN may be matched with an LPN who is interested in helping the CNA prepare for nursing school. You may have an employee who works well with people with Alzheimer's disease and their families. This individual could work as a mentor for other employees who would like to possess the same skills.

Some facilities use clinical ladder models to increase employee skills. Different levels of knowledge and ways to obtain and document the skills are identified. When an employee meets the requirements of one level or "rung" of the ladder, there often is a promotion. When employees have met the requirements for an advanced level, they often are recognized with a ceremony and a monetary award, an increase in pay or a set one-time dollar amount. Facilities have found that clinical ladders can assist with employee retention and improve employee morale. The benefit to the facility is better patient care. The improvement in care is a result of the facility seeking to prepare its own expert CNAs, LPNs, and RNs.

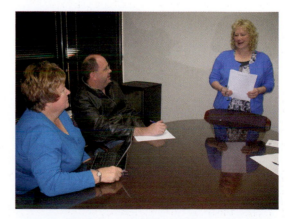

This LPN is providing an education session to staff to update their skills.

Safe, Effective Nursing Care

Working Effectively With Interprofessional Teams

Mr. Wise is a 69-year-old man recently admitted to a long-term care facility. He has been active all of his life but was recently in an automobile accident that left him paralyzed from the waist down. His wife is 10 years younger but she is unable to care for Mr. Wise at home because of her own health problems. When Mr. Wise is admitted, he is very upset and distraught. As the nurse goes in to begin the assessment, Mr. Wise is verbally abusive and screams at the nurse to leave him alone. He then turns to his wife and tells her to leave and never come back. He tells her she has abandoned him and he never wants to see her again. The wife begins crying uncontrollably but says she will not leave. Mr. Wise tells the nurse to help him prepare to return home immediately. The nurse has been on the job for only 3 weeks and does not feel that she is equipped to deal with a patient in this type of emotional distress. The nurse realizes that she has other members of the interprofessional team in the building and has identified that she will need some help with this patient.

Other members of the interprofessional team include her charge nurse, the physical therapist (PT), the nutritionist, the CNA, and the medical social worker (MSW). The nurse calls for help from the CNA and the MSW. Her rationale is that the CNA can help with the physical needs of this patient and the MSW can provided the emotional support and identify a support system for this family during this time of crisis. The nurse makes sure she identifies a caring CNA, even though this CNA is working in another wing of the facility. The CNA and MSW both arrive within minutes of one another.

The MSW is able to work with the patient and calm his fears. When the wife determines that the husband has settled down, she becomes more interactive and begins to help her husband settle into his new environment. The CNA begins to interact with the spouse and explains the layout of the building and the activities as she helps the spouse put away belongings and organize the room. Within a few minutes, the MSW has calmed the patient and begins talking with the spouse about community support that would be advantageous for her well-being.

In this situation, the nurse had the knowledge to recognize the contributions of other team members, in this case, the MSW. The nurse was able to request help from the MSW and demonstrated respect for the attributes that the MSW could bring to this situation as a team member in this patient care setting.

1. What would the outcome have been if the nurse had tried to handle this emotional family situation on her own?
2. Why do you think it was a good idea for the nurse to integrate the skills of the CNA and the MSW into this family's personal and emotional crisis?
3. How do you feel the nurse demonstrated respect for the professional attributes of the MSW?

Priority Setting

How do you highlight one priority among a group of highly important nursing skills? For instance, understanding good leadership and management, fine-tuning your delegation skills, implementing good decision making and critical thinking, setting priorities in safe patient care, implementing quality patient care, and following good communication skills are all significant parts of your job, which means they are all areas to prioritize.

To set a good example, a priority must be set. This chapter focuses on communication skills; the rationale for this is that becoming skilled at communication will highlight all of the other skills mentioned in this chapter. It comes into play when you implement good leadership, delegate, give instruction, and receive report; it is significant in accurately relaying the decisions you make, and it is essential for safe patient care. You need to learn good communication skills and incorporate them in every interaction associated with your job.

Please reread the sections in the chapter referring to these skills. Then consider how you can become proficient in using them. You may want to read more about them in management books in the library. Talk to your faculty person about them. Discuss them with nurses (RNs and LPNs) where you work or during your clinical experiences. Observe people in all settings to see if and how the skills are used. You may find that that many people do not use them. In these cases, problems may arise.

To be really good at active listening and assertive communication, you need to do what *does not* come naturally. You need to overcome your natural tendencies as a person. With attention to yourself and others, you can develop these skills, and they will be strengths to you throughout your career.

A CULTURE OF INCIVILITY

Before concluding this chapter on leadership, a brief discussion of a hostile work environment is necessary. While you may not be familiar with the terms used, you will probably recognize the behaviors.

"Civility" is described by Meires (2018) as professional behaviors including being polite, respectful, and cooperative with others. "**Incivility**" is used synonymously with bullying and lateral/horizontal violence to mean uncivil behaviors, including rudeness, body language such as eye rolling or refusal to make eye contact, and actions intending to belittle and intimidate others. Bullying and disruptive behaviors among staff prevent collaboration and teamwork, all of which lead to negative patient outcomes. Additionally, bullying negatively impacts nursing recruitment, retention, and job satisfaction. **Bullying** is described by Meires as consistent and repetitive actions and behaviors toward vulnerable individuals with the intention of intimidation, embarrassment, and isolation. It is difficult to imagine members of a caring profession treating others in this manner, but the occurrence is far too frequent. According to Edmonson, Bolick, and Lee (2017) and Blackstock, Bukola, and Cummings (2018), these behaviors may be due to nurses feeling undervalued and not respected by administration or physicians or because a majority of nurses as women may feel oppressed by male-dominated professions. Meires (2018) states those who bully may be immature or unstable or enjoy having power over another.

Pickering, Nurenberg, and Schiamberg (2017) examined bullying from the CNA viewpoint in the nursing home setting. The study conducted by these authors demonstrated that once the CNA accepted the presence of a hostile work environment as normal, he or she lost trust in the organization and in his or her ability to provide safe quality patient care.

Working without trust required the CNA to reform work expectations and activities leading to disengagement and detachment from doing the right thing and focusing on his or her own survival within the organization. As the primary providers of care in the nursing home, the CNAs working in a hostile work environment as part of this study acknowledged not only the unsafe patient safety outcomes resulting from their care, but also their own personal outcomes of increased absenteeism, turnover, injury, stress, and depression.

CRITICALLY EXAMINE THE FOLLOWING

Do bullying behaviors sound familiar to you? Have you been bullied or are you guilty of bullying behaviors towards others? Consider this scenario:

Hannah, a seasoned LPN, has returned to work after her husband lost his job. She attended a refresher course as she has been out of the work force for about ten years. Hannah is hired as the night shift charge nurse. Ellen, the director of nursing, and Susan, the day shift charge LPN, are good friends and between them have created a hostile work environment where new employees are targeted to see if they meet the expectations set by the organization. Hannah, as a new employee, becomes the target of their incivility. When Hannah gives report in the morning, Ellen and Susan make repeated negative comments about her decision making; their body language consists of eye rolling and smirking at each other as Hannah discusses her concerns for her patients. During one particularly hectic night shift, Ellen and Susan sat at the desk while Hannah and her CNA Robert attempted to complete their work. Hannah was told that giving report late or leaving work for the day shift to finish was totally unacceptable. After 2 months in this environment, Hannah begins calling in sick and eventually resigns her position.

Questions
1. Is this bullying? Why or why not?
2. As the nurse manager or the director of nursing, what is your role when you suspect a hostile work environment?
3. What do you see as the outcomes of working in a hostile work environment for patients? For staff?

Due to the prevalence of incivility and bullying in the workplace, it is important for a nurse manager to recognize the patterns of behavior and take necessary steps to alleviate the behaviors. Staff who are able to work in a positive work environment provide better care to their patients leading to better patient outcomes.

CASE STUDY SOLUTION

1. **Decision making:** You must first make decisions about how you will accomplish all the tasks you have. At this stage, you should prioritize your list, keeping patient safety at the forefront of all decisions. Look at your priority list to make sure you have done this.

2. **Delegation:** Taking 10 minutes to delegate tasks that you believe can safely be delegated will save a great deal of time and stress and will contribute greatly to the quality of care of your patients. Think about what can safely and quickly be delegated to others so that you, as the charge nurse, may assume the most important issues as you work through the priority list. Priorities that can safely be delegated, in this instance, include the following:

   a. Using your communication skills, ask the student instructor to assign her students to the patients on your unit. She knows where the charts are because she has been in your facility many times. Tell her to use the charts and to make sure each student will cover two to three patients under the instructor's direction. Make sure she follows up with you to report her assignments.

      Consider: If the policies in your facility allow for LPN students to dispense medications under the direction of their clinical instructor, then you are able to delegate this task. If not, you may want to consider calling in a MA-C to ensure the medications are dispensed safely and on time. However, consider that this decision will add to the day's expense but will also greatly add to the quality of patient care.

   b. Ask the new LPN to check on the night nurse. Have her report back to you on the night nurse's availability to participate in report. After the new LPN has completed this task, you may want to keep her at your side, to observe, while you complete patient care and follow through with your priority list.

      Consider: You must receive report as soon as possible so you will know of any other patient problems you may be facing. The LPN who you will be orienting should be involved in report, but she should not be responsible for taking the report and then passing the information on to you. You have not worked with her yet, and you do not know her skill level at this point. Your concern should always be patient safety.

   c. Using your communication skills, acknowledge with the CNA that you will interact with the patient and family member that has caused her stress. Let her know that she does not need to return to that patient at this time. Assure her that you understand how she feels but that you are in need of her professional help and follow through. Schedule some time later in the day to discuss this situation with her and to listen to her side of the story. Ask her to begin activities of daily living for all patients.

3. **Actions/implementation:** Now that you have efficiently made good decisions and safely delegated tasks, you have greatly decreased your stress and at the same time increased the quality and the safety of care that your patients will receive. The total amount of time you have taken to make these decisions and delegate these tasks is about 5 minutes.

   a. Because you are near the room of the irate family member, briefly step in again and communicate with the patient and the daughter. Let them know that you have an emergency and that you will return as soon as you have investigated and resolved this situation. Let them know this may take an hour and that you will bring the medication list with you when you come. This conversation should take no more than 2 to 3 minutes.

   b. No more than 10 minutes have passed since you walked in the door. You can now immediately and safely go to the new admission and complete an assessment of what has taken place. If the night nurse is available, ask to receive her input on this particular patient.

CASE STUDY SOLUTION—cont'd

Determine in your communication with the night nurse and the patient:

Is the patient coherent?

What was the assessment on admission?

Did the patient fall?

Complete a new assessment on this patient with attention to the report of a possible fracture. Call the physician with the results of the assessment and your determination of a possible fracture. Implement care as ordered by the physician. Some of this care may be delegated, depending on the outcome of the assessment.

c. Receive report from the night nurse so that you can efficiently begin your rounds. Send the night nurse home.

d. Confirm the student assignments and that patients' medications are being passed by the students and instructors or that you have an MA-C called in to help.

e. Begin your morning assessments with the patient of the irate family member and prepare to discuss the patient's prescribed medications and how they have been delivered. You will need to make sure that patient privacy and the Health Insurance Portability

and Accountability Act are not being violated with this family involvement.

f. Begin your new LPN's orientation by having her follow you through your morning assessments. You can ask questions and learn about her skills as you begin the day.

g. Complete your assessments and be prepared for your interdisciplinary meeting by 10 a.m.

h. After lunch, meet with your CNA, and use your leadership and management skills to initiate a productive conversation. As a manager, you can mentor your CNA by modeling behavior and communication skills that will assist the CNA to learn to interact with irate patients and family members.

i. Follow up with those to whom tasks have been delegated.

j. Sit down with your new LPN to discuss the process of orientation.

This case study is not unlike a situation that you may be presented with every day that you work. If you can become skilled at communication, decision making, and delegation, you will accomplish a greater level of success as you interact with your patients and co-workers.

Key Points

- Although the terms "leader" and "manager" often are used interchangeably, everyone has the potential to lead, while a manager usually denotes a person who is in a position of authority.
- The type of leadership style used by a manager may positively or negatively impact recruitment, retention, job satisfaction, and patient outcomes. The five leadership styles discussed in this chapter include authoritative, democratic, permissive, multicratic, and transformational. Each style has associated traits, and each may be appropriate in certain situations.
- Effective communication, including verbal and nonverbal language, is essential for nurses, especially those who care for elderly people. Assertive communication requires that a person being challenged not respond in an aggressive or angry manner to the situation. Instead, it is

necessary to resist the normal response and use the skills of communication to promote problem-solving. Active listening requires that a person being verbally attacked listens to what is being said. Because of the natural inclination to prepare a defense, listening is challenging.

- Appropriate decision making, planning care, prioritizing, and delegating are skills required by the LPN to ensure patient safety, quality of care, and outcomes reflecting patient and staff satisfaction. All of these skills take time to learn and become proficient in, and each is vital to being an effective manager.
- Decision making is one of the most important skills used in nursing. Sound clinical judgment is central to a patient's well-being and optimal outcome. The ability to assess a patient and identify all pertinent factors surrounding that assessment

are of primary significance when making patient-centered decisions.

- When setting priorities and making sound decisions, the LPN nurse manager must understand the importance of planning—the intelligent process of thinking based on facts and information, rather than on emotion and wishes. Planning is a process that never ends. It can be thought of as a hoop with notches where one stops and enters another phase of the planning process. It is a continuous process, much like a hoop, in that it does not stop once a decision is made.
- Delegation of routine tasks frees the manager to work on more complicated unit needs. Because delegation is crucial to effective management, you want to ensure you are doing it as efficiently as possible. When delegating to anyone, your responsibility as the manager is to identify if staff has the basic skills or education necessary to complete the assignment.
- Rounding can be an effective tool for managers to observe care; educate staff, patients, and family; and be a visible presence on the unit. Another way for the nurse manager to assess overall unit function is to periodically round on all staff and patients. Individual institutions may have policies as to when and how often rounding is to be done; ensure you know what your facility requires.

- Managing personnel may require hiring, observing, evaluating, and dismissing employees. Managers must understand legal ramifications of these actions as well as those of the institution.
- Working collaboratively with interdisciplinary teams has the potential to reduce errors, create patient-centered care, and reduce injury leading to increased patient, family, and staff satisfaction.
- Incivility and bullying in nursing are intentional acts intended to intimidate and harass others. The resultant hostile work environment negatively impacts recruitment and retention of staff as well as negatively affects patient safety.
- Each organization has an established process for evaluating employees. Avoiding potential evaluation problems, including leniency, recency, and the halo effect, should be a priority for nurse managers. Leniency errors occur when the manager looks the other way or wants to be buddies with all the employees. Recency errors occur when the manager does not keep accurate records of performance over a specified period of time and bases the evaluation on only what is remembered most recently. Halo errors occur when the manager allows an employee trait or behavior (positive or negative) to influence the entire evaluation. Any of these errors can lead to a poor employee evaluation and possibly poor employee performance.

Review Questions

1. As an LPN you must practice within the definition of your state's nurse practice act. The best way for you to determine whether the current job description is within the nurse practice act is to:
   1. Ask your co-workers.
   2. Read the current job description and compare to the nurse practice act for your state.
   3. Read the policies and procedure manual at your place of employment.
   4. Discuss it with the personnel office during the hiring interview.

2. The authoritarian style of management is not usually effective in the gerontological setting because:
   1. Authoritarian managers are not very person focused.
   2. Most employees need much more guidance to perform tasks correctly.
   3. It allows for a personable and caring approach to tasks, which is more time-consuming.
   4. Of the high number of emergencies in this setting.

3. As an LPN communicating with your patient while completing his assessment, you realize an important part of that assessment and the most honest form of communication is:
   1. Nonverbal communication.
   2. Verbal communications with facial movements.
   3. Sitting quietly and listening.
   4. Your patient education skills.

4. Generally, the best and safest patient care given to older people in all settings is based on:
   1. The family's wishes.
   2. The nurse manager's conflict management skills.
   3. The interdisciplinary team approach.
   4. The permissive management style being used.

5. You were hired 6 months ago as an LPN charge nurse for a skilled nursing facility. You are preparing for your first evaluation. You know that this performance review is not intended to:
   1. Improve the management of your workload.
   2. Criticize your overall performance.
   3. Discuss the manager's appraisal of your overall performance.
   4. Assist you to improve your patient care interactions.

6. As a nurse manager you should be cognizant of your interactions with all employees. If you want to be everyone's buddy or make sure everyone is your best friend, you would be demonstrating the:
   1. Halo error.
   2. Leniency error.
   3. Recency error.
   4. Partiality error.

7. The following behaviors are examples of incivility:
   1. Eye rolling.
   2. Use of sarcasm.
   3. Name calling.
   4. All of the above.

8. Transformational leadership is defined as
   1. Motivating others to exceed expectations based on trust and respect for the leader and his or her vision.
   2. Taking a hands-off approach to leadership with the expectation that staff will do the right thing.
   3. Taking the decision-making process out of the hands of staff so they can focus on the work to be done.
   4. Close observation of staff with the purpose of finding errors and mistakes.

ANSWERS 1. 2, 2. 3, 3. 4, 4. 3, 5. 2, 6. 2, 7. 4, 8. 1

CHAPTER 13
Infection

Tamara Dahlkemper

KEY TERMS

catheter-associated urinary tract
  infection
hepatitis C
immunization
pneumococcal disease
seasonal influenza
shingles
standard precautions
tetanus-diphtheria-pertussis (Tdap)
  vaccine
tuberculosis

CHAPTER CONCEPTS

Infection
Immunity

LEARNING OUTCOMES

1. Identify causes of infection in older adults.
2. Use appropriate environmental and hygienic
   measures that can reduce infectious diseases.
3. Develop a plan to assist an older adult in
   maintaining a healthy immune system.
4. Identify appropriate immunization protocols.
5. Discuss the role of the licensed practical nurse (LPN)
   in the management of infections in older adults.

CASE STUDY

Mr. J. is a 71-year-old homeless man who has been
living on the streets and in homeless shelters for over
10 years. He has been admitted to the hospital through
the emergency department due to a broken hip. Hip
replacement surgery was performed and Mr. J. is being
transferred to a rehabilitation facility until he is able to
walk well on his own and other living arrangements can
be arranged.

   On admission, Mr. J. was dehydrated and appeared
to be malnourished. He has a persistent cough that he
states he has had for several months. He has skin lesions
on his body and lice in his hair but otherwise is in good
health. He has a positive disposition and has been cooperative with the hospital staff. When asked, he does not
provide a very detailed health history but does admit to
a history of drug and alcohol use during his early adult
years. He denies use of either at this stage in his life.

Discussion

1. What concerns related to the concepts in this chapter
   should the LPN address for Mr. J.?
2. What immunizations should the nurse suggest that
   Mr. J. receive?

INTRODUCTION

Everyone wants to be healthy. Even a simple head cold is an irritating and inconvenient event in our lives. As a nurse, you know that there are many more serious infections than a head cold. When these infections attack older adults, the problems can be serious. This chapter is a challenge to you, the bedside nurse, to protect older adults knowledgeably from the reality of infection.

Some infections tend to increase with the process of aging and are related to the inability to perform activities of daily living or loss of independence. The physiological responses of older adults during an infectious illness differ from those of younger or middle-aged adults. The febrile response in older adults is diminished. The basal temperature in older adults is generally lower, so it is important to understand that a low-grade fever may indicate an infection in an older adult. The nurse needs to assess for an increase in temperature based on a person's baseline temperature. The older adult may also show signs of physical and mental decline before an increase in basal temperature occurs. In addition, the course of illnesses leading to recovery or death is different.

This chapter provides information on the prevention of infection and the treatment of infections when they occur. The following information and concepts are discussed:

- Maintaining a healthy immune system by participating in health-promoting activities
- Preventing infections with scheduled immunizations, keeping a clean environment, and following good hygiene
- Common infections

Infections can affect all the systems of the body and may be precipitated by chronic medical conditions.

As a nurse caring for older adults, you need to be aware of your own personal hygiene and become vigilant about washing your hands and taking proper care of soiled materials. **Standard precautions** should be used when there is a question about the spread of an infection. Infections can be carried from patient to patient on the hands of a nurse. As a dedicated caregiver, you want to avoid being a carrier of even the most innocent contaminant. The nursing role in the management of infection in older adults includes recognizing, reporting, and documenting signs and symptoms of infection, complying with

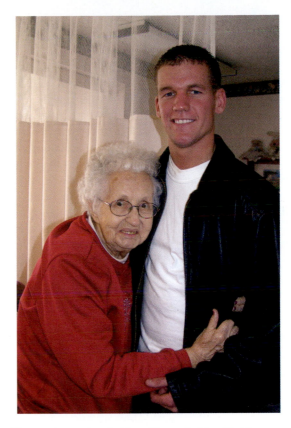

The great-grandson is 19 and in perfect health. His great-grandmother is 84 and should be cautious around anyone with an infectious disease because of her compromised immune system.

medical direction for care, and preventing the spread of infection.

TYPES OF INFECTIONS

Sexually Transmitted Diseases

Many health-care providers are uncomfortable when considering sexually transmitted diseases (STDs) in older adults. A myth of aging is that older people cannot participate in enjoyable sexual activity. The reality is that they can, and many do. With the development of erectile dysfunction medications and treatments for vaginal menopause signs and symptoms, there is the potential of increased sexual activity and sexually transmitted diseases in older persons.

Some people who have lived in monogamous relationships and have lost their companion may have sexual relations with one or more persons who have uncertain sexual histories. This factor can have a strong impact on an older adult's overall health. STDs about which you, as the LPN in the community, should have a working knowledge include syphilis; gonorrhea; chlamydiosis; hepatitis A, B, and C; HIV; genital warts; and other viral and bacterial infections. These diseases generally are discussed in basic medical/surgical classes. Their impact and treatment in older adults do not differ from that in younger adults.

As the nurse, you need to teach older adults who are sexually active with more than one partner the signs and symptoms of STDs and to seek medical treatment for them immediately. Older adults tend not to discuss sexual matters with younger people. This is a barrier that you need to overcome through caring and sensitive communication skills. Older adults at risk need to realize the variety of STDs and the symptoms of the most common ones. They should be able to report symptoms clearly so that the appropriate tests can be performed for accurate diagnosis. Common symptoms are pain, discharge from the penis or vagina, abdominal pain, and genital lesions. Your responsibility is to teach the older adults in your care about STDs, their signs and symptoms, how to get appropriate care, and how to have safe sex. The initial intervention that you, as the LPN, need to undertake is sex education. People aged 60 years and older generally have not had the benefit of formal sex education. An intensive but sensitive interview may indicate that the older adult does not have a full working knowledge of his or her own reproductive system even after having multiple children. This is the place to start if your assessment indicates that there is a knowledge deficit in this area. Be careful to not patronize older adults, or, in other words, do not treat them as though you are the "all-knowing" parent. Be a colleague and a friend. Explore the information together. Share only what is essential for good health unless the learner indicates a desire for more information. Allow the older adult to share the wisdom that comes through the experience of having and raising children.

The second educational concept that you need to teach sexually active older adults is safe sex. Many older people no longer feel a need to protect themselves sexually because they are not concerned about becoming pregnant. Your responsibility is to teach them that safe sex also means protection against STDs, most critically HIV/AIDS. Many older adults have never used a condom. Older adults often associate condoms with birth control, something about which they no longer feel concern. It may be uncomfortable to teach someone old enough to be your grandparent how to use one. The easiest technique

may be practicing putting a condom on a banana. It is acceptable to laugh and make the teaching fun. Laughter would assist the older adult who is uncomfortable with the exercise to relax and learn better. Make the point that the only truly safe sex is abstinence. Then emphasize that condoms are next in terms of safety and should always be used.

Obtaining a Sexual History

Prevention of STDs in older adults is the reason for obtaining a sexual history. Some older adults are at little or no risk for STDs, whereas others may be at high risk. Health education, appropriate treatments, and stopping the transmission of STDs begin with the identification of at-risk behavior.

A sexual history is an integral part of a complete patient history profile. The right questions need to be asked to elicit responses that give key information about risk factors and patient behaviors. Open-ended questions are more likely to give responses that have the most pertinent information. "Tell me about your sex life" would give much more information than simply asking, "Do you have sex?"

Patients must be reassured that their responses are confidential. Developing a confidential relationship aids the LPN in building a rapport of trust and confidence with the older adult. It is important to remember that the patient's values regarding acceptable sexual behavior may differ from yours, and you should not make personal judgments.

Some specific questions need to be asked and may cause you, as the interviewer, some discomfort.

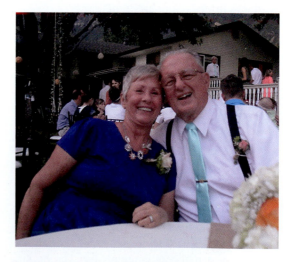

This couple, both in their early 70s, recently married. They should be educated about safe sex practices.

Questions such as "How many sexual partners have you had in the past 3 months?" or "Do you prefer to have sex with men, women, or both?" can seem intrusive. These answers are very important, however, when identifying potential risks for STDs. A complete sexual history should be included on the history form. Refer to chapter 7 for more information about sexually transmitted diseases.

HIV and AIDS

Individuals aged 50 years and older account for 50% of all people with HIV in the United States. Because older people often do not get tested for HIV on a regular basis, there may be even more cases than those that are currently known. Older adults may not receive a diagnosis until they are in a later stage of HIV infection or after the virus has progressed to AIDS (Centers for Disease Control and Prevention [CDC], 2018d).

Many factors contribute to the increasing risk of infection in older people. Older people in the United States generally know less about HIV/AIDS and STDs than younger people because they have not been the targets for educational and prevention messages. In addition, older people are less likely than younger people to talk about their sex lives or drug use with their primary care physician (PCP), and PCPs tend not to ask their older patients about sex or drug use. Finally, older people often mistake the symptoms of HIV/AIDS for the aches and pains of normal aging, so they are less likely to get tested (CDC, 2018d).

It is crucial that older adults understand that HIV/AIDS is a chronic disease but it can be managed. The main goal of HIV treatment with antiviral medication is twofold. The first goal is to decrease and slow the growth of the virus, and the second is to do this without causing extreme side effects, which can include fatigue, pneumonia, diarrhea, nausea or vomiting, dizziness, insomnia, skin rash, and dry mouth. Antiretroviral therapies (antiviral medication) have brought renewed hope for many people living with HIV. However, they do not offer a cure.

When caring for someone with HIV/AIDS, always use standard precautions. It is crucial that you follow the medication regimen closely and report any adverse reactions immediately. Good nutrition and hydration are also important.

THINK LIKE A NURSE

Remember, transmission of HIV/AIDS occurs through contact with an infected person's blood or body fluids. The virus dies quickly when outside the body. Holding a hand, hugging, or sharing close air space will not spread the disease. You will be protected from this disease while working with patients who are HIV/AIDS positive by using standard precautions: do not touch blood or body fluids unless you are wearing personal protective equipment.

How should you educate the patient and family regarding the transmission of HIV/AIDS?

The responsibility you have as the nurse is to educate the sexually active older adult in an effort to promote avoidance of all STDs, especially HIV/AIDS. If you are caring for a person with HIV/AIDS, you have a responsibility to assist him or her with management of the disease.

OTHER INFECTIONS

Due to a decreased immune system and other health concerns, older adults are prone to infection. This section discusses other infections that are of concern for older adults.

Tuberculosis

In the early part of the 20th century, **tuberculosis** (TB) was a major cause of death in the United States. In the 1940s, new drugs became available to treat TB. The United States, in contrast to many poorer countries, had the resources to treat all cases of TB, and the disease was almost eliminated in this country before the 1980s. Worldwide, TB is the cause of many illnesses and deaths, however. Resources for TB treatment have been lacking in poorer countries and continue to be problematic for world health organizations.

Few new cases of TB were reported in the 1970s in the United States because of national efforts to treat the disease. This lack of reported cases resulted in TB services being cut from government funding sources in the 1980s. However, soon after HIV was identified, new cases of TB began to occur in people infected with the virus. The increase in TB cases was also related to the immigration of individuals from other countries where TB is common, transmission of TB in group settings, and the development of drug-resistant strains (CDC, 2018i). In 2017, the overall TB case rate in the United States was 2.8 cases per 100,000 people, for a total of 9,100 cases. This is the lowest number of TB cases reported on record in the United States (CDC, 2018g).

Older adults have a higher probability for developing an active TB infection compared with when they were younger. In many cases, older adults were exposed but never developed the disease (latent TB). The TB bacterium may lie dormant in the body for many years and never cause active TB disease unless the immune system weakens, which can happen as people age (CDC, 2018h). The signs and symptoms of active TB disease are chest pain, coughing up blood or sputum, night sweats, weight loss, low-grade fever, and a cough lasting 3 weeks or longer. Due to Mr. J. living in a congregate environment and having a cough for several months, the LPN will want to suggest he be tested for TB and place him on infection protocol.

TB screening should be conducted on all nursing home residents to identify undiagnosed cases for treatment. TB is diagnosed with a TB skin test (TST) and TB blood tests. These tests only confirm that the individual has been infected with TB. Additional tests, such as a sputum culture and a chest x-ray, are needed to identify if the individual has TB disease. The LPN may be asked to collect a sputum specimen. The protocols at your facility dictate how the specimen should be gathered. Review the protocols and ask questions if you are unsure of the procedure. Staff members and other residents need to be protected from TB if a case is identified. Family members may also need to be protected.

As a nurse, you need to follow the medical orders closely and watch for signs and symptoms of complications with the drug protocols. The medication must be taken exactly as prescribed. It is possible that you will be asked to watch the older person take the medications to ensure that the pills are consumed. The medications may cause some side effects in the older person, which is why the patient may avoid taking the medication. Directly observed therapy (DOT) has been found to be successful in ensuring that the medications are being taken as directed. The LPN may do this or choose a responsible family member to observe the medication therapy.

Point of Interest

Drug-Resistant Organisms

The misuse of antibiotics has caused drug resistance. This means that the organism has become familiar with the antibiotic, which cannot now kill a specific organism. The organisms that infect our bodies have a great ability to change to survive. They become familiar with the antibiotics that are in the bloodstream. If there is not enough antibiotic in the body or if a wrong antibiotic is used, the organism can change its shape or chemistry so that the antibiotic cannot adhere to the organism and kill it. This is what drug resistance is.

Following is the best advice to decrease drug-resistant organisms:

1. Take antibiotics only when prescribed. It is just as important that if you start the antibiotic, you also finish every pill. Doing so ensures that the organism is killed.
2. Do not take antibiotics if you have a cold or the flu. They will not help. Antibiotics do not kill viruses, which are what cause colds and flu.
3. Wash your hands. This decreases the spread of drug-resistant organisms to other people who may have weakened immune systems that could easily be infected by the organism.
4. Do not ostracize people who have a drug-resistant organism. The risk of transmission is very low when proper personal protective equipment is worn during contact with the ill person's blood or body fluids.

As an LPN, you need to teach older adults with TB to wear a mask when in public or with people. You need to support the older person because the mask is uncomfortable to wear, difficult to use, and may cause the person to be sensitive about needing to wear the mask. The mask needs to be worn until sputum smears confirm that the person is no longer infectious.

Hospitals have special ventilation rooms for patients with TB to prevent the pathogen from being spread to other areas of the hospital. If the person is in a long-term care or assisted living facility, they should be moved to a private room away from other residents.

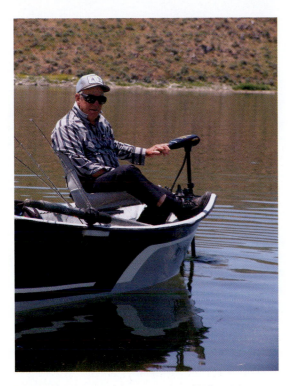

This 65-year-old man fishes year-round. When it is "mosquito season," he protects himself with a long-sleeved shirt and an upturned collar. It still is possible to get bitten by a mosquito, but he is minimizing the danger by being cautious.

West Nile Virus

West Nile virus (WNV) is an infection most commonly spread by mosquitoes. There are no vaccines to prevent or medications to treat WNV. The first case of WNV was reported in New York City in 1999; it has now spread across the United States. The symptoms are fever, chills, headache, aching bones, malaise, symptoms of respiratory infection, and muscle pain. Encephalitis or meningitis are complications of WNV (CDC, 2018e). Older adults are at greater risk for serious complications related to WNV. Individuals with cancer, hypertension, kidney disease, and diabetes are also at greater risk. Over-the-counter fever and pain relievers can be used for mild symptoms. Hospitalization with supportive treatments may be needed for more severe cases.

The LPN should advise older adults to protect themselves against mosquito bites by wearing long-sleeved tops and long pants and using insect repellent from dawn to dusk. Screens on windows and doors help keep the mosquitoes out of the house. In addition, because mosquitoes breed in standing water, all containers, such as a birdbath, should be refreshed often.

Hepatitis C

Hepatitis C is a liver infection caused by a virus. The virus causing hepatitis C is different than the viruses that cause hepatitis A and B. There is currently no vaccination for hepatitis C; however, research is being done to develop a vaccine. Hepatitis C can be an acute infection lasting a few weeks or a chronic infection lasting a lifetime. Most people with the acute infection go on to develop a chronic infection. Individuals with an acute infection may have mild symptoms that include fever, fatigue, joint pain, dark urine, clay colored stools, and jaundice. However, most people with hepatitis C do not know they are infected because they have no symptoms. Symptoms of chronic infection include chronic fatigue and mild to severe chronic liver disease. About 1 in 5 people with chronic hepatitis C infection develop cirrhosis, and a small number eventually develop liver cancer. The CDC recommends testing for all individuals born 1945 to 1965, the Baby Boomer generation, as well as current and former injection drug users. The CDC website lists other individuals who should be tested. Individuals with an acute infection should be monitored by their PCP, as there is no recommended treatment unless the infection becomes a chronic infection. Current treatment for a chronic infection includes 8 to 12 weeks of oral therapy with a cure rate of 90% (CDC, 2018f).

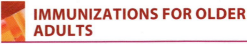

IMMUNIZATIONS FOR OLDER ADULTS

Immunization recommendations change as people age, and health conditions affect immune responses. The need for an older adult to be immunized is not always recognized. Immunization histories may not be part of the person's medical record, or the information simply may not be noted, which is why immunization histories are an important part of the assessment that you, as the LPN, will perform. Studies indicate that older adults are less likely to get immunizations because they do not see the benefit. The LPN must consider the need for the older adult to have continued protection from preventable disease and educate older adults on the importance of getting vaccinated.

Immunizations should be continued throughout life for vaccine-preventable diseases. Based on CDC guidelines, the following vaccinations are recommended for all older adults:

• Tdap
• Seasonal influenza
• Shingles
• Pneumococcal

Healthy People 2020

Objectives

• Reduce new invasive pneumococcal infections among adults aged 65 years and older.
• Reduce invasive antibiotic-resistant pneumococcal infections among adults aged 65 years and older.
• Increase the percentage of noninstitutionalized adults aged 65 years and older who are vaccinated annually against seasonal influenza.
• Increase the percentage of noninstitutionalized adults aged 65 years and older who are vaccinated against pneumococcal disease.

Source: https://www.healthypeople.gov/2020/topics-objectives/topic/immunization-and-infectious-diseases/objectives

Older adults who travel extensively will want to check with their primary care provider to see if they need additional vaccinations. Hepatitis A, hepatitis B, and yellow fever are recommended for most travelers.

These immunizations are generally available in PCP offices, senior centers, home health agencies, public health departments, and some pharmacies. Mr. J. will benefit from receiving the immunizations recommended by the CDC.

Tdap

Tetanus, diphtheria, and pertussis are serious diseases caused by bacteria. Diphtheria and pertussis are spread from person to person, whereas tetanus enters the body through cuts or wounds.

Tdap vaccines can help prevent these diseases. A single dose of Tdap is recommended for older adults who have not previously received the vaccine. Another vaccine, called Td, protects against tetanus and diphtheria but not pertussis. Td is recommended every 10 years for older adults who have had the Tdap vaccine.

CRITICALLY EXAMINE THE FOLLOWING

Some older adults do not understand the risks associated with not getting the immunizations recommended for their age group. After reading the information in this chapter, develop a short education program designed to teach older adults the importance of getting their immunizations. What additional resources will you use? How will you make the education session engaging for the older adults?

Seasonal Influenza Vaccine

More than 60% of hospitalizations that occur as a result of **seasonal influenza** occur in people 65 years old and older. It is also estimated that 70% of seasonal flu-related deaths occur in people over 65 years old (CDC, 2018b). The influenza or "flu" vaccine should be given each year to all adults, unless contraindicated. Older adults who have lung disease, diabetes, kidney disease, or other diseases that affect the immune system should be particularly encouraged to get the vaccine. The seasonal influenza vaccine should also be given to residents living in long-term care, assisted living, or other residential care facilities. Household contacts of high-risk older adults should also receive the influenza vaccination. The flu virus changes each year, so the formulation of the vaccine changes each year. Vaccines should be given starting around mid-October.

Shingles (Herpes Zoster) Vaccine

Shingles is a painful, localized skin rash (often with blisters) that is caused by the varicella-zoster virus, the same virus that causes chickenpox. Anyone who has had chickenpox can develop shingles. Shingles most commonly occurs in people aged 50 years old or older, people who have medical conditions that keep the immune system from working properly, people who receive immunosuppressive drugs, or people experiencing a great deal of stress. An estimated 1 million Americans get shingles every year, and about one-half of them are aged 60 years old or older. The CDC recommends that healthy adults aged 50 years and older receive the two-shot vaccine, Shingrix, 2 to 6 months apart. Zostavax may still be given to healthy adults aged 60 years and older or when a vaccination is needed and Shingrix is not available (CDC, 2018a). A common complication of shingles is postherpetic neuralgia (PHN). The severe pain caused by PHN can continue in some people long after their rash clears

Focused Learning Chart: Protocols for Pneumococcal Vaccine Administration

Who Receives It	*How It's Administered*	*What It Does*
Recommended for all adults age 65 and older	Intramuscular injections	PCV 13 protects against 13 organisms; PPSV 23 protects against 23 organisms
	Two vaccines: PCV 13 and PPSV 23	Markedly decreases death rate from pneumonia

up but will usually resolve in a few weeks or months. Older adults are at greater risk for PHN and long-term severe pain (CDC, 2018c) than younger people. The LPN assesses the need for the immunization and reports the findings. The PCP determines whether the immunization is needed.

Pneumococcal Vaccine

Pneumococcal disease occurs most frequently in older adults and those with a predisposing conditions such as pulmonary disease. Pneumonia is the most common pneumococcal infection in older adults requiring hospitalization. There are now two pneumococcal vaccines, the 13-valent pneumococcal conjugate vaccine (PCV 13) and the 23-valent pneumococcal polysaccharide vaccine (PPSV 23). The CDC recommends older adults get both vaccines. If an individual has not previously received a pneumococcal vaccine, the PCV 13 should be given first and then the PPSV 23 at least 1 year later. If an individual has already received one or two doses of PPSV 23, give the PCV 13 at least 1 year after the most recent dose. When chronic health conditions (lung, heart, kidney, liver disease; diabetes; alcoholism; cancer) are present, the vaccine should be considered at an earlier age (CDC Guidelines, 2017). The PCP determines when the vaccine should be given.

Patient Education

Older adults and their families should be taught the importance of maintaining current immunizations. The immunizations that all older adults should have based on the recommended schedule are Tdap, seasonal influenza, pneumococcal, and shingles. Older adults who travel frequently, especially outside the United States, should check with their PCP before traveling for information about additional vaccinations that may be needed.

Evidence-Based Practice

Rikin, S., Scott, V., Shea, S., LaRussa, P., & Stockwell, M. S. (2018). Influenza vaccination beliefs and practices in elderly primary care patients. *Journal of Community Health*, *43*(1), 201–206. https://doi.org/10.1007/s10900-017-0404-x

This study examined the relationship between vaccination behaviors and health beliefs related to influenza vaccinations in a sample of primarily Hispanic patients aged 65 years and older. The participants were asked about their perceptions of the effectiveness and safety of vaccinations. Of the 88% who completed the questionnaire, only 46.5% believed the influenza vaccination is effective and only 47% believe it is safe. Many stated concerns that the vaccination caused side effects, including acquiring the flu. Concerns also included a belief that the components of the vaccine are harmful. Others stated the vaccination is not necessary. A small number of participants expressed the belief that there are better ways than vaccination to prevent influenza.

The national rate of influenza immunization for individuals 65 years and older is only 63%. This may account for the fact that the majority of deaths and hospitalizations due to the influenza virus occurs in individuals 65 years and older. This study demonstrates the importance of educating older adults on the importance of the influenza vaccination and dispelling some of their concerns related to receiving the vaccination.

Question

As a nurse working in a community clinic, what can you do to increase the number of older adults receiving the flu vaccine?

MAINTAINING A HEALTHY IMMUNE SYSTEM

One of the purposes of the immune system is to protect the body from the invasion of harmful bacteria, fungi, viruses, parasites, and other microorganisms. As the body ages, lymphocyte function and antibody immune responses become delayed or inadequate and put the older adult at risk for infections. The following are ways to support the health of the immune system.

Nutrition

The LPN is responsible for assessing and monitoring an older person's nutritional status. This is an important aspect of maintaining a healthy immune system. (Review nutrition and the reasons for poor nutrition in chapter 8.) It is important to identify nutritional deficits and potential reasons for these deficits. The LPN must determine, through questioning and observing the person's nutritional patterns, why there may be nutritional deficits. Consider the nutritional status of Mr. J. Because he is homeless, he is most likely experiencing some nutritional deficits that will affect his immune function.

Lifestyle

The need for exercise, rest, and stress management and the need to avoid cigarette smoke and alcohol use are discussed in chapter 6. Compliance with these activities heightens the abilities of the immune system. As an LPN, you need to assess compliance or noncompliance with these activities frequently and educate the person as necessary. Knowing older adults' lifestyles, living conditions, and economic situations is important when assisting them in maintaining a healthy immune system.

Priority Setting

This chapter discusses many serious infections that can be transmitted from person to person. The overriding priority for this chapter is to always remember to wash your hands before and after every patient encounter.

THINK LIKE A NURSE

Infections and *hand hygiene* are words often used at the same time. Hand hygiene—washing your hands with soap, water, and friction for a minimum of 15 seconds—is the CDC recommendation. Teaching older adults this principle may protect them from many different infections. As a health-care provider, it is important to remember to do appropriate hand hygiene between patient care activities. In home health, extended care, or hospitals, there may be alcohol hand rubs. These products are safe to use and helpful in decreasing the spread of infections.

Chronic Medical Conditions

Chronic medical conditions have an effect on an older adult's immune system. Chapter 14 discusses chronic medical conditions and the potential for infections. A classic example is a person with diabetes. You need to educate the diabetic person to take precautions to prevent infections by wearing appropriate shoes, observing for lesions that do not heal, and caring for skin cuts and abrasions. Individuals with chronic obstructive pulmonary disease (COPD) are more susceptible to lung infections and need to be educated on the importance of frequent handwashing and avoiding individuals who are sick with a cold or the flu.

Urinary Tract Infections

Preventing urinary tract infections (UTIs) is an important aspect of preventive nursing. **Catheter-associated urinary tract infections (CAUTI)** are common in older adults needing catheters. If a catheter is needed, the best practice is to remove it as soon as safely possible. Chronic bacteremia is also common in older adults and is caused by colonized bacteria in the bladder. Generally, there are no symptoms with chronic bacteremia. Older adults should be encouraged to drink adequate fluids and to empty their bladders frequently. Incontinence may be the initial symptom of a UTI. If incontinence occurs, older persons should have their skin cleansed and soiled clothes replaced. Older adults' skin is sensitive and can break down, which increases the risk of infection. Changes in mental or physical status can also be a sign of a UTI and should be assessed by the nurse.

Respiratory Infections

Respiratory infections, especially pneumonia, may have a significant effect on an older adult. There are several risk factors that contribute to respiratory infections: decreased immune response, including age-related changes to the lungs, immobility, and increased incidence of hospitalization.

Pneumonia is one of the primary causes of death in the elderly population. Signs and symptoms of pneumonia can be altered in older adults, so patients should be watched closely to avoid a serious case of pneumonia.

Pneumococcal and influenza vaccines are encouraged in this population to prevent pneumonia and other respiratory infections. Encouraging mobility and proper nutrition and fluid intake can help decrease complications of respiratory infections. Mr J. will benefit from a nutritious diet and an adequate intake of fluids.

Integumentary System

Changes in the integumentary system accompany the process of aging. Many factors influence changes in the course of aging. Exposure to the sun, diet, heredity, and general health affect the skin. Pressure ulcers and their potential for infection are discussed in Chapter 16. The LPN should be aware of other skin infections. Redness, swelling, pain, lesions, and discoloration are some signs and symptoms of skin infections. As an LPN, you must report all signs and symptoms of a skin infection to the registered nurse.

Safe, Effective Nursing Care

Decrease Risk of Harm to Patients

Mr. Lowe is experiencing slight confusion and a decrease in physical strength as noted by his inability to get out of the chair on his own. He is also very unstable on his feet once he is standing. These are symptoms that are new for Mr. Lowe.

Changes in the mental and physical status of an older adult are a concern and should be assessed for an underlying cause in an effort to address the problem.

1. What could be causing the change in Mr. Lowe's mental and physical status?
2. As an LPN, what can you do to assist Mr. Lowe?

Point of Interest

According to the CDC, Standard Precautions should be used for all patients. This term means you treat everyone's blood and body fluids as if they are infectious.

Skin pathogens include the following microorganisms:

- Staphylococcal bacterial infections include impetigo, boils, carbuncles, and cellulitis.
- Streptococcal bacterial infections include impetigo and erysipelas.
- Fungal infections include the cause of "athlete's foot" and thickened nails on the fingers and toes.
- Viral infections include herpes zoster (shingles) and herpes simplex.
- Parasitic infections include scabies and lice.

It is impossible to protect people from the invasion of all harmful microorganisms, but an older adult with a healthy immune system will have a better recovery if an infection occurs. Adherence to wellness activities, plus additional measures, can prevent infections and increase positive outcomes.

Cultural Considerations

Susceptibility to disease and infection can be genetically determined so may have a different impact on particular cultures.

MAINTAINING A HEALTHY LIFESTYLE

Environmental Cleanliness
Household Pets

Household pets are a source of friendship and companionship for older adults. Older people need to be aware, however, that pets also can become a source of infection. Pets may become infected and transfer their disease to household members. Animal waste can become a source of infection if it is not properly handled. A pet needs health and medical consideration to protect the older adult from a disease carried by the pet. An assessment of the home always should include mention of household pets and how care of the pet is managed.

Kitchens and Bathrooms

Kitchens and bathrooms are great harbors of infections. Household assessments need to include bathroom inspection of towels, tooth care items, sinks, tubs, and toilets. Instructions by the LPN include not sharing personal hygiene items such as razors and tooth care articles. Kitchen assessments involve reviewing food preparation and food storage as discussed earlier. Personal cleanliness and hygiene may need frequent reinforced instructions. When instructing older adults about handwashing, the LPN should include cleaning under the fingernails.

Safe Food and Water

Food-borne diseases are very common in the United States. Millions of people become ill each year as a result of contaminated food, and thousands die. Microorganisms find food a great place to live and breed. The signs and symptoms of food-borne diseases may resemble a bad case of "stomach flu," and the older adult may delay seeking medical care. Most food-borne diseases have common signs and symptoms, which are abdominal pain, fever, vomiting, and diarrhea of sudden onset. Laboratory testing (stool culture) is required to identify the infecting organism.

In your role as the nurse, you will want to note the following in a suspected food-borne illness: the time that signs and symptoms occurred, what the person ate in the last few days, where the food was served, and whether other people became ill. This information should be reported to the local health department. The health department investigates all potential food-borne diseases, and they take appropriate actions. Food-borne infections can be prevented by good handwashing, using safe foods, and keeping food preparation areas sanitary. You need to instruct older adults preparing food to:

• Store food correctly.
• Protect food from insects, rodents, and animals.
• Cook food thoroughly.
• Eat cooked food immediately.
• Refrigerate uneaten food immediately.
• Reheat cooked foods thoroughly.
• Wash hands frequently.
• Keep food preparation areas clean.

Because of decreasing eyesight and sense of smell, some older adults may not be able to determine when food is spoiled, thus increasing their chances of becoming ill with a food-borne pathogen.

CASE STUDY SOLUTIONS

Mr. J. has been homeless for several years and most likely will go back to this lifestyle of living on the streets and in homeless shelters upon discharge. While he is in the hospital, several issues can be addressed to improve his future health:

1. It is important to address his skin lesions and make sure they are kept clean and dry. The PCP may want to culture the lesions to determine if they are caused by bacteria or fungus that needs to be treated.
2. Providing Mr. J. with good nutrition while in the hospital and rehab center will boost his immune system and help with the healing process.
3. Testing should be done to determine the cause of Mr. J.'s persistent cough. Because he has been living in homeless shelters, there is a chance he has contracted TB due to the congregate environment.

4. Mr. J. should also be considered for the following vaccinations:
   Seasonal influenza if Mr. J. is admitted between October and March
   PCV 13 and the PPSV 23 because of the high incidence of pneumonia is this age group
   Tdap, which will prevent the highly contagious pertussis
   Shingles, because of the high incidence of shingles in his age group. Also, living as a homeless person may be stressful.
5. Because of Mr. J.'s history of drug use, it is important for the LPN to discuss the need to be tested for HIV/AIDS.
6. Because of his age and his history of drug use, he should be tested for Hepatitis C.

   Mr. J. may not be open to receiving the testing and vaccinations as described above; however, providing him with these options is important to help maintain his health.

Key Points

- The nursing role in the management of infection in older adults includes recognizing, reporting, and documenting signs and symptoms of infection; complying with medical direction for care; and preventing the spread of infection.
- Many older adults are at risk of STDs if they continue to participate in sexual activity. Some adults engage in sexual activity with new partners who have a questionable sexual history. The incidence of HIV/AIDS in older adults has increased over the last several years. The LPN should perform a thorough sexual history and teach older adults about STDs and how to prevent them.
- Other infections older adults are exposed to include tuberculosis, hepatitis C, and WNV. Tuberculosis is common in living environments where many people reside in close proximity. It is recommended that adults born between the years 1945 and 1964 be tested for hepatitis C because many of these individuals could be infected with the virus and not know it. WNV is a less common infection but it can have a devastating impact on older adults due to the severity of symptoms.
- Immunization recommendations change as people age and should be continued throughout life for vaccine preventable diseases. The CDC recommends the following vaccinations for all older adults: Tdap, seasonal influenza, shingles, and pneumococcal. The immunizations are available through PCP offices, senior centers, home health agencies, public health departments, and some pharmacies.
- Infections in older adults are caused by exposure to bacteria and viruses. A weak immune system and some chronic conditions can make an older adult more susceptible to some infections. The physiological responses of older adults during an infectious illness differ from those of younger individuals.
- One of the purposes of the immune system is to protect the body from the invasion of harmful bacteria, viruses, and other microorganisms. Maintaining good nutrition is important for a good immune system. Maintaining a healthy lifestyle by getting plenty of exercise, rest, and managing stress also heightens the immune system's ability to function.

Review Questions

1. Mrs. R. is 80 years old and is in good health. On a recent visit, her daughter noticed that her mother seems confused and has decreased energy. Mrs. R. may have developed:
   1. Dementia.
   2. A urinary tract infection.
   3. An intolerance to food she recently ate.
   4. Insomnia.

2. This vaccination should be given annually to every resident in a long-term care facility.
   1. Influenza
   2. Pneumococcal
   3. Shingles
   4. Tdap

3. Mr. Z. is discussing his immunization history with the nurse. He mentions that at age 65 he received the PCV 13 vaccine and at age 66 he received the PPSV 23 vaccine. These are the only vaccines Mr. Z. needs to protect against pneumococcal disease.
   1. True
   2. False

4. You are admitting Mrs. J., 75 years old, to your rehabilitation facility after her knee replacement surgery. As part of the admission assessment you:
   1. Ask all of the assessment questions in front of the man she has introduced as her partner.
   2. Skip the sexual history part because you assume that at her age, she is not sexually active.
   3. Ask her partner to leave the room before asking her questions about her sexual history.
   4. Stop asking about her sexual history when she becomes embarrassed.

5. When discussing HIV/AIDS with an older adult,
   that person needs to understand:
   1. With newer drugs, HIV/AIDS can be cured.
   2. When taking the medications, you do not need
      to practice safe sex.
   3. If you are older than 65, you do not need to be
      concerned about contracting the disease.
   4. HIV/AIDS is incurable and is considered a
      chronic disease.

ANSWERS 1. 2, 2. 1, 3. 1, 4. 1, 3. 5, 4

CHAPTER 14
Common Medical Diagnoses

Kristiann Williams

KEY TERMS

acute condition
chronic condition
review of systems (ROS)

CHAPTER CONCEPTS

Metabolism
Mobility
Oxygenation
Perfusion
Sensory Perception

LEARNING OUTCOMES

1. Explain differences between acute and chronic stages of common medical problems in older adults.
2. Describe at least two common physiological changes in each body system that are normal aging changes.
3. Demonstrate nursing care appropriate for long-term care of an older adult who has one or more of the common pathologies discussed in this chapter.
4. Apply the concept of gerotranscendence to the common medical diagnoses of older adults.

CASE STUDY

Mr. Hughes is an 84-year-old man who has been married to his wife for 63 years. Mrs. Hughes has osteoarthritis and Mr. Hughes has been caring for her as her mobility has become increasingly limited over the past several years. Mr. Hughes has had hypertension (HTN) for over 40 years. Over the years, he has been on furosemide, a diuretic, and carvedilol, a beta blocker. He is currently on lisinopril (an angiotensin-converting enzyme inhibitor) and atenolol. His blood pressure typically runs in the 140s over 90s. He is 5'10" and weighs 250 pounds. He has been smoking cigarettes since the age of 15 and has gradually reduced his daily usage to 1 pack per day.

Together, Mr. and Mrs. Hughes live in a gated community where they are active in social activities. Their three children and numerous grandchildren live within 50 miles and visit them frequently. Recently, Mr. Hughes noticed some double vision along with headaches that persist on a daily basis. He sought an immediate eye exam. An internal eye exam showed an

Continued

CASE STUDY—cont'd

increase in ocular pressure and thickening of the vessels in his eyes. Previously noted bilateral cataracts were noted to be gradually worsening. A visit to his primary care provider (PCP) was encouraged and immediately sought out.

At his visit with his PCP, it was noted that his blood pressure was 192/114. While Mr. Hughes was talking to his PCP, he began speaking in non-sensical sentences (word salad). He was unable to tell the provider his name, current location, or date and was unable to move his left arm. Mr. Hughes was immediately taken to the local emergency department where it was determined that he had experienced a right-sided stroke.

Upon discussion with Mrs. Hughes, she revealed that Mr. Hughes has recently gained 30 pounds and had been inconsistent in taking his antihypertensive medications on a daily basis, due to the increased time to care for her needs. He has also been eating more fast food and after Mrs. Hughes has gone to bed, he would go out for an occasional ice cream.

After several days in the hospital and medication reevaluation, Mr. Hughes was transferred to an extended care facility, where he received physical therapy and speech rehabilitation for 2 weeks. He has residual weakness in his left arm, and has difficulty recognizing his family members. He is now returning home to have his wife provide care for him.

Case Study Discussion

1. What nursing approaches, especially monitoring through home care or physician office visits, can you suggest that may help to prevent additional strokes or complications?
2. What education can you provide to Mr. Hughes regarding factors that can lead to increased blood pressure?
3. What are some common complications that Mr. Hughes may experience?
4. What community resources are available to Mr. Hughes?

INTRODUCTION

You now are at the point in your education where you will learn how to enhance and personalize the bedside nursing care you will give to older people.

The points of emphasis are specifically on the physiology and psychology of older adults. You will recognize what makes gerontological nursing a specialty after reading this chapter and the following chapters. Be open to the uniqueness of giving holistic care (care that involves the entire person) to older adults. Frame the care that you give within a transpersonal caring format. The knowledge you will learn will be valuable to you throughout your entire career.

Older people often develop multiple health-care and medical problems that may complicate nursing and medical treatment plans. In contrast, younger people are more likely to see a physician or enter a hospital with a single health problem.

This chapter provides information in the following four areas:

- The differences between the acute and chronic states of a problem or medical diagnosis. More emphasis is placed on chronic rather than acute conditions because of the frequency of chronic problems in older adults.
- The differences between nursing care for acute and chronic medical conditions
- The effect of the normal changes of aging on medical symptoms. These symptoms are discussed in terms of the specific effect that aging has on a health problem.
- Application of the concept of gerotranscendence to common medical illnesses of older people

Priority Setting

This chapter provides an excellent explanation of chronic disease. The priority is for you to focus on the chronic disease information and learn and understand it. Because you will spend much of your career caring for older adults and because older adults statistically (on average) have two chronic diseases, you need to know about them. Learn the information in this chapter and build on it as you spend time in clinical areas. Ask questions of other nurses and the older persons with chronic diseases. Learn to understand how the diseases affect older people and their families, learn how to manage the illnesses, and learn how to assist the older person in managing the diseases.

Six body systems have been selected for discussion in this chapter. The changes in these systems are in older adults in any setting. Frequently seen medical conditions are included as examples of the disorders that affect each system. Often these conditions do not occur alone. For example, two or more cardiac problems may be present at the same time, and arthritis often occurs with other chronic conditions.

ACUTE VERSUS CHRONIC CONDITIONS

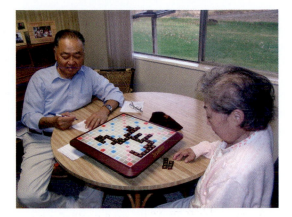

This woman has adapted to severe rheumatoid arthritis. She is unable to walk or straighten out her hands or legs, yet she lives a full and satisfying life.

An **acute condition** develops rapidly. The person experiencing an acute problem notices symptoms for a few minutes to less than 1 month. The acute symptoms may be caused by a previous chronic condition, such as congestive heart failure (CHF), or by a change in body function that is related to aging. For example, changes in kidney function could induce acute renal failure. An acute problem may also develop from an infection.

Research has shown that poor health does not have to be an inevitable consequence of aging. Older adults who practice healthy behaviors, take advantage of clinical preventive services, and continue to engage with family and friends are more likely to remain healthy, live independently, and incur fewer health-related costs. Important components to keeping older adults healthy are preventing chronic diseases and reducing associated complications.

A **chronic condition** is one that lasts 3 months or more. Many chronic diseases can be prevented with healthy lifestyle intervention. Chronic diseases tend to become more common with age.

About 80% of older adults have one chronic condition, and 50% have at least two. Chronic conditions commonly found in elderly individuals include: cardiovascular disease (including HTN), arthritis, diabetes, kidney disease, and mental health issues.

There are numerous ways to distinguish between acute and chronic medical conditions. Acute conditions may be thought of as requiring more immediate and often more sophisticated or technical levels of treatment. The goal with an acute condition is to cure the problem.

Chronic conditions develop over time and often are not noticed by the person with the problem until major deficits manifest. These conditions tend to require more help from the informal system of caregiving, specifically from the family or a home health nurse. Often an older adult develops a partnership with members of the informal system to gain more control over the chronic disease. Cure is often not the goal with chronic conditions. From a nursing standpoint, the goal is to provide care that is helpful in managing chronic diseases. This care should be focused on assisting the older adult to function at the highest possible level in the physical, social, psychological, and spiritual arenas of life. Achievement of this goal should provide a higher quality of life for the individual and decreased morbidity (disability). An alternative goal is to work with an individual to enable him or her to die with dignity; this is a realistic goal that needs to be acknowledged when working with people who have chronic, debilitating diseases. Chapter 10, which focuses on end-of-life care in the elderly person, can assist you in understanding this goal.

Nursing care requires observation of the patient's physical functioning. In the acute phase of illness, it is essential that the nurse note responses to medical treatments, such as medications or surgery. New signs and symptoms may arise because of such treatments. All changes must be reported because the new symptoms may be critical in determining whether to continue treatment or they may indicate complications from the medical interventions.

Nursing care for people with chronic diseases also requires the nurse to observe the person's physical functioning. In addition, it is important to have the observations of informal caregivers. The most critical information comes from the chronically ill person's observation of personal symptoms and overall condition. For treatment to be most effective, the person must be tuned in to the body's responses to treatment or to changes in total body function.

Various stressors may exacerbate a chronic but stable disease in the short and long term. Such stressors include uncertainty about the future, such as relocation or transition stress; starting a new treatment; or the development of an acute condition. For example, a person with emphysema may develop pneumonia, and although antibiotics may cure the acute condition, the antibiotics may cause a flare-up of the previously controlled chronic emphysema.

Many nurses and other health-care workers have difficulty working with people with chronic conditions. There is a tendency to look for timelines, place limits on how long the condition may last, or predict when it might get worse. It is crucial for you, the licensed practical nurse (LPN), to recognize that each patient is an individual and to know that each chronic condition has its own pattern. Some conditions, such as cancer, may get progressively worse. For a patient with a cerebrovascular accident (CVA), the recovery and return of ability depend on the part of the body affected. There is no accurate prediction or measure of recovery because of variable factors that differ from person to person. Other conditions may not change over months or years. This situation can be seen with multiple sclerosis, in which a person experiences periods of remission or absence of symptoms that last for a prolonged period of time.

A person with a chronic health problem, such as HTN, may need to learn to cope with a disease in which there are no visible signs or symptoms of pathology. Some people may not realize the disease is even present. Medications for HTN often have side effects that cause people to stop taking their drugs. Other people stop taking their medication for HTN when they feel good or believe the condition has resolved. This creates a very dangerous situation for the person. This situation can also occur with physical and emotional conditions and is something that the knowledgeable nurse frequently assesses and works to deter. Chronic diseases require long-term treatments such as medications or lifestyle changes.

Working with people with chronic conditions can be a challenge for the nurse. It is common for people with chronic diseases to become discouraged. This type of nursing care calls on your creativity to assist the older person to conserve time and energy to participate in activities that have meaning for the individual.

Focused Learning Chart: Understanding the Differences Between Acute and Chronic Diseases

Older adults have both acute and chronic diseases.

Acute	*Chronic*
Develop rapidly	Exist for at least 6 months
Need immediate care	80% of community living older adults have at least one chronic disease
Often more sophisticated care	Develop over time until major deficits are manifest
Goal is to cure the problem	Require assistance from informal caregivers (family, friends)
In older adults, the acute disease treatment may exacerbate one or more chronic diseases.	The goal is management, not cure.

Fatigue should be prevented, and ways must be found to help the chronically ill person learn to cope with loss and change. Use of a self-care model in providing nursing care can help patients maintain their remaining capabilities. The nurse, patient, and family form the team that is needed to encourage self-care. A crucial part of the team's function is maintaining good communication. This begins with an understanding of the history of the older person. One part of that history comes from a review of systems.

REVIEW OF SYSTEMS

To determine pathology and functional ability, a **review of systems** is used as part of the history and physical examination. This review covers all of the body systems in an orderly fashion. One purpose of the review of systems is to uncover symptoms that may be associated with the current health problem.

Another goal is to identify chronic conditions that may have persisted for years and to learn how the person has managed those conditions over time. The review of systems also is a method of gathering data that can help in deciding on the appropriate type of treatment for each individual. For example, some medications may be inappropriate if the person has problems with falling.

Healthy People 2020
Objectives
- Increase the proportion of older adults who use the "Welcome to Medicare" benefit.
- Increase the proportion of older adults who are up to date on a core set of clinical preventive services.
- Increase the proportion of older adults who receive Diabetes Self-Management Benefits.
- Reduce the proportion of older adults who have moderate to severe functional limitations.
- Increase the proportion of older adults with reduced physical or cognitive function who engage in light, moderate, or vigorous leisure-time physical activities.
- Increase the proportion of health-care workforce with geriatric certification.

Source: https://www.healthypeople.gov/2020/topics-objectives/topic/older-adults/objectives

The review of systems is especially useful for an older adult for the following reasons:

- Older people frequently have nonspecific, atypical symptoms. The review helps to identify possible causes for present problems. It is a method of defining the usual and unusual for the individual.
- Changes of aging may affect two or more body systems simultaneously. The review can help to show how an interaction between systems occurs.
- Older people often have a complex medical history. The review can help to tie the past into the present problem.

For the review of systems, each system and the usual questions asked are listed. Any positive response to a question is followed by other questions to determine the extent or duration of the problem and treatment, if any. It is desirable to have information about treatments used in the past and the effectiveness of those treatments. Treatments include medications bought over the counter (OTC) in addition to those prescribed by a health-care provider.

Pulmonary System
- History of frequent colds or upper respiratory infections?
- Cough? Productive or nonproductive of sputum?
- Appearance of sputum (not saliva)?
- Dyspnea, with exertion, changing position (orthopnea), or during the night (paroxysmal nocturnal dyspnea)?
- Immunization history (pneumococcal vaccine [Pneumovax], recombinant zoster vaccine [(Shingrix)], and influenza)?
- Exposure to anyone with tuberculosis and knowledge about the purified protein derivative (PPD) test for tuberculosis?

Cardiovascular System
- History of HTN?
- History of murmurs, irregular heartbeat, or palpitations?
- Fainting or falls, especially when changing position?
- Chest pain (at rest or after exercising) or presence of swelling in the legs?
- Easy bruising? Varicose veins? Anemia? Blood clots (if so, where)?

Gastrointestinal System
- Food and fluid intake: Typical 24-hour food intake? Number and size of glasses of water and other fluids? Who prepares the meals? Any food intolerances? Likes and dislikes? Vitamins taken? Use of alcohol or opioids? Use of OTC medications?
- Stomach or abdominal discomfort before or after meals?
- Problems with bowels and frequency of use of laxatives (what types)? Fecal incontinence, presence of hemorrhoids (any bleeding, pain, itching)?
- Nausea or vomiting (under what conditions)?

Musculoskeletal System
- Pain, stiffness, redness, swelling, or discomfort in joints (when and in what situations)?
- Pain or cramping in muscles (when and in what situations)?
- Weakness of arms or legs? History of broken bones or other injuries to muscles or bones?
- Ability to walk? Distance traveled before stopping and reason for stopping?

- Use of assistive devices such as cane or walker (if so, under what circumstances)?
- Type of daily exercise or activity?

Genitourinary System
- Difficulty holding urine and under what conditions?
- Burning, pain, or bleeding on urination?
- Sense of fullness in bladder even after urinating?

Women
- Number of pregnancies? Any complications?
- Symptoms associated with menopause?
- Vaginal drainage? Itching? Burning?
- If sexually active, any pain or discomfort?

Men
- Waking during the night to urinate? Dribbling after urinating or difficulty starting to urinate? Change in urine stream?
- If sexually active, any problems?

Neurological System
- Falls or fainting with or without dizziness? Steady or unsteady gait?
- Periods of amnesia or forgetfulness?
- Inability to hold onto objects?
- History of stroke or seizures?
- Difficulty with vision or hearing? Under what circumstances and frequency?
- Loss of feeling or numbness in legs or arms?
- Headaches?

Endocrine System
- History of increased thirst, hunger, or urination?
- Dry skin, loss, or thinning of hair?
- Intolerance to heat or cold?

Safe, Effective Nursing Care

Provide Patient-Centered Care

Ruby is a 76-year-old widow who has just been released from the hospital after falling at home. After careful observation and assessment, it has been determined that she does not have any broken bones and has been released to her home with the supervision of her family who lives nearby. She lives alone in her own home and has a daughter who lives two houses away.

She has several nieces and nephews who live in close proximity. She also has members of her church who check in with her frequently for any needs.

She has a 10-year history of type 2 diabetes and HTN. She is on sliding-scale insulin, which she administers after checking her blood sugar four times a day. Although she had bilateral cataract surgery 3 years ago, she has difficulty seeing the lines on her insulin syringe when she draws up the sliding-scale insulin. The risk of improper dosing is always present if a second person is not there to verify correct amounts. Because Ruby has fallen twice in the past 4 months, the family is considering moving her to another place where she can be more closely monitored.

Patient-centered care means recognizing the patient's needs and preferences while providing compassionate and coordinated care.

1. How can you support Ruby as she considers her options for staying at home or moving to an assisted living facility?
2. Describe Ruby's need for active involvement of her care.
3. How can you balance family concerns with honoring Ruby's wishes to remain in her home?

This review of systems provides only a baseline of information. As a physical examination is performed, the patient frequently remembers other symptoms or events to be added to the history. Often, the first contact with a patient does not provide all the information that may contribute to an understanding of the patient's health problems. The person may believe that symptoms were not important at the time, or the symptoms may simply have been forgotten, so the review remains incomplete. Consequently, the review of systems is always left open for additional information that may help with the planning and continuity of care.

CHRONIC ILLNESSES COMMONLY FOUND IN OLDER ADULTS

This section provides some background information about chronic conditions frequently found in older adults. The primary focus is on continuation of care rather than on immediate treatment and nursing care.

Cardiovascular Conditions

Coronary Artery Disease

The term *coronary artery disease* (CAD) indicates that the heart muscle is not receiving a blood supply adequate to meet its needs. CAD includes angina pectoris, myocardial ischemia and infarction, arrhythmias, CHF, valvular diseases, and HTN. Examples of three of these conditions are presented to show how some of the changes of aging may compound a person's ability to manage the condition. The first example includes angina and myocardial infarction (MI).

For some people, the first sign of CAD is a heart attack. The mortality rate for adults older than 70 years is about twice the rate for younger individuals. Cardiovascular disease is the leading cause of death and disability in older adults. For an older person, the symptoms of MI are often different from those symptoms of a younger person exhibiting a potential MI. Instead of crushing chest pain, there may be dyspnea, dizziness, weakness, abrupt confusion, fatigue, and upper abdominal pain. Chest pain occurs even less often in a person older than 85 years.

Because of the atypical symptoms, the diagnosis of myocardial ischemia or MI may be difficult to make in older people. The electrocardiogram (ECG) may not be as specific in diagnosing MI in older people as in younger people because of age-related changes such as ventricular hypertrophy. The cardiac enzymes phosphokinase (CPK), creatine kinase (CK), and troponin may not be elevated as much as in a younger person because of decreased muscle mass. Younger people usually have a more extensive MI, however, because of lack of collateral circulation. Nurses who work with older people need to be alert to the possibility of MI even when the usual signs do not appear.

Treatment for an older person who has experienced an MI may include coronary artery bypass surgery. Decreasing risk factors such as obesity, smoking, HTN, and diabetes can also decrease risks of a heart attack.

One goal of medical care is to avoid complications. CHF, arrhythmias, thrombi and emboli, and extension of the infarction are common complications. These may be prevented by close monitoring during the acute phase after an MI. The use of beta blockers, lipid-lowering therapies, and aspirin helps to decrease mortality.

Some people restrict their activity after MI and become less capable of self-care. Decreased activity can lead to *deconditioning*. This deconditioning may compound aging changes in the musculoskeletal system, such as decreased muscle mass and decreased muscle strength. The ability to balance activity and rest to avoid incapacity requires a strong cooperative effort among the patient, family members, and health-care personnel. Referral to cardiac rehabilitation may help the person to identify individual abilities and limitations and avoid deconditioning. Older people are capable of recovery and may return to their usual lifestyles, although sometimes a change in lifestyle may be required.

CHF

Most patients with CHF are older than 60 years. CHF is defined as the inability of the heart to pump blood to meet the metabolic demands of the body. The common causes of CHF in older adults include HTN, heart valve calcification, MI, CAD, cardiac hypertrophy, arrhythmias, thyroid disease, and anemia. An acute episode of CHF can be brought on by treatment for other conditions. Overaggressive intravenous fluid replacement (too much, too fast) and medications such as beta blockers are common causes of CHF. The symptoms of dyspnea and frequent nighttime wakening often lead to fatigue and decreased activity.

The goal of medical treatment is to reduce the workload on the heart and improve the ability of the heart to pump. Because patients with CHF have a weakened heart muscle, the pathology of CHF is decreased cardiac output. The use of drugs, such as digoxin, is a primary treatment. Digoxin, which is used to strengthen the force of the contraction of the heart, is most frequently used when atrial fibrillation occurs with CHF. Some older people have taken digoxin for many years. Periodic blood level evaluation of this drug is necessary to prevent toxicity and ensure that the drug is still required. Other drugs include diuretics and drugs that increase dilation of the blood vessels, such as angiotensin-converting enzyme inhibitors (ACEIs). A side effect with these drugs is falling, which results from a decrease in blood pressure with change in position (orthopnea).

Nursing responsibility in chronic CHF includes monitoring the older person for the following conditions:

- Presence of edema (swelling) in feet, legs, sacral area, lungs, abdomen, and around the eyes. Look for increased fluid in any dependent parts and weight gain, especially when appetite is decreased. Often, people gain weight because of fluid retention but lose actual body weight. This type of weight gain and loss can lead to decreased endurance and increased workload on the heart. A daily weight record is helpful to monitor fluctuations depending on severity or level of control of CHF.

- Blood pressure changes with change in position (postural hypotension). Blood pressure and pulse should be checked after 5 to 10 minutes of rest in a flat position, again within 1 minute of sitting, and again 1 minute after standing. Also ask the person whether dizziness occurs with these changes. A decrease of 20 mm Hg in blood pressure on changing position is significant. Patients need to be taught how to control balance before walking and how to use support equipment, such as a cane. The medication may need to be changed, or the patient may not be drinking sufficient fluid. Postural hypotension may result from a physiological change of aging in which the body does not respond to pressure changes. This is due to changes in pressure receptors in blood vessels. The cause of postural hypotension may be any or all three of the preceding possibilities.
- Maintaining a balance between rest and activity. This balance is crucial to prevent fatigue and accompanying inability in self-care. Most patients find that they benefit from a daily routine that allows for short periods of activity followed by rest. During the acute phase of CHF, activity should be minimal. An example is sitting in a chair for 30 minutes three times a day. As cardiac function improves, increased activity is possible. The activity level should be determined by the healthcare provider and closely monitored by the nurse.
- Maintaining an adequate diet to prevent loss of lean body mass. The patient's appetite may be decreased, or fatigue may be so great that five instead of three meals a day are needed. The DASH (Dietary Approaches to Stop Hypertension) diet of 1,500 mg/day of sodium may be prescribed, although many people do well on a diet with no added salt and no foods that are high in salt (National Heart, Lung, and Blood Institute, 2018). Decreased sodium intake may make food unappetizing and can cause anorexia. Use of spices instead of salt (e.g., cinnamon, thyme, ginger, garlic, lemon) and commercial salt substitutes may improve the taste of some foods.

Hypertension

A blood pressure below 120/80 mm Hg is considered normal. A blood pressure greater than 130/80 mm Hg is considered HTN for any age group (American Heart Association, 2018a). HTN is the leading cause of death and morbidity in the United States. The prevalence of HTN increases with age, and about 70% of adults older than age 65 are affected. Men, African Americans, diabetic patients, and obese people tend to be at greater risk. Most research now supports the need to treat a systolic blood pressure greater than 140 mm Hg and diastolic blood pressure greater than 90 mm Hg. Several factors associated with aging may predispose an older person to HTN. Stiffening of the aorta, increased cardiac afterload (the force needed to pump blood from the ventricle), and increased peripheral vascular resistance may be present. Changes in the baroreceptor reflexes may be indicated by fluctuation of blood pressure during physical activity or emotional experiences. Other causes of HTN may include changes in the kidney and endocrine system secondary to aging.

THINK LIKE A NURSE

When digoxin doses are too high, a common side effect is confusion. This is often mistaken for a progressive sign of aging. When there is a sudden change in personality or level of consciousness, what questions are pertinent to ask?

Blood pressure measurement is one of the most important parts of the physical examination. The following are some guidelines for obtaining an accurate blood pressure reading in older adults:

- Allow the person to sit quietly for 3 to 5 minutes before taking a blood pressure reading. Older adults, especially when physically deconditioned, require more time to adjust to a baseline function even after a minor stress, such as walking into an examination area.
- Select the cuff size appropriate to the person: the regular adult cuff may be too large or too small. Use of a pediatric cuff for people with small arms and a large adult or leg cuff for obese people is essential for accuracy. The cuff should be about 20% larger than the diameter of the arm.
- An auscultatory gap is often found with older adults. To avoid an inaccurate systolic reading,

palpate the brachial artery and inflate the cuff in increments of 10 mm Hg while palpating. When the pulse disappears, inflate the cuff another 20 to 30 mm Hg, and then listen for the sounds as you deflate the cuff. The first sound may be followed by a gap of 20 to 30 mm Hg before the sounds are again heard.

- If this is the first contact with the older adult, take readings on both arms to determine whether there are differences of more than 10 mm Hg. For example, if there is an arteriosclerotic plaque in the right subclavian artery, the blood pressure is lower in the right arm. The correct reading is then obtained from the left arm.
- Determination of orthostatic hypotension is needed, especially when monitoring the effect of antihypertensive drugs. (See previous note under CHF regarding technique.)
- If you have difficulty hearing the last sound for diastolic pressure, interpret the reading of a muffled sound as diastolic pressure. Make a note of this in your recording. One technique that can facilitate the diastolic reading is to elevate the arm above heart level.

Another nursing care technique for someone with HTN is monitoring medications to ensure the maintenance of regular doses. This monitoring also will tell you the person's willingness to continue taking the drugs. The usual reason for a person to discontinue the drug or alter the dosage schedule is the experience of unpleasant side effects. Specific side effects vary with the type of drug. Examples of side effects that may cause a person to stop taking the drug include constipation, drowsiness, depression, cough, dizziness related to orthostatic hypotension, anorexia, and, in men, impotence. In addition, some people stop taking diuretic medications if frequent trips to the bathroom interfere with their sleep or their daily activities.

When a person has had a consistent systolic pressure reading of 150 mm Hg or greater and then has a normal reading (120/80 mm Hg), further monitoring may be required. The decrease may be caused by side effects of medication. It also could be an indication of a heart attack. The usual symptoms of MI may not be present, but the person would be more fatigued and have less strength or energy to do things.

Teaching good health habits related to diet, weight loss, and exercise is also a nursing function.

Some people may be placed on dietary restrictions, such as no added salt, reduced cholesterol, or reduced calories. Severe restrictions usually are not needed, but basic teaching is needed to alert older adults and their families to factors that can help control blood pressure. If these measures are successful, medications may not be needed.

Efforts to reduce blood lipid levels in people older than 75 years of age are still considered questionable by some practitioners. Measurements of fasting lipid levels are used to determine cholesterol levels.

An older person may have more difficulty than a younger person in changing a lifetime pattern of eating. Use of a food diary may help with this change. Periodic contacts with nursing staff should check not only adherence to the diet, but also the person's reaction to the changes that have occurred. Emotional support provided in this way increases compliance with difficult dietary changes.

The use of regular exercise in controlling blood pressure is just as important for older people as it is for younger people. The health-care provider may prescribe aerobic exercise, especially walking or swimming, as an adjunct to control blood pressure and weight. Regular exercise may be just as beneficial as medication for some people. When people do not exercise regularly, they tend to start too fast. Instructions should be given for a minimum of 5 minutes of warm-up and stretching and a gradual increase in the amount of time spent in aerobic walking. Usually, the older adult can start with 10 minutes of aerobic walking two to three times a week. The time and frequency of aerobic activity can gradually be increased by 5 to 10 minutes each week. The person should be taught how to take a pulse to ensure that the pulse does not go beyond that person's maximum limit during the peak workout time. The maximum is based on resting heart rate and age. A cool-down period of at least 5 minutes after exercise also is needed.

Peripheral Vascular Disease

The maintenance of good vascular supply to the extremities is crucial for older people. When blood vessels are affected by arteriosclerosis and aging changes, the nutrition of tissues is impaired. Arteries and veins may be involved at the same time. A depleted oxygen supply results with retention of waste products in the body, which can cause muscle soreness.

THINK LIKE A NURSE

A common side effect when an ACEI is used to treat HTN is a nonproductive cough.

- If your patient presents with a sudden cough that was not precipitated by other cold symptoms, what interventions can you undertake?
- What important questions about the history of the cough can you ask?
- What physical assessment can you perform?

CRITICALLY EXAMINE THE FOLLOWING

Read the following patient care situation. Ponder how you would resolve the situation. Make some notes regarding what you decide and be prepared to share your thinking in class. Mrs. P. is your new home-health patient. She has been admitted and assessed by the registered nurse (RN), and your first visit is scheduled for this afternoon. Some of the things you think are significant from the RN's notes are that Mrs. P. is a 72-year-old morbidly obese woman who underwent right total knee surgery 9 days ago (3 days hospital; 6 days nursing home). She lives alone. Her home is on one level. She requires oxygen 24 hours a day because of right-sided heart failure with pulmonary HTN. She has been on antidepressants for most of her life; she finds them effective. Her HTN is managed with medication. The knee replacement was done because of severe degenerative osteoarthritis. A second total knee replacement is planned within the next 3 months. She has joint pain in shoulders and hips. She admits to being deconditioned because of chronic joint pain. The RN has asked you to evaluate Mrs. P. and outline a plan to counteract her deconditioned state so that her next knee surgery and her recovery from it will be easier. This requires some very creative critical thinking. Take time to consider this problem; ask others what they think would be effective; and think of Mrs. P. as a real person who needs your help and knowledge.

Evidence of decreased vascular function is indicated by skin ulcers resulting from venous stasis. Venous stasis is marked by changes in the skin, such as thinning and dryness or overgrowth of epidermis (outer layer of skin). A permanent brown discoloration may appear because of small hemorrhages (petechiae). Any slight trauma to the area can break the skin and begin an ulceration (open sore). Prompt treatment is needed to avoid infection. Even when an ulcer is healed, the area is always at risk for further breakdown. Concern about the condition may cause the person to limit activity. Functional problems—for example, limited ability to ambulate—may result.

Prevention of further trauma and interference with blood supply is the guide for nursing intervention.

Neurological Conditions
Stroke

The fourth leading cause of death for older adults is stroke. The term "brain attack" has been advocated to raise awareness of the need for rapid emergency treatment. A stroke can occur when there is limited or no blood flow to a part of the brain; it is a medical emergency and can cause permanent neurological damage and even death. Strokes happen despite increasing emphasis on prevention. Risk factors include old age, high blood pressure, previous stroke or transient ischemic attack (TIA), diabetes, high cholesterol, tobacco smoking, and atrial fibrillation (American Heart Association, 2018b). High blood pressure is the most important changeable risk factor of stroke. Stroke is a leading cause of serious long-term disability.

Strokes can be classified by type. Ischemic strokes, the most common type of stroke, occur when the blood supply to a part of the brain is suddenly interrupted. These are generally caused by a clot in the blood vessel. Hemorrhagic strokes occur when there is bleeding into the brain tissue or cranial vault. This can occur with brain trauma, aneurysms (weakening and bulging of a blood vessel), or uncontrolled HTN. Depending on the location of the stroke, there can be right- or left-sided weakness. If the stroke occurs in the right hemisphere of the brain, the left side is generally affected. If the stroke occurs in the left hemisphere, the right side is affected.

Patient Education

Teaching for Peripheral Vascular Disease
Keep legs elevated when sitting.
Avoid tight clothing such as nylon stockings.

Avoid extreme temperature changes.
Keep legs uncrossed when sitting.
Use cotton socks and properly fitting shoes.
Report any break in skin as soon as possible.
Avoid applying tape or salves to the area.

After the patient has been stabilized, usually in the hospital, planning for discharge and follow-up care is needed. Rehabilitation should begin as soon as possible, preferably in the hospital (refer to Mr. Hughes from the case study). Starting rehabilitation quickly helps prevent the development of some of the physical complications of a stroke. Two common complications are contractures and skin breakdown. Continued care aids in regaining pre-stroke abilities, providing emotional support, and maintaining physiological defense mechanisms, such as resistance to infections.

Classification of stroke on the basis of the involved hemisphere is important because it points to the type of nursing care required. The goals for care and the way the nurse interacts with the patient are particularly affected.

Frequently, a patient with a right hemisphere stroke exhibits the following characteristics:

• Difficulty recognizing faces
• Poor awareness of deficits caused by stroke
• Impulsivity
• Disorientation to place and time
• Impaired attention or memory
• Monotone and flat affect
• Difficulty with organization and problem-solving
• Difficulty retrieving words
• Weakness or paralysis on the left side of the body

A patient with a left hemisphere stroke tends to have more visible disabilities, such as:

• Extreme cautiousness
• Difficulty speaking
• Inability to express self verbally
• Inability to write words
• Inability to understand written words
• Weakness or paralysis on the right side of the body

Physical, occupational, and speech therapies should be included as part of the interdisciplinary team plan of care. Fatigue may require scheduled rest times, but a limit should be placed on the length of time allowed for rest.

Other losses also occur that are independent of the hemisphere involved. Neglect of one side of the body may first be exhibited in failure to eat food placed on one side of the tray or by failure to turn toward a visitor. Homonymous hemianopsia (loss of vision in the left or right visual field) (Fig. 14.1) or bitemporal hemianopsia (loss of the peripheral or temporal area of vision) may cause each of these symptoms. Therapy is to teach the person consciously to look at a "total picture" of self and surroundings.

Prevention of complications is a major component of post stroke care. After a stroke, a person is frequently at risk for infections (respiratory and urinary), falls, malnutrition, repeated strokes, and deconditioning secondary to lack of activity. Prevention of complications includes all of the following:

• Administering immunizations for pneumonia, influenza, shingles, and tetanus
• Maintaining regular bowel and bladder habits
• Monitoring fluid and food intake
• Monitoring medications
• Maintaining mobility and independence at optimal levels

Homonymous hemianopsia

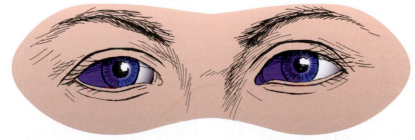

FIGURE 14.1 Homonymous hemianopsia results in the patient ignoring the entire side of the body that he or she cannot see because of the stroke.

THINK LIKE A NURSE

Patients who have had a right-sided stroke are a challenge for the LPN and the family. As the nurse, you have to help the patient and family cope with many frustrations. An area of potential conflict between the patient and caregivers is the patient's denial of disability or from impulsive behavior (acting without thinking). The patient may be unaware of the effect of this behavior, and the family must be constantly alert to the potential for injury to self or others. This type of behavior may persist throughout the remainder of the person's life. Think about Mr. and Mrs. Hughes in the case study. What are some ways the LPN can help them deal with similar changes Mr. Hughes is experiencing?

Older people tend to drink inadequate amounts of fluid. Teaching the older adult and family members ways to ensure consumption of 1,500 to 2,000 mL of water per day is useful. Some people fill a quart bottle with water every morning and drink from that throughout the day, periodically refilling it. When encouraging fluids, however, be sure the person does not have difficulty swallowing. People with swallowing difficulties after a stroke frequently have more difficulty with fluids than they do with swallowing solids. Thicker liquids such as pudding may be tolerated better than thin liquids.

The person's appetite may be affected by an inability to use a knife and fork. Occupational therapy should help with instruction on new ways for self-feeding. Meal plans may need to be altered to help the person lose weight or control sodium or cholesterol levels. Medications often are used to control HTN, cardiac arrhythmias, and blood clotting disorders. When a person begins to feel better, it is common to believe some medications are no longer needed. Compliance with medications must be frequently assessed. Accurate determination of blood pressure in the home or physician's office is essential. Listening to the apical heartbeat instead of relying on radial pulse is advisable. Laboratory work to follow prothrombin time and international normalized ratio (PT/INR) is critical (see Chapter 21). Following a set schedule to maintain a balance between rest and activity helps to minimize fatigue and to promote activity. Many older people who live at home may need continued follow-up after discharge from the hospital or nursing home. Home health care is important for the older adult to maintain optimal health.

Parkinson's Disease

Parkinson's disease (PD) occurs more often in men than women. The condition can begin as early as the mid-40s, but it usually appears between 60 and 80 years of age. PD is a chronic, progressive disease marked by slow movement, rigidity, unstable posture, and tremors at rest. There are some known causes for Parkinson-like symptoms, but in most cases of PD the cause is unknown.

The primary treatment for PD is medication. This condition also requires active involvement of the patient affected by the disease and the family. Education of the patient and family should be a primary objective for every nurse. Important information to be taught includes the following:

• Defining the disease and its problems
• Side effects and individual reactions to medications
• Methods to promote independence and activity while providing for safety

Some people with PD become very depressed and withdraw from social contacts. The person with PD can help to prevent depression by identifying times when fatigue occurs. The beneficial effect of medication may "wear off" close to the time for the next dose. Activity planned around these times of fatigue and decreased drug effect may help the person maintain physical and social function.

As the disease progresses, the person is at risk for several complications. Infections, gastrointestinal problems, and injury from falls are most common. Respiratory infections can occur when swallowing is affected. Aspiration of food and fluids can lead to pneumonia and malnutrition. Urinary tract infections may result from urinary retention and from inadequate fluid intake.

Constipation is a common gastrointestinal problem resulting from a lack of fiber-rich foods and fluids. Problems swallowing can lead to anorexia. Nausea and anorexia are common side effects of the medications used to treat PD. Consumption of semisolid foods or those with the consistency of pudding and foods with a high water content, such as fruits, may help.

A person with PD tends to be physically unstable. Falls can be prevented by the use of a cane or walker. Safety devices should be installed in the home, such as handholds in the bathroom and banisters in the stairway. Floor coverings and furniture should enable a barrier-free route for walking. Shoes that fit well, are lightweight, support the foot, and do not cause either slipping or too much friction are needed.

The goal is to maintain the person's function for as long as possible. A secondary goal is to support the family as they help to manage the daily activities of the elderly person. Coping with the changes that usually occur is difficult for most families. Referral to support groups and helping with problem-solving are two important nursing functions.

Sensory Losses

Many adults find that visual and hearing losses begin around 50 years of age. The eyeball changes shape for most people so that they become farsighted and require glasses for near vision, such as when reading. This aging change is referred to as *presbyopia*. Changes in the shape of the lens and a yellow discoloration may alter the person's ability to focus and to distinguish colors.

Three common pathological visual conditions experienced by older people include cataracts, glaucoma, and macular degeneration. Clouding of the lens, resulting in cataracts, is the most common pathological visual condition. Blurred vision and difficulty with nighttime driving may be the first clues of cataract formation. Outpatient surgery to remove the cloudy lens and replace it with an artificial lens is a common and safe treatment. Other eye conditions require more adjustment, however.

Glaucoma is one of the leading causes of blindness and results from increased pressure in the eye that damages the optic nerve. Central vision is usually retained, but peripheral vision is lost. People speak of having "tunnel vision." Glaucoma can be treated with surgery, eye drops or a combination of both. Any vision lost due to glaucoma is permanent and cannot be reversed even with surgery. All people older than 40 years of age should have a yearly examination for increased intraocular pressure (>22 mm Hg).

Macular degeneration destroys the point of maximum sight—the macula. Blurry vision is usually the first symptom that the older adult notices. Blindness does not result, but the person loses central vision. Peripheral vision is retained around that central blind spot. Macular degeneration can occur in one eye or both. Because the condition can occur in just one eye, frequently the symptoms are not noticed because the other eye can compensate for the loss of central vision. Increased magnification helps many people. Some people learn to adjust head positions to use peripheral vision. Use of zinc and vitamin A, C, and E supplements has been effective for some people in reducing the progression of macular degeneration in later stages.

Hearing loss increases with aging and is more common among men than women. This condition may be due to an aging change called *presbycusis* that occurs without previous injury or other known cause. Hearing difficulties lead to social and emotional consequences because communication with others deteriorates. Many people tend to talk more loudly to individuals who are hard of hearing. Speaking loudly results in sounds becoming more muddled, so that comprehension is worse. Some people are helped by the use of hearing aids, whereas others cannot be helped in this way because of the type or extent of hearing loss. Adjustment to a hearing aid may be difficult because of lack of finger dexterity. The inability to tune out distracting noises also may discourage individuals from using the aid.

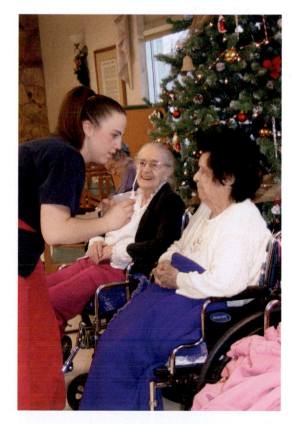

These women reside in a skilled nursing facility and have multiple chronic diseases. With the holistic care they receive in the facility, they are safe and satisfied with their lives.

People with visual or hearing loss should be informed about available services. Centers for the visually impaired in large cities can provide materials to assist people with using their remaining vision. Often, people can be taught ways to compensate for the loss. Audio amplifiers are available for hearing impaired individuals. These devices can provide greater amplification and are especially useful in open room areas.

Following are general guidelines for nurses working with visually impaired or hearing-impaired older adults:

- Face the person before beginning to speak. Avoid sitting in front of a window or light so there will not be any glare. Glare reduces the ability of a person to read lips.
- Speak clearly and slowly so that words are distinct.
- Try not to exaggerate your speaking voice.
- If possible, use a low pitch when speaking.
- Touch the person to indicate where you are.
- Identify yourself by name and explain why you are there.
- Keep the patient's glasses and hearing aid clean.
- Refer to local, state, or national resources for assistance (e.g., local centers for the visually impaired, audiologists, local Lions Clubs for help with glasses).

Pulmonary System
Chronic Obstructive Pulmonary Disease

Chronic obstructive pulmonary disease (COPD) is a condition resulting from exposure to irritants, most commonly cigarette smoke. Other irritants include breathing in chemical fumes, dust, air pollution, and secondhand smoke. Chronic bronchitis, asthma, and emphysema are included in this broad category. COPD is the third leading cause of death for people older than 65 years. The primary signs and symptoms are cough and shortness of breath. The lungs become hyperinflated, and the diaphragm flattens. The person must use abdominal and intercostal muscles (accessory muscles) to breathe. Use of these muscles requires more energy than use of the diaphragm.

A barrel chest is associated with COPD. A barrel chest is a condition when the person's sternum and ribs can be as wide front to back as they are side to side. This appearance may be due to increased residual volume of air because of destruction of the alveolar walls. In this condition, there is less lung surface for diffusion of gases. Severe kyphosis (rounding) of the back should not be confused with COPD.

There are two types of COPD: bronchitis and emphysema. Each type has distinct symptoms; however, the end result for all forms is chronic lung disease that has a strong negative impact on physiological and emotional function. Often, there is one event —usually an infection—that causes the person to recognize the chronic nature of the condition. There is no typical pattern to the disease process except that COPD is progressive, and serious complications do occur, especially repeated infections. Hypoxemia may result with any form of COPD.

The adjustments that a person with COPD has to make in lifestyle, habits, and work can be overwhelming. Prevention of complications is the primary goal of long-term care. Each person (and family member or significant other, when available) needs to have knowledge about the disease process and how to aid in self-care. Teaching self-care includes the following:

- Ways to prevent infections with balanced diet, balanced rest and activity, avoidance of situations in which spread of infection may occur, and use of influenza and pneumococcal immunizations
- How to avoid triggers that cause flare-up of symptoms
- How to recognize signs and symptoms of infection, such as increased cough, change in sputum, and decreased tolerance for activity
- Instruction in medication, including the use of oxygen, the purpose of each medication, and side effects to be expected
- How to keep track of the medication schedule and medications to avoid, such as cough suppressants
- Explaining the need for adequate hydration (2,000 mL/day unless other conditions, such as heart disease, rule this out)
- How to distinguish between anxiety and airway obstruction and measures to control both
- How to develop a support group or how to locate one

Evidence-Based Practice

O'Brien, J., Ottoboni, G., Tessari, A., & Setti, A. (2017). One bout of open skill exercise improves cross-modal perception and immediate memory in healthy older adults who habitually exercise. *PLoS ONE, 12*(6), 1–16. DOI: 10.1371/journal.pone.0178739.

As older adults age, memory skills tend to decline. In this study, older adults who routinely exercised for 60 to 80 minutes at a time showed an increase in memory-retaining skills, immediately after completing the exercise regime. Older adults who were less physically active did not show an increase in memory-retaining skills, although they did show improvement in memory immediately after completing a physical activity. Additional studies also support that the more physically active an older person is, the more likely they are to exhibit increased memory-retaining skills.

Questions

1. What are ways that older adults can increase their physical activity without causing muscle or joint injury?
2. How can older adults know how much they can tolerate exercising?
3. What are other ways that older adults can maintain their memory?

Musculoskeletal System
Osteoarthritis and Degenerative Joint Disease

Osteoarthritis is the most common chronic condition reported by older adults. The incidence of arthritis increases with aging. There are more than 100 types of arthritis. Destruction of the joint cartilage occurs, often followed by overproduction of tissue at the joint margins. The result is a visible enlargement of the joint, especially in the knees and fingers. The cause of the most common form, degenerative joint disease or primary osteoarthritis, is unknown. Primary arthritis is permanent and progressive, but signs and symptoms may appear or disappear at certain times or vary in intensity. Secondary osteoarthritis develops from a combination of physical stress on joints and a medical problem such as diabetes or inflammation. Gout and rheumatoid arthritis are examples of this form.

A patient with degenerative joint disease usually reports joint stiffness in the morning with limitation of motion and muscle aches, cramps, or spasms. The extent of these symptoms varies from person to person. Some people have very little joint pain or stiffness. Others may experience joint pain most of the day. There is no specific treatment.

The goals for treatment may include the following:

- Control of pain with nonsteroidal medications, such as ibuprofen
- Steroid injection into the affected joint
- Weight loss if the person is overweight
- Maintain activity
- Cope with physical and lifestyle changes
- Joint replacement

To reach these goals, it is usually helpful for the person to understand the nature of the condition and to avoid the use of ineffective treatments. It also is important to learn to identify events or activities that increase and decrease pain to promote self-care.

Another crucial aspect of care is to teach the older adult to use medications to prevent pain rather than to control pain after it has started, that is, take pain medication before activity or on a routine basis. Meal planning is another challenge. Meals should meet but not exceed caloric needs. (This can be a problem for people with low income, minimal sources of emotional support, or lack of energy or motivation to change eating habits.) The nurse should teach the patient and family to plan activities around the time of day when the person feels best and there is less pain.

A physical therapist can teach the proper use of moist heat, physical therapy exercises, and equipment (e.g., a walker) to decrease pain or stress on joints. A walker or other equipment may need to be examined to ensure that it is appropriate for the person's needs. The nurse should focus on teaching the older adult self-expression to maintain self-esteem, decrease depression, and promote social interaction. Referral to an arthritis support group and use of teaching materials from such a group may be helpful to older persons and their families.

Osteoporosis

Osteoporosis is the most common bone disease in the older adult. Osteoporosis is a disease in which bones become fragile and are more likely to fracture. Usually, the bone loses density, which is determined by the amount of calcium and minerals in the bone. Caucasian and Asian women who have small, thin frames are at highest risk. Men and women of all ethnic groups can develop osteoporosis. Women experience more rapid bone loss in their 50s than men do. The normal decrease in estrogen in women at the time of menopause and decrease in testosterone in men are leading causes of bone loss in the older adult (see Box 14.1 for other risk factors). By the late 60s, men

Box 14.1

Risk Factors for Osteoporosis

Positive family history for osteoporosis
Inactivity or immobility
Low calcium and vitamin D intake
Smoking
High intake of alcohol
High intake of caffeine
Long-term use of corticosteroids or anticonvulsant drugs
Low body weight
Weight loss surgery
Disease conditions: autoimmune disorders, diabetes, leukemia, hyperparathyroidism

and women lose bone mass at the same rate. The older adult may be unaware that he or she has osteoporosis until minimal trauma results in a fracture.

A major goal when working with someone with osteoporosis is to maintain safety. Injury resulting from a fall, especially a hip fracture, is one of the most frequent consequences. The resulting loss of mobility and restriction of activity create emotional problems and place the person at risk for other physical problems, such as skin breakdown and constipation. In addition, treatment is long and costly.

A major nursing responsibility is to teach the person and family to identify hazards in the home and community. Simple techniques that can be used to help maintain safety are the use of grab bars by the toilet in the tub or shower and the use of a tub chair for bathing. The house should be carefully examined for safety hazards such as "trippers" (e.g., scatter rugs, electric cords, uneven pavement, and pets). The person should be taught to maintain postural balance by rising slowly and avoiding sudden movement. Another area in which teaching is beneficial is the identification of risk factors—for example, limiting use of caffeine sources to one a day. Limiting the use of tobacco and alcohol may help decrease the progression of osteoporosis. Increasing the consumption of sources of calcium, such as fortified low-fat milk, yogurt, and cottage cheese, also increases the intake of vitamin D.

Metabolic and Endocrine Diseases
Type 2 Diabetes

Type 2 diabetes is becoming an epidemic. Diabetes is a condition in which the body does not properly process glucose for use as energy. Most of the food we eat is turned into glucose that our bodies can use for energy. The pancreas is an organ located by the stomach that makes a hormone called insulin. Insulin

is necessary to help glucose get into the cells of our bodies to be used for energy. When an individual has diabetes, the body either does not make enough insulin or cannot use its own insulin as well as it should. This causes glucose to build up in the blood. This is why many people refer to diabetes as "sugar diabetes."

Type 2 diabetes is becoming more prevalent in the United States. The Centers for Disease Control and Prevention (CDC) estimates that by the year 2050, one in three Americans will have type 2 diabetes if current trends continue. Currently one in ten adult Americans has diabetes (CDC, 2018).

In a condition called prediabetes, glucose levels are higher than normal, but not high enough to be considered diabetes. When a person is diagnosed with prediabetes, it alerts the individual that he or she is at risk for developing type 2 diabetes (see Box 14.2). Research shows that people with prediabetes can greatly reduce their risk of type 2 diabetes by losing weight and increasing their activity level.

Individuals diagnosed with prediabetes also are at higher risk for heart disease, stroke, and eye disease. Diabetes can cause serious health complications including heart disease, blindness, kidney failure, and the loss of feet or legs. Diabetes is the seventh leading cause of death in the United States (CDC, 2018).

THINK LIKE A NURSE

The symptoms of diabetes in the elderly can be masked, making the disease more difficult to diagnose. Warning signs such as increased thirst, frequent urination, and vision problems may be overlooked because of the common effects of aging on the body. Changes such as fatigue, weakness, mental confusion, incontinence, and other health complications related to diabetes are more often the presenting symptoms. In addition, it is not unusual for the older person to have high cholesterol levels along with elevated glucose levels.

What questions can be asked to determine changes in symptoms?

There is no cure for type 2 diabetes, but it usually can be controlled with diet alone. When the person is overweight, a reduced caloric intake coupled with regular exercise are recommended. Oral hypoglycemic drugs may be used if control is not achieved with diet and exercise. Some older adults may need insulin when adequate blood glucose level control is not achieved.

Box 14.2

Risk Factors for Type 2 Diabetes

Age 45 years or older

Prediabetes diagnosis

Overweight

Family history of type 2 diabetes

Physically active fewer than three times per week

History of having given birth to a baby who weighed more than 9 pounds

History of gestational diabetes

Certain ethnic groups (African American, Hispanic/Latino, American Indian)

The types of complications associated with diabetes mellitus, such as skin lesions and renal and neurological problems, also may be typical of aging. Teaching about skin care, protection of the feet, periodic eye examination, dental care, and recognition of infections is critical in maintaining proper control of diabetes. The nurse also needs to teach older adults with type 2 diabetes how to follow a regular schedule involving medication, diet, exercise, and blood glucose monitoring.

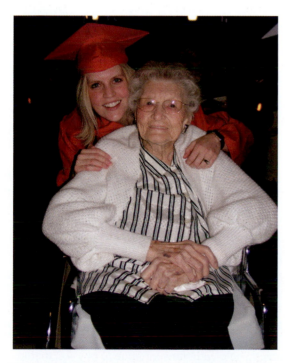

Older adults with chronic illnesses can live reasonably normal lives if they are willing to attend to the details of managing their disease. This woman was able to attend her granddaughter's college graduation because of her determination to live well with diabetes.

Cultural Considerations

Some cultures are more likely to develop chronic illnesses such as HTN, diabetes, and blood dyscrasias. The nurse should be aware of the possible cultural specific conditions so appropriate education and management of the condition can be addressed.

Hypothyroidism

Hypothyroidism is common, especially among older women. The presence of a low thyroid level is often overlooked because of the similarity between the symptoms of hypothyroidism and characteristics of aging. Symptoms of hypothyroidism, which are thought to be typical among older adults, are fatigue, memory loss, slowing of thought processes, dry skin, intolerance to cold, constipation, and thinning of hair. Symptoms can occur slowly over time.

Blood tests can show whether thyroid hormone levels are abnormal. Caregivers often attribute behavioral changes in an older person only to aging. Even small deficits of thyroxine or small increases in thyroid-stimulating hormone can result in slowed reactions. This should be a clear safety alert for every nurse. Patients also should be taught how to recognize signs and symptoms of overmedication or undermedication for this disease. It is especially important to monitor respiratory and cardiac function. People usually begin to notice improved function within a few days of starting treatment.

GEROTRANSCENDENCE

Each of the diseases discussed in this chapter requires a great deal of commitment and courage to manage and live with successfully. The people who are most likely to commit to self-management are those who have embraced the concept of gerotranscendence. Most individuals, however, do not understand the concept. Gerotranscendence is something that comes from within after living a life that successfully follows Erikson's developmental stages. A person who has gone through Erikson's stages has managed life well and with successful human interaction. Such individuals have loved and been loved, have avoided despair despite life's tragedies, and have been industrious and successful. Consequently, such people are ready for the losses of old age and the inevitability of death. Many psychologists say that the family and friends who can talk about death openly are the ones who are very close to each other. This comfort with oneself and with the inevitability of death is one aspect of gerotranscendence.

An older adult who has succeeded in Erikson's developmental plan can accept death because of a life well lived. The individual generally can continue living with singular or multiple acute and chronic diseases because there are few regrets in his or her life. Such people accept illness and work to manage it; they also accept the inevitability of death and plan for it.

Consider a 68-year-old woman with multiple serious chronic diseases. Within the last 3 months, she has been diagnosed with an aggressive cancer that has spread. She is undergoing chemotherapy and will also have radiation. She has purchased a burial plot, picked out and had a headstone put into place, and written her obituary. She is affluent and is now working on her will to update it. She has made a list of items that she wants to go to friends and each of her nieces and nephews. With those things done, she now plays with and makes plans to do things with her three grandchildren that include her only child and her husband. She has achieved gerotranscendence as she accepts her illnesses and the fact she will eventually die, and she has moved on to enjoy her life.

The way for older adults to achieve gerotranscendence is to have support from caring nurses like you throughout their lives. The way for you to achieve it later in your life is to be aware of Erikson's theory and apply it for yourself and to teach it to people who come into your life. It is worth the effort.

CASE STUDY SOLUTIONS

1. You should consider the desired effect of Mr. Hughes' antihypertensive medications and any over-the-counter drugs he may be taking. Consider the possible side effects of each, and whether there are any interactions among the medications. In addition, consider how frequently blood pressure needs to be checked (probably every 1 to 2 weeks after a medication is started; consider the use of a home health nurse to monitor this or use of a senior center if there is one where blood pressure monitoring can be done). Monitoring also should include keeping a diary of food eaten and looking at salt content and quantity of food and fluids. Even after a person has been on medications for some time, review of diet, activity, ability to take medications as prescribed, and whether the patient can continue to afford the medications (to avoid skipping doses) is needed. Encourage a follow-up with his PCP within 2 to 4 weeks to make sure that his medications are appropriate as his blood pressure is monitored.

2. You should discuss with Mr. Hughes the impact with Mr. Hughes that smoking has upon blood pressure. Smoking can cause the blood vessels to constrict, which can raise blood pressure. After many years of smoking, the blood vessels can become less flexible and unable to relax even after smoking cessation. The impact of an additional 30 pounds can also add to the increased blood pressure levels. Even a 20-minute walk around the block a couple of times a week can help keep him active. You can discuss the effects that prolonged smoking can have on the smaller vessels in his eyes and how it can lead to macular degeneration. Another area where Mr. Hughes may need assistance is medication management. Discuss the importance of taking his medication as ordered. What can he do to remember to take his daily medications? Can he set an alarm on his phone or watch to remind him?

3. Falls are common in older adults with weakness. You should discuss with Mr. Hughes that he should only get up with assistance. See if assistive devices can be placed in the tub and by the toilet. He may also be prone to choking if his swallowing has not resumed. Make sure that he has small bites of food and that he does not have foods that are difficult to chew. Thin liquids are often difficult to swallow. Teach Mrs. Hughes not to rush him through his meals.

Investigate the county agencies on aging, home health agencies, nutrition programs, transportation resources, and availability of neighbors or friends as well as family. Investigate if Mr. Hughes' family is available to assist with daily care. Are they able to assist with household duties and shopping duties to allow Mrs. Hughes some respite time? Is family available to help with transportation to physical therapy and doctor visits? Does the local health department have resources for smoking cessation?

Key Points

- Acute medical issues are those that last for a short period of time. Symptoms can occur for a few minutes and last less than a month. A chronic medical condition lasts 3 months or more. Some acute conditions can progress into chronic conditions.
- As a person ages, common changes occur as part of the aging process; vision and hearing diminish, muscles shrink, joints stiffen, blood vessels harden, digestion slows down, and memory can decrease.
- Nursing care appropriate for older adults includes observation of the patient's physical functioning. This may include responses to medical treatments, such as side effects of medication, and mental or physical decline.
- Older adults should be encouraged to be active participants in their care. This includes taking medications as appropriate, maintaining visits with their PCP, and accessing community and family resources.

- Review of systems is a method of looking at each of the body systems to note previous or current medical problems or issues. This includes the medical history and physical exam. Use of this method ensures that each system is addressed and that chronicity of conditions is determined and associated signs and symptoms are documented.
- Chronic illnesses commonly found in older adults can affect every body system. Some of these changes can be accelerated by lifestyle choices, such as poor nutrition, obesity, decrease of physical activity, and smoking. Many of these chronic illnesses occur along with other diseases, such as diabetes and macular degeneration.
- Gerotranscendence is the analysis of one's life lived as the inevitability of death looms nearer. It is the openness and the acceptance that despite the challenges of medical conditions, death is not to be feared but accepted as part of the life cycle.

Review Questions

1. Chronic health conditions differ from acute conditions in which of the following ways?
   1. Chronic conditions begin at an earlier age.
   2. Acute conditions tend to take time developing.
   3. Chronic conditions require active work by patient or family.
   4. Acute conditions occur briefly and resolve quickly.

2. A review of systems helps the nurse identify which of the following?
   1. Possible interaction among health-care problems
   2. Whether the person has been taking care of his or her health properly
   3. How much the patient can remember about past health history
   4. To whom the patient should be referred based on a system need

3. When a person has a right-sided stroke, one way to ensure the patient's continued attention to both sides of the body is to do which of the following?
   1. Observe for equal length of both arms.
   2. Observe the condition of the skin and mucous membranes on the affected side.
   3. Continue to teach the patient to strengthen the unaffected side and to avoid overuse of the affected extremities.
   4. Continue to approach the patient from the unaffected side to encourage communication.

4. A major concern with older adults who have chronic conditions such as osteoarthritis is lack of activity. Which of the following is an unwanted result of decreased activity?
   1. Diarrhea
   2. Poor hygiene
   3. Loss of sense of touch
   4. Deconditioning

5. An older person with a chronic condition such
   as HTN may not take prescribed medications
   routinely. The main reason for this is which
   of the following?
   1. Inability to remember a medication schedule
   2. Lack of symptoms that indicate blood
      pressure is high
   3. Fear of becoming dependent on the
      medication
   4. Undesired side effects of the medications

ANSWERS 1. 4, 2. 1, 3. 2, 4. 5, 2

CHAPTER 15
Physiological Assessment

Holli Sowerby

KEY TERMS

activities of daily living (ADLs)
auscultation
functional status
health assessment
holistic assessment
inspection
instrumental activities of daily living (IADLs)
palpation

CHAPTER CONCEPTS

Evidence-Based Practice
Patient-Centered Care
Safety
Communication

LEARNING OUTCOMES

1. Describe two unique aspects of physiological assessment for older adults.
2. Describe at least three normal aging changes for each body system.
3. List two tools that are commonly used to evaluate functional status.
4. Discuss the importance of nutrition to the physiological well-being of the older adult.

CASE STUDY

Miss S., an 85-year-old woman, has been added to your home health client list. She was recently hospitalized for nearly 1 week with an exacerbation of heart failure (HF). In addition to her HF, she also has diabetes. Her diabetes has been well controlled, but she received treatment with steroids in the hospital that have caused her to have an increase in her daily blood glucose levels. Miss S. is responding well to her medication regimen for the HF and will be receiving home health services for 4 to 5 weeks.

Discussion
1. What is your priority in assessing Miss S. today?
2. How will you meet the requirements of the priority assessment items?
3. What other points of concern should you address in your assessment?
4. How will you do that?

INTRODUCTION

Health assessment is a comprehensive evaluation of a patient's data, including the patient's physical, psychological, social, cultural, spiritual, and environmental information. Nurses involved in health assessment are not just simply collecting information about problems; the assessment must include identification of strengths, assets, potential risks, and potential areas of growth.

This chapter teaches how to do a **holistic assessment**. Holistic assessments go beyond the physical assessment and include all aspects of the older person's life. The ability to perform a holistic assessment requires a high level of thinking and a sophisticated ability to process information. This is your opportunity to learn and then to do something significant for the older adults in your care. This chapter outlines the parts of a physical, functional, discharge, and wellness assessment. The interrelationship between physical health, psychological well-being, and safety (Fig. 15.1) is highlighted. The licensed practical nurse (LPN) must be prepared to perform a complete and thorough holistic assessment of the older patient in an effort to improve the person's overall health and happiness.

PHYSICAL ASSESSMENT

The techniques for physical examination included in this chapter are not all-inclusive of the techniques used to conduct a total examination. This assessment outline assists you, however, in completing a head-to-toe physical examination of an older adult. It is important to remember to report any abnormal findings to the registered nurse (RN) or the physician.

Cultural Considerations

Diverse cultural backgrounds may affect many aspects of a physical assessment. The following are factors to consider when gathering assessment data:

• Health beliefs: In some cultures, people believe that talking about a possible poor health outcome will cause that outcome to occur.
• Health customs: In some cultures, family members play a large role in health-care decision making.
• Ethnic customs: Differing roles of women and men in society may determine who makes decisions about accepting and following through with medical treatments.
• Religious beliefs: Religious faith and spiritual beliefs may affect health-care seeking behavior and people's willingness to accept specific treatments or behavior changes.
• Dietary customs: Disease-related dietary advice will be difficult to follow if it does not conform to the foods or cooking methods used by the patient.
• Interpersonal customs: Eye contact or physical touch will be expected in some cultures and inappropriate or offensive in others (Agency for Healthcare Research and Quality, n.d.)

HISTORY

When taking a history on any system, there is information you need to have for an accurate record of the person's overall health. You need to know the person's:

• Exercise plan
• Eating patterns, including recent weight loss or gain
• Consumption of alcoholic beverages, caffeine, and water
• Sleep patterns
• Smoking history
• Stress management techniques

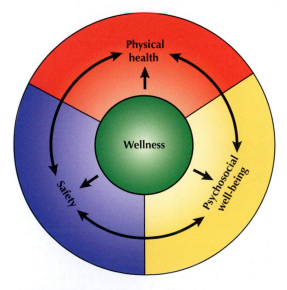

FIGURE 15.1 Interrelationship of physical health, psychosocial well-being, and safety.

- Sexual activity
- Medication record, including prescription and over-the-counter medications

---

Priority Setting

Learning how to perform a complete health assessment involves mastering many new skills. Here is one way to prioritize learning this new skill set:

1. Learn how to auscultate and palpate so that you can trust what you hear and feel. The only way to do this is to practice. It can take more than 50 practice assessments before one can trust what one is hearing or feeling.
2. After you have mastered the basic skills, you need to focus on the body one system at a time. For example, do heart assessments until you are really good. Blending the health history and integrated physical assessment allows nurses to identify patient problems and assets more accurately. This is part of the nursing process.

For Miss S., taking her medications appropriately is a serious matter. Any information about Miss S. and her use or misuse of the medications ordered to manage her HF must be reported to the RN immediately.

After you have obtained the previously listed information, you need to take a history and do an examination of the person's physiological systems. If you identify aspects of the assessment or history that you do not understand or know how to do, discuss your concerns in class or privately with the faculty person. In general, the history and physical examination of an older adult are similar to that of a middle-aged adult, but they also include specific aspects that relate to people who are growing older. It is important that you learn to adapt from one age group to another as you work in nursing.

The following information is presented in didactic manner for ease and efficiency in your study of the material. A nurse who can do an excellent history and assessment of a specialized group of people, such as older adults, is very desirable as an employee. It is likely that with continued practice, you will acquire the skills and knowledge to "pick up" on a subtle sign or symptom that may indicate a hidden problem, such as a "painless" heart attack, infection without a fever, or increased white blood count (WBC), all of which many older adults have. Subtle signs and symptoms are important to recognize because they may save a life.

The material in this chapter is divided into three basic skills for doing an assessment: history, inspection, and palpation (Wilkinson, Treas, Barnett, & Smith, 2016).

REVIEW OF SYSTEMS

Head, Neck, and Face
History
Evaluate the older adult's medical history for head injury, increased level of stress, thyroid dysfunction, neck injury, or infection.

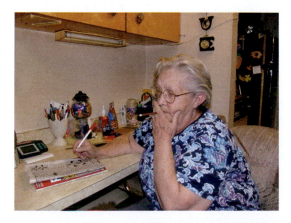

This woman smokes a pack of cigarettes a day and seldom leaves her house. Based on this information, what other questions should you ask her about her health as you take her history?

Safe, Effective Nursing Care

Improving Patient Care

At an interdisciplinary team (IDT) meeting, Dr. K. complained that the nurses were calling him at all hours with inappropriate requests. Before the nurse manager could respond, the pharmacist exclaimed that he was also getting unnecessary calls. When the nurse manager approached the physician and pharmacist for clarification, it seemed that the nurses were concerned about the well-being of a resident but were unable to communicate data to support their concerns. They would say things like, "the resident is acting funny" or "I don't know why but I have a funny feeling about how Mr. U. is doing."

The nurse manager called the nursing management team together to discuss this problem and possible solutions. The group decided the following:

1. They changed the reporting process. To help the nurses organize their thoughts and get all of the information they needed before they made a call, the group adopted Identification, Situation, Background, Assessment, and Recommendation (I-SBAR) as the reporting tool.
2. The nursing staff had a mandatory orientation and training on the use of I-SBAR. Online and printed worksheets were distributed to nurses as part of the training.
3. The staff used the I-SBAR for 2 weeks. At the end of 2 weeks, the nursing management team distributed a questionnaire asking the staff and other members of the IDT if there were any changes noted with the use of I-SBAR.

After the 2-week period, four of the nurses asked the management team to help them with physical assessment. They knew when a resident was agitated or anxious but felt ill equipped to perform an appropriate assessment. The nurse managers worked at the bedside with the nurses to help with not only assessment skills but also diagnostic reasoning. If a resident was short of breath or having difficulty breathing, the nurses were taught to not only take the resident's respiratory rate but to assess lung sounds; note when the difficulty breathing occurred (with activity or at rest); ask the resident whether he or she had any other symptoms; check capillary refill, oxygen saturation, pulse rate and rhythm, and blood pressure; and ask the resident whether he or she had ever had a similar problem and what were those circumstances.

This example shows how a change in process can definitely improve the practice of the staff and ultimately the care for a resident. It demonstrates the knowledge, skills, and attitude associated with quality improvement. The nursing management team demonstrated a commitment to quality care by looking at process and process improvement rather than simply pointing a finger at nurses who were not performing good assessments.

1. Why do you think the nurses came forward and asked for assistance with bedside assessments?
2. Can you identify a problem in your work setting that needs a process change to improve care?

Physical Examination

The assessment of the head and neck is the same for older adults as for younger people.

INSPECTION. Observe the older individual's head position. Note the size, shape, symmetry, and proportion of the head. If it appears abnormally large or small, measure the circumference or distance around the head. Evaluate hair distribution, pattern of baldness, and dryness of the scalp. Note if lice are found in the hair. The presence of lice demands immediate intervention. Assess the face for color, symmetry, and distribution of facial hair. Evaluate facial muscles by having the older adult demonstrate different facial expressions: raise eyebrows, close eyes, puff out cheeks, smile, show teeth, and frown. Note any wrinkles or dryness of the skin. Note the size of the neck. The trachea should be aligned with the midline of the suprasternal notch. Observe for symmetry of the neck muscles. Note venous distention, involuntary muscle tension, or swelling in the neck. Assess the active range of motion (ROM) of the neck by having the older adult tilt the head backward, forward, from side to side, and in a circular motion. ROM of the neck should be completed without limitation or pain.

PALPATION. Palpate the alignment of the trachea. Palpate the cervical muscles, and note any tenderness. Palpate the carotid pulses one at a time. What does the pulse feel like? Is it bounding? Weak? Or does it have a vibration-type movement? As the older adult moves the neck, palpate over the spinal area for crepitus. Crepitus is a slight grating sensation that occurs when you palpate, and it is not normal.

Abnormal findings include edema of the face (especially around eyes), involuntary facial movements (tic, tremor, droop), lack of symmetry, unusual size and contour, and tenderness.

Nose and Sinuses
History

Ask the older adult to describe any problems with the nose or sinuses. Note that epistaxis (nosebleed) is more common in older adults than in younger adults.

Physical Examination

INSPECTION. Observe the size, shape, and color of the nose. Note any flaring of the nostrils during breathing and any nasal drainage. Ask the older person to tilt the head so you can examine the nasal cavity for swelling, drainage, polyps, and bleeding. The nasal mucosa should be moist and dark pink. Frequently, men have an increased amount of nasal hair. Assess the movement of air through each nostril by occluding the nostril not being examined and asking the older adult to inhale and exhale through the nose. Assess the older adult's ability to smell by asking the person to identify different common smells (almond, vanilla, cinnamon, coffee). It is abnormal for the smell to be perceived differently in each nostril.

PALPATION. Palpate the nose for tenderness or masses. Abnormal findings include swelling of mucosa, bleeding, discharge, perforation, polyps, and deviation of nasal septum. It is abnormal to find nasal blockage, infection, crusting, and dryness.

Eyes
History
The nurse needs to discuss the following: vision changes, pain, excessive tearing or discharge, diplopia, infection, and cataracts. Ask whether the person wears glasses. When are the glasses worn? When was the last ophthalmic examination?

Physical Examination
INSPECTION. Assess the external eye and visual acuity. Examine the eyes for position and alignment. Note the symmetry of the eyebrows, eyelashes, pupils, and irises. Changes in the appearance of the eyelids can be due to systemic diseases such as hyperthyroidism, myasthenia gravis, or palsy. The eyes should be evaluated for redness, swelling, and discharge. Pupils should be equal in size unless they have been unequal throughout life or have become unequal as a result of surgery or trauma. They may react more slowly to light than they did in the person's youth. Normally, the pupils are black, equal in size, round, and smooth. If the older adult has cataracts, the pupils may appear cloudy.

Before testing visual acuity, the nurse should ensure that adequate light is available. If the older adult wears glasses, the lenses should be checked for cleanliness and alignment because those two factors can affect visual acuity. The line of the bifocals may cause double vision if the glasses are misaligned. Evaluate distant vision with a Snellen eye chart. Test each eye separately, with and without glasses. After testing separately, test the eyes together with and without glasses. Any person with 20/40 vision or less should be referred to a physician or nurse practitioner. To test near vision, use a newspaper or other conventional reading material; measure the distance from the face to the reading material. Have an alternate plan if the person cannot read. A possibility is to have the person look at a picture and describe the details to you.

Ears
HISTORY. The nurse needs to determine if hearing loss is having an effect on the older person's life. Does the older adult use any corrective devices, such as amplifiers or hearing aids? Following are some questions that can be used to elicit a history: Have you experienced pain from your ears? Have you had dizziness? In what situations? How long did it last? What relieved the dizziness? Have you had any discharge from your ears? What color? What consistency? Did it have an odor? Have you experienced a sudden or rapid change in your hearing? What were you doing when it occurred? Does it come and go?

Physical Examination
INSPECTION. Observe the older individual in conversation. Does the person lean forward or cup a hand to the ear to hear? Is a loud speaking voice used? Does the person request repetition of what has been said? If hearing loss is identified, speak to the person in a normal tone of voice and speak toward the better ear, if there is one. Assess the ear for size, shape, symmetry, redness, inflammation, swelling, discharge, and lesions.

PALPATION. The surface of the skin of the ear should have a smooth texture. Palpate around the ear and ask the older adult whether any pain or tenderness is present.

Mouth and Throat
History
The first aspect of history taking related to the mouth is to establish whether the older adult has any dental complaints. The following questions can be used to elicit a history:

Do you have any pain or discomfort? Are any of your teeth especially sensitive to hot or cold temperatures? Have you noticed any swelling in your mouth or throat? Do you have any difficulty chewing or swallowing? How does food taste? Is your mouth dry?

Do your dentures fit properly? Do you have any sores or lesions in your mouth or throat? How often do you brush your teeth, dentures, or tongue? Do you use dental floss? If so, how often? When was your last dental examination? What was the result? Do you clean your dentures at night in a cleaning solution?

Physical Examination

INSPECTION AND PALPATION. Inspection and palpation are used concurrently during the oral cavity examination. Use a gloved hand and a gauze pad to perform this part of the examination. If the older adult wears dentures, remove them before starting the examination. Evaluate the fit of the dentures to the gums or alveolar surfaces and the dentures themselves. Dentures are considered to fit improperly if there is inflammation and ulceration of the palate, mucosa, and alveolar ridges. Examine the dentures for cracks, missing pieces, and rough edges. Dentures should be stable and remain securely fixed during chewing. Underlying tissues should be pink and adhere tightly to the bone. There should not be food, debris, or excessive denture adhesive on the inside of the denture. If the older adult does not have dentures, examine the teeth. Note the number and position of teeth. Are they in good repair, or can you see cavities and broken teeth?

The gums should be pink, moist, and smooth. Inspect for signs of inflammation and lesions. The hard palate should be pale. The soft palate should be pink. Inspect for inflammation, lesions, pallor, and any purulent drainage or a white coating on the tongue. The uvula should be midline and red. It should move up as the older adult says "Ah." Tonsils, if present, should be small, pink, and symmetrical. Check the gag reflex with a tongue blade. The top and bottom of the tongue should be examined. A smooth, painful tongue may indicate vitamin B$_{12}$ deficiency. The tongue and mucous membranes should be pink, moist, and free of swelling and lesions. The tongue should relax on the floor of the mouth. Varicose veins on the bottom surface of the tongue are common. Ask the older adult to stick out the tongue to examine it. While you hold it out with a piece of gauze, inspect all sides of the tongue and the floor of the mouth. Report any white, scaly patches. The lips should be moist, smooth, and pink. Check the corners of the mouth for cracks. These cracks are a prime spot for *Candida* (yeast) infections.

Neurological System
History

Does the older adult have any problems with headaches? Shaking or trembling? Confusion or memory loss? In assessing the neurological system, the nurse also should ask if the older adult has experienced seizures. Is there an existing seizure disorder? What type of treatment has been received? What were the circumstances occurring before, during, and after the seizure?

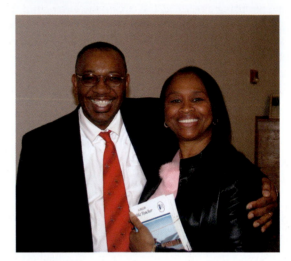

When taking a history on an older adult, it generally is helpful to obtain information from the family as well as the individual being assessed. An older adult may have problems accurately remembering events that happened a long time ago.

Physical Examination

INSPECTION. Examine the older adult's level of orientation. Is the person alert, lethargic, or nonresponsive? Oriented to place, time, and person? As the older adult answers questions, observe the face for symmetry of movement when smiling, talking, grimacing, or frowning. Evaluate the older adult's appearance throughout the examination. Is the person dressed appropriately? Is the person wearing multiple layers of clothing? If so, are they appropriate for the weather outdoors? Is there body odor? Does the person appear well groomed? Is the older adult's behavior appropriate? Evaluate the strength and symmetry of the older adult's upper and lower extremities. This is commonly done by asking the person to squeeze your hands. Ask the person to walk across the room and observe the gait for symmetry, balance, and coordination during ambulation. Note any weakness.

Peripheral Vascular System
History

Following are key history questions related to peripheral vascular functioning: Do you have diabetes? Do you wear garters or girdles? Do you wear ankle-, knee-, or thigh-high hosiery? When you take off your hosiery, is there an indentation in your leg that does not go away for several minutes? Do your shoes fit tightly? Do you have pain in your calves after walking? Do you ever experience pains, aches, numbness, or tingling in your calves, feet, buttocks, or legs? Are there any activities that you cannot do because of pains and aches in your extremities? What aggravates your pain? What relieves the pain? Does walking or climbing stairs cause pain? Do you ever notice change in the color of your extremities—red, blue, or pale? Have you noticed any hair loss over any part of your legs? Does your family have a history of problems with the legs? Do you sit for long periods with your legs crossed? Do you experience swelling of your legs at the end of the day? Does swelling return to normal in the morning?

Physical Examination

The physical examination of the peripheral vascular system includes **inspection**, **palpation**, and **auscultation**. The nurse should always compare one side of the body with the other when using these assessment methods.

INSPECTION. Skin color should be evaluated with the older adult lying down. Inspect the upper and lower extremities. Venous insufficiency is indicated if the legs are cyanotic when they are dependent (hanging down) or when petechiae or broken pigmentation is present on the skin over the legs. Chronic venous insufficiency is common in elderly people. If the legs become pale when they are elevated and turn dark red when they dangle, arterial insufficiency is indicated. The signs of chronic venous insufficiency are distended tortuous veins, hair loss, hyperpigmentation, cool or normal skin temperature, and pretibial edema or pedal edema that is worse during the day but improves at night when the older adult lies down to sleep. The signs of chronic arterial insufficiency include thin, shiny, atrophic skin; hair loss over feet and toes; thick and rigid toenails; and cool skin.

Edema of the legs and feet should be noted. The nurse may choose to record the width of the edematous area by using a measuring tape. When measuring the legs to assess edema, be sure to measure at the same place on each leg. If you wish to monitor changes in edema, lightly mark the location on the leg you are measuring with a felt-tipped marker and measure in the same place each day. Stasis ulcers are rare with varicose veins, but they commonly occur with deep vein insufficiency. Venous stasis ulcers are located on the sides of the ankles. Arterial ulcers may involve toes or places where the skin has been bumped or bruised.

PALPATION. Check the skin temperature of the older adult's arms and legs by using the back of your hand. Increased temperature can be caused by a localized response to inflammation. Cool temperature indicates decreased blood flow. Peripheral pulses should be evaluated by using the pads of the index and middle fingers. The pulse is evaluated for rate, rhythm, amplitude, and symmetry. Normal vessels feel smooth and resilient. In most older adults, increased resistance to compression may be palpated because of rigid and tortuous artery walls. The nurse should practice palpating the pulses of a young person and an older person to be able to differentiate the changes associated with aging. Pulses should be evaluated one at a time (carotid, brachial, radial, femoral, popliteal, and dorsalis pedis). They should be regular, strong, and equal bilaterally. Lack of symmetry between extremities indicates possible impaired circulation. If you have difficulty finding a pulse, feel throughout the area where it is expected to be and vary the pressure of your finger. Be sure you are not feeling your own pulse. The rate you feel should be different from your own heart rate. If you had difficulty finding a pulse, you can mark its location with a felt-tipped pen after it is found.

Cardiac System
History

Older adults should be asked questions to assess for cardiac disease risk factors, including smoking and exercise: Do you have any problems with dyspnea (shortness of breath)? Does your shortness of breath increase with activity (i.e., dyspnea on exertion)? Do you have chest pain? When does it occur? What are you doing when it occurs? Is the chest pain relieved by rest?

Physical Examination

INSPECTION. A cardiac physical examination procedure is the same for older and younger persons. The older adult should be evaluated while lying down, sitting up, and standing. Observe the neck and chest to detect any visible pulsations, lifts, or heaves. The heartbeat is usually not visible, but it may be if the individual is emaciated. It is abnormal to observe the heart beating on the chest wall of an older adult who is obese or of normal weight. Note any cough, shortness of breath, venous or abdominal distention, or cyanosis of mucous membranes and nailbeds. The legs, ankles, and feet should be observed for edema.

PALPATION. Feel the front of the chest over the heart for any thrills, heaves, or lifts. A thrill is a palpable vibration. A lift or heave is a pulsation that is more forceful than anticipated. There should be minimal changes in the pulse when the older adult changes positions between lying, sitting, and standing. Press on the nailbeds and observe for the return of a pink color; this is called capillary refill and should occur quickly. It is abnormal for refill to take longer than 2 seconds. Skin temperature should be palpated for unusual coolness or heat. The blood pressure should be checked using the orthostatic technique that you learned in Chapter 14. Orthostatic hypotension is a common problem with older adults.

AUSCULTATION. Older adults have more rapid and less distinct heartbeats. Many older persons live normal, everyday lives with chronic atrial fibrillation. Any irregularity of the heartbeat noted while listening to the heart should be reported to the RN or physician. Infrequent extra beats (ectopic) are fairly common. Another common abnormal finding is a heart murmur. A heart murmur is caused by thickened and rigid heart valves and decreased strength of myocardial contractions. It sounds like a hum or click and results from turbulent or backward flow of blood through the heart. If detected, it should be reported.

Focused Learning Chart: Assessment of Cardiac Risk Factors

Risk	Management
Advancing age	Understand medications
Being male	Smoking cessation
Women after menopause	Appropriate exercise plan
Obesity	Manage obesity
Elevated blood glucose levels (diabetes mellitus)	Decreased sodium intake
Elevated blood lipids (hyperlipidemia)	Low-fat diet
Elevated blood pressure (hypertension)	No constricting clothing
Sedentary lifestyle	
Smoking	

Respiratory System
History

Questions that are used to assess an older adult's respiratory status include the following: Do you have any difficulty breathing? Do you get short of breath with exercise or exertion? Do you have a cough? Is your cough dry or productive? What color and consistency is the mucus that you cough up? Is there any blood in the mucus?

Dyspnea or difficulty breathing is not a part of normal aging. It is often related to HF, pneumonia, anemia, and other lung diseases. It is present in only one-half of older persons with pneumonia. The first signs of pneumonia often include a nonspecific deterioration in health, such as slight cough, altered mental status, and tachycardia.

Ask the older adult if there is any history of lung disease. If so, what effect does it have on **activities of daily living (ADLs)**? Is oxygen used? Ask questions to determine if the older adult is using oxygen safely in the home. Other questions that can be used to elicit history of lung disease are as follows: Do you live in an area that has air pollution? Have you or any member of your family ever had tuberculosis? What is the date of your last chest x-ray study? Have you had the pneumonia vaccine (Pneumovax)? If so, when did you receive it? Have you had an influenza shot this year? Have you received one within the last year? Have you had a tuberculosis skin test? When?

Physical Examination

INSPECTION. In the older adult population, barrel chest, slight use of intercostal muscles, and slightly prolonged respirations may occur normally. If these signs and symptoms occur suddenly, they should be considered abnormal. The respiratory rate for normal older adults is 12 to 24 respirations per minute. A rate of 24 or greater is considered tachypnea. Observe for the use of accessory muscles and nasal flaring. A rate of less than 12 respirations per minute is considered bradypnea. Overt signs of lower oxygen levels resulting from bradypnea include decreased consciousness, confusion, and lethargy. The character of respirations also should be evaluated. A normal respiratory rate is even and unlabored. The older adult's skin, lips, and nail color should be inspected for cyanosis and pallor. Posture while sitting and standing should be noted. Posture affects the ability to breathe.

PALPATION. The anterior and posterior chest should be palpated for masses and tenderness of the ribs. The tracheal area should be palpated for any deviation.

AUSCULTATION. An older adult can become dizzy from hyperventilation if asked to take deep breaths for a long time. Allow the person periods of normal breathing between deep breaths. Listen fully to inspiration and expiration. Softer vesicular sounds and diminished breath sounds in the bases of the lungs are normal. Listen for abnormal (adventitious) sounds. These sounds are superimposed on the normal breath sounds. Crackles are often heard when the older adult has HF or pulmonary edema. Crackles result from air passing through moisture and sound like hair being rubbed between the fingers. Scattered crackles in dependent lung segments of some older adults should not be mistaken for bronchitis or HF. If the crackles disappear after coughing, they are not pathological. If they are present after coughing, pathology may be present. Wheezes are a whistling noise caused by air passing through a narrowed airway. This happens with bronchospasm and swelling of the bronchioles. It is commonly heard in chronic obstructive pulmonary disease (COPD) and in older adults with asthma. Pleural friction rub is due to inflammation between the membranes lining the chest cavity. It sounds like leather rubbing together.

Gastrointestinal System
History
In taking a gastrointestinal (GI) history, the nurse needs to focus on nutritional status, bowel habits, and medications. Ask the older adult or family member to give a 24-hour recall of the older person's diet. Evaluate the reported intake for nutritional balance. Is it full of fatty foods? Is it low in fiber? Does it have a high starch content? Calculate the amount of fluids the older adult drinks in a 24-hour period. The older adult needs 2,000 to 3,000 mL of fluids per day. Continue with more health history questions: How do you tolerate eating and drinking? Do you have problems with swallowing? Do you have the sensation that food is stuck in your throat? What is your bowel routine? Do you have abdominal pain? Do you use laxatives? Have you used laxatives in the past? How long did you use them? What kind of laxatives? How often were they used? Have you experienced any recent injury or infection?

Physical Examination
INSPECTION. Inspect the skin of the abdomen and note any lesions caused by rubbing of belts or corsets over the years. Check for fungal rashes in skin folds of adults who are obese or incapacitated. Does the abdomen look rigid? If so, refer the individual to the RN or physician. Abdominal rigidity can indicate bowel obstruction.

AUSCULTATION. Listen to the abdomen with your stethoscope. Mentally divide the abdomen into quadrants that intersect through the umbilicus. Auscultate each quadrant until you hear bowel sounds, or if there are no bowel sounds, listen continuously for 5 minutes. Bowel sounds are decreased in the older adult because of decreased gastric motility that accompanies normal aging. While the history was being taken, did the older adult complain of pain in the abdomen? Ask the older adult to point to the area of pain. Right lower quadrant pain may

Focused Learning Chart: Adventitious (Abnormal) Breath Sounds

	Crackles	*Wheezes*	*Plural Friction Rub*
Pathology:	HF or pulmonary edema	COPD Asthma	Inflammation between membranes lining chest cavity
Caused by:	Air passing through moisture	Air passing through narrowed airway	Inflammation
Sounds like:	Hair being rubbed through fingers	Whistling noise	Leather rubbing together
Report to RN if:	Coughing does not relieve crackles	Present	Present (is very painful)

indicate appendicitis. Left lower quadrant pain may indicate diverticulitis. Tenderness at the base of the xiphoid process may indicate stomach pain, hiatal hernia, or referred pain from the aorta. Palpation provides further information.

PALPATION. Relaxation of the abdominal muscles enhances palpation. If the older adult is obese, palpation may be difficult. If you palpate a mass in the abdomen, it could indicate diverticulitis, fecal impaction, mesenteric thrombosis, or cancer.

Integumentary System
History
History taking is the most important aspect of the skin assessment. The most common skin complaints are pain, pruritus (itching), paresthesia (numbness), and dermatitis. The nurse needs to find out as much as possible about any skin problem mentioned. Questions to ask include the following: Do you have any skin problems? What kind? How were they treated? Are you allergic to any drugs or environmental allergens? What are they? How long have you had the allergy? Have you been exposed to an infectious disease? What is your history of sun exposure? What is your skin care regimen? Evaluate all medications that the older adult is taking. Anything that can cause an allergic reaction, no matter how long the product has been used, should be discussed. Common allergens are soaps and topical medications.

Physical Examination
INSPECTION. Look at the older person's skin in a well-lit room. Skin folds should be evaluated for dampness, irritation, and fissures. Common skin folds are under the breasts and inguinal areas. Observe the scalp, behind the ears, the fingernails and toenails, genitalia, buttocks, and face. How clean is the older adult's skin? Is there an odor present? Assess skin color for variations that are not uniform and have changed since the previous examination. Note any pallor, jaundice, cyanosis, erythema, petechiae, and ecchymosis. Older adults with deeply pigmented skin tones should be evaluated for changes in color such as duskiness, graying, and blackish areas. Jaundice in a person of color should be evaluated on the hard palate and the soles of the hands and feet. Check pressure points over bony prominences, especially on individuals who are debilitated or immobilized. Pay particular attention to the areas over the scapulae, back of the head, earlobes, hips, heels, coccyx, and elbows.

The Braden scale is a common assessment tool used to evaluate the risk of pressure ulcer formation. This is a helpful assessment to complete on every older individual who enters a health-care setting. It provides baseline information on the older person's risk for pressure ulcer formation. Individuals at high risk should have preventive measures implemented from the start. The Braden scale (Fig. 15.2) also can be used for periodic assessment of the older person. If the older adult's risk for pressure ulcer development increases over time, new and more aggressive interventions for prevention should be implemented.

Evaluate the skin for lesions. Some lesions are normal. Table 15.1 describes normal and abnormal skin lesions. Note the consistency of the lesions. If there has been a change in color, consistency, edges, or growth, the lesion may have changed from normal to abnormal.

PALPATION. Check the skin for turgor. Gently pinch the skin on the forehead or anterior chest to see how quickly it returns to place. Poor turgor may be a normal aging change. It also could indicate dehydration or malnutrition or both. Palpate skin texture and note the temperature. Notice if the skin has become rough, dry, or coarse. Normally, the skin is smooth with some dryness. Check the skin temperature with the back of your hand. During this evaluation, note the symmetry of temperature and texture.

Patient Education
Patients should be taught to observe for any new skin lesions on their bodies or changes in existing lesions. This information should be shared with either their nurse or primary care physician.

Musculoskeletal System
History
The most common musculoskeletal complaints are related to the joints. Complaints include pain, stiffness, redness, limitation in movement, and joint deformity. If the older person complains of pain, determine where the pain originates and where it radiates. The most common soft tissue problem is pain in and around the shoulder joint. If the older adult has a sudden onset of low back pain, report it to the RN or physician. This pain could indicate a compression fracture of the spine.

Braden Scale
FOR PREDICTING PRESSURE SORE RISK

Patient's Name _____   Evaluator's Name _____   Date of Assessment

SENSORY PERCEPTION Ability to respond meaningfully to pressure-related discomfort	1. Completely Limited: Unresponsive to painful stimuli (does not moan, flinch, or grasp), due to diminished level of consciousness or sedation. OR Limited ability to feel pain over most of body surface.	2. Very Limited: Responds only to painful stimuli. Cannot communicate discomfort except by moaning or restlessness. OR Has a sensory impairment which limits the ability to feel pain or discomfort over ½ of body.	3. Slightly Limited: Responds to verbal commands, but cannot always communicate discomfort or need to be turned. OR Has some sensory impairment that limits ability to feel pain or discomfort in 1 or 2 extremities.	4. No Impairment: Responds to verbal commands. Has no sensory deficit that would limit ability to feel or voice pain or discomfort.
MOISTURE Degree to which skin is exposed to moisture	1. Constantly Moist: Skin is kept moist almost constantly by perspiration, urine, and so on. Dampness is detected every time patient is moved or turned.	2. Very Moist: Skin is often but not always moist. Linen must be changed at least once a shift.	3. Occasionally Moist: Skin is occasionally moist, requiring an extra linen change approximately once a day.	4. Rarely Moist: Skin is usually dry, linen requires changing only at routine intervals.
ACTIVITY Degree of physical activity	1. Bedfast: Confined to bed.	2. Chairfast: Ability to walk severely limited or nonexistent. Cannot bear own weight and/or must be assisted into chair or wheelchair.	3. Walks Occasionally: Walks occasionally during day, but for very short distances, with or without assistance. Spends majority of each shift in bed or chair.	4. Walks Frequently: Walks outside the room at least twice a day and inside room at least once every 2 hours during walking hours.

Continued

FIGURE 15.2 Braden scale for predicting pressure sore risk. (From Braden, B. J., & Bergstrom, N. [1992]. Pressure reduction. In G. Bulechek & J. McCloskey [eds.], *Nursing Interventions* [2nd ed., p. 63]. Philadelphia, PA: W. B. Saunders, with permission.)

	1. Completely Immobile:	2. Very Limited:	3. Slightly Limited:	4. No Limitations:
MOBILITY Ability to change and control body position	Does not make even slight changes in body or extremity position without assistance.	Makes occasional slight changes in body or extremity position but unable to make frequent or significant changes independently.	Makes frequent though slight changes in body or extremity position independently.	Makes major and frequent changes in position without assistance.

	1. Very Poor:	2. Probably Inadequate:	3. Adequate:	4. Excellent:
NUTRITION *Usual* food intake pattern	Never eats a complete meal. Rarely eats more than ½ of any food offered. Eats 2 servings or less of protein (meat or dairy products) per day. Takes fluids poorly. Does not take a liquid dietary supplement. OR Is NPO and/or maintained on clear liquids or IVs for more than 5 days.	Rarely eats a complete meal and generally eats only about ½ of any food offered. Protein intake includes only 3 servings of meat or dairy products per day. Occasionally will take a dietary supplement. OR Receives less than optimum amount of liquid diet or tube feeding.	Eats over ½ of most meals. Eats a total of 4 servings of protein (meat, dairy products) each day. Occasionally will refuse a meal, but will usually take a supplement if offered. OR Is on tube feeding or TPN regimen, which probably meets most of nutritional needs.	Eats most of every meal. Never refuses a meal. Usually eats a total of 4 or more servings of meat and dairy products. Occasionally eats between meals. Does not require supplementation.

	1. Problem:	2. Potential Problem:	3. No Apparent Problem:	
FRICTION AND SHEAR	Requires moderate to maximum assistance in moving. Complete lifting without sliding against sheets is impossible. Frequently slides down in bed or chair, requiring frequent repositioning with maximum assistance. Spasticity, contractures, or agitation leads to almost constant friction.	Moves feebly or requires minimum assistance. During a move, skin probably slides to some extent against sheets, chair, restraints, or other devices. Maintains relatively good position in chair or bed most of the time but occasionally slides down.	Moves in bed and in chair independently and has sufficient muscle strength to lift up completely during move. Maintains good position in bed or chair at all times.	

FIGURE 15.2—cont'd

Table 15.1
Normal and Abnormal Skin Lesions

Lesion	Description
Normal Skin Lesions	
Seborrheic keratosis	Raised; vary in size; tan to black; appear warty or greasy; frequently appear on trunk
Senile purpura	Vivid purple patch; well demarcated; eventually fades
Senile lentigines	Brown; irregularly shaped patches; age or liver spots; occur most frequently on back of hands, forearms, and face
Cherry angioma	Bright; ruby red elevated area; frequently found on trunk; common; insignificant; increase in size and number with age
Sebaceous hyperplasia	Yellowish, flat, solid elevations with central depression; looks like a small doughnut; common on face, forehead, and nose; more common in men
Abnormal Skin Lesions	
Senile or actinic keratosis	Precancerous; superficial patch covered by a persistent scale; common on sun-exposed areas
Squamous cell carcinoma	Firm, red-brown nodule; may arise from senile keratosis; common on sun-exposed areas and in fair-skinned individuals
Basal cell epithelioma	Starts as pearly colored solid elevation on face or ear; ulcerates leaving a crater with an elevated border and depressed center
Malignant melanoma	Brown-black lesion; may have flecks of red, white, or blue irregular border, irregular surface; arise from moles or appear as new pigmented, irregular lesion
Lentigo maligna melanoma	Less aggressive form of malignant melanoma specific to elderly adults; arise from lentigines that enlarge laterally

From McGovern, M., & Kuhn, J. K. (1992). Skin assessment of the elderly client. *Journal of Gerontological Nursing, 18*(8), 40–41, with permission.

Physical Examination

INSPECTION. If possible, observe the older adult while the person is participating in ADLs and **instrumental activities of daily living (IADLs)**. (See Functional Assessment section in this chapter.) Doing so allows the nurse to assess ROM, muscle mass, and level of independence in self-care. Some decline in ROM is expected. There is a general rigidity of the lower extremities.

Observe the older adult's ability to walk. Have the person ambulate a specified distance to determine endurance. It is normal for older men to have a slight anterior-flexion of the upper body while the arms and knees are slightly flexed. Note the kind of shoes worn by the older adult. Intervention is necessary if the person has an unstable gait yet wears high-heeled shoes. Have the older adult transfer in and out of the bed and chair, on and off the commode, and from the commode to the bathtub. Observe for symmetry of movement. Determine if the person needs assistance. Some older people may be independently mobile with the use of a wheelchair. Assess their ability to maneuver the wheelchair in the environment. Check the older adult's feet for lesions and deformity because these can interfere with gait and mobility. As with physical examination of all of the systems, report all abnormal findings of the musculoskeletal system to the RN or physician.

Reproductive System
History: Female Patient

Although questions about sexual functioning and the reproductive organs may be uncomfortable for the nurse and the older adult, it is important to ask them. Ask the older woman if she knows about breast self-examination. If not, education on the subject is needed. Although breast self-examination is no longer recommended, breast self-awareness is, and women are encouraged to be observant of any changes in their breasts. Inquire about symptoms of breast cancer. Does the person have any pain, nipple discharge, lumps, skin discoloration, or change in breast shape? Is there any family history of breast cancer or other cancerous conditions? Determine if the older woman has used estrogen or other medications that affect the breasts, such as digitalis, thyroid drugs, and antihypertensives. Has the older woman ever had an abnormal Papanicolaou (Pap) test result and if so, did she receive treatment? Has she been tested for human papillomavirus infection? Did she receive any medications for menopausal symptoms? Has there been any unusual bleeding since menopause?

Some common physical complaints that older women experience with intercourse include vaginal dryness, pain, and limited mobility from arthritis. These complaints should be addressed, and ways to deal with them should be suggested. Lubricants and using different positions during intercourse, such as the side-lying position, can help the older woman manage these concerns. Note the discussion in chapter 13 on sexually transmitted diseases.

History: Male Patient

The older man should be evaluated for symptoms of benign prostatic hyperplasia. Is there any change in the urinary stream? Any dribbling of urine? A sense that the bladder is not completely empty after urinating? Is there urinary frequency? Urgency? Burning during urination? Does the older man experience nocturia? How often? Review his medications and note whether he takes diuretics or an anticholinergic that might worsen benign prostatic hyperplasia. Does he realize the importance of checking his breasts periodically? Although male breast cancer is rare, it is possible for older men to develop breast cancer.

Physical Examination

INSPECTION. During the examination process, you should inspect the external genitalia on older male and female patients. Assess for skin or mucous membrane lesions, rashes, discoloration, hair loss, inflammation, discharge, asymmetry, and circumcision.

Urinary System
History

In gathering information about the urinary tract, the nurse needs to discover the chief complaint and the nature and extent of the older adult's underlying problem. The most common complaints are urgency to void, leakage when changing position, pain on urination, frequency of urination, voiding small amounts, and incontinence caused by coughing, sneezing, and laughing. The subject of urinary incontinence frequently causes the older adult to feel embarrassed. Incontinence may cause the older person to withdraw from usual social contact for fear of having an accident. It is also a major risk factor for pressure ulcer formation and urinary tract infections. Despite the difficulties and embarrassment that may be associated with discussing incontinence, it is a serious problem that can have multiple untoward effects.

If the older adult reports any complaints related to the urinary tract, determine the person's normal urinary and bowel habits before the symptoms began. Assess the past medical history for childbirths, previous surgeries involving the lower abdomen and pelvic floor, renal disease, and bladder cancer. Evaluate the older adult's medications. Diuretics and antiparkinsonian drugs can affect the urinary system. Periods of prolonged rest or immobility can cause urinary stasis. Urine that is allowed to pool in the bladder creates a favorable environment for the development of infection. To empty the bladder fully, it is important for the older adult to be able to use the sitting-with-legs-dependent position. Full bladder emptying may not be possible on a bedpan. Decreased fluid intake results in low urine volume and infrequent urination. This situation can create pooling of the urine and increase the risk for infection. It also can lead to dehydration, elevated blood glucose levels, and electrolyte imbalance. These conditions may manifest in the older adult through alterations in mental status.

Physical Examination

INSPECTION. Assess urine amount and color for the presence of any sediment.

PALPATION. Palpate the abdomen for distention of the bladder and signs of pelvic discomfort or masses.

CRITICALLY EXAMINE THE FOLLOWING

To complete a thorough assessment, you must use your critical thinking skills. The body systems are complex and dysfunction in one system can lead to dysfunction in other systems. For example, a patient who has a low blood pressure of 100/55 mm Hg may also have a problem with decreased kidney perfusion and may experience symptoms of orthostatic hypotension. You will need to investigate further by asking the patient about dizziness when they change position and decreased urinary output.

• What is another scenario in which a symptom in one body system affects another?
• List the other questions you will need to ask.

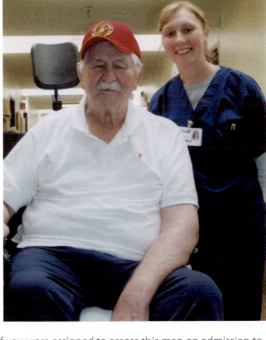

If you were assigned to assess this man on admission to the assisted living where you work, what observations could you make even before talking to him? His left arm is hanging without good positioning or apparent control. Does this man have a muscle or enervation problem in the arm, or has he possibly had a left-sided stroke? He is in a wheelchair. Why?

FUNCTIONAL ASSESSMENT

For an older adult, a functional assessment is as important as a physical assessment. Often, the older person demonstrates changes in function as the first or only sign indicating the onset of illness. Although the older person has many chronic illnesses, these typically are not problematic until function is affected. A functional assessment allows for the determination of a person's **functional status**.

Functional assessment encompasses a holistic approach to evaluating the older adult that includes physical, cognitive, and social function. Physical function comprises the individual's current health status in addition to how well the person performs ADLs and IADLs. Cognitive function includes the individual's memory, judgment, and thinking abilities. Cognitive function is discussed in chapter 18 and is not included in this section on functional assessment. Social function involves a psychosocial approach to determine how the individual interacts with the environment and with others.

Functional assessment involves evaluating the older adult to determine what the person can do (strengths) and cannot do (deficits). What the health-care team members see as a deficit may not correlate with what the older adult views as a problem. The older adult's true abilities, as assessed by the nurse, and the older adult's perception of these abilities must be considered.

Functional assessment assists in setting realistic goals. Cure as a goal is inappropriate for an older individual with chronic, irreversible conditions. The goal for such a patient would be to maximize functional strengths and compensate for deficits to achieve and maintain optimal independence in function.

In almost any health-care setting, the nurse is the health-care professional who spends the most time with the older adult. The nurse has many opportunities to observe the client's physical functioning. A decline in functional ability may represent a change in an underlying chronic disease or the onset of a new acute illness. Monitoring functional status helps track improvements and setbacks. It also indicates when additional services are needed. Use of a formal tool to evaluate functional status allows the nurse to validate, monitor, and communicate clearly clinical impressions to other members of the interdisciplinary health-care team.

Activities of Daily Living

The Katz ADL scale is widely used to assess ADLs. It is a well-rounded tool that is appropriate for use in most settings, including home, hospital, and nursing home. ADLs are the activities performed in taking care of oneself. The following areas are considered ADLs: bathing, dressing, toileting, feeding, ambulating or transferring, and continence. Direct observation is the most valid indicator in assessing ADLs. Watch the older adult perform ADLs and check for abnormal body movements. Rate the older adult on each of the ADL items of the Katz scale. Using the scale supplies specific information on how the older adult performs in each of the ADL areas, and the composite score can give you and other members of the interdisciplinary health-care team an overall view of the person's level of ability. The score also gives an objective means to monitor progress over time. Goals in each of the ADL areas can be set on the basis of scores on the scale.

THINK LIKE A NURSE

You are caring for a patient on home care services. The family states that the person is losing weight. What assessments can you do to identify the problem?

Instrumental Activities of Daily Living

IADLs include the ability to use the telephone, cook, shop, do laundry, manage finances, take medications, and prepare meals. These activities are needed to support independent living. Lawton's scale for IADLs is used widely (Fig. 15.3).

If possible, observe the older adult while he or she is performing IADLs. Look for abnormal body movements such as tremors or twitching for lack of balance or for poor vision. In addition to checking the person's ability to complete the IADL, it is important to assess the older adult with regard to safety. The older person may be able to cook a meal, but if the burner is left on, a serious safety concern exists.

In completing an IADL assessment, the nurse often must rely on reports from the older adult or family members. Keep in mind that individuals tend to overrate their abilities, and family members tend to underrate them.

Tools for assessing ADLs and IADLs are used to measure the older person's ability to do self-care and home-care tasks. They can be used to help identify needed services and to monitor the progress or deterioration of the older individual.

Evidence-Based Practice

Alberdi Aramendi, A., Weakley, A., Aztiria Goenaga, A., Schmitter-Edgecombe, M., & Cook, D. J. (2018). Automatic assessment of functional health decline in older adults based on smart home data. *Journal of Biomedical Informatics*, *81*, 119–130. doi:10.1016/j.jbi.2018.03.009

The researchers in this article were exploring new ways to help older adults live independently. Over an average of 2 years, the 29 participants agreed to have their activities tracked by *smart home technology*. Sensors placed in the participants' residence tracked behaviors such as sleep, cooking and eating, overnight patterns, in-home mobility patterns, and mobility and outings. Tracking this data allowed researchers to gather information about ADLs and IADLs in an unobtrusive way. Using this type of data may allow early detection of functional decline that could allow for earlier intervention from health-care professionals.

Questions
1. What functional assessment tools do you use in your care setting or the setting where you have clinical experiences?
2. Is the information gathered used to predict functional decline in your patients?

Social Function

Social function is how the older adult interacts with self, the environment, and others. It is the degree to which a person functions as a member of the community. Cultural and socioeconomic background and the older adult's environment define and limit social activities and relationships. Self-concept affects the older adult's ability to perform self-care activities. Psychological interventions may be necessary to enhance the older person's self-esteem before achieving independent functioning.

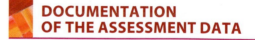

DOCUMENTATION OF THE ASSESSMENT DATA

It is challenging to have spent a long time collecting data only to find that when you sit down to document the assessment, words do not come. Just like

Instrumental Activities of Daily Living (IADL) Scale

Self-Rated Version Extracted from the Multilevel Assessment Instrument (MAI)

1. Can you use the telephone:
   without help, — 3
   with some help, or — 2
   are you completely unable to use the telephone? — 1

2. Can you get to places out of walking distance:
   without help, — 3
   with some help, or — 2
   are you completely unable to travel unless special arrangements are made? — 1

3. Can you go shopping for groceries:
   without help, — 3
   with some help, or — 2
   are you completely unable to do any shopping? — 1

4. Can you prepare your own meals:
   without help, — 3
   with some help, or — 2
   are you completely unable to prepare any meals? — 1

5. Can you do your own housework:
   without help, — 3
   with some help, or — 2
   are you completely unable to do any housework? — 1

6. Can you do your own handyman work:
   without help, — 3
   with some help, or — 2
   are you completely unable to do any handyman work? — 1

7. Can you do your own laundry:
   without help, — 3
   with some help, or — 2
   are you completely unable to do any laundry at all? — 1

8a. Do you take medicines or use any medications?
   (If yes, answer Question 8b) Yes — 1
   (If no, answer Question 8c) No — 2

8b. Do you take your own medicine:
   without help (in the right doses at the right time), — 3
   with some help (take medicine if someone prepares it for you and/or reminds you to take it), or — 2
   (are you/would you be) completely unable to take your own medicine? — 1

8c. If you had to take medicine, can you do it:
   without help (in the right doses at the right time), — 3
   with some help (take medicine if someone prepares it for you and/or reminds you to take it), or — 2
   (are you/would you be) completely unable to take your own medicine? — 1

9. Can you manage your own money:
   without help, — 3
   with some help, or — 2
   are you completely unable to handle money? — 1

SOURCE: Lawton MP, Brody EM. Assessment of older people: self maintaining and instrumental activities of daily living. *Gerontologist*. 1969;9:179–185. Reprinted with permission.
For additional information on administration and scoring refer to the following references:
1. Lawton MP. Scales to measure competence in everyday activities. *Psychopharm Bull*. 1988;24(4):609–614.
2. Lawton MP, Moss M, Fulcomer M, et al. A research and service-oriented Multilevel Assessment Instrument. *J Gerontol*. 1982;37:91–99.

FIGURE 15.3 Instrumental Activities of Daily Living Scale. (From Lawton, M. P., & Brody, E. M. [1969]. Assessment of older people: Self maintaining and instrumental activities of daily living. *Gerontologist*, 9, 179–185. Copyright © The Gerontological Society of America, with permission.)

in the beginning of the chapter, when practicing was discussed, documentation also requires practice. Electronic health records are helpful because the programming gives you options for documentation in the form of pop-up cues.

The Resident Assessment Instrument (RAI) discussed in Chapter 4 has very scripted documentation. When assessment data is entered into the RAI form, the program generates a plan of care, goals, and evaluation parameters.

CASE STUDY SOLUTIONS

In doing a holistic assessment, it is important that you review all the body systems and all of this patient's diagnoses. Managing Miss S.'s diabetes during her recovery period is as important as the management of her HF. According to the report, that is going well. You need to verify that her medical treatment is still managing her symptoms. HF is the priority concern because it is life-threatening and the reason she was admitted to the hospital. How will you assess Miss S. related to the HF? Following are some suggestions:

1. Assess for edema by checking her ankles, abdomen, lumbosacral area, and hands for swelling, and listen to her lungs for adventitious breath sounds.

2. Is she able to perform ADLs without dyspnea?
3. Does she understand her medication administration?
4. Is she weighing herself daily and recording those weights?

You will also need to consider her diabetes and how she is currently managing her blood glucose levels.

1. Has her diet changed?
2. Does she use injections to manage her diabetes, and if so, is there a sliding scale that can help compensate for her higher readings?
3. Is she still taking oral steroid medications?

Key Points

- To be an effective gerontological nurse, you need to develop skills in performing a holistic physical assessment and a functional assessment.
- Physical assessment skills are the foundation of good nursing and improve only with practice.
- Obtaining a thorough history is a vital part of a full assessment and can help you to provide better care for your patient. It should be included with a review of systems.
- There are many physiological changes that are age related and should be noted on the assessment of older adults. When assessing a patient, be sure to address all of the body systems.

- There are many ways to evaluate functional ability of older adults. The Katz ADL scale and Lawton IADL scale are tools that are widely used to assess functional status.
- Assessing nutritional status is an important part of a full assessment. Adequate nutrition is essential for health and for healing.
- Completing a functional assessment using a standardized tool can help you to work with the patient to set realistic and achievable goals.
- Documentation of assessments can be difficult if you have to write everything in paragraph format. Computer programs and data gathering forms can help to simplify and standardize documentation.

Review Questions

1. The following are normal aging changes except:
   1. Presbyopia, presbycusis.
   2. Urinary incontinence.
   3. Kyphosis, ptosis.
   4. Osteoporosis, arteriosclerosis.

2. Activities of daily living include:
   1. Shopping.
   2. Managing finances.
   3. Bathing.
   4. Using the telephone.

3. A common tool used for evaluating ADLs is:
   1. Lawton's scale.
   2. The mini-mental status examination.
   3. The Katz scale.
   4. 1 and 3.

4. A common symptom of myocardial infarction in an older adult is:
   1. Chest pain.
   2. Lethargy.
   3. Confusion.
   4. 2 and 3.

5. An important health problem that the nurse should help the older adult prevent is:
   1. Fecal impaction.
   2. Dehydration.
   3. Malnutrition.
   4. All of the above.

ANSWERS 1. 2, 2. 3, 3. 4, 4. 4, 5. 4

CHAPTER 16
Common Clinical Problems: Physiological

Tamara Dahlkemper

KEY TERMS

contracture
extrinsic factors
immobility
intrinsic factors
pressure ulcer
sarcopenia
urinary incontinence

CHAPTER CONCEPTS

Health Promotion
Mobility
Safety
Sleep and Rest
Tissue Integrity

LEARNING OUTCOMES

1. Describe how the nurse can assist in maintaining mobility for the older adult at risk for impaired mobility.
2. Define two categories of risk factors for falls in older people.
3. Identify two categories of incontinence.
4. Explain how prompted voiding and habit training schedules can be used by the nurse for prevention or reversal of incontinence.
5. Identify the mechanical and physiological risk factors for pressure ulcers.
6. Discuss the problems pertaining to adequate food intake in older people.
7. Describe two sleep disorders common to older adults.
8. Define iatrogenesis, and list common iatrogenic problems experienced by older persons.

CASE STUDY

Mrs. Z. is a 78-year-old widow who had total knee replacement surgery and was recently transferred to a rehab facility. Prior to the knee replacement, Mrs. Z. did not get much physical activity because of the pain she was experiencing. The goal in the rehab facility is to help her regain her strength so she will be able to go back to her home and live independently. Two days after her transfer, Mrs. Z. fell while trying to get out of bed to go to the bathroom by herself. She is now complaining of more intense pain in her surgical knee that requires stronger pain medication to provide comfort. She also does not want to participate in her physical therapy or get up to go to the bathroom because she is afraid of falling again. It has been 3 days

INTRODUCTION

With aging, each body system undergoes changes. These changes, although they do not usually result in illness or disease, cause health problems that are more prevalent in older people. As you learned in chapter 14, most people who are older than 65 years of age have multiple chronic conditions. As a result of normal aging changes combined with underlying chronic conditions, the older person has less physical reserve than a younger person to respond to the increased demand of an illness. With diminished physical reserve, the older adult is less capable of adapting to physical stressors and is at increased risk for clinical problems such as **immobility**, falls, incontinence, pressure ulcers, and alterations in nutrition and sleep. This chapter reviews the clinical problems that are common to older adults. In addition, effective management approaches, based on nursing diagnoses, are discussed.

ALTERATION IN MOBILITY

The process of aging, combined with the presence of chronic illness, places the older adult at risk for developing an alteration in mobility status. Immobility is a major medical disability for elderly adults and one that is frequently overlooked by health-care providers. Immobility often leads to numerous complications for older people in long-term care facilities, in the hospital, and in the community. Nursing care is essential to maintaining and improving an older adult's ability to be mobile.

Musculoskeletal System

Normal aging changes that occur in the musculoskeletal system increase the risk of developing problems related to mobility. The bones of an older person are less dense and more brittle, owing to changes in the formation of bone at the cellular level. As a result, older adults are likely to develop osteoporosis and subsequently be at risk for bone fractures.

With a fracture, mobility is restricted still further. Mechanical stresses, such as walking and standing, tend to stimulate the process of bone formation. When the body is immobilized, there is bone dissolution. This process is called *disuse osteoporosis*, and it makes the bones of the older person still more brittle and weak.

Generalized muscle weakness is also a normal aging process. This is usually related to a condition called **sarcopenia.** As people age, their muscle mass decreases, which causes weakness and loss of stamina. This weakness happens faster around age 75. The antigravity muscles are most affected by this change so that standing up can be difficult. In time, if muscles are not used, walking, balancing, and turning become severely impaired. *The loss of muscle mass is not only a symptom of generalized deterioration, but it is also a factor in the risk of falling.*

Priority Setting

The priority for this chapter is easy to identify. After you understand the content of this chapter, you need to assist every older adult to whom you give care to achieve his or her maximum physical ability. Keep that thought in mind and do not stray from it. By doing so, you will enhance the lives of all of the older people in your care.

The mobility of the joints is affected by the length and composition of the muscle fibers. When there is immobility, the muscles that bridge the joint shorten. With decreased muscle length and thickening of the joint cartilage (which is the connective tissue that surrounds the movable surfaces of the joint), the joints become stiff, which seriously affects the ability of the person to move.

Evidence-Based Practice

Najafi, Z., Kooshyar, H., Mazloom, R., & Azhari, A. (2018). The effect of fun physical activities on sarcopenia progression among elderly residents in nursing homes: a randomized controlled trial.

Journal of Caring Sciences, 7(3), 137–142. https://doi.org/10.15171/jcs.2018.022

The changes in muscle mass and strength associated with aging is known as sarcopenia. This condition can lead to an older adult's loss of mobility and independence. Studies have shown that exercise improves muscle mass and strength for older adults. Despite the known benefits a very low percentage of older adults engage in regular physical activity.

This study examined the effects of fun physical activities on the progression of sarcopenia for individuals living in nursing homes. Sarcopenia for each participant was measured using various assessment tools. Participants were divided into two groups of 35 individuals: the regular physical activity (RPA) group and the fun physical activity (FPA) group. Each group participated in physical activity for 20 minutes, 3 times per week for 8 weeks. The RPA group activity consisted of walking around the nursing home and stretching. The activity for the FPA group included balance, strength, endurance, and walking exercises using beach balls, stretch bands, and other fun exercise implements.

The results of the study showed the FPA group had an improvement in balance, the distance they were able to walk, and muscle strength.

Questions
1. What are some ideas for fun physical activities that could be added to an assisted living or long-term care facility's activity program?
2. What can nursing staff do to assist older adults to participate in regular physical activity?

Osteoarthritis, or degenerative joint disease, occurs most often in people aged 65 and older. It is marked by deterioration of the cartilage and formulation of new bone at the joint surfaces. With aging, the cartilage is less elastic, thicker, and more easily stretched. As a result, the joint is stiff, and there is decreased range of motion (ROM) of the joint. Over time, an older adult can lose the ability to mobilize efficiently as a result of stiffness in the joints. As joints are immobilized, **contractures** (a permanent contraction of the muscles that bridge the joint) can develop and limit mobilization further.

Cardiovascular System
Many of the changes in the cardiovascular system that accompany aging are closely related to inactivity. Similarly, these aging changes can be exacerbated, or become more severe, when there are prolonged periods of immobility.

Oxygen consumption and cardiac output are known to decrease with aging and may vary among older adults. This change is evident from the fact that the pulse rate of an older person does not increase in response to exercise as efficiently as in younger people. After physical exertion, the pulse takes longer to return to a normal level. The inefficient cardiac response to activity causes activity intolerance, but most older adults learn to adjust to the changes.

Respiratory System
As is true of all of the body systems, aging changes to the respiratory system put the older person at risk for complications when immobility is present. Normal anatomical changes in the aging body compromise

Focused Learning Chart: Alteration in Mobility Related to Aging

Respiratory System	Cardiovascular System	Musculoskeletal System
Decreased efficiency of gas exchange by alveoli	Decreased cardiac output	Generalized muscle weakness
Decreased vital capacity	Pulse rate does not increase efficiently with exercise	Osteoarthritis
Decreased elasticity of lung tissue	Decreased O_2 consumption	Bones more brittle (osteoporosis)
Structural compromise • Rigidity of rib cage • Kyphosis		Shortening of muscle fibers

lung function. Increased rigidity of the rib cage, kyphosis, and osteoporosis reduce the compliance of the chest wall, making it more difficult to inflate the lungs fully. The reduced compliance of the chest wall makes it more challenging for the older adult to maintain activity, and it increases the potential for complications caused by immobility. The lungs of most older adults have diminished vital capacity (the amount of air that can be expelled from the lungs after inspiration). Other changes include less efficient gas exchange by the alveoli and less elasticity of the lung tissue. The result is impaired ventilation and decreased blood supply to the lungs. Such changes not only may hinder the older person's ability to move, but, more importantly, they also place the older person at increased risk for developing atelectasis and pneumonia when immobilized.

Response to Illness

Chronic health problems may cause older people to restrict their movement. Poor eyesight may cause someone of any age to avoid activity because of fear of falling over an obstacle. Pain in the joints owing to arthritis or pain in the lower extremities owing to impaired circulation generally limits ambulation and causes older adults to become sedentary. Shortness of breath or angina secondary to chronic cardiovascular disease also may cause the individual to avoid activity.

Acute health problems can lead to immobility. The onset of an acute illness, whether or not it requires hospitalization, may lead to confinement in bed. Often, well-meaning family members and health-care providers encourage immobility. Bedrest often is ordered during hospitalization for an acute illness. In contrast to a younger person, an older adult who is on bedrest deteriorates rapidly and may develop irreversible complications. Although rest can promote healing, immobility promotes deterioration. Prolonged immobility is detrimental to the physical and mental health of a person of any age. When immobilized, the older person can develop complications such as contractures, pneumonia, thrombophlebitis, pressure ulcers, incontinence, constipation, dehydration, loss of appetite, and psychological problems related to sensory deprivation and depression. Although Mrs. Z. is experiencing increased discomfort, it is important to keep her mobile to prevent further complications.

Nursing Implications

Nurses as well as the older people to whom they give care need to be aware that promoting physical activity not only prevents complications, but also slows the rate of the aging process. In the hospital setting, the time for enforced bedrest needs to be limited as much as possible. As soon as it is medically safe to do so, the nurse needs to ensure that the patient is up and out of bed. If orders for bedrest are in effect, it is the nurse's responsibility to inquire whether such orders can be changed. Even transferring the person from a supine to a sitting position has beneficial effects. While on bedrest, older adults can be taught isometric and active ROM exercises. If the person is incapable of performing these exercises independently, the nurse must assist the patient in meeting this need through passive ROM exercises.

As soon as it is medically indicated, the older patient should be ambulated with assistance. This intervention is as important to the patient's health as receiving the proper medication or a dressing change. Nursing staff should support physical therapy services by ensuring that appropriate sturdy footwear, eyeglasses, and any assistive devices such as canes or walkers are available. Because of reimbursement issues, hospital stays are becoming shorter. As soon as the person is physiologically able, attempts to restore functional ability should begin.

As in the hospital setting, promoting functional mobility is central to the care of the older person at home or in a nursing home. The nursing home environment offers different possibilities for fostering mobility. In contrast to the hospital setting, where the presence of an acute condition may impede the nurse's attempts to restore function, the nursing home environment allows the nurse to monitor and promote mobility over an extended period. All residents should be considered for assisted walking unless the underlying chronic illness absolutely precludes such an activity. An older person who does not walk deteriorates even further and may eventually lose all ability to walk. Family members and other caregivers for the older adult who lives at home need to be taught the importance of mobility.

CRITICALLY EXAMINE THE FOLLOWING

Although immobility is a prevalent health problem, it often is not addressed in the care of the older adult. Identifying immobility as a patient-care problem and intervening to prevent it are central to nursing care of older persons. In addressing mobility needs, the licensed practical nurse (LPN) may prevent complications and shorten the length of time that the older person is in the hospital or rehabilitation facility.

Often nurses do not like to disturb patients when they are asleep or have visitors, to ambulate their patients or have them participate in physical therapy. After reading this chapter, what are your thoughts on the importance of ambulating patients? Will you modify your care related to the importance of mobility for your patients?

POTENTIAL FOR INJURY FROM FALLS

As with alteration in mobility, the potential for falls is closely related to many of the systemic changes that occur with aging. The aging of the musculoskeletal system, which may cause deterioration in mobility, also may increase the older person's risk for falling. More than one in four older adults fall each year and once a person falls, it doubles their chance of falling again. Falls can lead to mild or severe injuries. For older adults, falls can cause the highest percentage of deaths related to unintentional injuries (Centers for Disease Control and Prevention [CDC], 2018). As people age, the risk of being injured in a fall increases. The presence of chronic illness accompanying the aging process places all older adults at increased risk for falls (see Box 16.1).

Box 16.1

Medical Risk Factors Associated With Falls

Advanced age
Arthritis
Delirium
Dementia
Diabetes
Medication side effects
Muscle weakness
Postural hypotension
Parkinson's
Polypharmacy: more than four medications
Previous falls
Problems with balance and gait
Sleep disorders
Stoke
Visual and hearing impairment
   CDC (2017).
   Risk Factors for Falls. Retrieved from https://www.cdc.gov/steadi/pdf/STEADI-FactSheet-RiskFactors-508.pdf

When an older person falls, the person often becomes fearful of falling again. The older adult may limit activities and become more withdrawn and dependent on others, less mobile, and more at risk for future falls. Caregivers also may place restrictions on the older person's mobility to prevent another fall. At home, the family may admonish the older person to restrict activities so that a fall does not occur again. In the health-care setting, restraints should never be used to prevent the risk of another fall. These options do not promote health for the person.

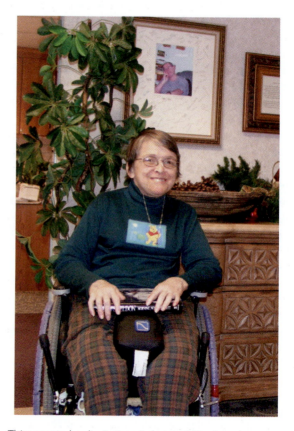

This woman has limitations in her mobility, but she can get around because she is in the right type of wheelchair for her needs. Her chair does allow her some physical activity.

Factors that predispose to falling are typically divided into two categories: intrinsic and extrinsic. **Intrinsic factors** include factors inherent to the individual, such as normal aging changes, deficiencies in health status, changes in mental status, immobility, and changes in functional ability. **Extrinsic factors** refer to environmental conditions, which may include poor lighting, slippery floors, inappropriate or poorly placed furnishings, and inadequate footwear. Falls among older adults often stem from the presence of intrinsic factors that hinder the older person's ability to manage the environment or from environmental conditions (extrinsic factors).

Intrinsic Factors

Age-related changes in posture, balance, gait, and vision predispose an older person to falls. Postural changes are common in older people and are due to a decline in strength and flexibility. In older adults, the head tends to be carried forward, the shoulders may be rounded, and the upper back may have a slight curvature, or kyphosis. Changes in posture and spinal alignment can affect balance and increase the risk of falls.

Posture and Balance

The body's ability to maintain its coordination in a standing position and to react to prevent a fall depends on coordination among the musculoskeletal system, the neurological system, and the visual system. Postural sway occurs when one or more of these three systems are not functioning at an optimal level. Balance problems are associated with postural sway, which can cause falls. Prolonged bedrest, aging changes, medications, and the presence of some chronic conditions are contributors to postural sway.

Postural reflexes play a role in fall prevention by responding to disturbances in balance during standing or walking. With aging, these reflexes become slower; older people are less able to "catch" themselves when they trip or begin to fall. Inactivity may result in a slower response to disturbances in balance.

Gait

With aging, the gross motor movements necessary for maintaining posture and gait, or walking, are altered. The gait of older people often is marked by decreased speed and step height; small, hesitant steps; diminished arm swing; and stooped posture. These changes are almost universal in people older than 80 years. The alterations in speed of movement and maintenance of upright posture adversely affect balance and often lead to a higher incidence of falls by older adults.

Vision

All older people experience changes in vision as part of the normal aging process. With aging, there is a decline in visual acuity, peripheral vision, depth perception, night vision, and tolerance for glare. The loss of vision that accompanies aging is a risk factor for falls because there is a decreased ability to focus on objects at a distance and to judge distances correctly. The result is that an older person may miss a step or trip over a curb. The decline in peripheral vision may cause an individual to trip over objects at the edge of the visual field. Visual deficits can compound a gait disability because vision is necessary to maintain stability while walking.

These normal, age-related changes in posture, gait, and vision, when compounded by the presence of an underlying chronic or acute illness, make falls the leading cause of death from injury in people older than 65 years. Because of the presence of these intrinsic factors, many older people are less capable of coping with the extrinsic factors that may be in the environment.

Extrinsic Factors

Most falls affecting older adults result from environmental factors. Such factors include clutter in rooms, inadequate lighting or glare, and unsafe furniture or equipment in the person's immediate area. Attempting to function in an area that is not designed to accommodate the aging person's needs can diminish the older person's confidence. The individual may begin to fear falling and may eventually become more sedentary. Such behavior leads to an eventual loss of function and an increased need to depend on others for activities of daily living.

Cultural Considerations

Cultural influences can either promote or hinder participation in physical activity. Some cultures believe in preventive health practices and incorporate healthy activities into their lives such as walking. Other cultures may understand the need for engaging in physical activity but older adults may not engage in activity due to the traditional values that consider physical activity inappropriate for older adults.

Nursing Implications

It is important for nurses to understand the role that intrinsic and extrinsic factors play in falls. The individual's ability to maneuver safely in the immediate environment is best monitored by the nurse. In the home and the institutional setting, most falls occur in the bedroom and the bathroom. It is important to assess the older person walking about the bedroom, getting into and out of bed, and getting on and off the toilet. Only by assessing the individual's ability to manage these daily activities in his or her own environment can you, the nurse, begin to anticipate needs and take steps to prevent a fall before it occurs.

Having assessed the older person's safety, the nurse, along with members of the interdisciplinary health-care team (IDT), should plan care according to the observed need. The nurse may observe that the older person cannot safely get on and off the toilet independently and may advise the individual not to attempt this maneuver unassisted. If the person is not cognitively intact, you may use a toileting schedule to discourage the individual from attempting self-toileting when you, the LPN, or other caregivers are not present to assist. If the older person cannot safely ambulate alone, the IDT may decide that physical therapy is indicated or that a program of daily assisted ambulation should be initiated.

Older adults who cannot safely stand or walk unassisted, but who may still attempt these actions, should not be left alone for extended periods. One idea is to bring the person out of the room so that staff members can observe the older adult. When someone who is not safe is left alone, mobility alarms would help the staff know when the individual is getting up unassisted. Mobility alarms can be attached to the bed and wheelchair. All members of the IDT need to remember to remove clutter and to maintain clear walking paths for older people, to adjust lighting to provide an optimal environment, and to wipe up spills from the floor as soon as they occur or are noticed.

ALTERATION IN ELIMINATION

Urinary Incontinence

Urinary incontinence, a problem that affects millions of Americans, is defined as an involuntary loss of urine that is sufficient to be a problem for the patient. It is most often seen in the elderly in general, with an increase in incidence in nursing home residents. The cost of caring for individuals with urinary incontinence can be expensive.

THINK LIKE A NURSE

You have been asked to present the educational section at the next staff meeting. Your nurse manager has requested that you develop a teaching plan for your colleagues regarding the importance of mobility in older adults. You have been asked to discuss two former patients who had mobility problems. As part of your lesson plan, write out the reasons an older person should be mobile. Identify ways mobility can be done successfully with the following patients:

1. An 87-year-old man with a fractured hip. He is deconditioned (a word from a previous chapter; do you remember it?) yet insists he can walk "by himself."
2. A 72-year-old woman who is "pleasantly confused" while recovering from a fractured femur. She is experiencing a great deal of pain and thinks you are her son.

Address both patients' ambulation plans.

Even greater than the economic cost are the psychological and social costs to the individual who is incontinent of urine. Incontinence is seen as a major reason older adults are placed in nursing homes (Holup, Hyer, Meng, & Volicer, 2017). People who are incontinent may feel embarrassed and socially isolated. They may withdraw from participation in social activities and become depressed. Incontinence is associated with the development of other health problems, such as skin breakdown, and urinary tract infections. Identifying the presence of urinary incontinence should be part of the nursing assessment.

Age-Related Changes Affecting Urinary Incontinence

Although incontinence is more prevalent in older people, it is not a normal aspect of aging. There are, however, numerous age-related changes that make the older person susceptible to developing incontinence. In older adults, the bladder capacity diminishes to about one-half that of younger adults. The diminished ability of the kidneys to concentrate urine makes urinary frequency and nocturia (excessive urination at night) common problems for the older person. In addition, many older people experience sudden and unexpected contractions of the detrusor muscle (the smooth muscle that makes up the outside wall of the bladder), which cause an urgent need to void. Changes in the central and autonomic nervous systems of the older person cause a decreased ability to contract the external sphincter of the bladder, which exacerbates urinary urgency further. Many postmenopausal women experience thinning and weakening of the muscles of the pelvic floor, a complex condition caused by many factors, including genetics, estrogen loss, and childbirth. In men, an enlarged prostate, often associated with aging, may lead to urinary retention, irritability of the detrusor muscle, and bladder spasms.

The urinary urgency that many older people experience often leads to incontinence in an institutional setting. When an older adult cannot go to the toilet independently or as often as needed, incontinence is likely to result. This situation is exacerbated further by the immobility that results from being ill or from needing medical interventions, such as intravenous therapy.

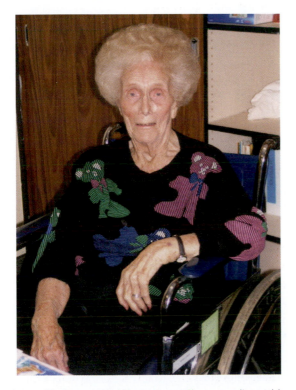

At age 83, this woman is incontinent. She wears disposable briefs, and the staff members keep her clean and free of urine odor.

Types of Urinary Incontinence

For the nurse to intervene in the management of incontinence, it is important to understand the underlying causes of incontinence.

Acute Incontinence

Acute or transient incontinence is incontinence that occurs because of the presence of a treatable medical condition, and it often resolves when the underlying illness is treated. The following mnemonic highlights the possible causes of acute incontinence:

D: Delirium
R: Restricted mobility
I: Infection, inflammation, impaction
P: Pharmaceutical, polyuria, psychological

Delirium is an acute confusional state that is brought on by an acute illness and that disrupts the physiological homeostasis in the older person. In a delirious state, the person is unaware of the need to void and does not have the capability to get to the toilet.

Restricted mobility, as already discussed, is a common cause of incontinence in elderly people. Individuals who are experiencing pain may be less likely to attend to urinary urges to avoid an increase in pain sensation. Individuals with physical limitations, such as Mrs. Z., are also at risk for incontinence.

Urinary tract infections cause frequency, urgency, and painful urination. This condition can lead to increased bladder contractions and incontinence. Many residents in long-term care have bacteria in their urine (bacteriuria), a condition that is asymptomatic and does not require treatment. When bacteriuria is accompanied by urinary incontinence, however, the person should be treated, and the effect of the treatment on the incontinence should be noted. Fecal impaction may obstruct the bladder outlet and may cause overflow urinary incontinence.

Many medications can cause urinary incontinence. Following is a list of drug groups that adversely affect an older person's ability to maintain continence:

• Sedatives/hypnotics
• Antipsychotics
• Narcotics
• Anticholinergics
• Diuretics
• Caffeine

Endocrine disorders that lead to hyperglycemia or hypercalcemia may cause urinary incontinence. Psychological causes that have been associated with urinary incontinence include depression and confusional states.

NURSING IMPLICATIONS. Most instances of bladder incontinence are transient and often reversible. In most cases, acute or transient incontinence can be resolved with treatment of the underlying illness or with discontinuation of a causative medication. Incontinence should never be accepted without first ascertaining that the older person has been assessed for underlying conditions and that treatment has been initiated.

Patient Education

Patients and family members should be taught that infrequent urinary incontinence that is not bothersome can lead to more frequent urinary incontinence and should be evaluated by their primary care provider (PCP).

Chronic Incontinence

There are several types of persistent or chronic incontinence. Incontinence is considered to be persistent if it continues after reversible causes have been ruled out or treated. In addition, persistent or chronic incontinence usually has a gradual onset, worsens over time, and occurs when there is a failure either to empty or to store urine. The four types of persistent or chronic incontinence are as follows:

Urge incontinence is the most common form of incontinence in older adults. In this type of incontinence, the individual feels the urge to go but does not have enough time to get to the toilet before the urine is released.

Stress incontinence occurs when a small amount of urine is released after there is a sudden increase in intra-abdominal pressure caused by coughing, sneezing, laughing, or lifting. This type of incontinence results when the bladder outlet sphincter is incompetent or weak. Stress incontinence is more common in women and is often a result of poor pelvic muscle tone and a shorter urethra.

Overflow incontinence is caused by impaired bladder emptying and overdistention of the bladder. When the bladder is not emptied sufficiently, the resident experiences frequent dribbling of urine.

Functional incontinence results when the individual is unable or unwilling to attend to toileting needs. In this situation, the bladder and urethra function normally, but cognitive, physical, psychological, or environmental impairments make

it difficult for the older person to get to the toilet. Inaccessible toilets, unavailable caregivers, depression, and inability to find the toilet all are possible causes of functional incontinence. Mrs. Z. is experiencing this type of incontinence and will need to be assisted to the toilet on a regular schedule.

Reflex incontinence occurs when the bladder contracts and leaks urine with no sense of urge. This form of incontinence is caused by damage to the nerves that warn the brain the bladder is filling. It is common in individuals with serious neurological disorders such as multiple sclerosis, and spinal cord and other injuries.

Mixed incontinence occurs when individuals experience more than one type of incontinence. Older women tend to have both stress and urge incontinence. Older men may also experience this type of incontinence due to surgery or removal of an enlarged prostate.

NURSING IMPLICATIONS. Treatment of urinary incontinence is based on the underlying cause. Medication intervention may be used to treat infection or stop abnormal bladder muscle contractions and tighten sphincter muscles. Surgical intervention is used to correct anatomical anomalies and remove obstructions. Behavioral interventions require that the health-care professional provide education and positive reinforcement to the older adult and family members. Behavioral interventions sometimes may be used in combination with medical or surgical interventions.

BEHAVIORAL INTERVENTIONS. Behavioral interventions, which are most often provided by nursing personnel, include the following:

• Bladder training (retraining)
• Habit training (timed voiding)
• Prompted voiding
• Pelvic muscle exercises

These techniques are most helpful with stress and urge incontinence.

Bladder retraining is used to restore the normal pattern of voiding by inhibiting or stimulating voiding. The goal is to lengthen the time between voidings. This is best done by instructing and assisting the individual to learn to suppress the urge to void in an attempt to increase the amount of urine the bladder can hold. This technique is used with individuals who are capable of understanding and remembering the instructions. Most bladder-retraining schedules begin with a schedule of toileting every 2 hours and gradually increase the amount of time between voidings to every 3 to 4 hours while awake.

Prompted voiding is different from bladder training in that the goal is not to increase bladder capacity, but rather to teach the incontinent person to be aware of toileting needs and to request assistance from the caregiver. In this technique, the person is asked to try to use the toilet at regular intervals and is praised for maintaining continence and using the toilet. The schedule that is followed usually involves toileting on awakening, after meals, at bedtime, and, if awake, at night. More voiding times can be added if the individual's voiding schedule indicates a need. This intervention works well with moderately confused people.

Habit training works best with cognitively impaired or confused people and requires the caregiver to take the patient to the toilet at regular intervals. The toileting schedule may be every 2 to 4 hours, or the caregiver may toilet the individual on awakening, after meals, midmorning and midafternoon, at bedtime, and at night, if awake.

Pelvic floor muscle exercises, also known as Kegel exercises, are used to alleviate stress incontinence. The goal of such exercises is to strengthen the pelvic floor muscles. Patients who are taught Kegel exercises must be cognitively intact and willing to participate in this exercise regimen. The exercise consists of the person contracting the pelvic floor muscles, holding the contraction for 3 to 4 seconds, and then relaxing the muscles. This should be done 15 times in succession at least three times per day, increasing to 10-second contractions each time. Once the person has met the increased seconds per contraction, a schedule of 10-second contractions and releases per day can be maintained.

In dealing with incontinence, nurses play a key role in education and treatment. Incontinence is not a normal part of aging but is more prevalent in elderly people. Many forms of incontinence are reversible, and all attempts should be made to assess, treat, and resolve incontinence when it is present.

Constipation

Bowel functioning and the avoidance of constipation are common concerns for older adults. Many older people were raised during a time when anything but a daily bowel movement was considered abnormal. The concern regarding this problem is appropriate because numerous age-related changes in the gastrointestinal system make constipation more likely.

It is probable that an older person has an extended gastrointestinal transit time as a result of slower peristalsis. More water is removed from the stool when it is in the colon for longer periods. The stool becomes harder and more difficult to pass. Immobility, decreased exercise, and a lack of fiber and water in the diet are common problems in older people, and these factors tend to exacerbate the tendency to become constipated. Certain drugs also may lead to constipation (see Box 16.2).

Immobility is particularly problematic in the maintenance of regular bowel movements. Muscular atrophy, which is a loss of tone in the muscles of the intestine, and generalized weakness of the muscles necessary for the expulsive mechanism of evacuation occur during periods of immobilization. The overuse of laxatives also causes a loss of muscle tone in the bowel.

Immobility not only affects the physiological functioning of the gastrointestinal system, but it also prevents the individual from interacting efficiently with the environment to meet the needs of the body. Factors such as strange environments, disruption of the usual elimination patterns, being forced to defecate in an unnatural position in unnatural surroundings (as occurs with the use of a bedpan), and suppressing the urge to defecate because of the inability to get to the toilet inhibit normal defecation.

Nursing Interventions

Nursing interventions aimed at prevention of constipation should be focused on establishing a regular pattern of bowel elimination that is not

---

B o x 1 6 . 2

Medications That Increase the Risk for Constipation

Antacids containing aluminum and calcium
Anticholinergics
Iron supplements
Antiemetics
Narcotics
Antidepressants
Diuretics
Antihypertensives
Anticonvulsants
Antispasmodics

associated with straining or discomfort. It is important for the older person's overall health to attempt to correct constipation without resorting to the use of laxatives. These interventions should include increasing physical activity, increasing water intake, increasing dietary fiber, and establishing a regular bowel routine. Regular exercise stimulates motility in the gut.

The older adult should be encouraged to drink 1,500 to 2,000 mL of fluids daily unless this is contraindicated by other health problems. Dietary fiber also plays an important role in the avoidance of constipation. Fiber holds water, making the stool softer and bulkier, which speeds the passage of stool through the intestine. It can be difficult to increase fiber in the diet of the older person because of lifelong dietary preferences and poor dentition. It may be helpful to consult a dietitian.

Assisting the patient to develop a regular bowel routine is an essential part of bowel maintenance and one in which the nurses play a pivotal role. In facilitating regular bowel routines, the nurse must assess how much, if any, assistance the person requires in getting safely to the toilet. The use of bedpans should be avoided whenever possible, but when they are used, the patient should be in an upright position unless this position is contraindicated. The nurse also needs to ensure that regular toileting times are maintained and that privacy is provided during toileting time.

ALTERATION IN SKIN INTEGRITY: PRESSURE ULCERS

A **pressure ulcer** is defined as any lesion caused by unrelieved pressure that results in damage to the underlying tissue. Pressure ulcers are an extremely serious health problem that can lead to pain, extended hospital stays, and further complications from infection. Older persons are particularly at risk, especially if they have multiple health problems. The development of pressure ulcers has been associated with the quality of health care and may signal overall poor care by the health-care system. Because pressure ulcers are, for the most part, preventable, maintaining adequate skin integrity is a quality-of-care issue for all nurses. Even more important than knowing the various treatment modalities is knowing how pressure ulcers develop. You need to become an expert in prevention techniques.

Risk Factors
Mechanical Risk Factors
Four mechanical factors that contribute to the development of pressure ulcers are pressure, shearing, friction, and moisture.

- *Pressure* ulcers usually occur over bony prominences such as the sacrum, ischium, trochanters, heels, elbows, and the back of the head, where normal tissue is squeezed between the internal pressure of the bone and an external source of pressure or friction, such as the chair or the bed. External pressure that lasts long enough and is sufficient enough to decrease blood flow results in inadequate oxygenation and nutrients to the area and the subsequent development of a pressure ulcer. Immobility is the most important risk factor in the development of pressure ulcers. Pressure of high intensity that is left unchecked for more than 2 hours can result in irreversible tissue damage.

- *Shearing* occurs when the head of the bed is elevated more than 30 degrees and the person slides toward the foot of the bed. In this situation, the skin over the sacrum does not move, whereas the subcutaneous tissue and gluteal vessels are stretched. Rupture of the blood vessels results. Subcutaneous fat, which lacks the ability to stretch, is particularly vulnerable to injury from shearing forces. Sores that develop on the sacrum, heels, and anterior tibial region are most probably a result of shearing. When shearing and pressure are both present, the amount of pressure necessary to cause tissue damage is half the amount that causes tissue damage when shearing is not present.

- *Friction* occurs when the skin is moved across the sheets, such as when the person is being pulled up rather than lifted up in the bed. The result of this motion is damage to the epidermis, which can lead to ulceration or a break in the skin. *Moisture* caused by perspiration or incontinence can increase the friction between the surface and the skin. Moisture also can cause maceration (softening of the skin), which weakens the skin and increases the risk of infection. In the presence of moisture resulting from urinary or fecal incontinence, the risk of pressure ulcer development on the sacrum and buttocks increases fivefold. Incontinence is a strong predictor of skin breakdown.

Physiological Risk Factors

In addition to mechanical forces, there are factors that are inherent to the individual that increase the risk of skin breakdown. Examples include aging skin, immobility, and malnutrition.

- *Aging skin* increases the likelihood of developing pressure ulcers because it is less resistant to the mechanical forces that can damage the skin. With advancing age, there is a decrease in the thickness of the cell layers of the epidermis, a flattening in the epidermal-dermal interface, and a loss of subcutaneous tissue. These changes cause impaired wound healing and decreased thermoregulation, causing the skin to become more fragile.
- *Immobility,* combined with the age-related changes of the skin, greatly increases the risk of pressure ulcer formation. Normally, spontaneous body movements that occur during sleep and throughout the day protect the skin from pressure. Many situations prevent the body from spontaneous movement, including physical disability, loss of sensation, presence of pain, or use of sedating drugs or anesthesia.
- *Malnutrition* is another physiological factor that can lead to pressure ulcer formation. Deficiencies in zinc, iron, vitamin C, and protein adversely affect the health of the skin. The more severe the malnutrition, the more severe the pressure ulcer. Malnutrition and the subsequent weight loss lead to loss of muscle mass and subcutaneous tissue. This diminishes the body's protective padding and increases the pressure over the bony prominences.

Safe, Effective Nursing Care

Promote Quality Outcomes for Patients

Providing quality care and ensuring positive outcomes for patients should be a priority for all nurses. Knowing how to find information by reading research articles and national guidelines regarding appropriate outcomes for the patient population you serve is a skill that is important in providing care to your patients. Taking that information and working with the health-care team to identify gaps between local and best practices and then helping to develop the processes to adopt best practices in your facility will improve outcomes for your patients. The Agency for Healthcare Research and Quality has developed a toolkit for preventing pressure ulcers in hospital settings. The toolkit can be found at http://www.ahrq.gov/professionals/systems/long-term-care/resources/pressure-ulcers/pressureulcertoolkit/putoolkit.pdf

1. How can the information in the tool kit be used to prevent pressure ulcers and improve patient outcomes in your patient population?
2. How will you share the information with the rest of the health-care team to involve them in preventing pressure ulcers in your facility?

Staging

Pressure ulcers are graded according to the degree of tissue damage. The staging of a pressure ulcer dictates the type of treatment to be implemented. Staging provides a means of describing an ulcer that allows for the ulcer to be monitored over time. Commonly used staging criteria are presented in the following list:

Stage I: Nonblanchable erythema of intact skin. (The skin is reddened, even in the absence of direct pressure.)

Stage II: Partial-thickness skin loss involving epidermis or dermis. The ulcer is superficial and manifests clinically as an abrasion, blister, or shallow crater.

Stage III: Full-thickness skin loss involving damage to or necrosis of subcutaneous tissue that may extend down to, but not through, the underlying fascia (fibrous membrane covering the muscles). The ulcer manifests clinically as a deep crater with or without undermining of adjacent tissue.

Stage IV: Full-thickness skin loss with extensive destruction, tissue necrosis, or damage to muscle, bone, or supporting structures (e.g., tendon or joint capsule). Undermining and sinus tracts also may be associated with stage IV pressure ulcers.

Prevention

Assessment of risk is a vital first step in prevention of pressure ulcers. If a person is found to be at risk for developing pressure ulcers, interventions to prevent skin breakdown can be initiated before an ulcer develops. Numerous assessment tools are available. Review the Braden Scale presented in Chapter 15.

Assessment should be done using the following criteria:

• Acute care: Assess on admission and every 24 hours or sooner if the patient's condition changes.
• Long term: Assess on admission and weekly for 4 weeks. Then assess every quarter or as the resident's condition changes.
• Home care: Assess on admission and on every nurse visit.

When an older adult is found to be at risk for alteration in skin integrity, preventive measures should be aimed at reducing pressure on bony prominences, preventing shear or friction, keeping skin clean and dry, and providing adequate nutrition and hydration. To reduce pressure, the person should be repositioned at least every 2 hours. This regular repositioning decreases the amount of time that pressure is exerted on any one body part. The appearance of reddened areas indicates that more frequent turning or other interventions may be indicated. When placing an older adult on either side, a wedge should be placed behind the person to prevent the person from lying directly on the trochanter (which is the bony prominence located below the neck of the femur).

Although at one time it was common practice to massage reddened areas over bony prominences, this is no longer recommended. Massage may exert pressure on the area and may cause further breakdown of the small capillaries. In some cases, it may be necessary to use pressure-relieving devices, such as air-filled, water-filled, or gel-filled chair pads or mattresses, and foam heel protectors and mattresses. The use of egg-crate mattresses, although common, does not provide sufficient pressure relief to prevent pressure ulcers. Walking programs and passive and active ROM exercises not only improve muscle strength and joint flexibility but also are important in the prevention of skin breakdown.

Patient Education

You are a home health nurse for a 79-year-old woman who is cared for by her husband with drop-in visits from three daughters. Sarah, the patient, is homebound because of general fatigue and postoperative total hip replacement. She can ambulate with a cane but is fearful and will not leave the house except on rare occasions. She says she is happy to be at home with her husband and not to have the arthritic hip pain. The problem is she is either in bed or a recliner chair most of the day and night. Her husband lifts her to and from the chair and bed when Sarah is "too tired to move herself."

You have noticed that Sarah's buttocks are reddened, as are her heels. Focus on a teaching plan for this couple. What do they need to know about pressure ulcers? What is the best way for you to share the hazards of immobility with Sarah? What can you do to prevent the stage I pressure ulcers from developing into something worse?

To reduce friction, persons should be lifted and not pulled when repositioned. The use of a lift sheet or a turn sheet is essential to distribute the person's weight evenly and avoid undue friction and stress on the skin. Shear can be reduced by decreasing the amount of time and frequency that the person's head is elevated above 30 degrees while in the bed. When out of bed and in a chair, the person should be repositioned at least every hour, and long-term sitting should be discouraged. While in the chair, the individual needs to be examined for appropriate posture and alignment because an inappropriate sitting posture can lead to pressure ulcers and increased shearing forces.

Although skin should be kept clean and dry to prevent pressure ulcers, older adults do not need to be bathed daily. Excessive bathing and rubbing can be drying and damaging to the skin. Using a mild cleansing agent that does not promote dryness and patting the skin dry are essentials of good skin care for the older person.

Treatment

Treating pressure ulcers is expensive and can extend the recovery and rehabilitation time. The treatment of pressure ulcers is extremely individualized, and it requires a team approach. Any suspicion of a pressure ulcer should be reported immediately to the RN so early treatment can begin. Nursing care is aimed at maintaining skin integrity by preventing irritation to the skin from friction and moisture.

Providing adequate nutrition and good hygiene are also important to assist with the healing process.

ALTERED NUTRITIONAL STATUS

Adequate nutrition is essential to the maintenance of health, prevention of disease, management of chronic illness, and recovery from acute illness. When the body is inadequately nourished, the individual is more likely to develop an illness and is less able to recover from illness. Caloric or protein malnutrition is a concern for older people.

To be adequately nourished, the body must have a sufficient intake of carbohydrates, fats, proteins, vitamins, minerals, and water. Difficulty obtaining appropriate nutrition can be a result of lack of knowledge about good nutrition, inadequate income or means of obtaining the appropriate foods, lack of socialization (which may lead to disinterest or overindulgence in food), or housing that is inadequate for storing and preparing nutritionally sound meals. The older person's diet is often lacking in calcium, vitamin C, riboflavin, niacin, and iron. A deficiency of any essential nutrient can cause changes to the body that, if left unchecked, can lead to illness. Chapter 8 covers additional information on nutrition of older adults.

Risk Factors

Anorexia (loss of appetite) is a major cause of inadequate nutritional intake in older people. Poor dentition, poorly fitting dentures, or lack of dentures may make it difficult for the individual to chew, and a soft or puree diet may be unappetizing. Diminished mobility makes it difficult for the older person to obtain and prepare food. A sedentary lifestyle also may lead to a decreased appetite. Polypharmacy, a common situation with elderly patients, can adversely affect appetite by altering taste sensation, impairing cognition and mood, or interfering with the absorption of nutrients. Other causes of anorexia in older adults may include the increased incidence of chronic illness, social isolation, depression, and unappetizing institutional foods.

Changes in the metabolism of older people translate into changes in nutritional requirements of the body. With aging, there is a decreased metabolic rate, and the body requires fewer calories for maintenance. Decreased mobility and the loss of muscle mass associated with aging also suggest that older people may need to decrease their caloric consumption.

Older adults use more energy, however, than younger people to do the same activities. If the individual is active, there may be a need to increase the caloric intake. With aging, the body does not metabolize protein as efficiently, so older people may need more protein in their diet.

Maintaining adequate nutrition in older persons who have a disease process poses a particular challenge to the nurse. People with advanced dementia may have weight loss even when there is an adequate intake of nutritional requirements. Neuroleptics, a commonly used class of drugs in patients with dementia, also may cause a loss of appetite. It has been postulated that there may be a disturbance in the metabolism of patients with advanced Alzheimer's disease, and this, too, may account for the unexplained weight loss in these patients. The term "failure to thrive" has been used to describe another entity associated with weight loss. Failure to thrive occurs when some elderly nursing home residents experience a gradual decline in physical and cognitive functioning associated with weight loss, withdrawing from food, withdrawing from human contact, and exhibiting signs of depression.

A significant problem for many older adults who have had a stroke or generalized weakness is aspiration, the inhalation of solids or liquids into the upper respiratory tract. This is a critical problem because of the serious consequences of an aspiration. It can cause pneumonia or death by choking. The symptoms of aspiration include a sudden severe cough or cyanosis while eating or drinking, voice changes, and increased respiratory rate after eating or drinking. The possibility of aspiration is increased with dysphagia (difficulty swallowing) and gastroesophageal reflux problems.

Assessment

Assessing the nutritional status of the older person can be a difficult task for the nurse. The recommended dietary allowance (RDA) that is established by the National Academy of Sciences Research Council is one way of monitoring how well an individual is meeting nutritional requirements. Additional nutrients that may be needed as a result of infection or chronic illness are not addressed by the RDA.

Complicating the assessment for malnutrition further are the changes of the aging body itself. Many physical manifestations of malnutrition are similar to changes that are associated with aging. These changes include dry, thin hair; dry, flaky skin; sunken eyes; dry oral mucosa; weight loss; and muscle weakness.

Using skinfold measures to estimate percentage of body fat may not yield accurate information because mean body mass (muscle tissue) decreases with age. Probably the most reliable indicator of adequate nutritional intake is a normal serum albumin level greater than 3.5 g/100 mL. Monitoring an individual's weight over time is also an appropriate means of recognizing alteration in nutritional status. A weight loss greater than 5% in the last month or 10% in the last 6 months is a concern and should be reported.

Nursing Implications

To reestablish adequate nutritional intake, healthcare providers should strive to maintain oral feedings with appropriate modifications. The diet may need to be made more palatable with foods that have different textures and flavors. Providing the individual's favorite foods whenever possible is also a good approach. Family members can be asked to provide favorite foods for the older person. Ensuring that the older person has dentures if needed and that they fit well and providing a diet that is appropriate for the person's dental status are imperative.

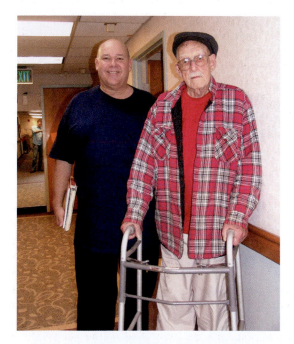

This father and son have lived together since the father's discharge from a rehab center. He was admitted for falling and for generalized weakness. Also, he was malnourished. The son enjoys cooking and caters to his father's wishes, which has improved the older man's health remarkably.

Everyone responds well to meals that are served in an attractive manner and in an environment that is relaxed and pleasant. Nursing staff should strive for this kind of atmosphere during mealtime by not raising their voices and trying to keep noisy dietary carts out of the eating area. Eyeglasses help the resident to see the food on the plate, and hearing aids allow the resident to socialize with tablemates during mealtime. It is important that the nurse ensure that the individual has whatever assistive devices are needed to make the eating experience a more pleasant one.

If the person's nutritional status does not improve despite these efforts, the nurse needs to consider other interventions. It may be necessary to offer more assistance with meals. The individual may need to be fed or have containers opened, or he or she may just need ongoing gentle encouragement throughout the meal to continue eating. Often, gently touching the arm or shoulder while encouraging feeding helps the older adult to attend to the task of eating. Touch is a caring behavior that indicates value and respect for the person being touched. Older people often are not touched or hugged frequently and generally respond positively to the act of being touched.

The dietitian should assist in deciding what, if any, supplements are needed. Liquid dietary supplements are best offered between meals so that the supplement is not substituted for the meal itself. The supplement can provide a large percentage of the RDA requirements but does not completely meet all dietary requirements.

Tube feedings and parenteral feedings can be used when all other attempts at oral feedings have failed. These methods have numerous complications, however. Striving to maintain adequate oral intake should be the goal of all nursing personnel. Adequate nutrition affects every aspect of the individual's health and well-being.

SLEEP PATTERN DISTURBANCES

Older people often complain of not getting enough sleep or not feeling well rested after sleeping. Sleep disturbances increase with age. It is estimated that sleep pattern disturbances affect one-half of people older than age 65 years who live at home and two-thirds of older people living in institutions.

Normal Sleep Patterns

A review of normal sleep patterns is necessary to understand the changes in sleep patterns that tend to occur with aging. There are five stages to normal sleep. Refer to chapter 9 if you need to review this material.

Age-Related Changes in Sleep Patterns

In the course of aging, people tend to sleep less than 8 hours per night. Older people have an impaired capacity to maintain sleep; sleep tends to be marked by more frequent and prolonged awakenings during the night. In addition, stage IV and rapid eye movement (REM) sleep diminish. In extreme old age, changes in cerebral blood flow and organic brain syndrome also are associated with a shortening of the REM stage of sleep.

The sleep patterns of older people can be disturbed by factors such as needing to void frequently during the night (nocturia) and changes in vision and hearing that cause incorrect perceptions of their immediate environment. These changes can lead to ineffective sleep or sleep deprivation. Sleep deprivation is marked by fatigue, tiredness, eye problems, muscle tremor, muscle weakness, diminished coordination and attention span, apathy, and depression.

Sleep Disorders

In addition to age-related changes in sleep patterns, some sleep disorders are common in older adults. Sleep apnea, a medical condition in which breathing stops for 10 seconds or longer numerous times throughout the night, is more common in older people. Untreated sleep apnea is associated with cognitive decline, cardiac disease, stroke, and decreased quality of life.

Another common sleep disorder for older adults is insomnia. Insomnia occurs when people have difficulty getting to sleep or remaining asleep, or they simply feel that they do not get enough sleep. Insomnia can be a result of medical and psychiatric conditions as well as use of certain medications.

Sundown Syndrome

Sundown syndrome is another disorder that affects many older people. Sundown syndrome is defined as the appearance or exacerbation of symptoms of confusion associated with the late afternoon or evening hours. This syndrome is marked by behaviors such as agitation, restlessness, confusion, wandering, and screaming that occur usually in the evening hours (sundown). Little is known about this disorder, which is a tremendous management problem for caregivers. Risk factors for sundown syndrome seem to be impaired mental status, dehydration, being awakened frequently during the night for nursing care, and recent relocation either to a new room or to the institution.

Nursing Interventions

Sleeping medications, tranquilizers, and sedatives are commonly used to promote sleep but should be avoided at all costs in older persons. Sedatives and barbiturates that depress the central nervous system may lead to other problems by depressing vital body functions, lowering basal metabolic rate, decreasing blood pressure, and causing mental confusion. Sleeping medications decrease spontaneous body movements that may lead to skin breakdown. Most of the medications used to promote sleep are not efficiently metabolized by the aging body, and the person may experience a hangover effect the next day. In addition, these drugs tend to cause blurred vision, dry mouth, and urinary retention. Because it is known that an elderly person cannot sleep as long as a younger person can, it is unreasonable to put an individual to bed at 8 p.m. and expect that person to stay in bed until 7 a.m. the next day.

There is much the nurse can do to promote sleep without resorting to the use of medications. Meeting the individual's comfort needs by offering back rubs or snacks such as warm milk, assisting with toileting needs, providing socks or an extra blanket to increase body temperature (which may be diminished in an older person), repositioning, and alleviating pain are just a few of the nursing interventions that may reduce insomnia. If these interventions do not promote sleep, it is prudent to allow the older person to come out of the bed and perhaps sit for a while in a comfortable chair near the nurses' station. This may reassure the individual of the surroundings and prevent attempts to get out of bed unassisted, perhaps risking a fall. During the daytime, increased physical activity may promote sleep. Refer to chapter 9 for more information on managing sleep issues for older adults.

IATROGENESIS

Iatrogenic disorders can be defined as disorders that a person acquires as a result of receiving treatment by a physician, nurse, or other member of the IDT. Iatrogenesis also can occur if the person does not receive treatment when it is indicated or receives incorrect treatment. An older person often presents with numerous chronic conditions that require complex interventions, numerous medications, and increased exposure to the health-care system; this puts older adults at increased risk of experiencing untoward effects of medical treatment. Iatrogenic disorders include the disorders previously discussed in this chapter: immobility, falls, incontinence, malnutrition, pressure ulcers, and disturbances in the sleep-wake cycle.

Common causes of iatrogenesis in the hospital are misuse or overuse of drugs, prolonged immobilization, nosocomial (hospital-acquired) infections, and malnutrition and dehydration secondary to preparation for diagnostic tests. In the nursing home, common iatrogenic disorders include immobilization, adverse drug reactions, falls, pressure ulcers, and nosocomial infections.

- Iatrogenic disorders are often cyclic in nature in that one disorder may quickly lead to another.

Consider the older person who is admitted to the hospital for abdominal discomfort. This person is unable to sleep and is prescribed a sleeping pill. Having taken this medication, the person is groggy when getting out of bed and sustains a fall. The staff, not wanting the patient to be hurt again, assigns a volunteer to sit with the person to remind him or her not to get up. The older person is now unable to get up and suffers from some of the adverse sequelae of immobility, such as incontinence, disorientation, and pressure ulcer formation. In time, the person's muscles become deconditioned, and the next time the patient is assisted out of bed, there is another fall, the person sustains a hip fracture, and the cycle continues. This scenario highlights how iatrogenic disorders can impact an older adult and why preventing such conditions from occurring is one of the roles of the LPN. Iatrogenesis can be prevented. Many of the clinical problems that the older person faces can be averted or alleviated with nursing interventions that are focused on improving and maintaining wellness and promoting function. Some of these interventions include maintaining proper nutrition, providing opportunities for physical activity, and monitoring sleep patterns to assure the older person is getting enough rest.

CASE STUDY SOLUTIONS

In this case study, there are several potential iatrogenic problems that the nursing staff should address:

1. It is not uncommon for individuals who fall to be worried about falling again, because subsequent falls are common in the older adult population. Mrs. Z. has several risk factors for a fall, such as diabetes, muscle weakness due to lack of physical activity prior to her surgery, and poor balance due to limited use of her surgical leg. It is best for her to continue getting up to the bathroom and to provide her some physical activity in addition to her physical therapy. Nurses should strongly encourage her to continue getting out of bed and should provide the assistance she needs.

2. The increase in pain medication and immobility is most likely the cause of her constipation. She

is also in a strange environment and is experiencing a change in her normal elimination pattern. Assessing when she normally has her bowel movements during the day and then providing assistance to the bathroom at that time will help her re-establish her elimination pattern. Encouraging her to drink more fluids during the day will help keep the stool soft. The nurse may also request a stool softener be ordered by the PCP.

3. Mrs. Z. is showing signs of skin breakdown due to urinary incontinence. Mrs. Z. is most likely experiencing functional incontinence because she is not able to get to the bathroom in a timely manner without assistance. It is important to assess if Mrs. Z. had problems with incontinence prior to her surgery to determine if there is another cause of the incontinence. Until she is able to get out of bed on her own, nursing staff should check with

CASE STUDY SOLUTIONS—cont'd

her every 2 to 3 hours to see if she needs help going to the bathroom. Mrs. Z.'s bed should be kept clean and dry. The nurse may also suggest that Mrs. Z. wear panty liners or briefs to help absorb urine leaks. If used, these items should be changed frequently. A Foley catheter should never be the first intervention used in

the presence of incontinence. An additional way to help alleviate skin breakdown is to make sure Mrs. Z. is maintaining proper nutrition. Assuring that she is getting a sufficient intake of carbohydrates, fats, proteins, vitamins, and minerals is important in maintaining a healthy immune system and in helping with the healing process.

Key Points

- The health-care needs of older adults are multiple and complex. Assessment and interventions aimed at correcting the illness, promoting function, and averting a subsequent decline should be initiated. LPNs can and should play a pivotal role in ensuring that the health-care needs of older persons are being met.
- The process of aging combined with the presence of chronic illness places older adults at risk for developing alterations in mobility. Immobility can lead to numerous complications, including fractures, muscle weakness, pneumonia, constipation, and pressure ulcers.
- The risk for falls is associated with many of the body changes related to aging. Older adults who have experienced a fall may become fearful of falling again and may limit their physical activity, increasing their dependence on others.
- Factors that predispose older adults to falling are typically divided into two categories: intrinsic and extrinsic. Intrinsic factors are those inherent to the individual, such as normal aging changes, deficiencies in health status, changes in mental status, and changes in functional ability. Extrinsic factors refer to environmental conditions such as clutter, slippery floors, poor lighting, and inadequate footwear.
- Urinary incontinence is a problem often seen in older adults with an increased incidence in nursing home residents. However, it is not a normal aspect of aging. Incontinence is associated with other health concerns such as skin breakdown and urinary tract infections. Incontinence can be acute or chronic.

- Acute incontinence occurs because of the presence of a treatable medical condition and often resolves when the underlying illness is treated. Chronic incontinence usually has a gradual onset or worsens over time. There are several types of chronic incontinence: urge, stress, overflow, functional, reflex, and mixed.
- Behavioral interventions to assist with incontinence can be provided by nurses. Prompted voiding is used to teach the incontinent person to be aware of toileting needs and to request assistance from the caregiver. A regular schedule is developed that works best for the patient. Habit training works best with cognitively impaired or confused people and requires the care provider to take the patient to the bathroom on a regular basis.
- Pressure ulcers are a serious problem that can lead to pain, extended hospital stays, and further complications from infection. Because pressure ulcers for the most part can be prevented, maintaining adequate skin integrity is a quality-of-care issue for nurses. Nurses should know how pressure ulcers develop and what techniques are best for prevention.
- Adequate nutrition is essential to the maintenance of health, prevention of disease, management of chronic illness, and recovery from acute illness. Caloric and protein malnutrition is a concern for older people. Risk factors for poor nutrition in older adults include loss of appetite, poor dentition, lack of socialization, increased incidence of chronic illness, and polypharmacy. Adequate nutrition affects every aspect of an individual's well-being.

- Sleep patterns in older people change with age and can be disturbed by factors such as getting up to go to the bathroom at night and issues with vision and hearing that change the perception of their environment. There are two sleep disorders common in older adults: insomnia and sleep apnea.

- Iatrogenesis can be prevented. Many of the clinical problems that the older person faces in health and in illness can be averted or alleviated with nursing interventions that are focused on improving and maintaining wellness and promoting function.

Review Questions

1. An example of an intrinsic risk factor for falls in the older person is:
   1. The use of diuretics.
   2. Weakened muscles in the lower extremities.
   3. Glaring lights in the hallway.
   4. The use of a cane.

2. To promote mobility in the older adult, the nurse should:
   1. Turn the patient every 2 hours.
   2. Encourage the patient to cough and take deep breaths.
   3. Ask the family to bring in the patient's walker from home.
   4. Assume that the physical therapist is helping the patient to walk.

3. The best way to promote urinary continence in the older person is to:
   1. Stop giving the diuretic because it causes the patient to have urinary urgency.
   2. Obtain a urine specimen for culture and sensitivity.
   3. Offer the bedpan every 2 hours.
   4. Assist the patient to the toilet in the morning, after meals, and at bedtime.

4. When seeing a reddened area on the patient's coccyx, the nurse would do all but one of the following interventions:
   1. Turn the patient every 2 hours.
   2. Ask the physician to order a medication to treat the skin.
   3. Help the patient to the toilet more frequently.
   4. Rub the area to increase circulation.

5. Which of the following is not an example of an iatrogenic disorder?
   1. Falling because of dizziness after receiving medication for pain relief
   2. Depression because of a stroke
   3. Incontinence because the patient could not find the bathroom
   4. Loss of weight because the patient cannot chew the food that is provided

ANSWERS 1. 2, 2. 3, 3. 4, 4. 4, 5. 2

CHAPTER 17
Psychological Assessment

Holli Sowerby

KEY TERMS

cognition
delirium
dementia
depression
gerotranscendence
level of consciousness
Theory of Human Caring

CHAPTER CONCEPTS

Assessment
Cognition
Health Promotion
Mood
Patient-Centered Care

LEARNING OUTCOMES

1. Identify three cognitive functions.
2. Use a standardized examination to screen for cognitive functioning.
3. Identify four uses of psychological assessments.
4. Describe the impact of depression on the mental status score.

CASE STUDY

Ms. F. is 81 years old and in general good health. Her family has become concerned for her safety and noted some minor problems with memory, a decline in her energy level, and an inability to take care of herself. After speaking with her and her doctor, her children met with their mother to discuss the possibility of moving her into an assisted living facility. Initially she was resistant to the idea but after several incidents involving missed medications, overmedication, and a small kitchen fire, she was convinced that it was a good decision. Together they visited several facilities and Ms. F. and her children found one they all liked. She moved in and was placed on a unit with other residents who functioned independently. A few months after admission, some of the residents began to remark to the staff that Ms. F. was ignoring some of their efforts to engage her in conversation. She started retreating to her room a little more. She seemed more withdrawn in general. She favored a chair off to herself rather than an available seat in a group of other residents.

Discussion
1. Based on this information, what is the first step you will take to identify the change in Ms. F.'s behavior?
2. What are the next steps you will take?

INTRODUCTION

Psychological assessments are essential tools in identifying the mental health of older adults in all health-care settings. Such assessments provide the basis for determining the psychological illness or wellness of a person as well as determining how much of a return to normal an individual can expect to achieve. Psychological assessments are important in any health-care setting, but especially when the focus is restorative care.

Restorative care, in its truest application, requires a body-mind-spirit connection. Relate this concept to Jean Watson's **Theory of Human Caring**—the two theories are conceptually the same, and it is hoped that they are beginning to have meaning for you in your practice. Nurses practicing within this framework are concerned with the physical indications that a person is declining, such as falling, incontinence, and immobility. Although behavioral or psychological indicators have received less prominence in terms of restorative care, they are equally important. Some examples of psychological indicators are failure to eat and a decline in functional level, such as severe memory loss or confusion without a physiological basis.

Although one can expect a certain amount of decline in older people who have vascular and central nervous system disease, it is important to identify the psychological areas of decline and recognize when interventions are essential. Maintenance of mental health and cognitive functioning is as important to restorative care as the maintenance of physiological processes. Nurses working with elderly people need to understand basic concepts of mental health and cognitive function so that they can participate in the care of the older adult more effectively. Assessment tools provide a brief, methodical approach to noting changes commonly found in individuals with cerebrovascular diseases, delirium, and dementia disorders.

MENTAL HEALTH

Over the years, clinicians in the field of mental health have tried to diagnose symptoms, traits, and patterns of behavior that identify disease. The view that identification and treatment of disease result in optimal health is known as the medical model. The simplest definition of mental health would be the absence of identifiable disease. Most people have short- or long-term psychological disorders at intervals throughout their lives; examples include grief over the death of someone close, post-traumatic stress disorder, or an eating disorder. A more comprehensive approach to mental health is to define the traits of the mentally healthy personality.

Practitioners use terms that have been formulated by theorists to describe and discuss psychological problems. Words such as *id, ego*, and *superego* are used by therapists who base their practice on Freud's theory. *Enmeshment* is a term used by some family therapists to describe interactions among family members that keep them dependent on each other. A therapist practicing within a Gestalt framework may focus on the feeling experiences of an individual.

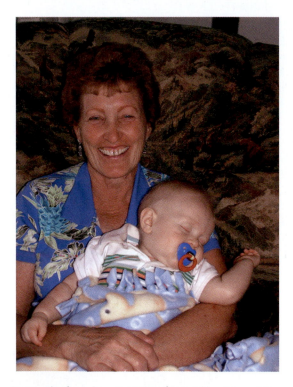

Review the four characteristics of mental health, and then look at this woman's face. You would need to interview her to determine whether it is true, but she does have the appearance of someone with purpose and meaning in her life.

The current trend is to identify wellness in mental health. **Gerotranscendence** is a theory of aging developed by Lars Tornstam (2005). The theory states that human development is a lifelong process that continues into old age and results in new perspectives

(Tornstam, 2005). Although it is difficult to define wellness, some characteristics have been described by psychologists, nurses, and physicians and are included in the following list of characteristics:

- A clear meaning and purpose in life
- A strong reality orientation
- An ability to cope creatively with life's situations
- A capability for open, creative relationships

Notice how these statements complement the concept of gerotranscendence? If an individual has achieved gerotranscendence, that person has increased personal life satisfaction, made a redefinition of self and relationships with others, and has become open to new and creative possibilities. Gerotranscendence is psychological well-being.

Priority Setting

The most important priority you can set when assessing older adults psychologically is to be able to do an effective mental assessment. You cannot fake an assessment and assume it will do any good for the person who is ill. Pick one of the assessments in this chapter and learn it well. Read about it in professional journals, talk to experts about how they perform the assessment, and look for a mentor. The mentor could be an experienced nurse or nurse practitioner. Let your mentor know that you want to be expert at doing the Mini-Mental State Examination, for example. Perhaps your mentor will talk to you about the things that he or she does, or perhaps your mentor will take you along as he or she does assessments. You cannot assess people unless you have developed the expert skill required to do an excellent assessment. Pick one tool and stick with it until you become proficient.

Mental health is not a product of good nurturing or of a life of positive experiences. There are individuals who function well in life—for example, they maintain a satisfying job and career, have a family, and make a contribution to their community—despite poor nurturing and environmental handicaps. Most views of mental health now embody a continuum of health and illness. This continuum is dynamic rather than static. Many situations have an impact on the functioning of an individual, including the following:

- The death of someone close
- Unemployment
- The birth of a child
- Relocation

Any individual, if sufficiently stressed, can show some signs of impairment. One concept refers to the continuum of functioning as a scale of the differences in people. Individuals who are higher on this scale require more stressors to impair their functioning than individuals who are lower on this scale, and they choose a life course based on thought and conviction rather than on impulse; they also show an ability to stand by a belief that is different from that of their peer group.

It is important for nurses working in gerontology to identify and promote positive mental health traits. Nurses can reinforce healthy traits and interactions in older persons. This is nursing care being given in the nursing model (Watson's theory) rather than the medical model. Because it is nursing model care, it is caring and holistic, which are strong traits of the profession of nursing and characteristics that you want to work to develop as a licensed practical nurse (LPN).

Cognition

Cognition is a mental activity concerned with processing information. It refers to a broad range of mental behaviors, including awareness, thinking, reasoning, and judgment. This process is very complex and involves many abilities or functions. Because it cannot be directly observed, many psychologists define cognition in cognitive functions. The cognitive functions can be conceptualized in numerous ways and can be defined as perceiving, thinking, remembering, communicating, orienting, calculating, and problem-solving (Cespón, Miniussi, & Pellicciari, 2018).

Perception

Psychologists believe that all behavior depends on how one sees oneself, the situation one is in, and the interaction between the two. Behavior changes as individuals become aware of details in their surroundings. Learning, problem-solving, remembering, and forgetting all are part of one's awareness of the environment. Effective communication with an older person depends on the nurse's ability to understand the perceptual world of that person. With such an understanding, the most bizarre behavior often becomes comprehensible.

The first phase of forming a perception is the ability to use the five senses to collect information about the environment. Frequently, older adults have impairments in the sense organs. In Chapter 2, you learned about the deficits in vision, hearing, touch, taste, and smell that may occur in older persons.

There is an emotional or feeling component to perception as well. Individuals take in information from the environment and form opinions about such information. Perceptions are normally evaluated against past experiences. An older adult may compare a meal eaten within the institutional setting with recollections of meals eaten with the person's own family. These recollections of past experiences are a part of forming perceptions.

Perceptual distortions also are known as hallucinations and delusional thinking. Although both may indicate a psychiatric illness in younger individuals, perceptual distortions are common in illnesses with **dementia,** an irreversible decline in mental function. Impaired memory and a natural distrust of a strange environment exaggerate this tendency in an institutionalized older person.

Orientation

Orientation refers to a person's awareness of self in the context of a particular time and place. Tests for orientation determine whether the persons being tested know their names, where they are, and the approximate time of day. Sometimes the expression "oriented times three" is used to indicate that an individual's orientation to time, place, and person is correct. Assessment of orientation is covered on every mental status examination. This is important information because a disturbance in orientation is one of the most frequent symptoms of brain disease. Awareness of time and place requires that individuals know where they are and can remember it. In this way, individuals keep in touch with ongoing history. Orientation depends on a person's ability to link each minute with the previous minute. Disorientation with respect to time is the first major confusion to occur as a result of dementia. Loss of a sense of place is likely to follow. Finally, the person loses the ability to recognize other people and, eventually, cannot remember who he or she is.

THINK LIKE A NURSE

You are caring for an 81-year-old woman who was just admitted to the medical unit where you work. The charge nurse asked you to do something about the woman because she is screaming, "Don't hurt me! Don't hurt me!" and thrashing out at the staff. Because you are experienced in gerontological nursing, you assess the woman to determine the problem rather than restrain or confine her because her behavior is inconvenient. Think in terms of orientation and list three reasons why this woman legitimately would be fearful. Then, list appropriate interventions. The first clue is in the section you just read on perception. The next clue is that the woman was just admitted and might be experiencing transitional stress. Be prepared to share your thinking in class.

Thinking

Every area of the brain is involved in the mental operation of thinking. The ancient Greeks believed there were higher and lower levels of thinking, a distinction that is still relevant. Higher level thinking includes the ability to form concepts and think in an abstract manner. Asking a person to interpret a proverb tests the person's ability to think abstractly. If a person interprets the proverb "a stitch in time saves nine" in a way that conveys that prompt attention to a problem prevents trouble in the future, the person's ability to think abstractly is considered intact. A concrete interpretation adheres closely to the exact meaning of the phrase. Concrete thinking is a lower mental ability. Someone with concrete thinking may answer the question about the proverb with something like, "If I make nine stitches, the cloth will hold."

Thinking processes have a hierarchical order. The lower mental abilities are more enduring and less affected by brain injuries and disease processes. The higher levels of thinking tend to be more fragile. At first glance, interpreting proverbs may seem a bit removed from a person's ability to function in the real world. The use of good judgment, the ability to think abstractly, and the capacity to reason are higher level abilities, however, that indicate the difference between independent and supervised living. To some extent, these abilities can be determined by proverb interpretation. In general, tests for abstract thinking are not included as part of the short tests of mental function.

Communicating

The only vehicle for assessing thinking processes in an individual is communication. People understand human thought when it is reflected in language. It is important to assess language problems because they are common in cerebrovascular and dementia disorders. Assessment of communication patterns, word order, and the general sense of a sentence provides a window into the dementia process. This is especially true with a person who has experienced a stroke. Sometimes people who have had a stroke have severe problems with communication. Small connecting words such as "if," "and," and "but" are missing. There are also several types of aphasia, which are impairments that affect an individual's ability to communicate.

Calculating

Calculating is a cognitive function that must be assessed carefully in terms of the person's intelligence and educational level. Poor performance may indicate dementia or delirium, anxiety, or depression. Serial 7s is one test that can determine a person's ability to calculate. The person is asked to subtract 7 from 100 and then to subtract 7 from that remainder, continuing five times. However, use of the Serial 7s by itself may not yield an accurate result. Consider the following situation: a nurse is interviewing a moderately to severely impaired patient with Alzheimer's disease. Although the patient is completely disoriented with regard to time and place and cannot recall the names of three objects seconds after they are told to him, he performs well on the serial 7 calculations. In seconds, he completes the operation and then turns to the nurse, announcing proudly that mathematics was always his favorite subject. This example highlights why you should assess all components of cognitive function.

CRITICALLY EXAMINE THE FOLLOWING

Whenever you are asked to complete these critical examination exercises, you are asked to think on a higher level. Has it seemed that way to you? Think back to your reactions in doing the critical thinking assignments. Did you avoid doing some? Were you irritated or upset at any of the assignments? Did you enjoy the challenge of doing them? Were you bored with them or did you view them as not being a challenge? Take some time and consider your reactions to these assignments. Consider how you felt when certain items were discussed in class. Did you benefit from the thinking of your classmates? Were your ideas and thinking valued by others? Take the time to write your reactions regarding the higher level thinking experiences. Be prepared to share them in class.

Problem-Solving

Problem-solving skills are essential to an individual's ability to function in any environment. Even people with dementia can exhibit aspects of problem-solving ability. Individuals in the early stages of Alzheimer's disease frequently make lists. Lists are coping devices that enable the recall of event sequences. When asked questions of orientation, some older people search for familiar cues in the environment. Examples of this behavior include the patient who was asked the date, spied a newspaper, and then winked and, smiling broadly, gave the correct answer. Another patient called out to a nursing assistant who was passing by the door. When the nursing assistant entered the room, the patient asked him for the date and promptly relayed this information to the nurse interviewer.

An individual's environment is filled with a multitude of clues that facilitate orientation, aid a failing memory, and maintain a stable perceptual field. Use of these clues enables older adults to maintain communication with nurses, other patients, and family members. Because a patient's environment is often filled with problem-solving clues, room changes and unit changes should be made infrequently and only after the most careful thought.

ASSESSMENT TOOLS AND HOW TO USE THEM

Mental status examinations are the most frequently used psychological assessments. Mental status assessment includes probing of the cognitive functions and **level of consciousness (LOC)**. In selecting a tool, it is important to remember that examinations with brief instruments are generally better tolerated by an elderly person. A short examination is much less tiring for an older person to sit through than a lengthy one. No brief instrument is a perfect detector of cognitive impairment, however.

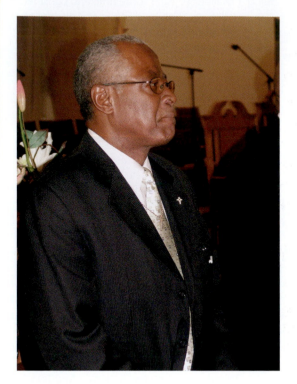

This man is a deacon in his church. This responsibility requires that he communicate, calculate, and problem-solve. He also needs a good memory to do his job well. Interviewing people about their activities gives you important information for a psychological assessment.

Screening tools initially may seem intimidating or cumbersome to use in clinical practice. Most tools are short and can be easily committed to memory after using them a few times. The following tests are commonly used and easy to learn and administer: Pfeiffer's Short Portable Mental Status Questionnaire (SPMSQ) (Pfeiffer, 1975), Folstein's Mini-Mental Status Examination (MMSE) (Folstein, Folstein, & McHugh, 1975), and the Mini-Cog (Mini-cog, n.d.). These scales are compared in Table 17.1 and are listed with a brief description in Box 17.1.

An important factor to consider in the scoring of all tests is that the educational level of the person being tested influences test results. An older adult with a lack of a formal education can score several points lower than an older person with greater deficits but more education. Some mental status tests have a method of scoring to correct for education.

There are important reasons for an LPN to gain skills in using assessment tools. A standardized test allows you, as the caregiver, to collect pertinent information in a short time. The collection of this information is organized and methodical. The initial test establishes a baseline and allows for comparison of changes over time.

Memory

Generally, the more active people have been, the better their overall memory is as they age. A dysfunction in memory occurs in almost all of the cognitive disorders common in older adults. Psychologists generally refer to two categories of memory: short-term memory (STM) and long-term memory (LTM). The time interval for measuring STM is seconds, whereas for LTM it is minutes and beyond. Many elderly persons demonstrate excellent long-term recall, although this recall may be rooted more in a belief than in fact; this is the nature of LTM. It means that the stories older persons tell of their childhood or young adulthood are stories based on their belief systems rather than on what actually happened. This attribute can be used effectively as a tool for reminiscence to strengthen a person's self-esteem.

Memory functions are extremely important to a person's ability to think. A deficit in STM means that a person is unable to recall some of the day's events. An older adult with severe impairment of STM experiences the routine of each day as a new experience. Such a person is trapped in an endless cycle of requesting basic information about the environment from strangers, such as "Where is my room?" or "When do we eat?"

Memory impairment limits the ability of a person to form a new idea or relate one fact with another. It is nearly impossible for memory-impaired individuals to organize new information into categories. A place where one can put something (a pair of glasses) for safe keeping may change several times a day. This makes a never-ending search for an important item an everyday event.

Screening for memory impairment is the most important part of any assessment for an elderly patient. The loss of STM is the first symptom of Alzheimer's disease. A stroke also may impair memory function, but in this case, the type and extent of impairment depends on the location of the damage in the brain. Other STM deficits may be due to depression. Individuals with depression are

Focused Learning Chart: Memory Function

Assessing memory function is the most important assessment when working with cognitively impaired adults.

In general, the more active people have been, the better their memory is as they age.

Long-term Memory (LTM)	Short-term Memory (STM)
Measure in minutes and beyond	Measure in seconds
Rooted in belief rather than fact	Unable to recall daily events: "Where is my room?"
	Without STM, a person is limited in forming new ideas or relating one fact to another.
	Loss of STM is symptomatic of Alzheimer's disease, cerebral vascular accident, and or depression.

Table 17.1
Mental Status Examinations

	Short Portable Mental Status Questionnaire	Mini-Mental State Exam	MINI-COG
Level of consciousness (LOC)		X	
Cognitive functions			
Remembering	X	X	X
Communicating			X
Problem-solving			X
Perceiving			
Thinking			
Orienting	X	X	
Calculating	X	X	
Corrects for education and culture	X		X
Number of questions	10	30	
Time required (minutes)	5	10	3

Modified from Gurland, B. J. (1987). The assessment of cognitive function in the elderly. *Clinical Geriatric Medicine, 3,* 53–63; and Waszynski, C. M. (2012). The Confusion Assessment Method (CAM), retrieved from http://consultgerirn.org/uploads/File/trythis/try_this_13.pdf.

inattentive to their environment. They often are preoccupied or self-absorbed. A decline in STM is an important finding on assessment and should prompt further investigation. The family of Ms. F. from the case study was concerned about her memory loss. This issue should be assessed further to determine whether it is an initial sign of a more severe problem. There are three steps in the memory process. Each step needs accurate assessment. The steps are reception (encoding), storage (retention),

Box 17.1

Brief Description of Common Screening Tools

The MMSE was developed by Folstein to be used with medical and psychiatric patients. Scores in the range of 9 to 12 indicate a high likelihood of dementia. Scores of 25 and higher are considered normal.

The *SPMSQ* was developed by Pfeiffer. This test is a little quicker to administer than Folstein's MMSE. Questions of orientation and memory are addressed, and there is one question concerning calculation. LOC is not assessed. An advantage over the MMSE is that there are specific directions for scoring this test to correct for education and race. A test score of 8 to 10 indicates severe intellectual impairment; 5 to 7, moderate impairment; 3 to 4, mild impairment; 0 to 2, intact status.

The Mini-Cog is a tool that can be used quickly to identify cognitive impairment and is best used to identify individuals needing more thorough evaluation. The first part of the test asks a patient to remember three common objects and then repeat those objects a few minutes later. The second part of the test asks a patient to draw all 12 numbers on a clock and place the hands at 10 minutes after 11:00. The clock must be drawn within 3 minutes. A correct response is all numbers drawn in the appropriate spot on the clock and the hands at the appropriate time. Refusal to draw the clock is scored as abnormal.

and retrieval (recall). Folstein's MMSE tests memory by asking the older adult to repeat three words after the nurse three times—for example, apple, ball, and lamp. The number of trials it takes for the older person to recall the three items is noted. Immediate repetition enables the nurse to determine whether the person has heard the three words correctly. After the older adult repeats the words accurately, the nurse requests that the person remember them. In 5 minutes, the nurse asks again for the older adult to recall the three words.

Orientation

All short mental status examinations include questions about orientation. Time orientation is tested by asking for the date (day, month, year, and day of the week) and the time of day. Because older adults often become quite skilled in using clues from the environment, it is important to remove newspapers or calendars that may help them find the answer. An older adult can sometimes have an accurate sense of time passing yet may not remember the exact date. The nurse may ask questions such as "How long has it been since you last saw me?" or "What was your last meal?"

Assessment of orientation in place generally begins with questions about the name or location of the place in which the person is being examined. The LPN needs to determine whether patients know the kind of place they are in—extended care facility or hospital. Short mental status examinations ask questions about the state, county, or country of residence. Many people with moderate

to severe dementia are unable to recall places. It may be more functional to question an older adult regarding the location of the bedroom or the dining room, for example, "Can you tell me where your room is?"

Assessing Delirium

Nurses sometimes have a difficult time recognizing **delirium** and often refer to it as confusion. Sudden onset is the most significant feature described by experts. Older individuals may develop delirium gradually, however, over the course of 2 or 3 days. An extended care facility resident was being assessed for delirium by the nurse. The resident, who was talking about snakes in her bed, suddenly stopped and turned to the nurse. "Your hands are very chapped," she said. "You should use gloves to do your housework. I always did." Then the resident returned to her delirious state.

Another feature of delirium is disorientation. One person may be mistaken for another. Sometimes an older adult imagines being at home or in another location. Other cognitive functions may become impaired. There also may be a disturbance in the sleep cycle. Many delirious elders are awake all night and then sleep during the day. A common tool used to assess for delirium is the Confusion Assessment Method. Once delirium is identified, the person should be reassessed every shift to assess if the person is still experiencing delirium (Hasemann, 2017). Assessment findings should be combined with results from the physical assessment and nursing observations.

Assessing Depression

Although research indicates that **depression** is no more prevalent in older people than it is in younger people, its manifestation is different and difficult to identify. It is important for you, as the nurse, to gain skills in the assessment of depression because of your focus on the quality of life for all people.

There is a heavy emotional cost to depression that ultimately affects the immune system, which can lead to physical illnesses and infections. Depression predicts the onset of disability almost as powerfully as disability predicts depression. Older individuals who are depressed are in a high-risk category for institutionalization because they are less motivated to care for their personal hygiene and nutrition. This lack of self-care increases their vulnerability to disease. In addition, depressed individuals are frequently withdrawn and socially isolated, and so they have weak support systems. The path to a nursing home for these individuals is apt to be very short and direct. It is possible that Ms. F. has depression and if diagnosed earlier and appropriately treated, she may have delayed admission to assisted living.

Some people older than 65 years of age are beginning to face some significant losses: economic, vocational, family supports, and friendships. Physical disabilities are frequently viewed as the beginning of the end. "If you have your health, you have everything," one grandmother reports. The loss of health signals a life of dependency for most older adults. Generally, the most impressive feature of depression is a feeling of sadness. To psychiatrists, the term clinical depression refers to a cluster of specific symptoms. These symptoms are clearly defined in a diagnostic manual called the *Diagnostic and Statistical Manual of Mental Disorders* (DSM).

Depression may be chronic or acute, and the symptoms may vary in intensity. Severe depression is thought to impair cognitive functioning at any age. Memory seems to be the function most influenced by depression, but there are many ways that memory can be affected. Information committed to memory when a person is depressed is likely to be biased. Other clinicians focus on the ability or lack of ability of older adults to attend to their environment as the indicator of a depression.

An assessment tool used to identify depression in older adults is the Geriatric Depression Scale, Short Form. This tool consists of 15 questions and can be used with patients who are physically ill or have mild to moderate dementia.

Evidence-Based Practice

Hasemann, W., Grossmann, F. F., Stadler, R., Bingisser, R., Breil, D., Hafner, M., … Nickel, C. H. (2017). Screening and detection of delirium in older ED patients: Performance of the modified confusion assessment method for the emergency department (mCAM-ED). A two-step tool. *Internal and Emergency Medicine, 13*(6), 915–922. doi:10.1007/s11739-017-1781-y

The purpose of this study was to develop a consistent delirium evaluation for a busy emergency department. Researchers determined that the modified confusion assessment method for emergency departments (mCAM-ED) was the screening tool they would use on all patients 65 years of age or older during an 11-day period. This tool is a two-step tool. First, the patient is screened for inattention by having them repeat the months backward (months backwards test). Second, interview questions adapted from both the Mental Status Questionnaire by Kahn and the comprehension test by Hart were asked. In total, 286 patients were screened using the tool and the average time it took to use the tool was 3.2 minutes on patients who were unimpaired. Screening patients that were found to have dementia or delirium took about twice as long. Researchers determined that this was a good method to quickly identify patients with dementia or delirium.

Questions
1. As an LPN working in a long-term care facility or home care, could you incorporate components of the mCAM-ED into your nursing assessments?
2. Would use of a standardized tool change the way in which you would provide care to your patients?

Patient Education

When using tools to assess older adults, it is important to educate them on why the tool is used. The nurse should explain to the older adult that it is an objective method to identify potential problems that may need to be addressed to improve their well-being and their nursing care.

WHEN TO ASSESS

Many hospitals and extended care facilities use some sort of standard mental status examination to screen for gross impairments on admission. This is an excellent practice. Although some initial confusion, agitation, or depression is often seen in older adults who are newly admitted because of transitional stress, this practice, if consistently done, helps staff to obtain a baseline of the person's overall cognitive function. The assessment can be repeated if the older adult exhibits acute changes in behavior, mental status, or functional level—for example, if there is a decline in activities of daily living (ADLs). Although screening tools are not diagnostic—that is, they do not point out the exact nature of the problem—they do show, factually, specific areas that have changed.

Validity and Reliability of Assessment Scales

Whenever a questionnaire is used in any clinical setting, psychologists are concerned about two questions: validity and reliability. Is the test question a valid question? For example, does the question really measure memory, orientation, or thinking? Validity is determined in trials that compare the consistency of results. Agreement is then reached by a panel of individuals who are experts in the content of the particular test questions used. The more experts who are involved in designing the process, the greater the validity of the test questions. Reliability is concerned with consistency. Would two nurses, each asking the same person the same questions, get the same answers? When the answer to this question is "yes," the test questions are reliable. All standard mental status questionnaires considered in this chapter are valid and reliable instruments. They have been used by a variety of experts for many years with consistent results. Because rating scales are designed to collect standard information about older persons in a methodical way, nurses should review the methods of using the rating scales together. This practice ensures that information is gathered in the same way. One nurse can interview an older adult while another nurse observes. Then they can reverse roles and compare the answers they received. Some experts recommend continuing this technique with 10 patients or until 80% of the ratings are the same.

ASSESSMENT TECHNIQUES

Older adults generally remain cooperative unless they perceive the questions asked as challenging their mental competence. Catastrophic reactions such as screaming or leaving the room angry can be precipitated when a person is pushed to perform beyond the person's competency. An older adult's refusal to answer questions should be accepted. This information in itself is significant. Older persons, aware of their cognitive impairments, may become defensive when their vulnerabilities are exposed. Attention to the following factors promotes the success of the psychological assessment.

Safe, Effective Nursing Care

Validate evidence-based research to incorporate into practice

As a nurse, it is important for you to recognize the importance of using assessment tools to guide your nursing care. Assessment tools can be used to identify changes in a person's ability from one period to another. They can also be used as a means of communication among health-care workers. Communicating specific information about the patient is important in providing patient-centered care. In the case of cognitive status, a tool can be used to identify changes in that person's cognitive abilities from shift to shift, and changes in the care plan specific to that patient can then be made. Potential safety concerns can also be identified. A nurse needs to become competent in using assessment tools to ensure reliability in the information that is gathered. Practicing using the tools on several patients is the best way to become proficient in using the tools.

Timing

The timing of an interview is an important factor in determining success. Regular staff members, especially nursing assistants in the nursing home setting, are especially skilled in knowing the best time to interview a resident. Allowing an older person to select a time may be the most effective way to gain cooperation.

Privacy

Privacy is very important. Questions that may seem routine to caregivers are often considered deeply revealing and very personal to older persons. All interviews should be conducted in the person's room or in a location that ensures confidentiality. When assessing Ms. F., it is important that you do the assessment in a private room with no family members present.

Elimination of Interruptions

Interruptions undermine the effectiveness of psychological assessments. They negatively affect a person's attention span, and they distract the nurse from focusing on the person being interviewed. Some interruptions are beyond your control as the nurse and occur regardless of the precautions taken. Reasonable efforts should be made to eliminate as many interruptions as possible because they have an impact on the reliability and validity of the assessment.

Positive Introduction of the Assessment

Introducing the psychological assessment in a positive and respectful manner is useful. Describing the test as "a lot of silly questions" may prompt the response that "If they are so silly, why should I answer them?" Let the older adult know that the information gained from this assessment will help the nurses in planning and providing care.

Point of Interest

As an LPN, you should develop polished skills with using assessment tools. Learn to use them well, practice on people many times, and then be prepared to share your skill and knowledge with the interdisciplinary team. This will make you a strong, positive asset to the place where you work.

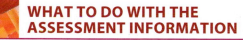

WHAT TO DO WITH THE ASSESSMENT INFORMATION

All information obtained from the older person must be used on the individual's behalf. This information should be dated and appear in an accessible place on the chart with a notation that this document must remain on the chart. Assessment information generally is not updated unless a person exhibits a behavioral problem or has a marked decline in functional level.

Applications in Clinical Practice

In the hospital or an extended care facility, psychological assessments may be used as one of the factors determining the unit assignment of a new resident on admission. They contribute to the identification of the person's strengths and potentials. When used in conjunction with the person's ability to perform ADLs, psychological assessments may point out the need for psychiatric evaluation. When a person's mental functioning seems much lower than the score of a psychological assessment might indicate, a mental illness is suspected.

Cultural Considerations

In many cultures, it is expected that family members will provide all care for older family members. Often, the caregiver is a spouse, who is also older. Evidence shows that caregivers of stroke survivors have an increased incidence of depression symptoms (Loh, Tan Zhang, & Ho, 2017). Untreated depression is a risk factor for the development of dementia. In cultures where the expectation is that family member will care for older members, a thorough depression screening of the caregiver is important to identify and treat depression in its early stages.

Psychological assessments can be used as a basis for care planning. This assessment is especially important when an older adult is able to compensate for their decreased functioning, leading staff members to conclude that the person is functioning at a higher level than is the case. Many individuals with dementia learn strategies to cover for losses in cognition. They may rely on list making, props in the environment, and social cues from others. Staff members sometimes can make excessive demands on older persons if they are unaware of cognitive deficits.

Psychological assessments can allow a broad determination of the effects of an intervention. For example, a person with sadness, who wishes to die, may be treated with an antidepressant. Effective treatment may enhance the abilities of depressed older persons to attend to their environment, improving memory and perception. On the mental status examination, such people may achieve higher scores in the area of recall. This information is useful to a consultant when a more extensive evaluation is considered necessary. It is helpful to be able to tell a consultant that an older adult has dropped 4 points on Folstein's MMSE because the examination was conducted 6 months earlier. It also is useful to note the specific area of decline—for instance, the area of decline is in orientation to time and place or in immediate recall.

Although older persons in the later stages of dementia present similarly regardless of disease process, the initial symptoms may clearly indicate one disease over another. The initial symptom of Alzheimer's disease is the gradual progressive decline in the ability to learn new information. The most significant early symptom of Pick's disease, a rare form of dementia that occurs in late middle age, is a change in personality. This is an important distinction.

Symptoms of dementia are a moving target that must be tracked. The tracking is done by frequent, well-recorded assessments. If an assessment tool has been used to establish a baseline in the early stages of the disease process, it may contribute to the diagnostic process.

Observations of a person's behavior and functional status are subjective and often inconsistently reported. It is difficult to get a clear idea of decline or progression over time without objective measures. Psychological assessments and other assessment tools provide the means for collecting factual information about older adults.

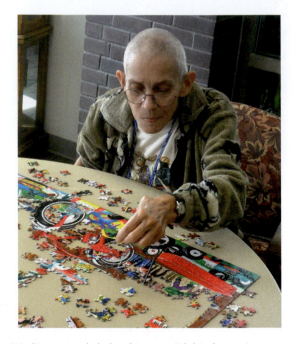

Working a puzzle helps this man with his depression.

Brief mental status examinations universally identify assessments of memory and orientation as the two features that provide the most information about an individual's cognitive functions. Assessments help establish a person's baseline functioning. They can be used to establish a diagnosis, plan care, and evaluate treatment efforts. Psychological assessments also enable the nurse to define problem areas in a more specific manner to consultants. Older adults cooperate well with assessments if the nurse is sensitive to timing, respects the person's privacy, limits interruptions, and presents the assessment tool in a positive manner.

CASE STUDY SOLUTIONS

1. The first step you should take is to talk to Ms. F. in a private setting to discuss the noted change in behavior. You want to hear directly from her what she is thinking and feeling. She may just feel the need to spend more time alone, or there may be some issues with the other residents that need to be resolved.
2. Complete a physical assessment to make sure she is not experiencing a physical condition that needs to be managed, such as pain. Also check to see when she had her last hearing examination in case she is having trouble hearing, thereby limiting her ability to participate in conversation. You will also want to complete the Geriatric Depression Scale to see whether she is experiencing some depression. The results of these assessments need to be reported to the registered nurse.

Key Points

- Cognitive function can be conceptualized in numerous ways and can be defined as perceiving, thinking, remembering, communicating, orienting, calculating, and problem-solving.
- Most psychological assessment tools are short and can be easily committed to memory after using them a few times. The following tests are commonly used and easy to learn and administer: Pfeiffer's Short Portable Mental Status Questionnaire (SPMSQ), Folstein's Mini-Mental Status Exam (MMSE), and the Mini-Cog.
- An initial screening for gross impairments should be done on admission. The assessment should be repeated if the older adult exhibits acute changes in behavior, mental status, or functional level.
- It is important to gather information about an individual's cognitive functions. Assessments help establish a person's baseline functioning. They can be used to establish a diagnosis, plan care, and evaluate treatment efforts. Psychological assessments also enable the nurse to define problem areas more specifically to consultants.
- Severe depression is thought to impair cognitive functioning at any age. Depression may be chronic or acute, and the symptoms may vary in intensity.
- Older adults will generally remain cooperative during psychological assessments unless they perceive the questions asked as challenging their mental competence. When performing assessments it is important to choose a time during the day that works best for the individual, provide privacy, eliminate interruptions, and provide a positive introduction to the assessment to be performed.
- Nurses who consistently encourage patients, and identify strengths in a factual way, are instrumental in improving the quality of life for older adults in their care.

Review Questions

1. A common tool used to assess delirium in older adults is:
   1. Mini-Cog.
   2. Geriatric Depression Scale.
   3. MMSE.
   4. CAM.

2. The nurse practitioner of a unit annually conducts an MMSE on all the residents. She informs you that Mrs. H.'s score in the area of orientation has dropped 2 points from last year. You suspect that the drop is due to:
   1. Delirium.
   2. Arthritis.
   3. Progression of dementia.
   4. Depression.

3. The activities department has alerted you to the fact that recently Mr. J. has not been interested in attending programs sponsored by their department. This morning, he complained to you that he believes that he is having problems with his memory. He did not eat breakfast and only picked at his lunch. He denies feeling depressed. You conduct an MMSE. There is a change in score from the admission MMSE conducted 3 months ago. His immediate recall of three objects on Folstein's MMSE has declined. You suspect:
   1. Delirium.
   2. Progression of dementia.
   3. A urinary tract infection.
   4. Depression.

4. Mrs. C. does not come out of her room for breakfast. The night shift staff members report that she was up all night and that she has a fever. You go to Mrs. C. to determine whether you can assist her. She seems to be asleep. When you touch her arm, she opens her eyes. She does not quite recognize you, her favorite nurse. She believes that it is bedtime and her main concern is that her husband (who has been dead for 20 years) is late coming home from work. When you leave the room, she returns to "sleep." Yesterday her MMSE score was 30/30. You know immediately that she is:
   1. Depressed.
   2. Having a massive stroke.
   3. Delirious.
   4. Confused, owing to dementia.

5. Important considerations when conducting psychological assessments are:
   1. Timing.
   2. Privacy and elimination of interruptions.
   3. Positive introduction of the assessment.
   4. All of the above.

ANSWERS 1. 4, 2. 3, 3. 4, 4. 3, 5. 4

CHAPTER 18

Common Clinical Problems: Psychological

Tamara Dahlkemper

KEY TERMS

anxiety
delirium
delusion
disorientation
hallucination
illusion
paranoia
somatization

CHAPTER CONCEPTS

Cognition
Health Promotion
Mood
Stress

LEARNING OUTCOMES

1. Recognize three general communication skills used when communicating with older adults.
2. Explain communication techniques that can be used for older adults with common psychological problems.
3. Describe how to manage difficult behaviors of older adults.
4. Identify three psychological conditions that can impact older adults.
5. Compare reality orientation, reminiscence, remotivation, resocialization, and validation techniques.
6. Select important information about psychotropic medications to include in teaching.

CASE STUDY

Mr. A. is an 80-year-old carpenter. He was also a master gardener and had a beautiful garden at his home. He lived with his wife in their home until 1 year ago, when he became too ill for his wife to manage his care alone. At that time, he became a resident of a skilled nursing facility in the town where he lives. He has been forgetful for several years and now wanders the halls looking for his garden and tries to use his eating utensils as a hammer. He becomes agitated when he is told that he cannot go back to his home. What actions can be taken to assist Mr. A.?

INTRODUCTION

Psychological problems are disturbances in mental or emotional health that occur as a result of external or internal stimuli. These problems are usually assessed by examining thought patterns, behaviors, and emotions. Because psychological difficulties are not as obvious as some physical problems that can be diagnosed by laboratory tests, it may be difficult to diagnose and properly treat older adults with these problems.

Almost any psychological problem that can occur with other age groups can occur with older adults as well. It is estimated that approximately 15% of the adult population aged 60 years and older have some type of mental health illness. The most common types of such illness include **anxiety**, cognitive impairments, and depression (World Health Organization, 2017). A few common psychological problems often observed in clinical situations are described in this chapter.

GENERAL GUIDELINES FOR COMMUNICATING WITH OLDER ADULTS

It is helpful to review some basic principles for good communication, particularly as they relate to communicating with an older person with a psychological disorder. It is important to practice the skills outlined throughout this chapter to develop your own style for working in a individualized way with each person in your care.

Forming Relationships With People Who Have a Psychological Disorder

Generally, relationships with patients progress through three stages. During each stage, there are concepts for you to recognize. At the beginning of a relationship, people can be uncomfortable. After all, they are sick, and you are new to them. As time goes on and trust is established, people enter a stage of the relationship that allows for more open communication that can be therapeutic in its purpose. The last stage of a relationship involves termination or saying goodbye. Problems in relationship-building can be prevented by understanding these normal stages.

Beginning a Relationship

People who have a psychological disorder may not be easy to get to know initially. They may have had problems starting relationships all of their lives and forming a relationship with a new nurse might be difficult. Some people with mental illnesses have trouble trusting others and find it difficult to trust a new nurse or a new roommate in a hospital or long-term care facility. There are some things that can be done

to help make the beginning of a relationship more comfortable.

If the person with a psychological disorder does not talk or becomes upset at first, do not take it personally. The person may be feeling uncomfortable and unsure of how you will react. You, as the nurse, can be creative in dealing with such issues, so it is important that you respond naturally. Some approaches to consider may be using humor to diffuse tension or discovering the person's interests, such as fly tying or crocheting, and asking him or her about it.

It's important to keep in mind the need to establish trust and not to reject the person. You may need to say to the individual, "It seems like you'd rather not talk right now. I'll come back in an hour and sit here (or at the desk, or at a table) just in case you want to talk to me then."

Priority Setting

When working with any person with a psychological disorder, the absolute priority is *safety*. As a licensed nurse, you are responsible for the safety of each person who is ill as well as the employees and visitors.

1. Some people with mental illness can hurt themselves. The most serious injury that can occur is suicide. The attempt at suicide can result in major injuries such as cuts at the wrist and falls. You must protect such people against their own self-destructive behavior. Suicidal people must be on a "suicide watch," which refers to additional staff caring for them in a smaller and more confined space. With the proper treatment—mainly medication—suicidal people recover, and their underlying condition, depression, is managed.

2. Some people with mental illness try to hurt others. It is their effort at gaining control of their out-of-control lives. Such people could start a physical fight with someone much weaker than themselves, could be verbally abusive, or could go to extremes to hurt others.

Because you are licensed, you are responsible for what happens on the unit. Be ever diligent; listen to the certified nursing assistants as they work closely with the patients; get to know the patients and develop a relationship of trust with them; then do your best to provide an environment of safety.

Developing a Relationship

Once you have developed a trusting relationship with an older adult, you are ready to be an instrument in the work of healing for a person with a psychological disorder. With the development of trust, the older person is able to share with you emotions such as fear and anger and the symptoms of more serious illnesses such as **delusions** or **hallucinations**. Your responsibility is to listen and guide the discussion.

If the older person has a serious disease, most of the verbal therapy is done in group or private sessions with a psychiatric health-care professional. Your responsibility is to listen, be genuine, and report anything unusual to the registered nurse (RN).

Ending a Relationship

Nurses begin and end relationships with many people every day. Sometimes this happens in small ways, such as taking a weekend off or going away for a conference or vacation. Sometimes it is more permanent, such as discharging a person to another facility or to the home, changing jobs, or saying goodbye to a person who is dying. During this phase of a relationship, people generally try to avoid the termination process. This often is exhibited when the patient ignores you and other staff members or acts out.

If a nurse is going away for a short time, the older adult may start demanding more attention by ringing the call light more frequently, becoming angry or irritated by small things, or not responding or talking. To prevent this from happening, it is best if the person knows as soon as possible when to expect the separation. Provide opportunities for the older adult to talk about it openly with you. If a permanent separation is approaching, some kind of formal farewell, such as a goodbye party, might be helpful. Taking pictures with patients and staff also can help ease the difficulty of a separation. If an older person is being discharged home, do not always assume it is a joyous occasion. Sometimes the situation at home is worse than being in an extended care facility or hospital. Even if a person is looking forward to going home, mixed feelings may exist about having to adjust to another new situation. Remember the difficulty of transitional stress.

It is not unusual for a patient who is ready to go home suddenly to become worse. If this happens, it may be a clue to you that the person is having problems with ending his or her present relationships. If you, as the nurse, talk about this openly by sharing feelings, such as "Things just aren't going to be the same around here without you, Mr. M.," the person may be more willing to discuss personal feelings.

Verbal Communication

Communication skills described in general nursing books also can be used successfully with older adults. Some skills are important to emphasize when working with elderly people who have psychological problems. The following discussion includes validation techniques, which are especially useful with disoriented individuals. Validation therapy is discussed in more detail later in the chapter.

Open Questions

Verbal communication can be helpful by using open instead of closed questions. A closed question is a question that can be answered with a simple "yes" or "no." An open question tends to encourage the person to talk more. Open questions are asked using such words as "who," "what," "where," "when," and "how." "Why" questions usually are not helpful, especially with someone who is disoriented. Some people with psychological disorders may be unable to answer a "why" question logically or rationally. If a resident in an extended care facility says she is looking for her mother, you may validate her by asking open questions, such as "What did your mother look like?" "What did you like to talk about with your mother?" "What did you and your mother do together?" If you were to ask, "Why do you want your mother?" the resident may be unable to tell you.

Giving Instructions

When giving directions, it is best to do so slowly, one step at a time. Individuals who are disoriented may be unable to perform any self-care activities unless they are prompted by very simple cues. Telling someone who is disoriented to brush his or her teeth may not get any results. If you tell the person to pick up the toothbrush, then pick up the toothpaste, then put the toothpaste on the brush, then put the brush in the mouth, and then brush up and down, the person may be able to do more than you originally thought.

Guided Choices

Some people may not respond to open questions as well as they do to guided choices. When asked, "What would you like to do today?" someone with a psychological problem may not know how to respond. When given a choice between two activities, with choices given one at a time, however, the person may be able to make a choice. An example of guided choices is: "Would you like to go to singing time today, or would you rather go for a walk outside?"

Empathy and Genuineness

When a nurse shows the desire to understand someone, it promotes more meaningful communication. Empathy can be expressed by maintaining eye contact, using a caring tone of voice, listening closely to what someone says, and making statements such as "This must be difficult for you," or "It sounds like you are having a rough time right now."

The opposite of empathy is patronizing a person. Using a tone of voice as if talking to a child is an example of being patronizing. This type of communication keeps the nurse from using empathy and is not helpful in communicating with older adults. Referring to an older person as "honey" or "dearie" is also patronizing and a hindrance to effective communication. Another example of patronizing behavior is referring to an older person in a report to another nurse as a "real cutie" or a "sweetheart."

It is important that the nurse be genuine when showing empathy. Being genuine means that nurses must truly represent themselves. Finding things you sincerely want to say to a person is more important than saying the right thing from a book.

Listening

Listening to someone includes listening to feelings, words, and behaviors. Sometimes people with emotional problems may forget or confuse the facts or use words that do not make sense. When this happens, it is especially important to listen to feelings instead of trying to get the facts straight. If a resident is incomprehensible but is speaking loudly and has tearful eyes, you might respond by saying, "This is extremely frustrating for you."

Another aspect of listening is to ensure the older adult can hear you. A review of the basic principles may help you. Start by placing yourself directly in front of the person. Stand so that there is not a bright light (e.g., a window on a sunny day) behind you so the person can read your lips as well as listen to you. Speak in a normal tone; do not shout even if the person cannot hear you. If you suspect the person is having difficulty hearing you, move closer to the person. Ask permission to move close to one of the person's ears and repeat what you were saying, in a normal tone. If the person seems comfortable with touch, place your hand on a shoulder and express nonverbal acceptance and caring with touch. Remember to smile and do not act rushed even if you are. You may find other successful methods for promoting the older adult's way of listening. If so, use them and share them with others.

Values and Culture

There are many different motivations for behavior during a conversation. Two that can enhance or interfere with effective communication are the values and culture of the nurse and the older adult. What one person sees as normal may be seen as unacceptable or offensive by a person who has different values or comes from a different cultural background. For example, a nurse who has been educated to value touch as a way of communicating concern and an older adult who perceives touch without permission as an invasion of privacy would have problems with the communication process.

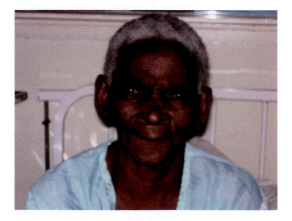

Do you recognize the cultural background of this man by looking at him? It is important to gather information quickly on cultures unfamiliar to you so that you can give caring, holistic health care.

Nurses know that older adults, as with other age groups, come from a wide variety of backgrounds with different cultural norms. In some cultures, it is acceptable to stand very close to people during conversations. A staff member who is unaware of this cultural difference may interpret such behavior as being intrusive. Another resident who values modesty may have difficulty talking openly about bowel and bladder problems. Some residents practice specialized medical rituals. To have meaningful communication with older adults, all caregivers need to understand and respect the various differences that can occur because of personal values and cultural behaviors. Being patient also is very important. Some nurses have to be available to the older person to whom they are assigned for several days before seeing a positive response. When the results do come and the nurse is able to communicate successfully with the older person, it is a very rewarding experience.

Nonverbal Communication

Psychologists say that nonverbal communication, such as tears or the inability to smile, is the most honest communication a person can make. To be an effective listener, you need to watch and listen to what is being said. Using direct eye contact and a caring tone of voice can help the communication process. Positioning the body at eye level also helps.

Touch

Touching is an important part of communicating with people. Many older people miss human contact and enjoy being touched. A person with a psychological disorder, however, may become frightened, withdrawn, or agitated if touched. When the nurse touches someone who has an emotional problem, it is a good idea to ask the person first if it would be all right. Saying "Would it be OK if I gave you a hug?" might be a way of asking for permission. Carefully note the response of the person to the question and the actual touch. Some people who are very withdrawn may respond only to touch.

Touch can be used to stimulate sensory memories as well. Different people respond to touch in different ways. Table 18.1 lists common responses to touch. A person who talks about his mother or says "Ma, ma, ma" repeatedly may respond well to stroking on the upper cheek. This stimulates the rooting reflex and can bring back memories of a loving mother. Stroking the upper arm from the shoulder to the elbow is perceived by many people as an expression of friendship. It feels comforting and safe to have someone touch in that way. If a patient is agitated, you can try stroking his or her upper arm while you talk quietly and gently to the patient.

Table 18.1

Common Responses of Disoriented Older Adults to Touch

Reminds Client of	Touch Technique
Mother	Palm of hand in a light circular motion on the upper cheek
Father	Fingertips, in a circular motion, medium pressure, on the back of the head
Spouse/ lover	Hand under the earlobe, curving along the chin, with both hands, a soft stroking motion downward along the jaw
Child	Cupped fingers on the back of the neck, with both hands, in a small circular motion
Brother or sister or good friend	Full hand on the shoulders and upper back by the shoulder blades; use full pressure in a rubbing movement
Animals or pets	Fingertips on the inside of the calf

From Feil, N. (1989). *Validation: the Feil method.* Cleveland, OH: Edward Feil Productions, pp. 47–48, with permission.

Cultural Considerations

What one person values as a way to communicate may be offensive to a person who has different values or comes from a different culture. A nurse who has been taught to use touch as a way to communicate compassion may have difficulty communicating with someone who culturally views touch as intrusive of their personal space.

Matching and Mirroring

Research has determined that it helps the communication process if a person can match or mirror another's behavior. Mirroring is doing exactly what the person is doing as if the person were looking into a mirror. Matching is using the same pattern or intensity of tone the person is using. This technique must be done in a respectful way and not as a way of making fun of the individual. If the nurse feels uncomfortable doing this, it is not genuine and does not help communication.

Matching and mirroring are nonverbal ways of helping someone know that you hear what he or she is saying. Matching of emotions can be done by labeling the emotion out loud and using the same intensity used by the older person. Mrs. C. may pound her fist on the arm of her wheelchair and say, "I hate them, I hate them, I hate them." Using matching and mirroring, the nurse would pound on the table with the same rhythm she is using and say, "You're angry, you're angry, you're angry," using the same intensity of emotion.

Universal Symbols

A universal symbol is an object in the present that represents something important from the past. Sometimes these symbols increase in importance for people who develop **disorientation** as they grow older. The symbol can be something that has meaning to the older person, such as a reminder of a hobby or life's work, or it can be a different type of symbol. Some typical symbols are listed in Table 18.2. An apron can be made with a large pocket in the front that can contain significant symbols. A gardener may touch gardening tools placed in the pocket of an apron and by doing this revive a memory of a time in life he enjoyed. As the gardener touches the tools, the nurse can encourage communication using these symbols of his previous life. Think about Mr. A. in the case study. Is this a technique that might help Mr. A.?

SPECIALIZED COMMUNICATION SKILLS

The hallmark of nursing care for persons with psychological problems is the ability to communicate effectively. In addition to the skills described earlier, there are other communication skills that can be used to make it easier to talk to older people with psychological disorders. Some standard communication skills and concepts from the Validation Method (Feil & Klerk-Rubin, 2012) are described in this section.

The Validation Method is a communication approach for relating to disoriented older adults, helping disoriented persons to express themselves. Sometimes communication with someone who is disoriented is blocked by the listener's need to have

Table 18.2
Universal Symbols and What They Can Mean

Symbol	Possible Meaning
Jewelry, clothing	Worth, identity
Shoe	Container, womb, male or female sex symbol
Purse	Female sex symbol, vagina, identity
Cane or fist	Penis, potency, power
Soft furniture	Safety, mother, home
Hard furniture	Father, God
Napkin, tissue	Earth, belonging, baby
Flat object	Identity
Food	Love, mother
Drink from a glass	Male power, potency
Any receptacle	Womb
Picking the nose	Sexual pleasure
Playing with feces	Early childhood pleasures

From Feil, N. (1989). *Validation: the Feil method.* Cleveland, OH: Edward Feil Productions, p. 73, with permission.

the disoriented person think or talk in a "logical" way. When the listener is able to put aside the need to communicate in a normal way, it becomes possible to communicate in other more effective ways. The listener becomes able to understand and validate the disoriented person's experiences.

Preferred Sense Words

All people relate to their surroundings through their senses. Most people respond more through one sense than through others. How a person talks can give an idea of that person's preferred sense. If Mrs. J. says, "I see what you mean. Look at this," she probably is a person who responds best to sight or visual words. Some people respond best to hearing or auditory words, and others respond best to words about feelings or movement (kinesthetic words). Table 18.3 lists commonly used visual, auditory, and kinesthetic words. The nurse can use the person's preferred sense

Table 18.3
Commonly Used Preferred Sense Words

Visual	Auditory	Kinesthetic
See	Listen	Feel
View	Hear	Grasp
Picture	Sound	Move
Look	Loud	Touch

to establish rapport. If an older adult says, "No one listens to me anymore," a response such as "What would you like for me to listen to, Mr. J.?" would receive a better response than "What would you like me to see, Mr. J.?"

Vague Pronouns

If a person is unable to fill in the details with enough facts to be understood, try using vague or ambiguous pronouns to help foster communication. Sometimes people refer to all women as "she" and all men as "he." If the nurse becomes too concerned about accurate details, the opportunity to communicate may be lost. Instead of worrying about the facts, such as who "he" or "she" is, try to focus on the feelings. If an older person says, "She's all alone. She can't stay there," you can respond, "You're worried about her. She's important to you." That type of sensitive response generally elicits more communication.

Speaking Slowly

Many people who have emotional problems have slowed thought processes. When this problem is combined with normal aging changes, it is very important for the nurse to use slightly slower speech and wait a little longer for the person to respond. Asking questions one at a time, instead of running several questions together, can also make it easier to talk to an older person with an emotional problem.

Asking the Extreme

When someone who is disoriented is upset about something he or she thinks happened, ask questions about the extremes of the situation. What is the worst? What is the best? Imagine the opposite. When is it better? When does it not happen? Suppose every night an elderly woman thinks some men are coming

to attack her. The nurse might ask, "When do they usually come? When are they not there? What helps you feel safe? What doesn't help you very much?" Often by looking at the extreme of a situation, the person can recognize what is happening in the "here and now."

Behavioral Changes

If a person with a psychological problem begins to display any unusual behaviors, it may be due to numerous different causes. Recent changes in relationships may contribute to increased wandering, shouting, and aggressive or withdrawn behaviors. These behaviors are common after a room or roommate change or when the person is becoming accustomed to new staff members. These behavioral changes also may indicate that a medication change needs close monitoring or that symptoms of the person's illness are becoming more acute.

Point of Interest

In all likelihood, you may be apprehensive about using the touch techniques just described. This is a test of courage of sorts. These touch techniques have a powerful impact on people with dementia. You need to have the courage to step into the situation and give the techniques a try. What if you use the rooting reflex touch on a resident and the person reacts loudly and with fear or anger? Don't walk away and say that technique never works. Instead, critically examine what has happened and consider what the mother of the older person did to cause such a strongly negative reaction so many years later. You have learned something important about the person by using this technique: The mother was not a positive influence in the older person's life, and the issues surrounding the mother may need to be resolved for the older adult.

When you are caring for a person who is exhibiting difficult behavior, you need to take special precautions. Be alert to any situation that would place you, the older adult, or other patients in danger. Report anything suspicious to the RN, and stay calm.

All persons with psychological disorders do not act in a dangerous way. Some sit quietly and never talk or move. This person needs your attention and expertise as well. Talk gently and kindly to the person. Sit with this quiet individual even if there is no conversation. Touch the person if it seems acceptable. All of these simple acts indicate acceptance of the person and are important for healing.

What should you do if an older adult is "yelling" at you? First, do not respond with anger. Stay calm. Be empathetic and kind. Listen to what is being said to identify what the problem really is. Get help if you need it. Be alert to what is going on throughout the unit and with the individuals in your care.

Some older adults with psychological disorders have hallucinations, delusions, and **illusions**. These are symptoms of serious mental illness. People exhibiting these symptoms may think that they are omnipotent, or they may see bugs crawling all over their arms, or they may think you are a princess and want to wait on you. When dealing with such issues, the first rule is to stay calm. The next most important thing is to tell the truth. Do not play into the symptom by saying, "Yes, I am Princess Laura," or something of that nature. Be caring, honest, and genuine with the person. If you feel uncomfortable or in danger, get help; this is never a wrong response.

Agitation

Agitation can occur as a result of physiological or psychological issues. Some people become agitated because of physical causes that result in delirium. Common psychological problems that can cause agitation are the manic phase of bipolar affective disorder, stress or anxiety, flashbacks from traumatic experiences, reactions following abuse, or dementia. When people become agitated, they also may become violent. Such violence can be directed toward themselves or others. Preventing agitation and managing it when it occurs can be accomplished by following a few simple principles, as follows:

• Watch for signs of agitation. Some people show signs of increasing irritability before a severe problem occurs. Others may have sudden, explosive outbursts. Notice if someone is talking very loudly, pacing more or faster, or making threatening comments to staff or others. Before an actual outburst occurs, try to keep the person talking to you by using some of the communication skills discussed in this chapter. With many people who are agitated, simply matching their breathing patterns or tone of voice is calming. With most people who are agitated, it is best to step back about 4 to 6 feet while talking with them. With disoriented elderly

people, the reverse may be true, especially if a sensory deficit is present. It may be more calming to move closer to maintain sustained eye contact and touch. This movement must be done cautiously to protect your own safety and that of others. If there is the possibility that other patients or visitors may be harmed, move them out of the way.

• If a person becomes physically aggressive, it is important to remember that the thumb is the weakest point of the hand. If a person has a hold on you, the way to remove yourself is by rotating away from the thumb of the person's hand. Most psychiatric facilities provide training sessions that allow you to practice dealing with these behaviors in a way that minimizes harm to yourself and protects the agitated person.

Dealing With Psychological Problems Caused by Stress

This section provides some general guidelines for dealing with older adults with psychological problems who are experiencing stressful situations. Making an

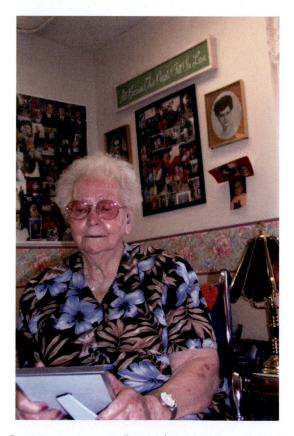

Reminiscence is an excellent tool to use to strengthen an older person's self-esteem.

extra effort to assign the same staff members to an older person in the hospital and extended care facilities may help to prevent emotional distress. A hospitalized patient may be assigned six different nurses during a 3-day stay. The sheer number of names to remember is difficult, but it is especially challenging for an older adult with emotional problems.

> **THINK LIKE A NURSE**
> A 78-year-old woman who is legally blind attempts to hit a staff member when she is being returned to bed. How will you respond to this situation?

In addition to the "normal" stress of being admitted to a hospital or extended care facility, an older person with psychological disorders has to deal with whatever illness caused the admission and the symptoms of the psychological illness. An example is a person who has hallucinations. Hallucinations are real to the person experiencing them, and they add a tremendous level of confusion to the daily life of the person. Hallucinations interfere with one's ability to perceive information accurately. The nurse's instructions or even a greeting may be misinterpreted; medications may look like spiders; walls and doorways may keep moving. The approach to such problems includes keeping the same caregiver with the patient throughout his or her stay. The nurse will begin to understand the behaviors of the older adult and be able to work within the limitations of the mental illness of the person.

It also helps when an older person's familiar belongings can be kept in the room; this promotes self-worth and helps to prevent disorientation. Small objects and pictures can be placed near the older person during a hospitalization to prevent the disorientation that can accompany stressful changes during an illness. Playing taped music of familiar songs generally is better than television viewing in preventing sensory overload. These are just a few examples of simple nursing interventions that can be used to prevent psychological problems caused by stress in older adults.

Violent Behavior

If an older adult starts to act violently, the nurse must remember to protect the individual from their own behavior at all times. The nurse needs to call for help and, as a member of a team, decide what the intervention should be. Do not raise your voice; stay calm. These are the basic rules for handling someone who is violent.

Some violent behavior can be life-threatening. If you are in that type of situation, slowly gather any endangered patients and take them to safety. There is no formula for what to do in every possible situation. Simply stay calm and safeguard the patients and yourself.

> **THINK LIKE A NURSE**
> Mrs. C. starts yelling and shouting, "Call the police, call the police," while she is throwing items at her roommate. How will you respond to this situation?

Safe, Effective Nursing Care

Respecting Patient Needs

Mr. J. walks into the visitor's area, unzips his trousers, and begins to masturbate. The nurse gently approaches him to get his attention by moving in close and speaking to him and calling him by name. He then quietly leads Mr. J. to his room, makes sure that he is safe, and gives him privacy to do whatever he wishes sexually.

As a nurse, it is important to understand that some confused patients will act out sexually.

1. When seeing this behavior, does it make you uncomfortable?
2. What are your thoughts about this patient's behavior?
3. Did the nurse handle the situations appropriately?
4. How would you handle it differently?

Sexual Acting Out

Acting out feelings of anxiety may take many forms. Sometimes older adults with dementia lose social controls and express sexual feelings openly. Some people, such as individuals in the early stages of Alzheimer's disease, have an increased desire for sexual activity. People with other types of psychological problems, such as bipolar affective disorder, show sexual feelings in ways that are socially inappropriate. Dealing with these behaviors is almost always difficult, no matter how experienced the nurse is. Always consider if the acting out is an expression of the need for affection and touch. Notice any factors that seem to trigger the behavior to intervene before the behavior occurs.

SELECTED PSYCHOLOGICAL CONDITIONS

Depression

Depression in later life is usually triggered by a life event such as illness, a change in the living situation, or loss of a loved one (see Table 18.4). It can also be a relapse of depression earlier in life. Depression is common in people who have one or more chronic condition. These chronic conditions include heart disease, stroke, cancer, arthritis, Alzheimer's disease, and Parkinson's disease. Although depression in older adults is underdiagnosed, it is the most treatable psychological disorder.

When the effects of the losses of aging are combined with the effects of physical risk factors, it is clear why many elderly people are depressed. The good news is that most people who have depression can be helped by antidepressants and psychotherapy. Antidepressants that are used to treat depression are generally effective.

Tricyclic antidepressants were widely prescribed in the past and are still effective for many people. Tricyclic antidepressants may cause anticholinergic side effects such as constipation, urinary retention, hypotension, and tachycardia. With the advent of selective serotonin reuptake inhibitors, safer treatment options are available for people who have depression.

Table 18.4
Risk Factors for Depression

Medications
Grieving
Loneliness
Alcohol and substance abuse
Changes in environment
Previous episodes of depression
Low socioeconomic status
Loss of independence
Loss of functional status
Chronic medical illness or disability

Medications are an important part of treating depression but are most successful when used in conjunction with other types of therapy. Psychotherapy with a therapist educated to work with older adults can help the person develop coping skills for dealing with depression.

Along with psychotherapy and antidepressants, older adults should maintain good health habits, as this can have a positive impact on mood. Older adults should be encouraged to participate in regular physical activity and maintain a nutritional diet. For older adults with physical limitations, it may be difficult to participate in regular activity. Likewise, older adults with physical limitations or financial issues may find it difficult to provide a nutritious diet. The nurse should assess an older adult's needs and provide opportunities for some form of activity and a healthy diet for the older adults in their care.

Depression and Confusion in the Elderly Person

Assessing someone who is depressed is complicated by factors that occur as a result of normal aging. Chapter 17 describes how to assess someone with depression and how to use standard measures of depression. Some of the behaviors seen in people with depression may be very similar to behaviors seen with other problems that are common in older people. Individuals who are depressed may not care about their surroundings and begin to be disoriented and confused as they draw inward. It can be very difficult to know whether the mental slowing and memory loss attributed to depression are actually caused by the depression or represent changes commonly found in the early stages of dementia. Many elderly people who have depression are thought to have dementia and are not treated for their depression (see Table 18.5).

Depression and Suicide

Assessing for the risk of suicide is essential for someone who is depressed. The suicide rate among older adults is high. It may not seem likely that an older person would have thoughts about suicide, but it happens too frequently. If an older person says something like "I just don't want to live anymore," the tendency may be to discount the person and say, "Oh, you don't mean that," or "You'll feel better tomorrow, you're just having a bad day." If

Table 18.5
Differences Among Delirium, Dementia, and Depression

	Delirium	*Dementia*	*Depression*
Onset	Rapid	Slow	Rapid
Duration	Short	Long	Short or long
Night symptoms	May worsen	Frequently worsen	Usually do not worsen
Cognitive functions	Variable	Stable	Variable
Physical causes	Common	None	Possible
Recent changes	Common	None or minimal	Common
Suicidal ideation	Rare	Rare	Common
Low self-esteem	Rare	Rare	Common
History of psychiatric symptoms	Not usually	Rare	Common
Mood	Labile	Labile	Depressed
Behavior	Labile	Labile	Slowed thought and motor processes

a person expresses a wish to die, has a major change in life, or begins to give away cherished possessions, these can be signs that the person may be planning suicide.

Asking people whether they are having thoughts about killing themselves is not "putting the thought into their heads." Many people are relieved to talk to someone about suicide if asked in a calm, matter-of-fact manner. Finding out whether the person has a plan and what it is are essential pieces of information. If a homebound older adult describes a hoard of potassium supplements or cardiac medications that are readily available, and if the person's conversation indicates a plan to take the medication after the nurse leaves, the situation requires immediate action. Persons who say they do not want to live but have not thought about how they would end their lives are at a much lower risk for an immediate suicide attempt than persons who have a plan. Many incidents of so-called noncompliance with medications are actually intentional attempts to overdose. If an older adult is having thoughts about suicide, listen carefully, intervene immediately if necessary, and refer the person for treatment.

CRITICALLY EXAMINE THE FOLLOWING

Many people believe that depression is not an actual illness and that the depressed person just needs to deal with it and get on with life. What are your thoughts about individuals who suffer from depression? Do you have anyone in your life who has depression? How has it impacted their life and those around them? After learning about depression, have you changed your views?

Failure to Thrive

The term *failure to thrive* is most often applied to young children who do not grow and develop as expected. Some older persons who are depressed also may have failure to thrive or a giving-up complex. This may be the case when the older person no longer makes an effort to continue with life, such as by refusing to eat, refusing medications, or choosing to resist or refuse treatment for health problems. If there is not an intervention that involves the interdisciplinary team and the family, the older adult may die in this situation.

Delirium and Dementia

Because depression can cause confusion and disorientation, it can be difficult to determine whether the older person has a problem with delirium, dementia, or depression (see Table 18.5). Many factors influence a person's ability to think clearly.

Emotional stress and change can cause anyone to have difficulty remembering scheduled appointments or to be distracted easily from activities of daily living, such as turning off the burner when cooking. Sometimes physical factors such as illness, insufficient oxygen, or high or low blood glucose levels may cause a person to show signs of confusion. A person who has a problem with disorientation can be found in any setting. When a person becomes disoriented, the caregivers may become resigned to the problem and consider this to be a normal part of the aging process. That is not a correct assumption. Clarification of the differences between delirium and dementia can provide guidance for effective intervention in both situations.

Delirium

Delirium refers to a situation in which an older person has a rapid change in behavior and thinking ability. Mental status changes that occur with this acute problem usually affect an individual's ability to recall where he or she is, what day or time it is, or even the individual's own name. Delirium may cause agitation or rapidly changing moods. Someone who is delirious commonly has an anxious facial expression. Short-term memory may or may not be intact. With delirium, the older adult pays little attention to surroundings or may respond slowly to new surroundings.

A person with delirium usually talks in a rambling way that does not make sense. The individual may have difficulty staying awake, or the individual could have increased activity and be awake all the time. Sensory and perceptual disorders, such as hallucinations and delusions, may be present. A person with delirium may perceive that a nurse holding a syringe has a knife or that a baby is crying when no baby is there. Changes in thought content and process also may be present. Fixed ideas or beliefs as well as disjointed or flighty thoughts may be evident.

Delirium can result from various physiological causes and can be reversed. Malnutrition, electrolyte imbalance, infection, change in blood glucose, hypoxia, drug reactions, pain, sensory deficit, and dehydration are common causes of delirium. Delirium can also result from excessive environmental noise, unfamiliar surroundings or people, use of restraints, and excessive bedrest. It is important to determine what is causing the delirium because the sooner the problem can be treated, the sooner the delirium resolves. Refer to chapter 17 for information on assessing for delirium.

When an older adult has a period of delirium, it can be very upsetting for the family and nursing staff. Explaining what is happening to all involved can help reduce stress and make it easier for everyone to handle the problem behaviors that occur.

THINK LIKE A NURSE

A 75-year-old man who has just had surgery develops delirium, is agitated, and tries to pull out his nasogastric tube. How will you respond to this situation?

Patient Education

An important part of providing patient education is also educating family members. When an individual is experiencing delirium, it can be stressful for family members who may not understand why their loved one is behaving in such a manner. The nurse should inform the family that the behavior is temporary and once the underlying reason for the delirium is addressed, the behavior will stop.

Family members should be encouraged to maintain a quiet environment and limit the number of visitors during an episode of delirium. The goal is to provide a stress-free environment for the older adult.

Dementia

The symptom of dementia is usually defined as the loss of intellectual abilities to the extent that it interferes with normal activities of daily living. Dementia is characterized by problems with cognitive ability, personality changes, memory impairment, decreased intellectual functioning, and changed judgment and mood.

Dementia usually occurs gradually, over months or years, and is the result of deterioration of the brain. Neurological diseases such as Pick's disease or Huntington's disease can cause this damage, or the damage can be the result of vascular problems such as multi-infarct dementia. Advanced AIDS also has an associated dementia. The most common type of dementia is associated with Alzheimer's disease. It is estimated that in the future dementia will outweigh heart disease and cancer as a major health problem. This estimate is based on the growing number of elderly people in the population and the strong correlation between aging and Alzheimer's disease.

Because dementia is such a significant concern, new approaches to dealing with this problem are being examined. Validation therapy is a way of communicating with people who have dementia (Feil & Klerk-Rubin, 2012). Validation means respecting the feelings of the person and confirming that, from the individual's perspective, the experience is true.

The Validation Method discussed earlier in the chapter is being used in many countries for people who are disoriented to decrease stress, promote self-esteem and communication, reduce use of chemical and physical restraint, and make it possible to sustain independent living for a longer period.

Evidence-Based Practice

Abrams, R. C., Nathanson, M., Silver, S., Ramirez, M., Toner, J. A., & Teresi, J. A. (2017). A training program to enhance recognition of depression in nursing homes, assisted living, and other long-term care settings: Description and evaluation. *Gerontology & Geriatrics Education, 38*(3), 325–345. https://doi.org/10.1080/02701960.2015.1115980

Studies have shown that depression rates of older adults living in long-term care facilities is higher than those of individuals living in the community. However, many residents go undiagnosed for depression because frontline staff are unable to distinguish between behaviors of normal aging and symptoms of cognitive impairment including depression. Staff education on depression has been shown to improve outcomes for residents.

This study evaluated the benefits of an educational program designed to educate nursing and social work staff about tools needed to identify individuals and communicate with individuals with depression and the essentials of depression treatment. The program consisted of three educational modules about depression; pretests and posttests were given to each participant. Scores from the pretests and posttests showed that participants gained increased information about the recognition, detection, and treatment strategies for residents at risk for depression.

Questions
1. What additional information do you need to feel confident in recognizing depression in residents living in an assisted living or long-term care facility?
2. What tools can you use to assess for depression in this population?

STAGES OF DISORIENTATION. Naomi Feil (2012) has described four stages of disorientation that occur with people who are "old-old" (older than 80 years of age). Disorientation is a term used by Feil to describe symptoms associated with late-onset Alzheimer's disease. These changes occur in people who have had fairly normal lives until they reach their 80s, when they begin to show signs of disorientation. The stages are malorientation, time confusion, repetitive motion, and vegetation.

Malorientation. Malorientation is the first stage of disorientation. People who are maloriented may initially appear as if nothing is wrong with them. These people may be oriented as to where they are and who the president of the United States is, but they are beginning to forget information important for maintaining normal activities of daily living. They may try to cover up their memory loss by making up excuses. They do not like to be around people who are disoriented because they are threatened by their own memory loss. They deny their feelings and blame other people for their problems.

People who are maloriented respond best to open questions about facts, not feelings. It is important to hold on to acceptable social roles and rules for people who are maloriented. Encouraging someone who has been a teacher to lead the Pledge of Allegiance may be a way of helping maintain dignity and promote self-esteem. Often, the technique of using commonly preferred sense words assists this person to relate to the caregiver. It is best to listen to a maloriented person until you identify what the person's preferred sense is and then address the person with words that represent that sense. For example, someone who often says, "Oh, yes, I see what you mean," probably is a visual person and may respond to visual words better than to other choices (see Table 18.3).

Time Confusion. As people become more disoriented, they withdraw more from the real world and retreat into their own inner world. During this stage, people lose a sense of real time and respond to an inner sense of time.

A person may think about his or her mother (who is dead) and because past time has fused with present time talk about her as if she was present. Because the nurse feels a need to orient the time-confused person, he or she might say something like, "Your mother is dead; you can't go to see her." This only agitates and distresses the individual, who has no real need to stay in a painful present reality. Using the validation approach, the nurse would move close, use touch, and say, "You miss your mother. What color eyes did she have? Blue or brown?" This is an effort to stimulate pleasant thoughts and memories for the person. There are several different methods of touching a person with dementia that are designed to evoke feelings about a loved one. See Table 18.1 to review common forms of touch.

Repetitive Motion. If people with dementia continue to retreat from present reality, they may enter the stage of repetitive motion. During this stage, movements or sounds are repeated constantly. Usually, speech is limited to single-syllable words, and eye contact is made only after someone touches and talks to the person. The use of touch with these people is very important. Individuals with repetitive motion are often ignored emotionally, with caregivers providing physical care only. Validation techniques of sustained eye contact, stroking, and touching can help reach people in this stage of disorientation and prevent the final stage, which is that of vegetation. When persons are in the repetitive motion stage, they often communicate through universal symbols. These people use objects to represent thoughts. A common example is carefully folding and holding or caressing a napkin, which could represent a baby. Other examples are given in Table 18.2.

Vegetation. The final stage of disorientation and withdrawal is vegetation. In this stage, very little movement or sound is noted. Eye contact is very rare. Using touch and familiar music can help reach a person in this stage.

ALZHEIMER'S DISEASE. Alzheimer's disease is an irreversible, progressive brain disease. It involves parts of the brain that control thought, memory, and language, and can profoundly affect a person's ability to carry out daily activities. In most people

Focused Learning Chart: Stages of Disorientation in Persons With Dementia

Malorientation	*Time Confusion*	*Repetitive Motion*	*Vegetation*
1st stage	2nd stage	3rd stage	4th stage
Appear normal	Ambulatory, but confused	Generally nonambulatory	Bedridden
Forgetful regarding day-to-day information	Withdrawn from real world and retreat to own inner world	Retreat from present reality	Vegetative state
Make excuses to cover up memory loss.	Respond to inner sense of time (childhood, newly married).	Use objects to represent thoughts; make sounds, not words, or just single-syllable words.	No words or eye contact and very little movement
Ask open questions about fact, not feelings; use commonly preferred sense words (Table 18.3).		Use touch (Table 18.1) and universal symbols (Table 18.2).	Use touch and familiar music to comfort.

with Alzheimer's disease, symptoms first appear after age 60 and the risk increases with age. Alzheimer's disease is the most common cause of dementia among the elderly. Currently, as many as 5.7 million Americans of all ages have Alzheimer's disease; 5.5 million are older than age 65. It is expected that by 2050, the total number of individuals with Alzheimer's disease will increase to almost 14 million (Alzheimer's Association, 2018). Although younger people may develop Alzheimer's disease, it is much less common. Nearly one-half of those aged 85 years and older may have the disease. It is important to note, however, that Alzheimer's disease is not a normal part of the aging process.

Plaques and protein tangles that develop in the brain are two of the main features of Alzheimer's disease that are responsible for the changes in cognitive abilities. There probably is not one single cause of the disease, but several factors that can affect each person differently. Age is the most important known risk factor for Alzheimer's disease. Family history is another risk factor. Scientists are also researching the role that high blood pressure, increased levels of cholesterol, and blood glucose play in developing Alzheimer's disease.

Lack of communication between the neurons may cause inappropriate or demanding behavior. For example, a patient may not understand the need for appropriate toileting needs. They may not remember the steps about how to undress to bathe. Often, the elderly adult with Alzheimer's disease may become combative or uncooperative. The anger can be a mask for his confusion and anxiety. The person may constantly follow his spouse or caregiver and fret when the person is out of sight. The world can be strange and terrifying to a person who cannot remember the past or predict the future. Having a trusted and familiar caregiver close by may be the only thing that provides security and peace of mind. Having a set routine also helps the person cope with the uncertainty. Many patients do not like to be in unfamiliar environments and will often refuse to leave the comforts of their home or room. Understanding for the person with Alzheimer's disease and his or her frustrations with the loss of control of behavior and physical abilities is very important.

Although medication and brain exercises can help manage symptoms in some people, currently there is no cure for this devastating disease. Researchers are continuing to examine the evidence for physical, mental, and social activities as protective factors against Alzheimer's disease.

Paranoia

Some people with emotional problems fear that other people are trying to hurt them. Such paranoid ideas are an indication of problems the person may have with trusting others. This **paranoia** can occur with several forms of dementia, Parkinson's disease, or other psychological disorders. Paranoia is an early symptom of Alzheimer's disease. People who are paranoid often seem very convincing and logical. Developing trust is the priority with someone who is paranoid. Being consistent and reliable in all that you do with the person can be the best way to develop trust. Do not make promises you cannot keep. If you say you will do something, following up with the paranoid person is especially important. It is also important to identify potential stressful situations and alleviate the situation when possible to decrease anxiety. It is particularly important to avoid putting medicines in food or drink without the paranoid person's knowledge.

Substance Abuse

Health-care workers who are working with people who have chemical dependency problems recognize that there are a growing number of older adults with substance abuse problems. Because many older people are treated for a wide variety of physical problems, sometimes they receive prescription drugs from several different sources. The availability of prescription drugs contributes to the problem of drug abuse among older persons.

Alcoholism is another problem for many elderly adults. Many of the same reasons that people use substances to self-medicate (e.g., depression, losses, loneliness) in other stages of life are even more of a problem for elderly people. Because many memory lapses found with substance abuse are similar to the memory lapses in the early stages of dementia, substance abuse may not be discovered until it is advanced. Sometimes families have difficulty confronting older family members about substance abuse problems. The denial of a problem, which is characteristic of most substance abuse problems, is especially difficult to deal with when working with older adults. This situation creates a problem with the treatment process. If a substance abuse problem is suspected, it is best to contact trained professionals to assist with interventions.

DEVELOPMENTAL DISABILITIES

Historically, people who had developmental disabilities did not live to an old age. With advances in health care, more individuals who have developmental disabilities, such as Down syndrome, are living longer. There is evidence that as individuals with Down syndrome grow older, they are at high risk of developing younger-onset Alzheimer's disease.

Individuals with developmental disabilities may have some of the problem behaviors that have been identified in this chapter. Principles for setting limits on behavior include the following:

- Recognize the person's feelings and encourage expression of them.
- State the limit clearly.
- Point out ways that behavior can be expressed within the limits and what is outside the limits.
- Allow the person to express anger at having limits placed on him or her.

GROUPS FOR THE ELDERLY

Many older adults with psychological problems can benefit from group interactions. Some types of group therapy that have been used successfully with older persons are discussed next.

Reminiscence

Based on memories of similar events or experiences, many older adults form bonds in groups. Stimulating memories of childhood or early adulthood can serve to improve feelings of self-worth and provide an opportunity to review their lives. Memories may stimulate laughter and happiness or other emotions and serve as a way of coping with present circumstances. Groups can be conducted around an important event, such as Pearl Harbor Day. Common, shared experiences, such as early school days, can be recalled to promote socialization and provide mental stimulation. Reminiscence also can be used individually as a means of helping people process any unfinished business in their lives.

A very structured form of reminiscence is the life review process. This process provides an opportunity for evaluation and integration of life experiences. People in more advanced stages of disorientation are unable to benefit from this type of therapy.

Remotivation

To improve interest in and quality of life, remotivation techniques can be used. The emphasis with remotivation is the use of real objects to stimulate senses and provide new motivation in life and the surrounding world. Pictures, plants, animals, or sounds can be used to encourage group interaction. Because Mr. A. enjoyed gardening as a hobby, he may benefit from a group garden. Holidays, birthdays, or hobbies can be used to focus on participating in the here and now. The focus is on factual information as opposed to exploration of feelings. These groups work best with people who have depression or early stages of disorientation.

Resocialization

Encouraging residents to assume social roles can stimulate feelings of increased self-esteem. The focus for this group is on social roles and not on problem-solving. Discussion may occur about previous social gatherings and how people behaved during these events. The emphasis is on the present and on the discussion of factual information.

Many older adults with psychological problems can benefit from group interactions. Group members are assigned roles, such as the greeter, or to serve each other refreshments. Feelings are not the focus of resocialization groups, which can be helpful for mildly disoriented individuals.

Reality Orientation

The goal of reality orientation is to help residents become oriented to present reality. Constant reminders about the present—that is, where they are and what day it is—are given. Current events on the television or in the newspaper can be used as topics to stimulate discussions. The season of the year, holidays, and the weather are other topics to promote orientation to reality. These groups are focused on keeping people oriented to present reality and are not usually very effective with people who have more than mild disorientation.

Validation

Validation groups combine some of the other types of techniques with group problem-solving and a focus on support. Members are assigned roles, sing familiar songs, serve each other refreshments, and reminisce about the past. Movement is encouraged during group activities. The group is presented with a problem to

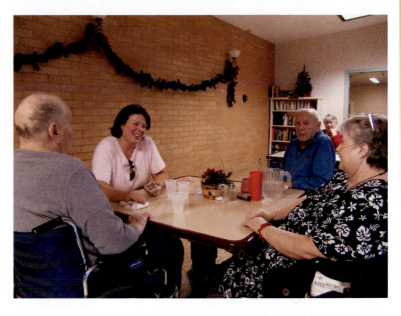

This group of older adults is being led in a resocialization group. Many older adults with psychological problems benefit from group interaction.

solve. Resolving losses and expressing feelings are emphasized. Validation groups are most effective for people who have moderate disorientation.

PSYCHOTROPIC MEDICATIONS

As with all medications, adaptation is necessary when using psychotropic medications with an older adult. Teaching the older person and his or her family about the reason for the medication, side effects, toxic effects, and what to do if a dose is missed are very important when psychotropic drugs are used.

Many psychotropic drugs require time—sometimes several weeks—before a therapeutic effect is achieved. This waiting period may be longer for some older people. Older people may show more signs of toxicity at lower-than-usual doses because their ability to excrete the drug is impaired, resulting in a buildup of the drug in the bloodstream. Older people also could be more difficult to treat because of side effects that occur secondary to the difference in distribution and excretion of drugs in the aging body.

Psychotropic medications work in the brain in various ways. Most medications work by helping to change the level of neurotransmitters or chemicals in the brain. It is hoped that reestablishing a more normal balance will help the person have fewer psychological problems. Because these drugs work on the brain, it is important to use them only for psychological problems and not just because the resident has behaviors that irritate other people. Before any drugs are used to sedate a person with problem behaviors, all other types of nursing interventions must be used along with documentation of the interventions.

Because of physical health problems, some medications used to treat mental health problems may be contraindicated or may require careful administration in the older patient.

PHYSICAL AND MENTAL HEALTH

Because there is such a strong relationship between physical and mental health, many professionals believe that all diseases have physical and emotional aspects. Some older people grew up in a time when it was frowned on to admit that mental illness existed, but it was more socially acceptable to have a physical problem.

This expression of emotional problems through physical complaints is called **somatization**. If a stressful situation is encountered, the person who uses somatization may develop a backache, headache, or stomachache to avoid dealing with problems. This does not mean the ache is "all in the head," but it may mean that the person finds it easier or more acceptable to have a physical pain than an emotional one. For someone who has done this for 80 or 90 years of life, it may be difficult or impossible to change this way of coping. The nurse can help the patient learn to meet needs more directly by encouraging the person to talk about feelings openly.

PATIENT RIGHTS AND LEGAL RESPONSIBILITIES

The current standard of care in health-care facilities is that the older person has the right to the least restrictive form of treatment. Federal and state regulating agencies have specific regulations protecting these rights. In most states, treatment can be administered involuntarily only if a danger exists to the individual or to others. The length of time allowed for this type of treatment varies from state to state but is usually only a few days. If a longer treatment schedule is required and the older person is unwilling to consent or unable, an application for guardianship may be made; the person's rights to make personal decisions are taken away and assigned to a guardian. This procedure may be necessary for people with some types of mental illness, including dementia.

When agitated behaviors become severe, the nurse has to make a decision about how to handle the problem. Points that must be considered are the patient's right to the least restrictive treatment environment and the legal issues related to the use of chemical and physical restraints. If an older adult has an episode in which increased symptoms of bipolar affective disorder or schizophrenia are exhibited, an antipsychotic drug is likely to be more effective than it would be for someone with dementia or delirium. Before giving a chemical restraint, it is necessary to try talking to the person as well as using behavioral interventions. When all else fails, physical restraints may be necessary on rare occasions. If using physical restraints, remember the following safety precautions:

1. Use the least restrictive device.
2. Check on the person often.
3. Remove the restraints every 2 hours for a brief period.

CASE STUDY SOLUTIONS

Working with the entire nursing staff, a plan is developed for using validation therapy with Mr. A. When he asks about his home or garden, the staff ask him open questions about facts such as, "What color are the flowers in your garden?" "What did you like to grow in your garden?" An apron with a pocket is obtained and a small trowel and gardening gloves are placed in the pocket. His toolbox is brought into his room along with other familiar objects from his home, such as pictures of his garden. The staff has put him in charge of a small garden outside the facility where he spends several hours a day working in the soil. The staff also have provided an area where with assistance he is able to use his hammer to hammer large nails into a piece of wood. Individual sessions of validation are scheduled 20 minutes a day, three times a week, by the activities staff.

Over a 6-week period, the staff notices that Mr. A. spends quiet, productive time in the garden area and using his hammer. He carries his toolbox with him most of the time but does not use its contents. With the use of these validation techniques, he is no longer agitated.

Key Points

- Understanding basic principles of communication can be helpful when communicating with older adults with psychological conditions. Using open-ended questions, giving instructions in small steps, listening, and demonstrating empathy and compassion are all skills that the nurse should practice and use. Developing a trusting relationship with patients or residents will help with the communication process.
- Additional communication skills that can be used when communicating with individuals with psychological conditions include using preferred sense words and vague pronouns, speaking slowly, and asking the extreme. Using "sense words" may help the nurse establish better rapport with an individual. Using vague pronouns helps a person when they are unable to communicate the details of a situation or story. It is always important for nurses to speak slowly and wait longer for a response when talking to someone with slow thought processes. By asking about the extremes of a

situation, a person can recognize what is happening in the here and now.

- It is not uncommon for people with psychological conditions to display unusual behaviors. These behaviors may include agitation, violence, and sexual acting out. Each of these behaviors must be handled specific to the individual. The nurse should assess the situation and determine the appropriate interventions.

- Many older adults with psychological conditions can benefit from group interactions. Reminiscence therapy stimulates memories from younger years and can provide improved feelings of self-worth. Remotivation uses real objects to stimulate senses to improve a person's interest in life and quality of life. Resocialization encourages individuals to assume social roles to stimulate feelings of increased self-esteem. Reality orientation helps a person become oriented to present reality. Validation combines some of these types of techniques with group problem-solving with the focus on supporting the individual.

- There are several psychological conditions that can affect older adults including depression, dementia, delirium, paranoia, and substance abuse. Each condition has their own set of symptoms and treatments. The nurse must have knowledge about each condition and be able to recommend appropriate nursing interventions to improve quality of life for older adults experiencing these conditions.

- As with all medications, adaptation is necessary when using psychotropic medications with older adults. The older person and his or her family should be taught the reason for the medication, side effects, toxic effects, and what to do if a dose is missed. Many psychotropic medications require several weeks before a therapeutic effect is achieved.

- Individuals with developmental disabilities are living longer. When managing behavioral problems, it is important to recognize the person's feelings and encourage expression of them, state clear limits, and allow the person to express anger at having limits placed on him or her.

- The expression of emotional problems through physical complaints is called somatization. When a person is experiencing a stressful situation, they may complain of a backache, headache, or stomachache because they feel that it is more acceptable to have a physical pain than an emotional one.

- When caring for individuals expressing behavioral problems such as agitation, the nurse should manage the situation with the least restrictive method. Physical and chemical restraints should be used only on rare occasions in extreme situations.

Review Questions

1. The best intervention for an elderly resident of a skilled nursing facility who has paranoia is:
   1. To encourage him to lead a large group in singing.
   2. To plan one-on-one activities with staff and other residents.
   3. To invite the resident to sit on the residents' council of the skilled nursing facility.
   4. To have the resident join a weekly bingo group.

2. An elderly homebound person taking medication for a psychological problem needs to know which of the following?
   1. If dizziness occurs, notify the nurse.
   2. It may take several weeks to get the desired effect.
   3. Report any changes in vision.
   4. All of the above.

3. Validation techniques are best described as:
   1. A way of helping someone resolve past experiences.
   2. Helping someone find new meaning in growing older.
   3. A reminder of a painful present reality.
   4. Bringing someone from the past into the present world.

4. A hospitalized older adult shows signs of depression. The best intervention is which of the following?
   1. Ignore the person's feelings because they are a normal part of aging.
   2. Tell the person to cheer up because things are not so bad.
   3. Do not allow the person to talk about being sad because that makes it worse.
   4. Encourage the person to discuss feelings openly because it helps to talk about problems.

5. When teaching older adults or their families about the use of psychotropic drugs, one of the most important concepts to teach is:
   1. The meaning of the different colors of the medications.
   2. The stress psychotropic drugs put on the kidneys.
   3. To anticipate the chronic lightheadedness that most people experience.
   4. Not to expect the full effect of the drug for several weeks.

ANSWERS 1. 2, 2. 4, 3. 1, 4. 5, 5. 4

CHAPTER 19

Rehabilitation and Restorative Care

Tamara Dahlkemper

KEY TERMS

functionality
rehabilitation goal
rehabilitation
restorative care

CHAPTER CONCEPTS

Health Promotion
Patient-Centered Care

LEARNING OUTCOMES

1. Define the concepts of rehabilitation and restorative nursing in a holistic framework.
2. Apply the goals for implementing rehabilitative and restorative care.
3. Identify the clinical implications of restorative care in walking programs, continence training, and feeding and self-help programs.

CASE STUDY

At age 65, Mr. M. had an incapacitating stroke and is in a rehabilitation facility participating in a rehabilitation program. He is able to communicate verbally and with gestures, but he is unable to move his right arm and his right leg is very weak. He is having a difficult time feeding himself because the stroke affected his dominant hand. He is having problems with urinary incontinence and constipation. Mrs. M. is very upset because Mr. M. is sleeping all of the time and refusing to work with the physical and occupational therapists.

Mr. and Mrs. M. are both concerned about how he will function when he gets home to his two-level home. Mr. M. recently retired and he and his wife plan to travel as soon as possible.

Discussion

As the LPN working with the interdisciplinary team (IDT), what are the care focus priorities for Mr. and Mrs. M.?

INTRODUCTION

Nurses strive to promote the health of older adults. Generally, nursing care involves assisting older persons in overcoming the symptoms of an acute health problem or the worsening of a chronic condition. Nurses use medications, treatments, and referrals to help the individual overcome physical, psychological, social, and spiritual illness. In the acute care setting, nurses assist older adults through the crisis of illness and discharge them back into the community to their homes or a supportive living environment. The goal of gerontological nursing care is to assist older adults to attain the highest level of health possible. Assessment of their general health and ability to meet their personal needs are considerations during the discharge process. Sometimes older adults are no longer physically or emotionally able to return safely to their homes. The licensed practical nurse (LPN) plays a significant role for older adults who need restorative care.

This chapter presents an overview of gerontological nursing concepts based on rehabilitative and restorative care. Rehabilitative and restorative nursing care surpasses the traditional custodial approach that prevailed in the care of older adults before the initiation of the 1990 Omnibus Budget Reconciliation Act (OBRA) regulations. Data collection for residents in extended care facilities is done on the minimum data set (MDS) (see chapter 4) and emphasizes restorative care of older adults as a major priority of care.

As people age, they experience increased incidence of chronic disease processes such as hypertension, diabetes, osteoarthritis, and heart failure; these processes can lead to disabilities such as mobility issues and activity intolerance. With the elderly population increasing, nurses are called on to provide rehabilitative and restorative care to older people in health-care facilities and community settings.

UNDERSTANDING REHABILITATION AND RESTORATIVE CONCEPTS

Rehabilitation is the process of teaching and training individuals to achieve their highest level of independent function (Stott & Quinn, 2017). People are most familiar with rehabilitation programs for spinal cord injuries. For older adults, rehabilitation often is prescribed for paralysis after a stroke or deformity from rheumatoid arthritis and after joint replacement surgery for severe degenerative joint disease. Rehabilitative care is a multidisciplinary care model. Physical therapists, occupational therapists, speech therapists, dietitians, respiratory therapists, recreation therapists, social workers, psychologists, nurses, and rehabilitation physicians all are members of rehabilitation care teams. The priority for Mr. M. and his wife is to get them networked with the IDT. In an IDT meeting, Mr. and Mrs. M. are participants in a clinical conference in which the rehabilitative team reviews Mr. M.'s case and allows him to make informed decisions on how to proceed with the goal of discharge.

Priority Setting

When dealing with rehabilitation and restorative care, there are three priorities for you:

1. Get to know the person admitted to the unit and the person's family and significant others. To make the rehabilitation and restorative program meaningful for the person receiving treatment, you need to know the person's personal goals and dreams. Because people are not brought to a rehabilitation and restorative care unit in a life-and-death crisis, you have time to meet this priority. Take the time to identify the person's goals and share them with the rest of the IDT team.

2. Use your knowledge and skills as a nurse to prevent disabling consequences (i.e., footdrop, contractures, pressure ulcers, depression) while carrying out rehabilitative and restorative programs.

3. It is assumed that you will carefully follow all physicians' orders. The third priority goes beyond doing what is legally and morally required of you, such as following orders. It is to support the people in your care as they go through the challenges of a rehabilitative or restoration program. It is difficult and demanding. Your support can make a significant difference in the outcome for each individual.

Rehabilitation is initiated after an extensive assessment of an individual's physical, emotional, spiritual, and functional assets and liabilities. To develop a rehabilitative plan, assessment information and the resources available to assist the individual are reviewed. Often, an individual does not need all available services. The team is restructured to include the necessary health-care team members. This team works with individuals and their families to develop goals and to decide the best way to work toward the goals. Mr. M. has a significant physical disability to his right arm and leg. The nurses, physical therapists, and occupational therapist will evaluate not only the right-sided weakness but also how the weakness affects Mr. M.'s ability to perform activities of daily living (ADLs), walk, climb stairs, and manage instrumental ADLs (IADLs).

Selecting a short- or long-term living environment is one of the first choices that a rehabilitation team must make. Every care environment has the potential to be a place for rehabilitation. Limiting factors often are insufficient family support, environmental safety, insurance reimbursement, and access to the rehabilitation team. An older adult with a total hip replacement may want to go home, but home has an upstairs bathroom, and there is no one available to prepare meals. A man may be recovering well from knee surgery and wants to have intensive inpatient therapy, but his insurance company does not approve the cost. An elderly woman may want to go to her rural community hospital for rehabilitation after a stroke, but the services she needs are unavailable in that community. The rehabilitation team works to help the person access support services and find the most appropriate environment for the rehabilitation process.

Restorative care is related to rehabilitation. It has the same goal—to assist older people with reaching their highest functional ability. The major difference is the intense involvement of the entire health-care team. Because of the direct involvement of therapists and other health-care professionals, rehabilitation is an expensive service. Restorative care is initiated after an older person has reached the rehabilitative goal or has not shown any further improvement. The health-care team is involved in designing restorative care plans but is not directly involved in the implementation. An older person who is in a rehabilitation program after a stroke would have the benefit of a physical therapist to learn exercise, safe walking, and transferring techniques. The older adult continues to need assistance with exercises and walking, but a nurse or a nursing assistant encourages the person to do as much as possible independently and assists him or her only if necessary.

Rehabilitation provides individuals with intensive short-term strengthening and retraining, whereas restorative care continues the process over time. Older adults often have a major health crisis and go through intensive therapy and training only to move to an environment where everything is done for them, and the benefits of the therapy are lost. Examples of restorative programs are ambulation, personal care, feeding, and toileting. The challenge for the nursing team is to continue to promote high levels of independent function. It is faster to transfer a person into a wheelchair and push the person to the dining room for breakfast, but that is not promoting independence. Promoting independence in care and use of adaptive equipment can encourage Mr. and Mrs. M. to work with the IDT to meet short- and long-term rehabilitation goals.

This same concept of needing to hurry is associated with high incidences of incontinence. It is often perceived as faster to change an older adult's briefs and bedclothes than to anticipate the need for voiding and walking the person to the bathroom. With rehabilitative and restorative nursing care, "faster" is not the goal.

The same principle applies to eating and personal care. Have you ever watched someone struggle to put a shirt on a paralyzed arm? Watching that struggle is uncomfortable because nurses know they could help that person get the shirt on faster and without as much stress and strain. It is very difficult to watch someone try to eat independently when they have a disability and to see the stress and frustration that can occur. Yet that older person deserves the right to feel the satisfaction of accomplishing a task or meeting a personal goal.

The concepts of rehabilitation and restorative care are crucial to promoting an older adult's optimal level of function. The focus of rehabilitative and restorative care is to maximize the abilities and functions of older adults to ensure the highest level of independence and quality of life. Rehabilitation and restorative care are not isolated treatments with limited application. They embody a broad set of principles to incorporate into every facet of nursing care in all settings.

Within the context of the IDT effort and after clinical conferences with the team to determine what plan is to be designed, LPNs, working cooperatively with the registered nurse (RN), prepare the rehabilitation goals and nursing care plan. In this capacity, the LPN's role becomes one of practitioner, educator, counselor, case manager, researcher, and consultant.

NURSING ROLES

Bedside Caregiver

As caregivers, LPNs provide direct care to older adults until the skills necessary for self-care have been developed by the individual. Nurses need to give older adults positive reinforcement, encouragement, hope, and an opportunity to develop and use their physical and social skills.

Educator

When serving in the role of educator, nurses provide older people and their families with information related to the disability and its treatment and management. Included in the education plan should be health measures to obtain and retain function and to prevent further disability. Effective outcomes are more likely to occur when older adults and their families are included in the process of determining the goals of rehabilitation and restoration of function and treatment. It is important for older adults and the family or other caregivers to recognize that they are responsible for the decisions made and actions that result from those decisions. This is a predominant principle of rehabilitative and restorative care.

Counselor

As counselors, nurses assist elderly people with describing, analyzing, and responding to the current situation that makes rehabilitation or restorative care necessary. Counseling is the process of helping people solve and cope effectively with their problems. Counseling disabled people and their families is an ongoing process that requires supportive behaviors from the entire IDT. LPNs, after establishing trust and rapport with the older adult and the family, need to focus on assisting them in dealing with their grief over the losses imposed by the older person's current disability. The opportunity to express personal feelings assists the elderly person in developing coping skills related to the event of trauma that made rehabilitation and restorative therapy necessary. The LPN should counsel disabled elderly persons and their families to respond to the feelings of loss, frustration, and anger that they generally feel. It is important to express and deal with such feelings as a family.

Advocate

When assuming the role of advocate, LPNs use their influence and power as health-care professionals to bring about necessary changes for the older person and the family's well-being. That advocacy allows the rehabilitation and restorative care to have maximum effect. The LPN's interventions aid the older adult and the family members in obtaining necessary community-based services; the community-based services assist older disabled adults in maintaining their status as fully functioning, independent individuals within the constraints of the limitations imposed by the disability. Such interventions may include the use of assistive or adaptive devices such as crutches, a walker, a plate guard, and a padded spoon.

Case Manager

Generally, an RN is the case manager for disabled persons. In some situations, the LPN is asked to serve in that role. The case manager role places the LPN as a central figure working with the total health-care team throughout the entire episode of illness. The major focus for a case manager is to resolve actual problems and prevent potential problems for the aging person. The treatment plan, once agreed on by the IDT, is under the supervision of the licensed nurses (RNs and LPNs) working in conjunction with each older adult and family. When the plan is agreed on, a contract is entered into by the individual, family members, and nurse. This contract allows the plan to be implemented with clear communication with each person involved. This management may take place in a hospital or extended care facilities and continue into the community where home-based care is provided.

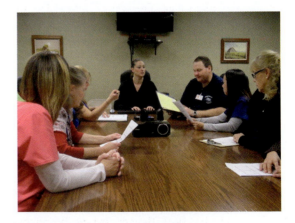

This LPN is meeting with the IDT to plan care for the residents in her care.

Researcher

Many LPNs work in conjunction with RNs and a qualified nurse researcher to gather data on the rehabilitation and restorative care of older adults. Many questions remain unanswered regarding rehabilitative and restorative care of older adults in numerous areas. Each area provides a rich arena for research. Some research interests are the following:

- Management of behavioral symptoms
- Feelings about placing disabled family members outside the home and into an institution for care on a permanent basis
- Barriers that prevent the use of respite and daycare services
- Accurate measures of caregiver burden
- Effective coping strategies used by caregivers
- Types of educational and support programs needed to assist caregivers
- Services needed to individualize care at different stages of an illness or injury

Point of Interest

Refer to the chapter on end-of-life issues (chapter 10). Review Kübler-Ross's five stages of grief. The older adult and the family will be going through these stages related to the physiological, emotional, or functional losses they are experiencing.

All of these clinical questions need to be raised when older individuals experience a traumatic episode and require nursing care. The nurse is responsible for raising questions regarding the specific needs of the older individuals and seeking systematic answers through research. A research approach helps build a body of knowledge regarding rehabilitation and restorative care.

GOALS OF REHABILITATION AND RESTORATIVE CARE

A **rehabilitation goal** is defined as a written statement of desired behavioral outcomes from which steps or strategies may be designed to achieve that desired end. Goals provide direction. They are the measuring tool for an effective plan of care. For example, "I will buy a car today" is a statement of the desired outcome. A defined series of steps needs to be taken before accomplishing that goal. Some of the steps are establishing a means to pay for the car, deciding what type of car to buy, finding out the selling price of cars at various car dealers, checking on insurance, and buying the car.

From the time of injury or disability, the efforts of all health-care professionals involved in care of the older adult are to be focused on the ultimate goal: the highest level of personal independence possible within the limitations imposed by the injury. In setting goals, LPNs assess the older person to determine what assets of mind, body, and spirit are present that would aid in the accomplishment of the goal. For instance, can the person ambulate sufficiently to make trips to the bathroom, dining room, and physical therapy department? The LPN might ask the following questions:

- Is the person able to communicate needs verbally?
- Can the person feed himself or herself?
- What are the goals of the older adult?

The information derived from the assessment is important in determining realistic and achievable goals for each individual. For lifelong quality of living, the components of a successful rehabilitation and restorative program must include the following goals, which should be individualized toward increasing the function and performance of the individual:

- Independence and self-care
- Mobility
- Involvement in activities—social, civic, family, church, and recreation
- Fulfillment of life's goals
- Holistic approach to living with a disability

You must be knowledgeable in evaluating the current holistic status of the older adult. For older adults, major changes in three areas are crucial to the success of a rehabilitation and restorative care program. Changes must be noted in physical, functional, and psychological status. Each of these areas can greatly affect the ability of the older adult to carry out the goals identified in the plan of care.

Physical Changes Affecting Restorative Care

Numerous physical changes may be present when an older adult sustains an injury or trauma necessitating rehabilitation. Existing health problems must be considered in planning rehabilitative and restorative care, as follows:

- Musculoskeletal changes secondary to past fractures, osteoporosis, arthritis, osteoarthritis, muscular dystrophy, or loss of strength in arms and legs can create mobility difficulties. Such situations can occur because of muscle atrophy, decreased bone mass, loss of subcutaneous fat, and decreased flexibility of the joints and limbs.

- Cardiovascular changes secondary to diminished cardiac output, irregular heart rate, and increased blood pressure readings can result in diminished circulation that does not bring sufficient oxygen to the body. Such conditions often cause a lack of activity because of fatigue. Cardiac changes may be the result of thickening of heart valves, thickening of blood vessels, or delayed response to stress.
- Respiratory changes related to diminished respiratory rates can create ventilation challenges for the older person and may be caused by long-standing asthma, obstructive lung disease, emphysema, tuberculosis, upper respiratory illnesses, limited rib cage expansion, atrophy of respiratory muscles, decreased arterial oxygen tension, decreased vital capacity, and diminished cough.
- Renal and digestive tract changes create elimination difficulties that may impair implementation of a restorative program. These changes may include decreased peristalsis of the intestinal tract that results in constipation or diarrhea, decreased intestinal enzyme levels that reduce the ability to digest foods properly, decreased bladder capacity resulting in incontinence or retention of residual urine, and diminished glomerular filtration in the kidney. The latter may result in edematous lower limbs that make it difficult for the older person to ambulate comfortably.
- Cognitive impairment inhibits the ability to participate in rehabilitation and restorative care (Mizrahi et al., 2018).
- Perceptual changes may be exhibited by loss of visual acuity, diminished hearing, decreased sense of taste, lower sensitivity to touch, and decreased proprioception (spatial sensitivity or awareness of where things are in the available space).

Functional Changes Affecting Rehabilitative and Restorative Care

Environmental factors can impact functional status and may include the following:

- Inability to negotiate stairs in the home
- Functional implications of acute or chronic disease processes
- Physical factors, such as limited range of motion (ROM), strength, and endurance
- Inability to consume sufficient nutrients to maintain optimal health
- Inability to cook food, clean a home, or complete the laundry and other crucial chores

THINK LIKE A NURSE

When LPNs are involved in research, they are asked to gather data for the principal investigator. This is an opportunity you should take. You will learn from the principal investigator, will be able to spend time with older adults while gathering data, and will have pride in the finished research project.

These functional changes need to be assessed by a nurse so that realistic goals can be established.

Psychological Changes Affecting Rehabilitative and Restorative Care

The psychological status of an older adult is a crucial component of any rehabilitation and restorative care program. When the older person possesses psychological well-being, there is a strong motivation to work toward the highest possible level of function. When older people feel needed and wanted by family, friends, and associates, they generally possess self-esteem and a positive self-image—two critical factors in developing a high degree of motivation to proceed with the restorative care program. Mr. M. is obviously having difficulty coping with the disability and the rehabilitation program. Often a psychologist or psychotherapist is part of the IDT. The mental health specialist can help Mr. M. develop positive coping skills and motivation for rehabilitation.

Focused Learning Chart: Holistic Functional Assessment

Psychological	Physiological	Sociological
Memory	ADLs	Interaction with others
Judgement	IADLs	Family support
Thinking ability	Current health status	Involvement in the community

Patient Education

The nurse should teach patients and family members the importance of self-care as it relates to rehabilitative and restorative care. Patients should be instructed to do as much of their care as possible. Although doing most of their care by themselves may be difficult and even painful at times, it is critical to meeting their goals.

DEVELOPING GOALS FOR REHABILITATIVE AND RESTORATIVE CARE

When developing goals for rehabilitative and restorative care, LPNs need to complete a full nursing assessment under the guidance of the RN. The nursing assessment should include a database with the following elements:

- Patient history that includes the older adult's past medical conditions, psychological impairments, hospitalizations, and previous injuries (see chapter 15)
- Physical assessment of all body systems (see chapter 15)
- Functional assessment to check for functional ability and mobility (see chapter 15)
- Mental status and psychological parameters that may be present, such as depression or anxiety (see chapter 17)
- A spiritual assessment to determine any spiritual needs or deficits that may be a deterrent to good rehabilitation progress

Following the assessment, the LPN and RN work together as a team to analyze the data and prioritize rehabilitative and restorative goals for the older person. The following principles of holistic nursing care should be the guidelines for identifying goals:

- When the older adult enters the hospital or nursing facility, rehabilitation must begin immediately.
- Proper body alignment is to be maintained at all times.
- Pressure ulcers are to be prevented on all body parts.
- Rehabilitation is to be implemented concurrently with the illness, whether chronic or acute, temporary or permanent, or disabling or nondisabling.
- Joint function must be kept free through proper exercise and ROM.

- Convalescence is a gradual process and may extend over a considerable period of time for the older person.
- Nurses must understand the person's self-concept and feelings of dependency and isolation, if they exist.
- The time period for rehabilitation depends on the person's psychological acceptance of the condition and his or her physical condition.
- People born with disabilities usually have less difficulty accepting their condition than persons who acquire disabilities later in life.
- More severe emotional reactions are produced when accidents are traumatic.
- Loss and its meaning vary with every person.
- Any personality problems that may be exhibited are generally the result of the person's personality characteristics before disability.
- The usual initial reactions to physical injury are shock, fear, disbelief, and anxiety.
- Periods of grief occur when loss of any physical ability is experienced.
- Depression, anger, and denial may be present.
- Values are examined and limitations are put in perspective over time.
- Time is essential for acceptance.
- The family needs emotional support and comfort during the acute phase of the trauma or illness.
- All information should be given to the family and older adult, including information about resources for rehabilitation services and economic assistance.
- The nurse or social worker should be familiar with community agencies that can help.

Cultural Considerations

An older adult's perception about aging and their day-to-day ability to function are culturally specific. Nurses should consider this when developing patient goals.

Evidence-Based Practice

Ritchie, R., Wood, S., Martin, F. C., & Jones, G. D. (2017). Impact of an educational training program on restorative care practice of nursing assistants working with hospitalized older patients. *Journal of Clinical Outcomes Management, 24*(9), 425–432.

Studies have shown restorative care can help individuals improve independence by restoring and maintaining function. In hospitals and other acute care settings, functional decline and deconditioning regularly occur as a result of exposure to the hospital environment, and these changes are independent of the patient's medical condition on admission. In the hospital setting, certified nursing assistants provide the majority of care to patients and are in an ideal position to also provide restorative care. In extended care facilities, restorative care has resulted in favorable outcomes.

This study, conducted in the United Kingdom, evaluated the benefits of providing a restorative education program to nursing assistants (NA) with the goal of increasing restorative care in hospital settings. The program included information on the risks of hospitalization, benefits of mobilization, examples of restorative care, and the skills necessary to provide restorative care. The program also included scheduled training sessions on the units. The results of the study showed an increase in the amount of restorative care provided by NAs.

Questions

1. Based on your experience working as or with a certified nursing assistant, what skills need to be taught or better emphasized to improve restorative care in acute or long-term care settings?

IMPLEMENTATION OF GOALS IN REHABILITATIVE AND RESTORATIVE CARE

Goal 1: Maintenance of Joint Function

The implementation of planned care for older people requires that a holistic approach be adopted. The major concern in implementing care is the prevention of deformities through passive exercises that keep joints movable, promote venous return and lymphatic flow, and help prevent excessive demineralization of bones. This goal and care depend on the physician's orders that identify the extent of the exercise program to be implemented. By means of a thorough assessment of the physical condition of the older adult and the specific illness and prognosis for recovery, nurses assume responsibility for the passive exercise program. Such

a program may include ROM activities in which each joint is put through the normal activities of which it is capable—supine, prone, lateral, medial, anterior, and posterior positions. This approach maintains the functionality of the joints and reduces the risk of contractures, strictures, and limitation of activity. By implementing passive ROM, nurses assist the injured person to resume independence of function and perform at optimal levels.

Healthy People 2020

Objective: Reduce proportion of adults with functional limitations

Goal 2: Active Exercise

Active exercise is designed to improve function and performance. It may include transferring from bed to chair, ambulating with assistive devices, using crutches properly, knowing how to maneuver the wheelchair, using hand-eye coordination, and using assistive devices that promote independent living in a normal manner. In each of these activities, nurses, in the role of teachers, help motivate the person to be as active in personal care as possible. Always follow the physician's orders for active exercise. A physical therapist is an excellent resource for these activities as well.

Goal 3: Bladder Continence

In some situations, it is necessary for the LPN to initiate bladder-training programs. Achievement of continence avoids the use of indwelling catheters. Bladder training aids in reducing the chance for urinary tract infections and increases self-esteem. Retraining is based on the development of clear patterns of communication between staff, the older adult, and the family regarding the schedule for toileting (usually every 2 hours). During retraining, the bladder is emptied at set times throughout the day. Limiting fluids after 6:00 p.m. so that the bladder can retain urine throughout the night is another strategy. Periodic catheterization may be employed to develop reflex emptying when the sensation for voiding is diminished or absent.

Goal 4: Bowel Continence

In addition to bladder training, it is important to employ bowel-training techniques if they are needed. Bowel training requires the establishment of a routine

Box 19.1

Spiritual Assessment

You are working with the RN to do a holistic assessment on an 80-year-old victim of a motor vehicle accident. Sister Agnes, a Catholic nun, was walking to prayers when she was hit by a speeding car. She has multiple fractures that will keep her in bed for days. She is in pain, and the RN is working to resolve her discomfort. You are working with the RN to complete the spiritual assessment.

Spirituality discussions make some people uncomfortable. If that is true for you, please work on your skills in this area to overcome such feelings. When considering this discussion with Sister Agnes, you already know two significant things about her that will influence your interview. First, because she is a nun, you can feel reassured that she is a spiritual person and will welcome the discussion. The second thing you know is counterproductive to the first. She is in pain and will not feel like having a lengthy discussion. What two questions could

you ask Sister Agnes that would give you the basic information you need without causing her undue distress?

Thoughtfully write your questions and come to class prepared to share them. Below are two sample questions that may help you shape your questions for this activity.

1. Do you believe in a higher power or God? *Note:* For a Muslim, the higher power would be Allah; for an agnostic, it would simply be a higher power. For Sister Agnes, her response probably would be that she believes in God.
2. What can I do for you or with you while you are here to assist you in meeting your spiritual needs? *Note:* Some people may want you to pray with them, others may want religious artifacts in the room, and others may want a visit from their spiritual leader. Other people will want nothing.

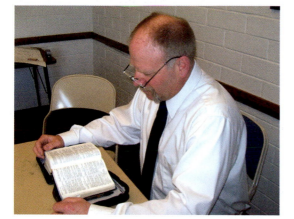

A holistic assessment includes asking about the older adult's spirituality. Religion has a significant role in the lives of most older people. It is important to know about their spiritual needs and strive to meet them. This man takes great comfort in reading his scriptures. To do so, the scriptures need to be easily accessible, there should be good lighting, and he needs his glasses.

older adult. If constipation does occur, it may be necessary to provide medication to soften the stool and allow the bowel contents to move into the lower colon area for elimination. It also is helpful in bowel-training programs to request that the older adult use the toilet instead of the bedpan to facilitate bowel elimination. This is not always possible. Rectal suppositories are useful when initiating a bowel-training program. Enemas are rarely used as part of a bowel-training program.

Safe, Effective Nursing Care

Meeting the Individual Needs of Patients
You work in a long-term care rehabilitation facility. Recently, the adult children of a patient have come to the nurse manager to make a complaint. Every time one of the children comes to visit their mother, she is holding hands and talking in a quiet and intimate manner with a male resident. The children want the time together stopped. The nurse manager has asked you to look into the situation. When you ask the resident about her male friend, she shares that she has never met such a kind man. She shares, "We were both very lonely. No one gets excited about rehabilitation for knee and hip replacement but we may have never met if we did not have surgery." You report your

for emptying the bowel daily. Often, this occurs normally in the morning approximately 20 minutes after breakfast. The intake of food stimulates the duodenocolic reflex, which assists in bowel elimination. A diet consisting of whole-grain breads, cereals, fresh fruits, whole bran, and increased fluid intake is helpful in providing the bulk and fluid needed for effective bowel training. This approach also reduces the complication of constipation in the findings back to the charge nurse, and she schedules a care conference with the IDT, the resident, and the resident's children.

During the care conference the children become emotional and challenge the resident's behavior as "childish" and disrespectful of their father who passed away 6 years ago. The resident becomes tearful. The RN, LPN, and social worker use therapeutic communication techniques to diffuse the emotionally charged challenges of the children and encourage the resident to discuss her feelings about the situation and her feelings about the fellow resident. The geriatrician goes on to explain the seriousness of loneliness and discusses with the children the therapeutic value of friendships, touch, and intimacy.

Think about it: The focus of teamwork and collaboration is positive outcomes for the resident. Through education about and demonstration of respect for the resident and her expression of affection to a fellow resident, the team is attempting to educate the children about the resident's rights and the positive benefits to expressing affection.

Patient-centered care really describes the behavior of the nurse, by going to the resident and asking her direct questions about the children's concerns, along with advocating for her in the IDT meetings.

Is there additional information you need to gather? If so, what is it? How important is sexual expression for older adults? Is it being expressed appropriately in this situation? Please carefully ponder your response and be prepared to share your thinking in class.

Goal 5: Appropriate Sexual Expression

When implementing a holistic plan of care, the LPN must be aware of the older adult's intimacy needs. This means building in time during the rehabilitation and restorative care process for partners to have privacy.

Goal 6: Psychosocial and Spiritual Well-Being

It is crucial to include interventions that address the psychosocial and spiritual needs of older adults. Communicating, increasing self-concept and self-esteem,

treating the person with dignity and respect, and meeting spiritual needs are essential to holistic nursing care. Examples could include uninterrupted time to pray, arrangements for visits from the local clergy, and allowing religious artifacts in the room.

Final Thought About Implementing Goals

The implementation of care measures should focus on the older adult's previous coping skills. It is important that older adults become partners in the care regimen by sharing knowledge and adaptability. The goals are established by the older person, the family, and the nurse as a member of the IDT based on the assessment data. When the goal is stated in specific, measurable terms, evaluation of the progress and outcome of care are easily measured. The terms of the goal are to be put in the framework of self-care and self-responsibility.

ASSESSMENT OF GOALS

Goals are assessed at intervals—sometimes daily, sometimes weekly, sometimes monthly—depending on the goal to be accomplished. When the goals have been stated in observable, measurable terms, the assessment of their achievement is relatively easy. In the course of the disease or traumatic injury, in-depth documentation is important for noting the patient's progress. A systematic approach to fulfill all the stated goals assures the patient, family, and health-care team that a holistic approach has been incorporated into the older adult's care.

Goals Specific to Elderly Adults

Restorative nursing goals specific to older adults include the following:

- Improvement of function
- Delay of deterioration
- Accommodation to dysfunction
- Comfort in the dying process

Improvement of Function

Functionality is defined as the ability to continue to live one's preferred lifestyle without disruption. In other words, each older adult can live independently, do ADLs and IADLs, be mobile, and have self-care ability. To live independently suggests that there is no need for physical assistance or supervision from another person. Goal assessment on a daily or weekly basis is essential to good care.

To improve function, it is necessary to take into account the impact of the older person's social and environmental situation, the functional implications of acute or chronic disease processes, and the physical factors that may influence function. By combining these factors, a picture of the capability of older adults to live and function should emerge for the health-care team.

ROM exercises are exercises performed routinely to preserve the function of the joints and muscles. It is crucial that this maintenance function be performed correctly and on a schedule so that no deterioration of the physical status of the person occurs. The nurse, under the direction of the physical therapist, does this activity or instructs another health-care team member to carry out the activity correctly.

Improving the strength of the muscles necessitates that some resistance be exerted so that the muscle works hard to maintain or improve its function. Resistance is often accomplished through the use of weights or by pushing against an object to provide resistance. The actual testing of the muscle strength and endurance is done by the physical therapist, and a plan of exercise is identified. This plan must be carried out meticulously so that every muscle and its function are duly exercised, and strength and endurance are improved.

Mobility is identified in various stages, depending on the type of injury or disease present in the older adult. The progression is usually from bed mobility, through transfer activities, to wheelchair or ambulatory locomotion. Transfer includes getting from bed to a chair and back to bed, on and off a toilet, and in and out of a bathtub or car. These activities involve standing, sitting, pivoting, turning, or side-slide movement (sliding from bed to chair using a transfer board). To promote function in mobility involves locomotion or moving from one point to another. Older adults may need to use a wheelchair, so the ability to propel and maneuver the wheelchair is important. Wheelchair use involves the development of arm strength with the use of weights or other forms of strength building. Other assistive devices such as crutches, braces, and splints may be needed to assist in locomotion. To help the individual reach optimal function, instruction needs to be given in the best approaches to maintaining balance and endurance and in the use of devices to prevent falls.

When the goal is to improve function, there is a positive outcome orientation. For example, if the nursing diagnosis is stated:

- Body image disturbance: Functional—self-esteem disturbance related to function limitations, role and lifestyle change.

Then the goal should be written:

- The older adult will verbalize positive statements about self.
- The older adult will identify and demonstrate appropriate strategies to deal with functional limitations.

Some of these strategies could be the ability to manipulate buttons and zippers, to tie shoelaces, and to put on underwear. If the older adult is unable to perform these functions, devices such as long-handled reachers, button hooks, and elastic shoelaces may allow the person to perform more independently.

In helping older people retain functional ability and avoid deterioration, it is important to be aware of the disease processes that may interfere with their ability to achieve independent living. Such limiting problems most often involve cardiorespiratory, neurological, or musculoskeletal systems. Many of these conditions may impose significant functional limitations on the person. All of these factors must be kept in mind when implementing goals for rehabilitative and restorative care for the elderly person. Dedication to the restorative care plan helps older people keep motivated and engage in the purposeful and varied activities that promote function and performance.

CRITICALLY EXAMINE THE FOLLOWING

You are taking care of Mrs. R. who was recently admitted to the rehab facility following total hip replacement surgery on her right side. She is still having trouble bearing weight on the surgical side and walking. The rehabilitation team plans to meet to discuss her goals.

Consider Mrs. R.'s rehab needs and write goals for her rehab program. Remember, goals need to be observable and measurable.

Delay of Deterioration

A primary goal of rehabilitative and restorative nursing is the delay of deterioration in all functional aspects. If bouts of depression are noted on admission and during the course of treatment, the RN should be notified and a psychiatric consultation requested if it is determined to be appropriate for the individual. Depression signals initial deterioration of motivation. Helping the person maintain a spirit of hopefulness is one way to assist in the delay of deterioration.

Another approach to ensure delay of deterioration is to ensure that the nursing care plan calls for exercise of all mobile bodily parts—legs, arms, fingers, toes, neck, hips, and knees. Movement of all of these joints is essential in the maintenance of a healthy state. No nurse should ever allow a contracture to occur. Use of pillows, a footboard to prevent footdrop, and resting splints for wrists and fingers aids in proper alignment of the body to maintain function and delay deterioration. Properly aligned and supported body parts assume their natural posture and position. Passive ROM exercises for all joints can delay deterioration to a great extent. Caution must be exercised, however. If care is not used in moving the joints, soft tissue injury can result from undue stretching of the muscles and joints; this could cause additional injury and slow the rate of recovery, or it could cause great pain when the person becomes active again.

Another priority concern is the prevention of pressure ulcers. Excellent skin care should be a daily part of nursing care for all persons. This is especially important for elderly people who have impaired nutritional status. Pressure ulcers may develop over any bony prominence and on the occiput, ear parts, sacrum, and greater trochanter. Special devices to cushion these parts need to be used as a preventive measure, such as special pillows, donuts, gauze dressings, and special mattresses (circulating water or air). Turning the person every 2 hours is the best preventive measure to ensure skin integrity. When turning the person, the support of limbs and back for good body alignment is essential to keep weakened muscles from further deterioration.

Cognitively impaired elderly persons need individualized nursing care. These people need appropriate sensory stimulation to maintain their contact with the world. Putting the person in a position where others can be seen and the careful use of the radio and TV can help stimulate cognitive functions and lessen the possibility of further deterioration.

To delay deterioration, older adults should participate in out-of-bed activities as soon as they have achieved a medically stable condition. First, they should dangle their feet for several minutes to gain a sense of balance. When this activity is tolerated, the nurse should help the older adult to stand by the side of the bed with whatever assistive device is needed (e.g., a walker or cane). Finally, the person should be assisted to walk to a chair and sit with proper support for approximately 15 minutes at a time. You, as an LPN, are essential for providing the appropriate encouragement to the individual.

Accommodation to Dysfunction

The goal of helping elderly people accommodate to dysfunction requires a great deal of motivation on the nurse's part. It is essential for the LPN to listen attentively and actively to the personal fears, hopes, thoughts, feelings, and values that are expressed by the person who is adjusting to the deficits sustained during an accident, injury, or stroke. Nurses should be aware that a rehabilitation program is primarily a learning and training process. Each person must have the ability to absorb new information on how to use personal potential and how to practice new skills. If a person has sustained an injury that created a footdrop

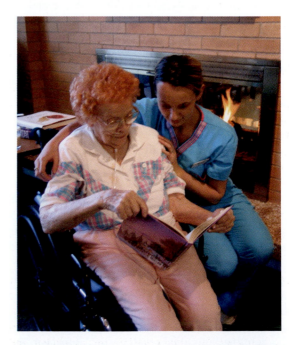

This woman was admitted to the skilled nursing facility in a weakened condition. The first goal is to prevent her from deteriorating any further. As you can see, she now can be up in a wheelchair for short periods.

gait, the individual must learn to accommodate walking by lifting the foot intentionally so that it remains flat as weight is shifted from one side of the body to the other. This action requires major concentration until the old adage "practice makes perfect" becomes second nature to the walker. The nurse's role is to encourage the person to keep working for the highest outcome possible.

Holistic wellness occurs for the older adult receiving restorative care when:

• The psychological self-image of the person incorporates personal limitations into a healthy and acceptable image.
• Social activities and interactions with friends and family continue to be a major part of the person's life.
• The person exhibits gerotranscendence by accepting the new lifestyle with joy, peace, and gratitude for the remaining strengths of his or her personhood.

These are the elements to be found when the goal of accommodation to dysfunction is achieved. As the grief and sense of loss diminish, older people adopt a healthier view so that life, once again, is worth living for them.

Comfort in the Dying Process

Restorative nursing may include providing comfort measures and palliative care to elderly people. Palliative care means providing the care requested by the older person in advance directives and a living will. The individual's decisions must be honored by the nurse and family members. In an advance directive, the older adult may have requested that no food or water be given after it has been determined that no benefits would be derived from such comfort measures. Life-sustaining technologies such as intravenous solutions or use of a ventilator also may be terminated if no positive outcome is predicted. All of these wishes are to be followed, using the Code of Ethics for Nurses.

Nurses are to be supportive of the advance directive wishes of terminally ill older adults and their family members. Nurses must be accountable to support advance directive decisions and facilitate implementation of the individual's wishes. All care decisions are to be carried out in a compassionate and caring manner. Nurses need to approach care of the dying older adult with reverence for body, mind, and spirit as the dying adult approaches end of life. The nurse should attend to the dying person with dignity and respect. Chapter 10 contains more information on end-of-life issues.

CLINICAL IMPLICATIONS OF REHABILITATIVE AND RESTORATIVE CARE

Using the framework of the restorative care principles and guidelines that were cited earlier in this chapter, four clinical rehabilitative programs for older adults are outlined:

• Walking programs
• Bladder and bowel continence training
• Feeding and self-feeding programs
• Self-care—ADL programs

Walking Programs

Mobility is crucial to optimal functioning for older people. To be mobile means that the individual enjoys the satisfaction of independence in living. Nurses play a key role in providing motivation for a walking program. Depending on the type of assistive device needed by the older adult to aid in gait control, the nurse follows the directions given by the RN, primary care provider, or physical therapist. Excellent foot care is critical to maintaining a walking program. Also, properly fitting shoes are important to establish proper posture while walking. Mr. M. may require referrals to community resources, home care services, and durable medical supply companies to assist him in obtaining medical equipment for home use and even receiving nursing care in the home.

The older adult may need braces or crutches to walk. Leg and back braces are devices that are used to support body weight, limit involuntary movements, or prevent and correct deformities. Crutches are devices that may be necessary to help the person learn to walk again in a normal manner. Crutches may be used temporarily or permanently, depending on the type of injury sustained during the trauma.

For successful crutch walking, it is important to strengthen the muscle groups used in this activity. This strengthening should begin as soon as the physician believes that the older adult has recovered sufficiently to consider walking. Strengthening exercises should be provided while the person is still confined to bed. These exercises include the muscles of the arms, shoulders, chest, and back. Before ambulation, the older adult should be taught how to move from the bed to the chair and should be capable of performing this movement without assistance. Older people who need assistance to learn to stand, balance themselves, and ambulate again sometimes experience difficulty. Having patience as a nurse is an important quality.

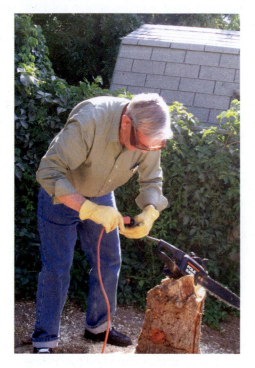

As people grow older, they need to keep moving. This 85-year-old man has spent most of his life working outdoors. He will never go to a gym because "they are for sissies!" He keeps busy with outdoor projects. They keep him moving, and provide him with satisfaction and a purpose in life.

Important points in crutch walking include correct measurements for crutches so that they fit properly. Crutches need to have heavy rubber tips to prevent the crutch from sliding. The crutches need to be moved in a rhythmic way that propels the person forward. Crutches should have padding on the underarm piece so that weight is not placed on the radial nerve. The handhold on the crutches may have padding to reduce irritation there as well. The nurse should emphasize good posture for a person who is crutch walking: The head should be held high, and the pelvis should be kept over the feet for excellent balance. Crutch walking is best taught in several short lessons to reduce fatigue in the older adult. When ambulation begins, it is important to have an attendant in front

and in back of the person to provide stability and to reduce anxiety about possible falls.

Several types of gaits may be used in crutch walking, depending on the type of injury and the physician's orders. They are as follows:

- *Four-point gait*: The person bears weight on both feet and has four-point contact with the floor (both crutches and both feet).
- *Two-point gait*: There are two points of contact with the floor (crutches only).
- *Swing-to gait*: Crutches are placed ahead of the person, and, with weight on the crutches, the body swings through to the crutches.
- *Three-point gait*: Partial weight-bearing is permitted.

As the older adult practices the walking program outlined earlier, the person should master sufficient ADLs to be independent. This independence includes being able to get up and down steps and in and out of cars. It is important for nurses to be very familiar with all assistive devices used in walking programs.

Walking programs also are initiated for older adults without assistive devices. Walking for the older adult is an excellent physical fitness activity. It provides cardiovascular fitness and aerobic exercise. Walking for 20 to 30 minutes, three times a week, has been supported by research as a way to maintain good physical fitness and conditioning. Walking should be a lifelong program to promote wellness and joy in living.

Continence Training

A second major clinical challenge is maintenance of bladder and bowel continence in a traumatized, disabled older adult. An older adult who is the recipient of good nursing care should not experience urinary or bowel incontinence. The use of an indwelling catheter is ineffective bladder management. Urinary infection can result within 24 hours of catheter insertion. Catheter insertion also lowers the self-esteem and self-concept of the person trying to regain control of a traumatized life.

Bladder retraining is generally successful when a regular time schedule is established for emptying the bladder. Retraining of the bladder takes patience on the part of the older adult and the nurse. For more information on bladder training, refer to chapter 16.

A similar program for bowel training should be initiated soon after admission. As noted earlier, increasing the patient's fiber and fluid intake and a regular toileting regimen promotes bowel elimination on a regular schedule. If constipation does occur, stool softeners are the treatment of choice to resolve this problem. The use of enemas is not part of a retraining program. Enemas should be used only in an emergency.

Feeding and Self-Feeding Programs

The clinical challenge of maintaining nutrition adequate for tissue repair and health demands a high level of skill on the part of the LPN. In the early stages of rehabilitative and restorative nursing, the older adult may need to be fed through a nasogastric or enteral feeding tube. A specially formulated calorie-specific formula is administered through the feeding tube in either bolus feedings or continuous drip infusion.

As the older adult progresses in recovery, he or she may need to be placed on a feeding program in which manual assistance by the LPN or nursing assistant is needed until the person has sufficient strength for self-feeding. Older adults should be fed at regular mealtimes, and snacks should be provided. Promoting the older person to a self-feeding program is a definite sign of progress. Encouragement should be given by the nurse so that the older adult consumes sufficient calories to have adequate nutrition to meet the energy demands of rehabilitation.

Self-Promoting Behaviors and ADLs

Independence in personal care is a challenge for older adults with disabilities that affect their ROM, mobility, strength, coordination, and dexterity. It is important that members of the nursing care team allow older adults to have time to perform aspects of their own care independently. Occupational therapists can provide assistive equipment that makes self-care easier. Built-up handles for toothbrushes and hairbrushes are easier for older adults to hold. A chair in the tub or shower may allow a weak individual to be able to bathe independently. Lowered sinks, counters, and mirrors might allow a wheelchair-bound person to sit up near the sink to wash and perform other personal care. Specially designed plastic devices with long handles to insert inside a person's socks and long-handled shoehorns allow older people who are unable to bend over to put on their own socks and shoes. Clothing with Velcro fasteners is easier to fasten and unfasten when dressing. Adjustments in the care environment and education of all personal care staff are essential to the success of self-care ADL programs.

CASE STUDY SOLUTIONS

1. Mr. and Mrs. M. need to understand that rehabilitation is a gradual process and may last an extended period of time, but every effort will be made to help Mr. M. regain his function. However, there are no guarantees that Mr. M. will regain the same level of function that he had prior to the stroke.

2. The LPN arranges for Mr. M. and his wife to become participants in a clinical conference in which the rehabilitative team reviews Mr. M.'s case and allows him to make informed decisions on how to proceed with his rehabilitation. It is important to include both Mr. and Mrs. M. in this process.

3. Until Mr. M. is getting regular activity, he needs to be encouraged to drink fluids regularly to help with his constipation. The LPN may also want to suggest that he be started on a stool softener.

4. The LPN also is concerned about Mr. M.'s despondency. She documents Mr. M.'s behavior and informs the RN about his psychological state. Together, the nurses talk with Mr. M.

about his depression and seek his approval to obtain a psychiatric consultation. This problem is then referred to a mental health professional.

5. A bladder retraining program should be implemented to prevent incontinence. This can be accomplished by helping Mr. M. to the bathroom on a regular schedule.

6. Mr. M. is encouraged to eat nutritious meals so that his tissue can make repairs and to prevent pressure ulcers. He needs sufficient energy from his nutritional intake to do his exercises and walking program properly.

7. Activities are scheduled for him so that Mr. M. can regain his social skills and interact with people without embarrassment and hesitation.

8. In anticipation of Mr. M.'s discharge from the rehab facility, the LPN will want to work with the physical and occupational therapists to determine the equipment he will need when he gets home. The social worker will also be helpful in identifying community resources available to help Mr. and Mrs. M. when he gets home.

Key Points

- Rehabilitation is the process of teaching and training individuals to achieve their highest level of independent function. Restorative care is initiated after the person has reached the rehabilitative goal or has not shown any further improvement. Both types of care are provided by IDTs that include nurses, physical therapists, occupational therapists, recreational therapists, social workers, psychologists, and rehabilitation physicians.
- The nurse fulfills several roles when working within the context of rehabilitation and restorative care. The roles include: bedside caregiver, educator, counselor, advocate, case manager, and researcher. By fulfilling the responsibilities of these roles, the nurse ensures the patient and family understand the goals of the rehab program and have the education needed to make decisions regarding the patient's care.
- When developing rehabilitation goals, the nurse must be knowledgeable in evaluating the current holistic status of the older adult. Changes must be noted in physical, functional, and psychological status. Each of these areas can affect the ability of the older adult to carry out the goals identified in the plan of care.
- The implementation of planned care for older adults requires a holistic approach. Every effort should be made to maintain joint function with the use of ROM activities and active exercise as tolerated. Interventions that maintain bladder and bowel continence should be set up. The older adult's psychological and spiritual well-being should be assessed and the identified needs met.
- Rehabilitation goals are assessed at intervals depending on the goal to be accomplished. When the goals have been stated in observable and measurable terms, the assessment of their achievement is relatively easy.
- Within the framework of restorative care, there are four clinical rehabilitation programs for older adults. The programs include walking, continence training, feeding and self-feeding, and self-promoting behaviors. Walking programs provide the mobility needed to maintain good function. Older adults are taught to use devices to help with mobility such as walkers, canes, and braces. During the recovery process a patient may need help with feedings that is provided by nursing staff. As the patient improves, they will be promoted to a self-feeding program. Independence in personal care is important for older adults. It is important that members of the nursing care team allow older adults the time they need to perform aspects of their own care independently.

Review Questions

1. The aim of rehabilitation for older adults is to:
   1. Engage in limited ADLs.
   2. Deny function and performance that existed before the incident.
   3. Keep food and fluids at a level so that energy and strength are minimized.
   4. Restore an individual to his or her former or best possible function.

2. Which of the following directives most closely coincides with the desired goals of a successful rehabilitation program?
   1. Keep physical changes at a minimum and promote self-esteem.
   2. Promote independence and self-care, along with mobility and a holistic approach to living with the disability.
   3. Promote involvement in limited activities and ROM exercises.
   4. Promote the fulfillment of the patient's life goals despite mobility problems.

3. Principles of rehabilitation include the most important step in nursing care, which is:
   1. Doing passive ROM.
   2. Understanding the patient's self-concept and encouraging feelings of dependency.
   3. Beginning rehabilitation immediately on the patient's admission.
   4. Giving selective information to the family.

4. Rehabilitation goals specific to older adults include:
   1. ROM exercises, transfer skills from bed to chair, dependency on enema usage.
   2. Improvement of function, delay of deterioration, development of codependent behavior.
   3. Accommodation to dysfunction, comfort in the dying process, accommodation to an indwelling catheter.
   4. Delay of deterioration, improvement of function, accommodation to dysfunction, comfort in the dying process.

5. In continence training for bladder control, the nurse should:
   1. Increase fluids, especially during the evening hours, and toilet the patient every 4 hours.
   2. Restrict fluids during the nighttime hours and toilet the patient at his or her request.
   3. Increase fluids during the daytime hours and toilet the patient every 1,000 mL.
   4. Increase fluids during the daytime hours and toilet the patient every 2 hours.

ANSWERS 1. 4, 2. 2, 3. 3, 4. 4, 5. 4

CHAPTER 20
Pharmacology

Rieneke Holman

LEARNING OUTCOMES

1. Discuss how anatomic and physiologic changes of aging impact the safety of pharmacotherapeutics for older adults.
2. Define polypharmacy.
3. Describe common pharmacology issues that licensed practical nurses (LPNs) should be aware of to improve the safety and effectiveness of pharmacotherapeutics for older adults.
4. Describe the pharmacologic management of pain for older adults.
5. Describe interventions the LPN can implement to promote safe medication use by older adults.
6. Collaborate with other health-care professionals to implement Beers criteria.
7. Develop a nursing care plan that addresses pharmacotherapeutics for older adults.

CASE STUDY

Mrs. C. has been recently discharged to home from a rehabilitation facility. She was admitted to the rehab facility following a fall from which she did not sustain any fractures but has been experiencing increased weakness and fatigue. Mrs. C. was diagnosed with heart failure many years ago and now has trouble getting herself to the bathroom. Her medication regimen is as follows:

- Lisinopril, 20 mg, once a day by mouth for heart failure
- Carvedilol, 25 mg, twice a day by mouth for heart failure
- Furosemide, 20 mg, twice a day by mouth for heart failure
- Potassium chloride, 50 mEq, twice a day by mouth for potassium replacement

CASE STUDY—cont'd

- Spironolactone, 25 mg, once a day by mouth for heart failure
- Simvastatin, 20 mg, once a day by mouth for hyperlipidemia
- Clopidogrel, 75 mg, once a day by mouth for anticoagulation
- Levodopa, 250 mg, four times a day by mouth for Parkinson's disease

Mrs. C. is 86 years old, lives with her husband, and has a daughter who is very involved in her care. She has macular degeneration and is virtually blind in both eyes but can navigate through her home when all the lights are on. She has been complaining of extreme fatigue and weakness and is worried about getting herself to the bathroom from her living room chair. Home physical therapy and nursing visits were ordered for Mrs. C. upon discharge from the rehab facility. You are the nurse assigned to visit her.

Mrs. C. denies using any illicit drugs, alcohol, or tobacco. When asked about all her medications, she explained she takes one baby aspirin a day, one fish oil pill a day, and she drinks a glass of water mixed with a "tablespoon" of turmeric every day. She insists it "helps her heart."

Discussion

1. What are your priorities during your home visit?
2. What nursing diagnoses might be appropriate for Mrs. C. at this time?
3. What role does Mrs. C.'s macular degeneration play in her pharmacotherapy?
4. What can the nurse do to encourage Mrs. C. to be compliant?

INTRODUCTION

Since ancient times, humans have used substances to cure or alleviate physical and mental illnesses. Herbal remedies have been used in many cultures for thousands of years. People have learned to extract and modify chemicals from plants and animals to create medicines used to treat nearly every condition. Today medicines are synthesized and studied for use in the general population. Western medicine relies heavily on medications as part of treating illness and disease. As the population ages, people will live longer and therefore need more medications to treat chronic diseases. Modern advances in health care, including the continuous creation of new drugs, has contributed to longer and improved quality of life for older adults. A person will use more medications as an older adult than in any other stage of life. The combination of physiologic aging, presence of chronic diseases, and the use of multiple medications creates the need for special pharmacologic considerations by the LPN. Mrs. C. takes many medications to manage her chronic diseases and will most likely need them for the rest of her life. The nurse must take a lot into consideration when caring for Mrs. C. to provide safe and competent care in relation to her medications. This chapter examines **pharmacology** considerations specific to older adults.

ANATOMIC AND PHYSIOLOGIC CHANGES AFFECTING PHARMACOTHERAPEUTICS

Pharmacotherapeutics is a broad term used by health-care professionals related to medication administration. The term refers to the use of medications to prevent and treat the signs and symptoms of diseases and other health-related conditions. Pharmacotherapeutics includes such concepts as how medications work in the body, how they are to be administered, expected therapeutic and adverse effects, appropriate nursing assessments and evaluations, and adequate patient teaching. Nurses must have a working knowledge of these concepts to safely administer medications to clients.

Sensory Changes

Anatomic and physiologic changes that occur with aging can affect the vision, hearing, and touch in older adults. These changes can adversely affect a person's ability to take medications correctly. Nurses need to be aware of these changes and provide appropriate interventions to ensure safe and effective medication use.

Changes in Vision

Anatomic and physiologic changes to the eye due to aging include hardening and yellowing of the lens, weakening of the iris muscle, and decreased sensitivity of cone cells in the retina. These changes have implications for safe medication use because of the increased difficulty focusing on small print, seeing in low light, and differentiating some colors.

As an individual ages, presbyopia becomes more pronounced. Presbyopia is the inability to focus up close, which makes it difficult to read small print. The small text on medication labels may be impossible for an older adult to read. The inability to read a medication label correctly can lead to significant medication errors that can have serious consequences. To help avoid medication errors and their accompanying adverse effects, nurses can use a variety of interventions. If an older adult is self-administering medications, the nurse should assess whether the client can accurately read and interpret the medication labels. If a nurse is providing written educational materials about medications, it is wise to ensure the font is large. In addition, large printed tags attached to medication bottles may be helpful, and nurses can encourage the use of magnifying glasses or reading glasses.

Mrs. C. is not only experiencing normal eye changes, but she has also been diagnosed with macular degeneration. What further implications does this diagnosis have on Mrs. C.'s ability to safely take medications? What different interventions might the nurse use to ensure safe medication use? To address Mrs. C.'s vision issues related to medications, the nurse must start with assessment. How much of Mrs. C.'s vision is affected? Is she totally blind? What other senses has she honed to help her in her environment? If Mrs. C. is totally blind, what resources does she have to help her with her medications? Does she require a family member or home health nurse to aid in medication administration?

The iris muscle, like all other muscles in the body, becomes weaker with aging. The iris muscle has decreased ability to contract and therefore decreased ability to increase the size of the pupil. Older people are more sensitive to low light environments than younger people, and often need more light to be able to see clearly. When providing written instructions, be sure to provide the maximum amount of ambient light. Similarly, encourage older adults to use a lot of light when reading medication labels or preparing medications to prevent errors.

As the cone cells in the retina become less sensitive, it creates a challenge for older adults to differentiate certain colors, especially blues, purples, greens, and browns. This may create a problem when a nurse says, "take the blue pill in the morning, and the green one at night." To help prevent errors related to pill color, teach the older adult to differentiate pills by size and shape.

Changes in Hearing

Older adults often experience presbycusis, or decreased hearing due to aging. The changes in the inner ear and auditory nerve usually occur in both ears and cause a gradual decrease in hearing acuity, especially with high-pitched sounds. Hearing loss can affect the client's ability to hear and understand medication instructions. The nurse should assess whether hearing loss is an issue because some older adults will nod their heads or express agreement, even when they did not hear what was said. To accurately assess hearing loss, the nurse can ask the client to repeat what was said or explain to someone else the teaching that occurred.

When hearing loss is present, the nurse may use several interventions to increase the effectiveness of verbal instructions. When speaking to an older adult with decreased hearing, always face them so they can read your lips; speak in a slow, audible manner without shouting; and use a low-pitched voice. Be sure to speak to the client in a quiet room with minimal background noise and provide written instructions for reinforcement. To be sure medication education has been received and understood, always ask the client to repeat the instructions or give a demonstration.

Changes in Touch and Dexterity

Due to changes in the skin and nerves as they age, older people experience decreased sensitivity to touch. Disease processes such as diabetic neuropathy often exacerbate this issue. In addition, decreased muscle strength and arthritic joints can significantly decrease hand dexterity in older adults. These changes in touch sensation and dexterity can lead to problems with self-administering medications. Decreased touch sensitivity may hinder the ability to pick up small pills, and decreased dexterity can create a significant challenge in opening containers such as childproof bottles and individual bubble packs.

Nurses can help older adults experiencing problems with touch and dexterity. Nurses can request or encourage the client to request nonchildproof lids for pill bottles. Nurses can also assist by opening difficult pill packages and placing medications in easy-to-open flip top pillboxes. Nurses can also teach family members or care givers to fill pillboxes, making it easier for the older adult to self-administer their medications.

Cognitive Changes

Normal physiologic effects of aging also include the brain and nervous system. The size of the brain decreases, as do the number of nerve cells. These changes lead to difficulties with memory, which can greatly impact the safety of medication use. Older adults sometimes have trouble remembering whether they have taken their medications. This may potentially lead to underdosing or overdosing. Changes in cognition also affect understanding and remembering medication instructions. Multiple medications with varying dosing schedules can be difficult to manage for an older person, and medical jargon may be difficult to understand.

Another physiologic change to the central nervous system (CNS) occurs in the blood-brain barrier, which becomes less efficient as we age, allowing more drugs to penetrate the CNS. Drugs that cross the blood-brain barrier in older adults can affect mood, level of consciousness, and cognition. Changes in these three CNS functions can inhibit a person's willingness and ability to take medications, as well as create problems in other aspects of daily life.

Helping to overcome cognitive challenges is an important task of the nurse. Providing simple instructions in lay terms, repeating information, and giving written instructions can all help support an older person's cognitive function. Another nursing intervention is to assist in setting up weekly pillboxes that allow medications to be placed in a separate section for each day of the week and time of day. Use of pill boxes may help simplify confusing drug regimens. Finally, the nurse must assess whether the client is safe to perform self-administration of medications, and if not, needs to recruit assistance from family or other caregivers.

Pharmacokinetic Changes

Drug manufacturers create medications based on healthy pharmacokinetic processes. Most medications exert their therapeutic effects by being introduced into the bloodstream (absorption), travelling to the appropriate cells (distribution), and binding to cell receptors. To minimize adverse effects, drugs need to be broken down (metabolism) and removed from (excretion) the body. These four processes are altered in older adults due to the anatomic and physiologic changes of aging.

Absorption

Medications are absorbed in various ways, depending on their routes of administration. Oral administration is one of the most common routes used for older adults. Gastrointestinal (GI) changes of aging cause alterations in the absorption of oral drugs. Decreased gastric emptying, decreased GI motility, and decreased blood flow to the GI tract all cause medications to be absorbed more slowly, but more completely. Sometimes delayed gastric emptying can cause nausea and vomiting, which can potentially affect **medication compliance**. Another factor affecting absorption in the GI tract is decreased stomach acidity. Medications that are highly acidic, such as aspirin, have a more difficult time being absorbed in the low acid environment of an older adult's stomach. Nurses can plan on oral medications having a slower onset because of the changes in absorption, especially if medications are given with food, which is a common practice with older adults.

Distribution

Once a medication is absorbed into the bloodstream, it then travels throughout the body and is distributed to different tissues and eventually the target cells. Decreased cardiac output in older

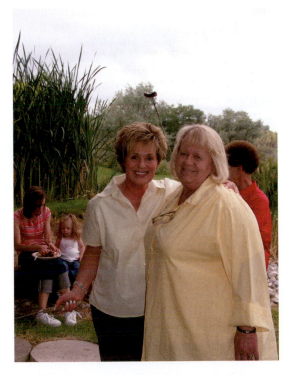

Both of these women take medications daily. Because they are compliant and follow their drug regimen correctly, they are able to live their lives to the fullest. They both agree that their health is improved because of the medications they take.

adults causes a general slowing of distribution to body tissues. Several other factors also affect the distribution of drugs, such as the proportion of body fat to water, total body fluid, and the amount of plasma proteins. Older adults have a higher proportion of fat to water than younger people. This causes fat-soluble medications to be stored longer in the tissues, which can cause adverse effects. Since older adults have less total body water, water soluble drugs tend to be more concentrated and may cause more severe effects. Another significant change in older adults is the decrease of plasma proteins due to the decrease in liver function. Drugs that are highly protein-bound, such as warfarin, rely on binding with plasma proteins to exert a therapeutic effect at therapeutic doses. When there are fewer protein-binding sites, more free drug is available in the bloodstream, and therefore can cause adverse effects, or even toxicity. Nurses must be aware of these changes in distribution to be alert for medication adverse effects.

Metabolism

Many different tissues can metabolize drugs, but the major organ responsible for metabolism of drugs is the liver. As a person ages, the liver decreases in size and function. The hepatic enzymes required for metabolizing medications can decrease with age. As a result of this change, drugs may take longer to be broken down and thus remain active longer in the bloodstream. The decrease of metabolism of drugs can lead to adverse effects. As drugs remain in the body, they can accumulate to toxic levels. The nurse should monitor the older adult more closely for adverse effects of medications, and when adverse effects are noted, suggestions made to the prescriber for decreased doses or longer times between doses.

Excretion

Although drugs can be excreted in different ways, the kidneys are the main organs that clear medications from the body. Like the liver, kidney function diminishes with age. As blood flow to the kidneys and glomerular filtration rates decrease, the filtration of drugs from the bloodstream also decreases. Again, this leaves medications in the body longer with the potential to accumulate to dangerous levels. Kidney function labs should be closely monitored when a client is using a medication that could impair renal function.

COMMON PHARMACOLOGY ISSUES FOR OLDER ADULTS

Polypharmacy and Chronic Illness

In addition to normal physiologic changes, older adults experience illnesses as well. The longer a person lives, the more likely he or she will be to develop one or more chronic diseases. The term comorbidity is used when a person has two or more chronic illnesses. Chronic diseases common to older adults are hypertension, heart disease, arthritis, and diabetes. Each of these diseases may be treated with one or more medications. For example, Mrs. C. is prescribed an angiotensin-converting-enzyme inhibitor, a beta blocker, a loop diuretic, a potassium-sparing diuretic, and a potassium supplement, all for heart failure. She also takes medications for other diseases such as Parkinson's disease and hyperlipidemia. If Mrs. C. also has diabetes and depression, several additional medications may be added to the list. In addition, if Mrs. C. is diagnosed with a urinary tract infection, one or more antibiotics may be added. Mrs. C. also takes a number of over-the-counter (OTC) medications, vitamins, and natural remedies. It is important for the nurse to remember that although these medications are not prescribed, they still have the potential to interact and create adverse effects for Mrs. C.

Cultural Considerations

People of many different cultures use herbal and other nonpharmacologic remedies to maintain health and treat illness. Herbal remedies can be purchased online or in small markets. Often, people will see traditional practitioners who will prescribe and dispense herbs or other remedies. Nurses must remember to ask all clients about use of herbal or other nonpharmacologic treatments when they complete a medication history since some herbs can interact with medications.

It is easy to see how an older adult can develop a long list of medications that are used to manage their illnesses. The likelihood that all the different medications are to be taken at the same time, once a day is very small. Complicated drug regimens increase the chances of a drug error. For example, Mrs. C. must remember which medications need to be taken twice a day versus once a day, and which ones need to be taken in the morning versus ones taken at night. Another factor of polypharmacy that nurses must consider is that clients have many prescribers who may not be aware of all the different medications the client takes. For example, Mrs. C. sees her cardiologist for her heart failure medications, her neurologist for her Parkinson's disease medication, and her general practitioner for her anticoagulant medication. Each provider may be unaware of the other unless Mrs. C. shares that information. In addition, Mrs. C. may use different pharmacies to get her medications. She may use the pharmacy in her general practitioner's clinic due to convenience, and she may use the pharmacy near her home for her heart failure medications. Each pharmacy has no record of Mrs. C.'s medications from the other pharmacy, and therefore, the pharmacist at each location cannot provide adequate monitoring and teaching about all the medications Mrs. C. takes. An important nursing intervention to prevent **adverse drug reactions** (ADRs) from drug-drug interactions is to encourage the client to keep a list of their medications with them at all times, provide the list to each care provider, and choose one pharmacy for the dispensing of all prescribed medications.

Healthy People 2020

Goal

Ensure the safe use of medical products.

One of the main goals for Healthy People 2020 is to improve the safety of medical products, including medications. One of the emerging issues in the improvement of medication safety is the creation of a national health information database that would include electronic medical records and electronic prescribing systems. This is an important step in improving the safety of medications in older adults who experience polypharmacy and deal with multiple prescribers and pharmacies.

In addition to the concern of drug errors due to a complicated medication regimen, the LPN should have a heightened awareness of ADRs related to a client's polypharmacy. ADRs caused by drug-drug interactions usually occur when one drug interferes with the **pharmacokinetics** of another drug. For example, if drug A prevents the excretion of drug B,

then drug B will have an opportunity to build up in the body and cause adverse effects, perhaps to the level of toxicity. Another example of altered pharmacokinetics is when two highly protein-bound drugs are used together. When two or more highly protein-bound drugs are used at the same time, they compete for plasma protein binding sites (of which an older adult has less) and the result is more circulating free drug. When there is more free drug circulating in a client's bloodstream, it is more likely the client will experience adverse effects. Clients who take more than one highly protein-bound drug should have lowered doses of those drugs. Nurses should be sensitive to clients' complaints of adverse effects, especially when new medications are added to the regimen. In addition, nurses serve as a crucial member of the health-care team by reporting adverse effects to prescribers and suggesting changes in dosage when adverse effects occur. It is important to remember it is not within the licensed nurse's scope to prescribe or alter prescriptions, but open conversations about a clients' drug regimen are certainly within the nurse's scope and an expected part of the nurse's practice.

Issues With Compliance

Often, when nurses think of older adults being noncompliant with medications, they think only of patients who willingly refuse to take medications. However, unwillingness to take medications is only one aspect of noncompliance. The other aspect involves a patient's ability to remain compliant with medications. This scenario would apply to the willingness aspect of taking medications. LPNs should be aware of willingness and ability issues when assessing client medication compliance. In addition, a wise nurse realizes noncompliance may be intentional or unintentional. Clients may choose to alter dosages of medications, or they may simply forget to take them.

Adverse Effects

Many older adults stop taking or reduce the dosage of medications to avoid adverse effects. Even for people with impaired cognition, such as those with Alzheimer's disease, it does not take long to associate medications with the unpleasant feeling of nausea after every dose. Nausea is a very common adverse effect of many medications and is often caused by the medication irritating the stomach lining. Recommending medications be taken with food, if not otherwise contraindicated, can help alleviate the nausea associated with many medications. If a medication cannot be taken with food, encourage the client to take it with a full glass of water (at least 8 ounces). This will help the medication flush through the stomach faster and hopefully decrease the experienced nausea. Other adverse effects that may affect compliance of medications are sleepiness, anxiousness, lightheadedness, and frequent urination. Table 20.1 lists common medications and their associated adverse effects. If Mrs. C. is planning on a shopping outing with her daughter, she may choose not to take her diuretic that day because she does not want to have to worry about going to the bathroom in the stores. For a person with heart failure, avoidance of taking the prescribed diuretic can have serious consequences on the disease process.

Point of Interest

Increasingly, older adults are familiar with the internet and have the means to travel. It is common for older adults to purchase medications either online, or by traveling out of the country. Border towns in Mexico and Canada are popular sites for older adults to stock up on medications. A major factor is decreased cost. However, drug manufacturers outside of the United States are not required to meet the same safety and purity standards. Customers may find they have bought medications with inaccurate or misleading dosages, impure active ingredients, or even placebos.

Table 20.1

Drugs and Their Adverse Effects That Contribute to Noncompliance in Older Adults

Effect	*Drugs*
Drugs that cause dry mouth	Anticholinergics, antidiarrheals, antiemetics, antipsychotics, muscle relaxants, antihistamines, antiparkinsonian medications
Drugs associated with ulcer formation	Adrenocorticotropic hormones, aspirin, ibuprofen, indomethacin, iron
Drugs that alter absorption of nutrients	Colchicine, neomycin, isoniazid, cholestyramine, orlistat, antacids, sucralfate
Drugs that promote constipation	Aluminum-containing and calcium-containing antacids, narcotic analgesics, anticholinergics, iron, tricyclic antidepressants
Drugs that promote diarrhea	Antacids, antiulcer medications, antibiotics, antihypertensive medications, cholinergics
Drugs that may cause liver damage	Acetaminophen, analgesics, anesthetics, antibiotics (especially penicillin and sulfa), antineoplastics, cardiovascular drugs, oral antihyperglycemics, steroids, statins
Drugs that may cause central nervous system depression	Antihistamines, antipsychotics, anxiolytics, cardiac glycosides, narcotics, sedatives/hypnotics
Drugs that may cause heart dysrhythmias	Antidepressants, cardiac glycosides, phenytoin
Drugs that may cause kidney damage	Aminoglycosides, antibiotics, colchicine, ibuprofen
Drugs that may cause electrolyte imbalances	Corticosteroids, diuretics, electrolytes
Drugs that may cause blood dyscrasias	Antineoplastics, antipsychotics

Financial Issues

Financial difficulties affect the ability aspect of medication compliance. Many people are willing to take their prescribed medications, but they are unable to afford them. Older adults who are on fixed incomes, especially those in low-income areas, may not have the financial means to purchase drugs. Commonly used drugs, such as insulin, can be expensive. Older adults on lower incomes will use varied strategies to save money when taking medications. Some common strategies are to split pills in half, only take pills every other day instead of every day, wait to get prescriptions filled until there is enough money saved up, or simply not get prescriptions filled. Older adults may also share medications with each other in attempts to help one another, or they may stop taking their medication once their symptoms have disappeared and save the unused portion for later use. These can be dangerous practices and create a challenge for the nurse. Although the LPN has no control over a client's financial situation, the nurse can provide education on how medications work and why it is important to take the medications as directed. In addition, the nurse can be an important link between the client and much-needed resources by referring the client to a social worker or case manager. For example, setting a financially disadvantaged client up with an assisted meal program has been shown to significantly decrease medication noncompliance (Srinivasan & Pooler, 2018).

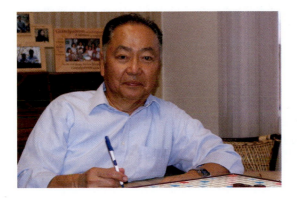

This man's wife has rheumatoid arthritis. He feels concern over being able to pay for the medication necessary for her to move as little as she does. His commitment is to his wife, however, and the quality of her life. He says he always has made it work, and he will in the future as well.

> ### THINK LIKE A NURSE
>
> Mr. and Mrs. H. "snowbird" in Yuma, Arizona, every year. During the winter months, they live in a community in Arizona near a Mexican border town. They have found medications to be much less expensive in Mexico and make specific trips there to purchase medications. What teaching can you do with Mr. and Mrs. H. about this practice?

Drug Misuse

As previously discussed, issues with medication compliance in older adults can be caused by many factors such as drug adverse effects and financial difficulties. Although medication noncompliance is not an issue specific to older adults, they are especially susceptible to misuse. The LPN needs to be aware of the many ways older people misuse medications, such as contraindicated use, erratic use, underuse, and overuse.

Contraindicated use can be a problem when a client has several different health-care providers prescribing medications that are not safely taken together. If the client also uses several pharmacies, the safety of all the client's medications taken together will never be assessed. This may lead to unsafe drug-drug interactions, which is a potential cause for emergency care. Other contributing factors of contraindicated use are foods and home remedies. Some drugs can have significant adverse effects when combined with certain foods or herbs. For example, if the herbal remedy, kava, is used in combination with other CNS depressants, the result is excessive CNS depression, which could have disastrous consequences. To combat the effects of contraindicated use, the nurse can provide thorough teaching in verbal and written forms to help older adults be aware of dangerous drug-drug, drug-food, or drug-herb interactions. In addition, nurses should always encourage clients to use one pharmacy and share all medication information with all providers.

Another type of misuse is erratic use, which means the medication is not used on a consistent basis. This is commonly seen in people who have cognitive or memory problems, or in people who cannot afford their medications. Erratic use prevents the maintenance of therapeutic blood levels. Forgetting to take a stool softener for two days may not have dire consequences, but forgetting to take an antiepileptic drug may cause severe seizure activity, or forgetting to take a diuretic may cause fluid overload. The nurse can help prevent erratic use by creating a system in which the older adult can track daily medication use. Using a calendar or a smartphone app can be useful in helping an older client to remember their daily medications. The nurse also can suggest that the client take their medication at the same time as other daily activities. For example, it may be more useful to tell a client to take their medication every morning with breakfast, rather than to take it at 7:00 a.m. every day because the client may not be awake at 7:00 a.m. every day, but always eats breakfast every day. Another tactic is to teach the client to turn their pill bottles upside down or put them away in the cupboard after each time they take them. Then, each morning, the client turns the pill bottles right side up or takes them out of the cupboard for the next day's doses. The nurse can also assist in setting up a weekly pill box and teach the client or a family member how to fill it each week.

Underuse is frequently a problem related to finances, but it can also be associated with other reasons. Underuse is when a client consistently takes fewer or smaller doses than prescribed. As previously discussed, some low-income clients may not be able to afford their monthly medications and may split doses or take doses every other day to save money. They assume "taking some medication is better than none." Another reason clients may underuse medications is because of undesired effects. For example, Mrs. C. complains that "she just doesn't feel good" when she takes her full dose of simvastatin every day. She admits she takes a half dose every day because she feels better and she still feels like she is getting the benefits of the medication. The nurse can be helpful in decreasing underuse by ensuring clients get help with resources to pay for medications and by also encouraging clients to discuss any unwanted side effects with their providers. Nurses can explain that a dosage adjustment or change in medication is a viable solution to maintaining compliance while also avoiding adverse effects.

The last way drugs can be misused by older adults is overuse. Overuse usually occurs when a client believes "if one pill is good, then two are better" or if a client believes the medication will be useful for something other than what it is indicated. If Mrs. C. realizes the furosemide that she takes causes her to lose weight and significantly decreases the swelling in her ankles and legs, she may decide to take double doses thinking the effects will be even greater. What she may not know is that excessive furosemide can cause extreme dehydration and potassium loss, which is dangerous for the heart. Again, thorough teaching of the effects, and adverse effects, of medications is an important responsibility of the LPN.

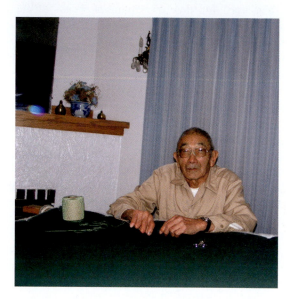

The problem of polypharmacy is challenging for older adults. This man has multiple chronic diseases. The medication prescribed for him from his three physicians adds up to 22 pills each morning and 12 at night. It worries him, and he wants help in organizing the medications. Where would you refer him if he were your neighbor or family member?

Drug Abuse

Drug abuse is not generally associated with older adults, yet they are not immune to this phenomenon. Just like in the general population, older adults can abuse all kinds of medications. This section will discuss a few of the more commonly abused medications by older adults.

Laxative Abuse

Due to the normal changes of aging that occur in the GI tract, older adults may not have bowel movements every day. In addition, many older adults take medications such as anticholinergics and opioids that slow the bowel. Some older people take this as a sign of distress and feel the need to stimulate their bowels with laxatives. Laxatives are a common drug abused by older adults. Some people may use laxatives every day or even several times a day. Elderly people sometimes forget when they have bowel movements and use more laxatives in efforts to stimulate more bowel function.

The abuse of laxatives can cause many problems. Excessive use of laxatives can damage the intestinal walls, which can affect their musculature and their ability to absorb water, nutrients, and medications. Decreased water absorption can lead to dehydration, decreased nutrient absorption can lead to malnutrition and poor wound healing, and decreased medication absorption can lead to decreased or absent therapeutic effects. Laxative abuse also can cause diarrhea, which can create electrolyte and fluid imbalances. These imbalances can be dangerous, especially for people who already suffer from kidney or cardiovascular disease.

The nurse can aid in decreasing laxative abuse by monitoring bowel movements, providing patient teaching about healthy bowel habits, and encouraging nonpharmacologic methods to stimulate bowel movements, such as increased fluid intake, the consumption of high-fiber foods, and an increase in physical activity. If necessary, bowel training can be initiated, and referrals can be made if psychologic interventions are needed.

Antibiotic Abuse

Antibiotics work well for bacterial infections, but they have become severely overused. Prescribers are becoming more aware of the dangers of antibiotic overuse. However, some prescribers are unwilling to "argue" with a client who insists on being prescribed an antibiotic for an inappropriate use, such as a viral infection of cold or flu. Many older adults are not aware of the differences between bacterial and viral infections and do not realize antibiotics are ineffective against cold and flu infections. This lack of knowledge also causes elderly people to seek out and "stockpile" antibiotics. A common practice of older adults who buy their medications out of the country is to purchase many antibiotics, even without prescriptions. When Mrs. C. was newly diagnosed with heart failure, she was healthy enough to travel, and lived in Arizona every winter. She and her husband would purchase many "Z-Paks" (azithromycin) and store them at their home. Mrs. C. stated that she likes having the Z-Paks because she uses one whenever she gets a cold.

Antibiotic abuse has led to antibiotic-resistant strains. Many of the antibiotics we have are no longer effective against bacterial infections. Antibiotic resistance is an important issue in skilled nursing facilities where health-care acquired infections are more prevalent. In addition to antibiotic resistance, antibiotic use can harm the client, especially if the antibiotic is from a broad-spectrum class. Broad-spectrum antibiotics can kill the "healthy" bacteria of the client, leading to such problems as diarrhea, yeast infections, and even clostridium difficile infections.

Research has shown that nurses are knowledgeable about inappropriate uses of antibiotics (Kistler et al., 2017). The nurse can help clients avoid antibiotic abuse by teaching about the differences between bacterial and viral infections, ensuring proper use of antibiotics, and encouraging techniques to avoid infections, such as good hand hygiene. As an integral part of the health-care team, the LPN is also responsible for advocating for the client when a prescriber inappropriately prescribes antibiotics.

Evidence-Based Practice

Cochran, G., Rosen, D., McCarthy, R. M., & Engel, R. J. (2017). Risk factors for symptoms of prescription opioid misuse: Do older adults differ from younger adult patients? *Journal of Gerontological Social Work, 60*(6-7), 443–457. doi: 10.1080/01634372.2017.1327469

It may be common knowledge that the United States is facing a serious opioid epidemic, but how the epidemic affects older adults is largely unknown. Although the epidemic is being widely researched within the general population, the authors of this study wanted specifically to examine risk factors of opioid abuse in adults aged 65 and older.

The researchers surveyed 318 adults filling opioid prescriptions and categorized them by age. Participants were asked about symptoms and risk factors of opioid misuse, including opioid-seeking behaviors, illicit drug use, alcohol abuse, depression symptoms, posttraumatic stress (PTSD) symptoms, general health, and pain.

Within the group of participants aged 65 and older, the only significant risk factor for opioid overuse was illicit drug use within the past year. For the 50–64 age group, opioid misuse was correlated with PTSD symptoms and illicit drug use. Ironically, pain and depression were not risk factors for opioid misuse.

The authors concluded that health-care providers must routinely assess clients seeking opioids for risk factors such as illicit drug use and PTSD that may indicate opioid misuse. Clinicians must also be aware of services designed to help people at risk for these behaviors.

Finally, the researchers outlined the dangers of opioid use for older adults due to changes in physiology and pharmacokinetics. They noted that opioid dosing times for older adults need to be more spread out, rather than closer together.

Question

What health history questions should a nurse ask a client who is newly prescribed opioids for pain?

OTC and Home Remedies Abuse

Monitoring OTC drugs and home remedies is a difficult task. Many people abuse substances that can be found in a spice rack or pantry shelf. For example, some older adults use baking soda (sodium bicarbonate) as an antacid for stomach or chest discomfort. Because baking soda is a base, excessive use of this product can lead to serious acid-base imbalance. Some older adults abuse OTC medications for pain or sleep such as acetaminophen (Tylenol) or diphenhydramine (Benadryl, Motrin PM). Although acetaminophen is a safe drug when taken in therapeutic doses, acetaminophen toxicity is the leading cause of acute liver failure in the United States (Mayo Clinic, 2019). The abuse of diphenhydramine can cause problems such as dry mouth, decreased urination, and even cognitive dysfunction due to its anticholinergic effects.

Nurses need to be vigilant about assessing for the use of home remedies and OTC medications in older adults. Thorough medication histories must be taken, and nurses need to ask specifically about all drugs used, even if they are not prescribed. LPNs must remain knowledgeable about home remedies, herbs, and OTC medications to provide teaching and safe care to older adults.

Alcohol Abuse

Alcohol abuse is not unique to younger adults. Older adults battle alcohol abuse as well and often have more severe consequences. Alcohol abuse causes many problems for older adults taking medications. Alcohol interferes with the pharmacokinetics of many medications, usually making them more toxic

due to decreased metabolism. If an older adult has had a long history of alcohol abuse, the liver also may have decreased plasma protein output, which has implications for highly protein-bound drugs. Alcohol abuse can also adversely affect acid-base balance, fluid and electrolyte balance, and blood sugar maintenance. Changes in these balances can hinder the pharmacotherapeutic effects of many drugs. Not only does alcohol have physiologic consequences for medications, but alcohol also impairs cognition, affecting thinking and judgment. Alterations in thinking and judgement can cause older adults to be noncompliant with their medication regimen. Lastly, it is important to remember that alcohol is a CNS depressant. When combined with other CNS depressants such as benzodiazepines or narcotics, the results can be deadly.

PHARMACOLOGIC MANAGEMENT OF PAIN FOR OLDER ADULTS

One of the most common health complaints of older adults is pain. Two common causes of pain in the elderly are arthritis and neuropathy. Arthritis occurs as the cartilage between bones wears down after years of use. When the cushion between the bones deteriorates, it causes an inflammatory effect causing pain and swelling. Neuropathy, on the other hand, is not necessarily a normal event of aging but often accompanies other chronic diseases such as diabetes. Neuropathies occur when nerves become damaged or inflamed. Treating pain in older adults is extremely important for maintaining mobility and activities of daily living. For example, an older adult living in a skilled nursing facility will not want to walk to the dining room if he is experiencing severe arthritic back pain. LPNs should be adept at assessing for pain, administering treatments, and evaluating pain therapies.

Non-narcotic Pain Management

Older adults who experience mild to moderate pain do not need an analgesic such as morphine. Instead, there are several non-narcotic options, and many are over the counter. These medications are considered safe when taken at therapeutic doses and are generally inexpensive. Some non-narcotic options for pain management are acetaminophen, aspirin, and ibuprofen or other nonsteroidal anti-inflammatory drugs

(NSAIDs). Although acetaminophen is effective at treating pain and fever, ibuprofen and the other NSAIDs are effective at treating pain, fever, and inflammation and often provide better pain relief. However, many older adults cannot take NSAIDs because of other medications they are taking or because of disease processes they have. For example, older adults taking the anticoagulant warfarin cannot take NSAIDs due to the increased risk of bleeding. NSAIDs are also affiliated with gastrointestinal bleeding. Individuals with existing peptic ulcer disease or those on medications that can cause gastrointestinal bleeding or ulcers (corticosteroids) should not take NSAIDs for pain.

The nursing responsibilities related to nonnarcotic pain management in older adults mainly involve monitoring and education. Although the OTC pain medications are generally considered safe, they do have maximum daily dosages. When these dosages are exceeded, they can have severe consequences such as liver or kidney damage. It is the responsibility of the LPN to monitor all medications containing acetaminophen, aspirin, and ibuprofen, because many combination medications contain these ingredients. For example, Ultracet is a combination of tramadol and acetaminophen. If a client is taking Ultracet regularly, and then takes Tylenol in addition, the maximum dose of acetaminophen per day is easily reached. Nurses must teach clients about maximum OTC drug doses, and to take note of their daily OTC drug intake.

Nonpharmacologic Pain Management

Nurses should use several tools, including medications, for managing older clients' pain. In addition to administering and teaching about medications, nurses should be familiar with nonpharmacologic pain modalities, such the use of heat or cold, massage, elevation, music therapy, distraction, and imagery. Nurses should be aware of options provided by other practitioners such as acupuncture, acupressure, and electronic stimulation. Pharmacologic and nonpharmacologic therapies can be used together to provide excellent pain relief.

Narcotic Pain Management

Despite the current opioid epidemic, nurses should not be reluctant to adequately treat pain with narcotic analgesics, especially in short-term, acute care settings. Even in long-term skilled nursing facilities,

narcotics are commonly used to treat pain in older adults. Morphine, hydrocodone, and oxycodone are all commonly used narcotic analgesics. Some older adults need long-acting narcotics such as a fentanyl transdermal patch or sustained release morphine for chronic pain. A commonly used medication to manage chronic pain in the elderly population is a mixed narcotic–nonnarcotic analgesic called tramadol. Tramadol is less likely than other narcotics to cause the adverse effects of respiratory depression and dependence.

Although narcotics are effective drugs at treating moderate to severe pain, they are not without adverse effects. The nurse must be vigilant at monitoring for respiratory depression (especially in the beginning of treatment), constipation, and orthostatic hypotension and implement interventions to prevent constipation and falls from orthostatic hypotension. In addition, nurses must be familiar with the antidote for opioids: naloxone. Nurses need to monitor for therapeutic effects and provide patient teaching about adverse effects and the potential for tolerance and dependence.

NURSING CONSIDERATIONS FOR SAFE PHARMACOTHERAPEUTICS OF OLDER ADULTS

Nurses play an important role in protecting older adults from adverse drug effects, either by safe administration, effective teaching, or by advocating for their safety. Although most older adults are independent with their medication administration, the nurse is a vital partner in maintaining good health and providing valuable guidance. This section will outline several practical ways a nurse can promote safe medication use and use Beers criteria to work with other health-care providers in ensuring optimal client care.

Practical Recommendations for Nursing Care

In addition to the numerous recommendations for nursing interventions listed throughout this chapter, the LPN also can perform the following actions to promote safe medication use in older adults:

1. Discard any discontinued or expired medications. Review all necessary medications with the older client or their family members and encourage them to dispose safely of any medications

not being used to simplify the drug regimen and avoid confusion, and therefore medication errors.

2. List all of the client's medications, prescribers, and pharmacies and encourage the client to keep copies of the list to share with each provider. In addition, encourage the client to transfer all medication prescriptions to one pharmacy to enhance medication reconciliation and therefore safer medication use.

3. Coordinate medication administration with daily activities such as meal times. Also, take into consideration sleep and activity habits such as nap and bedtimes. By coordinating medication administration with established patterns, it improves compliance.

4. Encourage the older adult to discuss adverse effects. Nurses can also teach ways to minimize those effects or talk to their prescriber about them. This is another strategy to enhance compliance.

5. Use and encourage nonpharmacologic therapies. Nurses can use therapies such as those discussed in the pain management section of this chapter. But that list is not exhaustive. Other options for alternative treatments are elevation for swollen extremities, warm milk for encouraging sleep, or lavender aromatherapy to promote calmness. Any alternative that can promote wellness and decrease the number of medications for the client is a step in a safer direction.

Point of Interest

It is important to never flush unused medications down the toilet, dispose of them in the sink, or throw them away in the garbage. Even seemingly harmless drugs can be life-threatening to a child or cause a problem in the water supply. Teach the older client or family member to dispose of medications at local drug disposal locations, which are often local pharmacies. City and county services often have drug take back information as well. The U.S. Drug Enforcement Administration (DEA) holds an annual prescription drug take back day, listed on their website: https://takebackday.dea.gov/. The website also provides a search for local take back locations: https://apps.deadiversion.usdoj.gov/pubdispsearch/spring/main?execution=e2s1

Safe, Effective Nursing Care

Safe, Effective Medication Use in Older Adults
Providing patient-centered care

• Consider the client's preferences for pain management.
• Consider the client's preferences for use of nonpharmacologic treatments.
• Consider the client's eating and sleeping habits when administering medications.
• Assess client educational needs and preferences prior to doing medication teaching.
• Use family and other caregivers to reinforce medication education.

Working in Interprofessional Teams
• Maintain open communication with the client's prescriber(s).
• Provide the prescriber information about the client's response to medications.
• Communicate medication-related lab results to the provider.
• Use the prescriber or pharmacist for medication-related questions.
• Encourage the client to share information about all medications taken with all prescribers and pharmacists.

Employing Evidence-Based Practice
• Use current resources when teaching about medications.
• Use current research when teaching about the combination of medications and alternative treatments such as herbs.

Beers Criteria

Another intervention nurses can use to increase the safety of medication for older adults is to be familiar with and use Beers criteria. Beers criteria (American Geriatrics Society, 2015) are an evidence-based list of medications that are inappropriate for older adults, based on research studies. The criteria were originally established in 1991 and have been through four revisions, with the latest one occurring in 2015. The current revision expanded to five categories of potentially inappropriate medications (PIMs) for older adults. The five categories are:

1. Potentially inappropriate medications for most older adults
2. Medications to avoid for use by older adults with certain diseases or syndromes

3. Medications to be used with caution
4. Medications with important non-anti-infective drug–drug interactions
5. Non-anti-infective medications to be avoided in older adults or have dosages adjusted depending on renal function

The criteria were purposefully designed to encourage a team approach to medication management for older adults. This approach includes the LPN as an important member of the team in monitoring for adverse effects and advocating for the older client. Although Beers criteria is the responsibility of the prescriber, the nurse should also be familiar with the criteria to promote safer medication use in older adults. The nurse can compile the client's medication list, assess for any adverse effects, and share the information with the registered nurse or the prescriber. The nurse caring for the older adult can request a Beers criteria medication review with the health-care team, if one has not already been completed. By doing this, the nurse performs an important advocacy role. Reviews completed by the prescriber, pharmacist, and nurse can help simplify the medication regimen, as well as protect the older client from adverse effects.

PHARMACOTHERAPEUTICS OF OLDER ADULTS AND THE NURSING PROCESS

Similar to any other type of nursing care, the nursing process should be applied to pharmacotherapeutics of older adults. The steps of the nursing process, as outlined in chapter 4, consist of assessment, diagnosis, planning, implementation, and evaluation.

Assessment

CRITICALLY EXAMINE THE FOLLOWING

You are a home health nurse for a company that serves a low-income area of your city. The majority of your clients are older adults with several chronic disease that require medication. In addition to monitoring medication use, part of your responsibilities include evaluating laboratory values. In the course of the 2 years you have been working for this company, you have noticed many of the older adults have serum albumin levels below the normal range (3.5 to 5.5). As the nurse, use critical thinking to answer the following questions:

1. What do you anticipate is (are) the cause(s) of the low albumin levels?
2. What is the impact of low albumin levels on the pharmacotherapy of your clients?

Prior to administering any medications, the nurse must do a thorough assessment, including a health history and current medication assessment. Ask about past and current diseases or illnesses, especially liver and kidney function since they play such a major role in pharmacokinetics. When asking about the person's medication history, be sure to specifically ask about all types of medications, including prescribed, OTC, herbs, and illicit drugs. Always remember to ask about the person's allergies. If the person reports having an allergy, an important follow-up question is "What did the medication do to you?" Differentiating between nausea and a true anaphylactic response is important to note.

The nurse must also perform a thorough physical examination, including an assessment of sensory status. What is the person's nutrition and hydration status? Is the person obese? These factors influence pharmacokinetics, and therefore drug efficacy. Does the person have impaired hearing or vision? Is the person able to open pill bottles? Will modified containers be necessary? Will any impairments create anticipated medication errors? The answers to these questions will contribute important information to the nurse's potential plan of care.

An assessment should also include reviewing the client's cognitive status and potential for compliance. Is the client confused? Can the client be trusted to safely self-administer medications? Can the person understand the nurse's teaching? Ask the client to explain what they know about medication indications, dosages, and adverse effects. Investigate whether the person takes the correct doses of medications at the correct times and ask whether there are any reasons why the person might avoid taking their medication.

Finally, assess the client's social support. Are there family members or caregivers that can be involved in medication administration if necessary? Does the client need a family member or caregiver for transportation to prescribers' offices or pharmacies? The client's social support can be involved in the nurse's teaching, which will also improve compliance.

Focused Learning Chart: Key Questions When Completing a Medication History Assessment

Medications	Physical	Psychosocial
What prescription medications do you take?	Do you have any allergies to any medications? If so, which ones?	Do you know what all your medications are for?
What OTC medications do you take?	What reactions do you have to medications you are allergic to?	Do you need help taking any of your medications?
What herbal or natural remedies do you use?	Do you have any chronic health diseases, especially problems with the liver or kidneys?	Can you afford to purchase all of your prescribed medications?
Do you use any recreational drugs or substances?		

Diagnosis

The following nursing diagnoses pertain to pharmacotherapy of older adults:

- Deficient knowledge related to new medication regimen
- Risk for falls related to orthostatic hypotension from antihypertensive medication
- Noncompliance related to inability to purchase medication
- Constipation related to opioid use for pain

Planning

Patient Education

The SENC competencies can be incorporated into medication education in several ways. First, when you provide the client education about pharmacotherapy, try to put yourself in their shoes. This strongly promotes client-centered care. Remember that though you may be very familiar with the medications, the client most likely is not. Think back to your pharmacology course and remember how overwhelmed you were at all the information you received. Your client probably feels the same way. There is a lot to remember about safe medication administration, so be sure to accommodate your client's needs to the best of your ability and tailor your teaching specifically to each client.

When providing medication information to clients, always use evidence-based resources. If you can, keep a current nursing drug guide handy and share your references with your clients. Incorporating technological advances is also easy because there are many excellent digital resources to aid in your teaching. Several accurate and reliable medication apps are updated regularly. Apps and online resources such as the Centers for Disease Control and Prevention website can be useful tools in providing evidence-based teaching. Many older adults use the internet, so part of your teaching should include which websites are reliable and which are not. In general, websites that end in .com should be avoided because they can have ulterior motives and may contain biased information. Websites that end in .gov, .edu, or .org are usually nonbiased and contain reliable information.

Lastly, remember you are a part of a health-care team, and other health-care professionals can assist you in providing accurate medication education. Do not be afraid to acknowledge your limitations. If you do not know something about a medication, admit it and ask others for help. Pharmacists and prescribers are excellent resources for needed information. In addition, encourage the older client to ask questions of the prescriber and pharmacist.

When thinking about planning related to pharmacotherapy of older adults, you need to ask yourself two questions: "What do I need to accomplish?" and more importantly, "What do I want the older adult to accomplish?" If your overall goal is to administer medications safely, consider all aspects necessary to accomplish that goal. Perhaps you are doing a morning medication pass on a busy skilled nursing facility hall. What are all the items you need to complete the task safely and efficiently? Be sure to have all the necessary medications. Review each client's medication administration record for accuracy and completeness. Be sure you have the supplies you may need such as medication administration cups, syringes, and needles, and any food or drink used to assist in giving medications. Plan how and when you will complete your documentation. With all of these steps, ensure you are incorporating best practice and your facility policies and procedures. Giving some thought to these types of plans can make your medication administration go much more smoothly and help you anticipate and prioritize needs for nursing care.

Maybe your goal is to teach an older client about a new medication. Planning involves *when* and *how* you are going to accomplish the teaching. Consider the best time of day for your client to receive information. Bedtime may not be a suitable teaching time because older adults may be too sleepy to understand and remember the information. Another thing to consider for timing of teaching is when the family or caregivers will be with the client. Waiting to provide teaching until the spouse or other caregivers are present is wise. When considering *how* you will accomplish your teaching, think about the client's learning needs and abilities. Will you need to provide handouts in addition to verbal teaching? Will you need an interpreter because the client speaks very little English? Are there visual or hearing disabilities to consider? Do you have all the equipment you need? If you plan to teach insulin administration, for example, do you have the necessary syringes, needles, and a sharps container for needle disposal? Again, thinking through the process prior to implementation can save a lot of time and frustration in the end.

The most important question regarding planning is "What do I want or need for the older adult to accomplish?" What are your goals for the client? Do you want them to verbalize their understanding of why they are taking certain medications? Do you need them to demonstrate safe insulin self-administration? Plan to provide adequate patience and time for practice. Be sure the client has everything they need to be successful in accomplishing the goals.

Implementation

Implementation related to pharmacotherapy involves three things: administering the medication, teaching the client about the medication, and documenting medication administration and client teaching. Administering medication may sound simple, but there are many things to consider to ensure safe and effective care. Always use the five rights of medication administration to be sure you are giving the right medication to the right client at the right time and in the right dose and route. It could be dangerous for your client to receive oral potassium drops in the eye by mistake. When giving oral medications, remember that extended-release and enteric-coated capsules and tablets should never be crushed, opened, or chewed. If the older adult cannot swallow pills, the nurse can consult with the prescriber to change the medication form or route. Intramuscular injections should be given in the ventrogluteal site. The deltoid and vastus lateralis sites should be used as a last resort owing to their decreased mass and blood flow. One important exception is the annual flu shot, which is given in the deltoid. Intravenous therapy should be monitored closely in older adults. Fluid overload could be detrimental and exacerbate conditions such as heart failure, hypertension, and kidney disease.

Client teaching is an important part of implementing medication administration. Make it a routine part of your practice to be continually providing your client information about their medications. Confirm client understanding by having them repeat back the teaching, explain the information to someone else, or by having them demonstrate any administration-related skills. Finally, always remember to document the teaching you provided, and the client's response to the teaching, including their understanding of the information. For example, the home health nurse pays a visit to Mrs. C. and learns Mrs. C.'s husband has been giving Mrs. C. her levodopa as two pills twice a day, instead of one pill four times a day. He figured it was easier to give it only twice a day, and she was still getting the right number of pills throughout the day. Mrs. C.'s daughter stopped by during the nurse's visit and mentioned Mrs. C. had been smacking her lips and tongue a lot lately, which was unusual. The nurse realizes Mrs. C. is being overdosed on levodopa twice a day and is exhibiting a type of tardive dyskinesia, which is an adverse effect of levodopa. The nurse teaches Mrs. C. and her two family members about the relationship between the lip smacking and the levodopa administration. The nurse stresses the importance of following the medication order as it is written to avoid adverse effects. The nurse documents the teaching given, including what was said, who was present, and that Mrs. C. and her family stated understanding.

Evaluation

Point of Interest

You are the intake nurse at an urgent care clinic and are assessing an older man who is accompanied by his wife. He is complaining of severe coughing, chest pain, and lethargy. As part of your intake assessment, you ask the client about his medications, but neither he nor his wife can remember them. One suggestion you can make is the "grocery bag" option. Have the wife, or other family member, go home and place all of the client's medications into a grocery bag. Tell them to be sure to include any OTC medications or home remedies, including herbals and vitamins. Reassure the family member they will get all the medications back. Once you have all the medications, make a list. Be sure to ask the client and his wife how he takes each medication and compare that to what is ordered on the label. You may be surprised that many of the medications are not being taken as prescribed. By using the "grocery bag" method, you can create an accurate list of medications and assess how they are actually being used.

Evaluation of pharmacotherapy is a crucial part of the nursing process for providing excellent care. Many aspects of medication administration need to be evaluated. Ask the client about any effects of the medication, including the therapeutic effects, any adverse effects, and side effects. As a part of evaluating medication effects, the nurse is also responsible for monitoring blood levels and laboratory values as required with some medications. The client's willingness and ability to be compliant should be evaluated. As in the example of Mrs. C. and her inappropriate levodopa administration, be sure to ask the client and any caregivers when and how they are actually taking their medications. Use a matter-of-fact, nonjudgmental tone and attitude to elicit the most accurate information from the client. Finally, evaluate the client's understanding of the medication and the client's response to any teaching that is given. Again, the best way to truly evaluate a client's understanding is to have them repeat any information given, teach the information to someone else, or demonstrate any newly learned skill. Evaluation is important because it informs the continuing cycle of the nursing process, and it is an important part of the SENC competency of providing safe, quality client care.

CASE STUDY SOLUTIONS

1. Introduce yourself and complete a full assessment. Perform a physical assessment, home assessment, social support assessment, health history, and medication history. Ask about the role Mrs. C.'s husband and daughter play in her care. Inquire about financial resources and the ability to visit the doctor and obtain her medications. Assess compliance by comparing all of Mrs. C.'s pill bottle labels with how she says she actually takes her medications.

2. The following nursing diagnoses are appropriate for Mrs. C.:
   - Risk for falls related to weakness and medications
   - Ineffective health management related to complicated drug regimen
   - Deficient knowledge related to multiple medications
   - Noncompliance related to complicated drug regimen

3. Macular degeneration has caused Mrs. C. to go blind in both eyes. This sensory impairment can be dangerous when taking medications. Mrs. C. may be totally dependent on her husband to help with her medications, in which case the nurse should assess Mrs. C.'s husband's understanding of her drug medication and assess his compliance as well. In addition, Mrs. C. will not be able to read any teaching materials you provide her. Your teaching will strictly need to be verbal, but you can provide written materials for her husband and daughter.

4. As the nurse, you can help Mrs. C. be compliant with her drug regimen by assessing her current system of managing her drug regimen. The nurse should make recommendations such as creating a master list of all medications to share with prescribers and pharmacists, using only one pharmacy to fill all medications, and encouraging Mrs. C. to take medications with

CASE STUDY SOLUTIONS—cont'd

routine activities such as meals or before naps. Ensure Mrs. C. has a pill box that can be easily accessed and teach her husband and daughter how to fill it. The nurse can find out if the baby aspirin and fish oil were recommended by her prescriber, and if not, to discontinue to simplify her medication regimen. The nurse should also research the effects of turmeric and determine if there are any significant interactions with her prescribed medications. The nurse can share her findings with Mrs. C. and her family. Lastly, the nurse should enlist Mrs. C.'s husband and daughter to help with compliance. Provide teaching and written instructions for all family members that are involved in Mrs. C.'s care.

Key Points

- Older adults experience normal anatomic and physiologic changes due to aging. These changes affect sensory function, cognition, and pharmacokinetics of drugs, which could ultimately affect the safety of pharmacotherapy in older adults.
- Older adults are at higher risk for polypharmacy due to having multiple disease processes. Polypharmacy increases the risk of adverse effects of drugs.
- Some older adults have problems with compliance for a variety of reasons. Clients need to be willing and able to take their medications as prescribed. One compliance issue is the misuse of medications.
- Drug abuse is not unique to younger adults. Some older adults abuse drugs such as laxatives, antibiotics, OTC medications, and alcohol.
- Pain management is an important part of pharmacotherapy for older adults. Older clients can be treated with narcotics, non-narcotics, and even nonpharmacologic therapies to manage pain.
- Nurses can do many practical things to ensure safe and effective pharmacotherapy. Some interventions include discarding expired or discontinued medications, helping the client create a list of all medications, prescribers, and pharmacies and encouraging the use of only one pharmacy, coordinating medication administration with daily routines, encouraging discussion about medication adverse effects, and using nonpharmacologic therapies.
- The nurse should be familiar with Beers criteria. Nurses play an important role on the health-care team by being a client advocate and encouraging Beers criteria reviews of client medications.
- The nursing process is applied to pharmacotherapy, like any other aspect of nursing care. The nursing process consists of assessment, diagnosis, planning, implementation, and evaluation.

Review Questions

1. What effect do laxatives have on absorption of drugs in the older adult's GI tract?
   1. Absorption is blocked.
   2. Absorption is more complete.
   3. Absorption is decreased.
   4. Absorption is not changed by laxatives.

2. What is the definition of polypharmacy?
   1. The use of multiple pharmacies to fill prescriptions
   2. The use of multiple drugs for diseases
   3. Taking more than one pill at a time
   4. Receiving prescriptions from many different care providers

3. Mr. W. and his granddaughter are discussing Mr. W.'s medication regimen with the nurse during a medication history. Mr. W.'s granddaughter explains Mr. W. cuts his pills in half to make them last longer. Which of the following methods of drug misuse is Mr. W.'s granddaughter describing?
   1. Contraindicated use
   2. Erratic use
   3. Over use
   4. Under use

4. Due to the current opioid epidemic in the United States, narcotics are never used for pain in older adults. True or False?
   1. True
   2. False

5. The nurse notices Mrs. A. has been exhibiting severe drowsiness and confusion since the start of a new medication. The nurse researches the new medication and discovers it is on the Beers list for inappropriate medications for older adults. What course of action should the nurse take at this time?
   1. The nurse should continue to give the medication and ask Mrs. A.'s care provider for a medication to decrease drowsiness.
   2. The nurse should file a complaint against the prescriber that ordered the inappropriate medication.
   3. The nurse should call for a meeting with the prescriber and pharmacist to conduct a Beers criteria review on Mrs. A.'s medications.
   4. The nurse should quit working at that facility due to the incompetence of the prescriber.

6. When applying the nursing process to pharmacotherapy, what three things are included in the implementation stage?
   1. Giving the medication, teaching about the medication, charting medication administration
   2. Completing a health history, medication history, physical assessment
   3. Using the correct site for intramuscular injections, giving water with oral medications, monitoring intravenous therapy
   4. Using good lighting, speaking slowly and loudly, facing the client

ANSWERS 1. 3, 2. 2, 3. 4, 4. 2, 5. 3, 6. 1

CHAPTER 21
Laboratory Values

Deborah Judd

KEY TERMS

albumin
asymptomatic bacteriuria
diagnostic tests
glycolated hemoglobin (HbA1c)
hemoconcentration
international normalized ratio (INR)
leukocyte esterase
QuantiFERON TB
screening tests
urine microalbumin

CHAPTER CONCEPTS

Patient-Centered Care

LEARNING OUTCOMES

1. Identify laboratory tests that are important indicators of health and disease in older adults.
2. Apply an understanding of laboratory tests to the health of older adults.
3. Identify medications that should be monitored.
4. Describe nursing actions appropriate for abnormal laboratory values.

CASE STUDY

Mrs. J. is a 76-year-old woman who lives in an assisted living facility. She has been a widow for 7 years. She eats one meal per day in the community cafeteria if she wants and then uses her mini kitchen in the apartment for other meals. She generally uses prepackaged foods or snacks such as yogurt and bananas.

Mrs. J. has had intermittent urinary frequency and urgency without dysuria and mild incontinence for 4 to 6 weeks. She was provided oxybutynin 3 weeks ago for the new incontinence. She has been successfully treated for symptomatic UTIs in the past. She now complains of not feeling well for about 5 days and reports to her daughter that her energy level is decreased.

She has nocturia, decreased appetite, and new onset of dizziness, forgetfulness, and inability to stay focused. "I feel dizzy and maybe confused."

She reports "falling twice" in the last 2 days but did not hit the ground because she "caught herself on the sofa."

Mrs. J. has been on hypertension medications for about 12 years and was diagnosed with diabetes 3 years ago. She has mild osteoporosis. She had been walking

Continued

CASE STUDY—cont'd

the sidewalks and paths in the garden area daily but doesn't seem to have enough energy to do that now.

Mrs. J. takes the following medications.

- Glucophage (metformin), 100 mg by mouth twice a day
- Lisinopril, 10 mg by mouth once a day
- Hydrochlorothiazide, 25 mg by mouth every morning
- Clonidine, 0.1 mg, 1/2 to 1 tablet by mouth as needed; blood pressure (BP) >>150/95
- Aleve, 200 mg twice a day by mouth as needed for aches and pains
- Aspirin, 81 mg as needed by mouth once a day
- Multivitamin, over the counter (OTC) by mouth once a day
- Calcium, 600 mg twice a day for bones
- Vitamin D_3, 1,200 IU by mouth once every morning

Allergies: Penicillin

Mrs. J. and her daughter go to the emergency department for evaluation due to her recent falls, increased fatigue, dizziness, and concentration changes.

Physical Assessment

General: BP: 108/60: previously 132/76, HR: 88, R: 20, T: 99.6

Height: 5 feet 6 inches; weight: 115 pounds: previously 128 pounds

Pale, older woman unsteady on her feet. Apparent malaise and fatigue compared to previous visits. No apparent distress. Cooperative. Well-groomed.

ENT: No dentures; mild dental plaque and gum irritation noted. Otherwise ears, nose, and throat within normal limits.

Neurological: Pupils equal and reactive to light. Cranial nerves grossly intact. Thought processes slower than previous visits. Follows commands. Alert and oriented during the visit, but is unsure of the date, day, or time.

Cardiovascular: Apical pulse—regular rate and rhythm. Peripheral pulses normal. No palpitations noted.

Lungs: Clear to auscultation

Abdomen/flank/pelvis: Soft, nontender with hypoactive bowel sounds all quadrants.

Negative costovertebral angle (CVA) tenderness. No pelvic pain or masses noted with palpation.

Musculoskeletal: Slow and deliberate movements without obvious deformity. Stiffness upon arising. Gait slow and deliberate. Upper and lower extremities: strength 3/5 bilaterally, decreased due to fatigue. Patient reports some hip pain and stiffness when she walks in the exam room.

Laboratory Results

Urinalysis results:

Color: Amber with slightly cloudy appearance and no obvious sediment

Odor: Strong, pungent odor

Nitrite: Positive

Leukocyte esterase: Positive

pH: 7.1

Specific gravity: >1.030

Protein: Trace

Glucose: Positive

Ketones: Negative

Blood: Trace

Urine microscopic examination:

Bacteria: Positive >5/HPF

WBCs: >10–12/HPF

RBCs: 3–5/HPF

Discussion Questions

1. What potential concerns do you have based on Mrs. J.'s history, physical exam, current health problems, and urinalysis results?
2. What other laboratory tests might be ordered to assess Mrs. J.'s health status?
3. What nursing actions or education might you provide for Mrs. J.?

INTRODUCTION

Laboratory testing is a useful tool for nurses who care for aging patients in various health-care settings. There are many useful tests to assist the licensed practical nurse (LPN) in providing safe, quality nursing care for older adults. Laboratory tests are often ordered on admission to a hospital or nursing home, or for older adults when visiting a primary care provider in an outpatient clinic. LPNs may also collect blood specimens in other settings, such as home health or hospice care, for evaluation in a laboratory at a later date. As an LPN, you have studied laboratory values and their meanings in your medical and surgical nursing classes. As a practicing LPN, you will need to learn how to use laboratory resources at the facility where you work to interpret laboratory values of older adults correctly. The purpose of this chapter is not to repeat that information but rather provide you with a ready reference for common and significant diagnostic lab tests for elderly people along with specific and pertinent information for aging patients. Rationale for testing is reviewed generally. In addition to this resource, advancing medical technology allows you easy access to internet resources where general laboratory testing information and the meaning of those laboratory values are readily available. Internet resources are listed at the end of this chapter.

SIGNIFICANCE OF LABORATORY VALUES IN OLDER ADULT PATIENTS

Laboratory tests are a routine part of the health examination for all people. For many tests, the normal ranges are different for elderly people than for people younger than age 65 years. For other tests, there is no change with age. Older adults may have greater deviations from normal laboratory range values when under stress, and return to normal levels is often slower in elderly people than in younger people. Laboratory tests are used to determine medical conditions and influence interventions. The diagnosis and treatment of these conditions result in substantial improvement in health, even in elderly individuals with multiple health problems.

It is important for the LPN to understand that laboratory tests may be ordered as part of a periodic older adult examination for screening or diagnostic purposes. The Patient Education box lists routine older adult screening recommendations. These recommendations support the national Healthy People 2020 goals. **Screening tests** are defined as laboratory tests performed on people without signs and symptoms of a specific health problem or diagnosis to determine whether there is evidence to support risk for certain conditions (e.g., cervical cancer screening). Screening tests are generally believed to be a cost-effective method to identify potential disease and lead to definitive potential cases for follow-up interventions. **Diagnostic tests** are performed to establish a diagnosis and are ordered based on the presence of specific symptom clusters and recent subjective/objective report of a positive screening test result.

Laboratory diagnostic testing is often less expensive than more complex diagnostic testing regimens such as radiology imaging.

PATIENT EDUCATION

As a nurse, you should teach your older adult patients and their families the importance of routine screenings. The following lists some of the routine screenings for older adults as recommended by the U.S. Preventive Services Task Force (USPSTF):

• Serum glucose for people aged 40 to 70 years
• Blood pressure screening
• Depression screening
• Latent tuberculosis (TB): For individuals at increased risk
• Osteoporosis screening (bone measurement testing): Women aged 65 years and older
• Hepatitis C: One-time screening test for patients born between 1945 and 1965. Those at high risk for infection should be screened as needed.
• Colorectal cancer: Screening with various methods should begin at age 50 years and continue until age 75 years. For individuals aged 76 to 85 years, the decision to screen is based on patient's overall health and prior screening history.
• Breast cancer screening: Biennial screening mammography for women aged 50 to 74 years.
• Cervical cancer screening: Not recommended in women older than 65 years who have had adequate prior screening and are not otherwise at high risk for cervical cancer.

Healthy People 2020

Objectives

Increase the proportion of adults with diabetes who have a glycosylated hemoglobin measurement at least twice a year.

Increase the proportion of persons with diagnosed diabetes who obtain an annual urinary microalbumin measurement.

Relationship to Clinical Status

The LPN should not consider laboratory findings in isolation, especially when caring for often frail older adults seen in clinical settings. The elderly person's gender, dietary pattern, activity level, tobacco use, alcohol intake, current medications, and aggressive medical or nursing interventions may alter laboratory findings. It is essential that you consider all facets of the individual's health and habits when you review the laboratory results. For example, abnormal laboratory values may indicate a physiological stressor such as dehydration or a medication side effect rather than illness.

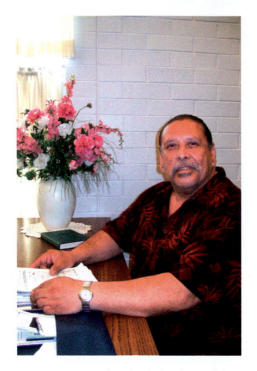

It is important to remember that behind every laboratory procedure there is a human being who might be anxious about the procedure itself or the results of the procedure.

COMMON ROUTINE TESTS

Several laboratory tests are performed routinely on elderly people. The physician or nurse practitioner may request other tests based on the results of routine testing. These laboratory tests are often part of an outpatient well older adult screening. They are used as diagnostic tools to assess and determine medical diagnoses and to monitor health status related to those diagnoses. It is important for LPNs to understand common lab tests and reasons for them. Less common tests may require the nurse to verify information related to the test via technology or printed resources.

A routine laboratory evaluation generally consists of the following:

- Complete blood cell count (CBC)
- CMP: This is also called a Chem 7 or Chem 14 test depending on the lab components measured for the patient. It includes the following tests:
  - Serum glucose
  - Serum creatinine level
  - Serum blood urea nitrogen (BUN)
  - Serum electrolytes: Sodium (Na), potassium (K), calcium (Ca), bicarbonate (HCO), magnesium (Mg), chloride (Cl), phosphate (HPO_4)
- Thyroid function tests
  - Thyroid-stimulating hormone (TSH)
  - Thyroxine (free T4)
  - Total triiodothyronine (free T3)
- Urinalysis (dipstick and microscopic testing)
- Stool guaiac test (occult blood)

The following section discusses the most common laboratory tests ordered and their meanings for older adults. The values shown under headings are normal reference values from *Davis's Comprehensive Handbook of Laboratory and Diagnostic Tests with Nursing Implications* (7th ed.) As an LPN, you should refer to the reference intervals used by the clinical laboratory where you work for the most precise reference ranges.

Urinalysis
Normal Reference Values

Appearance	Clear yellow/straw
Specific gravity	1.005–1.035
pH	4.5–8.0

General Information
The urinalysis is one of most common point-of-care and diagnostic lab tests performed. It allows providers to assess a patient for various potential health issues. Normal urine in an elderly person should test negative for glucose, ketones, blood, bilirubin, **leukocyte esterase**, protein, nitrates, and crystals or stones (calculi). The leukocyte esterase value in the urinalysis indicates an inflammatory response initiated by the presence of leukocytes (WBC) from infection or irritation. If both the leukocyte esterase and nitrite test results are positive, the patient is diagnosed with a UTI. Traces of protein may be present as people age.

Normal microscopic examination of the urine includes zero to three red blood cells (RBCs), zero to four white blood cells (WBCs), a few epithelial cells, and a few crystals per high-power field (HPF) on microscopic examination. Elderly people commonly have the presence of 0 to 3 hyaline casts on low-power field. In addition, 10% to 50% of older people have **asymptomatic bacteriuria** (presence of bacteria in the urine without symptoms). Refer to Table 22.1 for urinalysis specifics.

Table 21.1
Urinalysis Dipstick Screen

Urinary Substance Tested	Reference Value	Significance of the Reference Value
Color	Yellow, amber	Some medications change urine color.
Appearance Odor	Clear Ammonia-based	Pus, casts, blood, bilirubin can change color or appearance of urine (less clear to cloudy).
	Foul or fruity	Dehydration or lower fluid intake concentrates urine (color or odor change noted). Bacteria and other excreted wastes affect urine odor sometimes.
pH	4.0–8.0	Vegetarian diet (fruit and vegetables) elevates pH (alkaline). High-protein diet (meat and eggs) lowers pH (acidic). Acidic: diarrhea; diabetes mellitus; respiratory acidosis; COPD or asthma; metabolic acidosis Alkaline: vomiting, gastric suction; diuretics; UTI; metabolic alkalosis; respiratory alkalosis
Specific gravity	Adult: 1.001–1.035	Low: renal failure; diuresis; hypothermia; overhydration
	Elders: range lowers from decreased ability to concentrate urine	High: dehydration; water restriction; vomiting; diarrhea
Protein	Negative	Positive protein: diabetes mellitus; congestive heart failure; systemic lupus; malignant hypertension
Glucose	Negative	Positive glucose: diabetes mellitus; Cushing's syndrome; severe stress; drug interactions
Ketones	Should be negative	Positive ketones: uncontrolled diabetes mellitus; starvation; high-protein diet; excessive aspirin use; dehydration; diabetic ketoacidosis
Nitrites	Negative	Positive nitrites: leukocyte esterase and bacteria
Bacteria	Negative	Pyuria = WBC >10 (probable UTI) Asymptomatic bacteriuria = WBC <10

Continued

Table 21.1

Urinalysis Dipstick Screen—cont'd

Urinary Substance Tested	Reference Value	Significance of the Reference Value
	Elders: May be positive without reported symptoms Older female: More common bacteria >70 years	Probable UTI
Leukocyte esterase	Negative	Identifies enzyme activity of WBCs (bacterial presence)
Bilirubin	0.1–1.0 unit/dL	Positive bilirubin and urobilinogen: hepatic disease (liver; gallbladder; biliary tract)
Urobilinogen	Negative	Positive urobilinogen: Hemolytic process; UTIs
Blood	Adult: negative	Positive blood: cystitis or prostatitis; renal trauma; kidney stones

COPD, chronic obstructive pulmonary disease; UTI, urinary tract infection; WBC, white blood cell.

Nursing Implications

• As you care for older adults, you can encourage adequate and appropriate nutrition and fluid intake. LPNs can discuss bladder hygiene, including frequent hand-washing, regular urine elimination, and proper use of toilet paper (front to back).
• Usually a midstream, clean-catch specimen is requested.
• All urine collected for culture or sensitivity studies must be in a sterile container and should be refrigerated within 10 minutes of collection. If left an hour or more at room temperature, pH changes occur. Normal occurring bacteria can split urea into ammonia and the urine becomes alkaline (higher pH).
• First-morning and fasting urine specimens are collected when the individual awakens. This morning specimen is the most concentrated urine of the day. Analysis of this fasting urine for protein, nitrite, glucose, and urinary sediment is most accurate at this time.

Evidence-Based Practice

Alpay, Y., Aykin, N., Korkmaz, P., Gulduren, H. M., & Caglan, F. C. (2018). Urinary tract infections in the geriatric patients. *Pakistan Journal of Medicine, 34*(1), 67–72.

UTI among older adults is the second most common infection and it is the second leading cause for an antibiotic prescription. The history of UTI is the most common predictor of its development in older adults. As the body ages, there are reductions in lymphocytes (WBC) in the bone marrow, which decreases the ability to fight infectious organisms. Decreased fluid and nutritional intake, chronic disease, and possible increase in cross-contamination of fecal matter influences the prevalence of UTIs in older adults. New evidence indicates that those with UTIs have an increased risk for falls and that level of consciousness changes without obvious reason may be related to an undiagnosed UTI.

This study examined several aspects of UTIs in the elderly population including clinical findings, complicating factors, and diagnostic approaches. The study was conducted over a 3-year period in a hospital setting. The most common signs and symptoms of UTI in the sample were dysuria (pain on urination), abdominal pain, incontinence, nausea, vomiting, and cognitive changes.

The study identified that urine dipstick testing along with clinical status can serve as the first level of screening. The study also determined that older adults should receive immediate treatment due to the potential for complications and mortality related to UTI.

Questions

1. How does this evidence influence the way LPNs might advocate for quality care of older adults related to potential UTIs?

- A screening urine containing bacteria, protein, leukocyte esterase, nitrites, or blood should be cultured. A microscopic examination of the urine also may be done to assess for crystals or stones, casts, epithelial cells, or other urine sediment (solid matter) (see Box 21.1).
- For all urinary testing and specimen collection, you will need to instruct the patient on why each test is being ordered (screening or diagnostic).

- All random urine specimens need at least 10 mL of urine for analysis; sometimes you will need more volume.
- It is important for you to provide water to hydrate the patient if he or she is unable to void unless there is a reason that would alter the test results.
- LPNs should be aware of medications that can change urine color.

UTI is a specific health issue common in elderly people. The highest incidence of reported UTIs is in long-term care facilities. This is in part because urinary tract pathogens become resistant to antibiotics in nursing homes. Incontinence of urine and stool, poor hygiene, and an age-related decreased immune response are other contributing factors.

1. Typical UTI symptoms are:
   Frequency
   Burning
   Hematuria
2. UTI in an older person often presents differently:
   Nocturia
   Incontinence
   Confusion
   Anorexia
   Lethargy or noticeable level of consciousness (LOC) change

Box 21.1

24-Hour Urine Specimens

A 24-hour urine specimen is collected to study a variety of urinary sediments and substances. It is often ordered based on a routine urinalysis or a comprehensive metabolic panel (CMP) blood test.

The most common 24-hour urine tests are ordered to assess renal function. The urine collected is evaluated for creatinine, BUN, protein, and sometimes calcium, potassium, phosphate, or sodium (electrolytes). The GFR and creatinine clearance values are determined using a specific formula. A serum creatinine level is needed to calculate the values, and it is drawn on the day the urine specimen is returned.

Nursing Implications

You will be responsible for providing the patient with a container to collect the urine in, along with instructions

on how to collect the specific urine specimen requested. A 24-hour urine specimen measures the average excretion for substances eliminated in variable amounts during the day.

Proper collection of a 24-hour urine requires that the first void of the day be discarded and the time noted. Urine is collected until the next day's first morning void at or before the designated start time the day before. If one urine specimen during the 24 hours is discarded or spilled, the test will not be accurate. All urine needs to be refrigerated until it is returned to the laboratory.

It is important for you to remind those persons collecting the urine specimen to make sure they drink adequate fluids and do not exercise heavily or have excessive protein intake because that alters the test results.

24-Hour Urine Microalbumin

Values of a 24-hour urine test can vary 30% to 40% when the time of the urine collection is not designated as 24 hours, if the first voiding is not discarded, and the specimen is not properly stored as directed. The following normal reference values are based on adherence to the aforementioned standard protocol parameters and recommended testing methodology.

Normal Reference Values

Normal: <30 mcg/L
Microalbuminuria: 30–300 mcg/L
Macroalbuminuria: >300 mcg/L
On a standard urine dipstick, 10 to 20 mg/dL is the minimal detection limit of protein.

General Information

The **urine microalbumin** test is used to determine the level of albumin (a blood protein) in the urine. It is ordered to determine microvascular kidney damage in people with diabetes or hypertension who are at risk for developing kidney disease (especially in patients whose diabetes is uncontrolled). If protein is present on a urinalysis dipstick, a 24-hour urine collection is ordered. The 24-hour urine test measures the ratio of **albumin** (a group of simple proteins) to **creatinine** (the waste product of muscle breakdown) in the specimen. The results reflect changes in renal function that allows proteins to leak from the small filtration tubules in the kidney. When there is an increase in blood urea nitrogen (BUN) or creatinine in a serum blood test and positive protein in the urine, this test is ordered to assess renal status. Individuals with diabetes should have this test performed annually. In patients with diabetes, a serum estimated glomerular filtration rate (GFR) is requested when the serum creatinine blood sample is requested.

Nursing Implications

Urine collection for a 24-hour urine test begins after the first morning void on day 1 and is collected until after the first morning void of the following day. The patient is instructed to collect urine as they normally urinate throughout day 1. Patients may be provided a urine container for the toilet to collect the urine. The specimen must be refrigerated and is returned as soon as possible to the lab. When the patient returns to the lab with the urine container, a blood specimen is collected to measure creatinine and sometimes BUN and glucose.

Stool for Occult Blood (Stool Guaiac)

Normal Reference Value

Negative result: Absence of test solution (reagent) color

General Information

Assessment of a stool specimen for blood is a relatively easy and inexpensive laboratory test to identify the presence of blood in the stool or gastrointestinal (GI) tract. Bleeding is common in older people, especially in individuals taking aspirin-containing medications and nonsteroidal anti-inflammatory drugs (NSAIDs). It is estimated that about 2.5 mL of blood per day appears in the stool. Hemorrhoids and colorectal cancer are the most common causes of minor bleeding in elderly people.

Abnormal bleeding from the GI tract may be either occult (hidden) or obvious by observation. Minor bleeding can decrease hemoglobin and hematocrit and cause symptoms of fatigue and weakness. The fecal occult blood test can be used for colorectal cancer screening when performed at home on a yearly basis. A fecal occult blood test also can indicate the presence of GI blood; however, it is not specific for determining the source of that blood. A stool hemoccult test may be done during a clinic visit or at home as directed.

Nursing Implications

- There are various tests for fecal occult blood, all requiring the contact of a reagent with a stool specimen.
- A single stool smear can be obtained with a gloved hand during a rectal examination as part of a digital rectal examination (DRE) to check the prostate gland in a male patient or during a female pelvic examination or Pap test.
- A positive test result, indicated by color (usually blue), occurs when there is more than the normal amount of GI blood present.
- The presence of hemorrhoids, common in elderly individuals, especially if there is chronic constipation, can result in a positive stool guaiac result.
- It is recommended that at least three separate random stool specimens be collected when the specimen is tested at home. For each stool sample collected, a small amount of stool is applied to the test card that is from at least two areas of each stool.
- You should instruct the person to avoid red meats, vitamin C intake, iron supplements, and

aspirin for 2 to 3 days before testing to avoid invalidating the results.

- You should always check the manufacturer's directions and suggestions on how to perform the test.

Tuberculosis Testing

Extended care facilities, assisted living, resident homes, and rehabilitation centers have a TB infection risk five times greater than that of nonresident older adults. For elderly adults in extended care facilities, the Centers for Disease Control and Prevention (CDC) now recommends either the intradermal purified protein derivative (PPD) 2-step test (TST) or the **QuantiFERON TB** blood test. The blood test measures the presence of the tubercle bacillus in an individual. It determines if an antigen/antibody reaction has occurred from exposure to the bacteria.

MYCOBACTERIUM TUBERCULOSIS. The intradermal purified protein derivative (PPD) test is the standard TB screening test for older adults. In the event of an outbreak, a 2-step PPD or QuantiFERON test may be ordered as an optional diagnostic test. QuantiFERON is not frequently used as a screening test because it is cost prohibitive.

Normal Reference Values

PPD Skin Testing Assessment:

Negative result	<6 mm of induration
Borderline positive	6–10 mm of induration
Positive result	>10 mm of induration

QuantiFERON TB Gold test:

Positive TB antigen value:	>0.35 IU/mL
Negative TB antigen value:	<0.35 IU/mL

General Information

The tuberculin skin test (PPD) is still the most commonly used screening method for the detection of TB. Up to 25% of older adults who are clinically ill with TB show no reaction (<10 mm of induration) to intradermal injections of 1 mL of tuberculin solution. Anergy (lack of reaction to specific antigens) is common in older adults due to decreased ability to initiate an inflammatory response to the intradermal tuberculin solution. For this reason, the CDC now recommends a second intradermal PPD

test 1 to 3 weeks after the first one (two-step testing, or TST) for older adults. It is recommended that older adult residents in an assisted living, extended care, or retirement community be screened with a 2-step PPD skin test on admission and when there is suspected exposure of TB thereafter in the facility. The 2-step PPD test is performed as follows:

STEP 1:

Placement: A small amount of fluid (tuberculin) is injected under the skin of the lower arm.
The testing site is assessed 48 to 72 hours after placement.
Results of Step 1 of the TST are documented.

STEP 2:

Repeat PPD testing procedure 1 to 3 weeks following step 1.

The CDC issues information by state on the prevalence and frequency of TB and screening recommendations are determined by state regulations and risk for TB exposure. Currently, the CDC reports that incidence of TB infection is low in many states. Based on the most current evidence, annual screening is no longer universally recommended. However, there is no risk to older adults if they receive a single PPD test annually. Some facilities will require annual screening, although it is no longer recommended by the CDC. As an LPN, you will notice that TB testing policies vary from one facility to another. Treatment with antituberculosis medication is effective in congregate living situations when necessary and reduces the risk of epidemic infection.

QuantiFERON is a blood test that detects active or latent TB. The results are generally reported as positive or negative. A positive test result does not mean the older adult has active TB, but rather indicates exposure and the presence of an antigen/antibody reaction. As with a positive PPD skin test result, a chest x-ray is required to verify disease status and an additional sputum sample is recommended. QuantiFERON is not the recommended screening test for older adults but is now being used more frequently. The cost of the QuntiFERON test ranges from $100 to $250.

Nursing Implications

Older adults who have a positive reaction to the PPD test often have no clinical evidence of infection. They require further assessment when the test is positive. If the patient has had a previously positive PPD test, chest x-ray is required for TB assessment. LPNs should verify the timing of the 2-step TB skin placements and document the results of each placement and test results.

CRITICALLY EXAMINE THE FOLLOWING

During the next several weeks in a clinical setting, review the lab results for your assigned patients. Consider the following questions:

• What lab tests are ordered and why?
• What treatments were added or changed related to the test results?
• What additional lab tests can you recommend for your patients and why?

HEMATOLOGIC (BLOOD) TESTING

Blood is the body fluid that transports nutrients, cells, electrolytes, and metabolic wastes. Most laboratory tests analyze specified components of the blood with reference values determined as a normal range based on random and verified typical public samples. Reference values vary slightly depending on the laboratory used and its accepted reference range. LPNs use laboratory tests to aid in safe, quality care because many elderly patients present with vague signs or symptoms that are seen in a variety of common chronic diseases.

One of the most common laboratory or hematologic tests to determine the cellular elements of the blood is the complete blood count (CBC). This test is often used along with a metabolic profile to determine overall health status. Plasma or serum refers to the fluid substance of the blood. Plasma actually contains fibrinogen, a clotting substance, whereas serum is the fluid without fibrinogen.

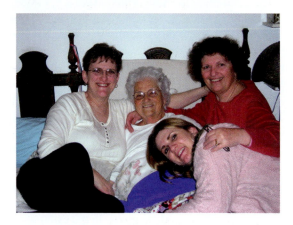

These women are glad their mother performs routine screenings each year.

Today, laboratory machines perform most routine CBC analysis. The term differential (diff) refers to the different types of cells examined in the blood count: erythrocytes, or RBCs, and leukocytes, or WBCs. When a CBC with auto differential (diff) is ordered, the cellular components are determined with technology rather than manually as was done in the past. There are times when the physician or nurse practitioner may order a blood smear or CBC with manual differential. Generally, there are no apparent age-related changes in reference values for the CBC laboratory test. It is important to remember that blood counts may vary with altitude and **hemoconcentration** (an increase in the number of red blood cells).

The CMP is used to assess blood values inclusive of common electrolytes, liver enzymes, renal function indicators, glucose, overall protein, and albumin. Additional common blood tests ordered for elderly adults include vitamin B_{12}, folic acid, TSH, calcium and phosphorus, magnesium, uric acid, immune globulins, lipoproteins (lipid profile), and coagulation studies. Coagulation studies include prothrombin time (PT), partial thromboplastin time (PTT), and **international normalized ratio** (INR), a standardized measurement of oral anticoagulation.

Complete Blood Count (CBC)

The CBC includes RBC count, hemoglobin, hematocrit, and RBC indices; WBC count; platelet count; and sometimes a differential. Values for the CBC do not change with age.

RBC Count
Normal Reference Values

Male	4.7–6.1 million cells/mcL
Female	4.2–5.4 million cells/mcL

General Information

The RBC count is a useful hematological test to diagnose anemia, polycythemia, cardiac or renal disease, and other bone marrow abnormalities in combination with other blood or urine tests.

There are six differentiated RBC markers in a CBC:

1. Total number of RBCs
2. Hemoglobin (Hgb)
3. Hematocrit (HCT)
4. Mean corpuscle volume (MCV)
5. Mean corpuscle hemoglobin (MHC)
6. Mean corpuscle hemoglobin concentration (MCHV).

The last three markers are the characteristics of individual RBCs.

Decreased RBC Count

Anemia
Fluid overload
Kidney problems
Bone marrow invasion of other cells or tumors
Recent hemorrhage
Chronic illness
Autoimmune diseases
Increased RBC Count
Polycythemia (altitude related)
Dehydration
Hypoxia
Congestive heart failure
Impaired pulmonary ventilation
Abnormal hemoglobin
Significant physical training (i.e., marathon races; more elders are participating in them)

Hemoglobin
Normal Reference Values

Male	13.8–17.2 g/dL
Female	12.1–15.1 g/dL

General Information

Normal Hgb levels are maintained throughout life in healthy individuals. Hemoglobin concentration in whole blood parallels the RBC count, meaning that as the number of RBCs increase, so does Hgb, and vice versa. For elderly adults who already experience decreased energy levels associated with general aging and chronic disease, lower Hgb level affects oxygen binding and overall cellular and physical energy.

Increased Hemoglobin

Polycythemia
Dehydration
High altitude
Chronic obstructive pulmonary disease (COPD) or other obstructive lung disease

Decreased Hemoglobin

Anemia
Dietary iron deficiency and/or poor iron absorption
Recent hemorrhage (GI bleeding is a common reason in elders)
Fluid retention causing hemodilution kidney disease

Hematocrit
Normal Reference Values

Male	$47.0 \pm 5.0\%$
Female	$42.0 \pm 5.0\%$

General Information

Hematocrit measures the percentage by volume of packed RBCs in whole blood. It is determined by spinning the blood; the heavier RBCs settle to the bottom. The value is a percentage (ratio) of cells to serum.

Decreased Hematocrit

Anemia
Hemodilution
Bone marrow disease
Kidney disease
Rheumatoid arthritis
Liver disease (cirrhosis)
Relationship to aging and decrease in intrinsic factor in seventh to ninth decade of life

Increased Hematocrit

Polycythemia
Significant volume depletion occurs with associated BUN and creatinine.

RBC Indices
Normal Reference Values
Mean corpuscular volume (MCV) (RBC size)
Male   78–100 fL
Female   79–102 fL
Mean corpuscular hemoglobin (MCH; RBC color/Hgb): 25%–35% content
Mean corpuscular hemoglobin concentration (MCHC; RBC color/Hgb): 31%–37% content

General Information
RBC indices aid in the diagnosis and classification of anemias by providing information about the size, hemoglobin concentration, and hemoglobin weight of an average RBC.

Nursing Implications
You will need to be aware of your patient's RBC count along with his or her Hgb and Hct levels to understand if the patient is at risk for venous thrombosis from elevated values. Clot formation and pain most commonly occur in the lower leg (calf area). This is termed a deep vein thrombosis (DVT). Use of anti-embolism stockings, also called TED (thrombo-embolic deterrent) hose promote better circulation. You may be required to assist patients with TED hose use. If bedrest is ordered for a patient in your care, you will need to ensure the patient follows recommendations for prevention of DVT (e.g., elevation of the affected limb, use of compression stockings, etc.).

If RBC, Hgb, and Hct are low, patients will most likely have symptoms of fatigue. The physician may order iron supplementation and you will want to educate the patient on ways to conserve energy. If levels are extremely low, a blood or packed red blood cell (PBRC) transfusion may be ordered by the physician.

WBC Count
Normal Reference Values
4,500–10,000 cells/mcL

General Information
The WBC count is used to identify infectious or inflammatory processes, evaluate the need for further tests, and to monitor the older person's response to chemotherapy or radiation therapy. The WBC count decreases with age because of an overall reduction in lymphocyte cells. The major implication of fewer lymphocytes is a decreased ability to resist and fight infection.

Decreased WBC Count (Leukopenia)
Bone marrow depression from primary disease such as leukemia, myeloma, and other tumors
Reactions to antineoplastic agents or other toxins
Viral infections, such as influenza and infectious hepatitis, which are more common in older adults
Sepsis
Radiation treatments
Drug use, including phenytoin, NSAIDs, and metronidazole
General nutritional deficiency

Increased WBC Count (Leukocytosis)
Infection
Inflammation
Tissue necrosis
Leukemia
Excessive exercise
Stress (common in elderly individuals due to physiological as well as emotional stress, which can be related to finances, loneliness, and functional decreases, among other things)

WBC Differential
There are five kinds of WBCs: neutrophils, lymphocytes, monocytes, eosinophils, and basophils. Each WBC cell type functions as part of the body's defense system against infectious or other foreign substances. WBC types are most often expressed as the percentage (%) or ratio of the individual WBC type per 100 WBC cells.

In older adults, an infection may not be accompanied by an increase in the number of WBCs. The WBC differential is necessary to detect and diagnose

Box 21.2
White Blood Cell Cellular Functions
- Neutrophils: Reflect general phagocytosis of bacteria and foreign substances and control inflammation
- Eosinophils: Reflect allergic responses, parasitic infection, and autoimmune diseases
- Basophils: Reflect acute allergic response, stress reactions, and bone marrow disease
- Lymphocytes: Reflect infections, systemic lupus, response to chemotherapy or radiation, leukemia, and infectious hepatitis
- Monocytes: Reflect tuberculosis, chronic infections or inflammatory disease, and response to drug therapy

disease. It often is collected along with other blood or urine tests.

Normal Reference Values
Neutrophils: 1.6–6.7 K/mcL or 55%–70%
Eosinophils: 0.0–0.5 K/mcL or 1%–5%
Basophils: 0.0–0.3 K/mcL or 0%–3%
Lymphocytes: 1.2–3.4 K/mcL or 16%–46%
Monocytes: 0.2–1.0 K/mcL or 4%–11%

General Information
The WBC differential helps determine the severity of an infection, detect allergic reactions and parasitic infections, identify various types of leukemia, and assess the individual's capacity to resist and overcome infection.

Neutrophils can be differentiated to include bands, which are immature neutrophils, and segmented neutrophils known as segs, which are mature neutrophils. These values are important for cancer patients, individuals undergoing treatments that suppress bone marrow, and for elderly patients who are prone to infection and who often do not manifest the same signs or symptoms of infection as younger adults. An increase in bands requires further investigation. Neutropenia is a significant syndrome with specific nursing considerations for the LPN.

Platelet Count
Normal Reference Values
130,000–400,000/mcL

General Information
Thrombocytes, or platelets, are cellular fragments found in the blood and are necessary for clotting. A clot forms as the cells aggregate or join together to form a plug necessary for clot formation and hemostasis. Platelets contribute to phospholipid activity in the coagulation process.

Decreased Platelet Count (Thrombocytopenia)
Hemorrhage
Bone marrow disease
Chemotherapy or radiation
Prescribed anticoagulation therapy
Folic acid or vitamin B_{12} deficiency
Disseminated intravascular coagulation (DIC)
Idiopathic thrombocytopenia
Systemic lupus

Drugs (furosemide, indomethacin, penicillin, phenytoin, quinidine sulfate, salicylates, thiazides, tricyclic antidepressants, and others)
Destruction resulting from immune disorders, radiation, or mechanical injury

Increased Platelet Count (Thrombocytosis)
Iron deficiency anemia
Hemorrhage: Splenectomy
Rheumatoid arthritis
Polycythemia vera
Malignancy or other tumor formation
High altitudes
Persistent cold temperature
Strenuous exercise

Erythrocyte Sedimentation Rate
Normal Reference Values
A slight increase is noted for normal reference value in the fifth to sixth decades.

Male <50 years old: 0–9 mm/hr
Male >60 years old: 1–20 mm/hr
Female <50 years old: 1–20 mm/hr
Female >60 years old: 1–30 mm/hr

General Information
The erythrocyte sedimentation rate (ESR), also known as the sed rate, is a useful hematology test to measure how fast RBCs settle into the bottom of a laboratory tube with gravity over one hour. The faster the cells descend, the smaller the RBC size; the slower the descent, the larger the RBCs.

The value of the ESR is that it is an inexpensive lab test that is easily obtained when a CBC is drawn. The ESR is not a specific test, meaning that without other laboratory values it may be difficult to know the source of the inflammatory process. It does indicate changes in fibrin, reactive proteins, and autoimmune globulins leading to better quality of care as the reasons for the elevations are explored. Serial ESR evaluations monitor resolution of infection, inflammation, or vasculitis.

Increased ESR
Polymyalgia or fibromyalgia syndromes
Temporal arteritis (common in the elderly)
Rheumatoid versus osteoarthritis differential
Chronic inflammatory disease
Infection
Malignancy
Vascular collagen disease

Decreased ESR
Sickle cell anemia
Liver disease
Polycythemia
Elevated blood glucose

Folic Acid and Vitamin B$_{12}$
Normal Reference Values
Folic acid: 3.1–17.5 ng/mL
Vitamin B$_{12}$: >250 ng/mL
200–250 ng/mL: Acceptable range in older adults
   unless symptomatic

General Information
Folic acid, a vitamin B complex element, is necessary for RBC and WBC function. Folic acid decrease indicates protein malnutrition, anemia, and liver or renal disease. Alcohol use and other prescribed drugs can decrease this vitamin as well.

Vitamin B$_{12}$ is necessary for full development of the RBC. A decrease in B$_{12}$ level is associated with gastric malabsorption and gastric disease. Aging is not believed to be a factor for vitamin B$_{12}$ decrease; however, there is more pernicious anemia as people age.

If anemia is present, an iron level and/or total iron-binding capacity (TIBC) may be ordered to assess overall health status, especially in patients with chronic disease.

Increased Folic Acid
Overuse of dietary supplement(s)
Leukemia
Vegan/vegetarian diet
Vitamin B$_{12}$ deficiency

Decreased Folic Acid
Poor nutrition (common in older adults)
Anorexia
Malabsorption
Celiac disease
Crohn's disease
Cholestasis
Lymphoma
Pancreatic cancer
Pernicious anemia
Bowel resection
Liver disease

Nursing Implications
A deficiency of these vitamins affects overall energy and is often associated with macrocytic anemia.

Vitamin B$_{12}$ is required for optimum RBC development. Some studies suggest that a deficit of these vitamins contributes to dementia and Alzheimer's disease.

Metformin, a common oral drug for diabetes, may decrease folic acid and vitamin B$_{12}$. It is important that patients with diabetes have these serum levels checked at least every other year.

Homocysteine, an inflammatory substance associated with coronary artery disease and cardiac events, is reduced if there are adequate levels of vitamin B$_{12}$, folic acid, and vitamin B$_6$. When they are elevated, this plasma substance level should be checked.

Coagulation Tests
PT
NORMAL REFERENCE VALUES
Normal: 11.2–13.2 sec with INR of 1.0
Therapeutic: 1.5–2.0 times normal control

PTT or Activated PTT (APTT)
NORMAL REFERENCE VALUES
PTT normal: 22.1–43.1 sec
APTT normal: 25–36 sec
Therapeutic target for both: 1.5–2.5 times normal
   control

INR
NORMAL REFERENCE VALUES
Normal: 1.0–1.50 with the ideal value as close
   to 1 as possible
Therapeutic target: 2.0–3.0 (ideally 2.5)

General Information
Prothrombin, or factor II, aids in the clotting process. The PT test measures prothrombin. It is used to diagnose many bleeding disorders and the effectiveness of anticoagulation therapy. PT is determined before initiation of warfarin therapy and then daily until maintenance dosage is established. Thereafter, PT determinations are made at 1- to 4-week intervals, depending on the stability of the person's therapeutic level. It may be checked weekly if there is variability or difficulty maintaining the ideal reference values. There is no clinical diagnostic significance for a low PT other than diet or pharmacology considerations; there are very rare malignancies that alter the PT and promote thrombophlebitis.

The PTT test verifies blood consistency and appropriate anticoagulation for heparin products. The

PTT test is primarily for assessment of therapeutic heparin interventions. It can be useful in identifying bleeding disorders, which change plasma clotting factors and indicate deficits of the body's intrinsic system (i.e., hemophilia or systemic lupus). Abnormal values (high) usually are the result of liver disease, especially cirrhosis; vitamin K deficiency; or changes in gastric absorption (lack of bile salts) or long-term antibiotic therapy, which changes normal GI bacteria.

The INR blood test verifies the results of the PT. The INR blood test verifies the results of the PT test; it is the "standard" value from one lab to another regardless of the lab location.

When administering anticoagulation therapy, the nurse should ensure that the following interventions are performed:

• Many drugs have a potentiating or inhibiting effect on warfarin, so all medications being taken by an individual taking warfarin such as sulfonamides, digoxin, and cephalosporins should be monitored. Patients should avoid aspirin or NSAIDS. All medications must be reviewed. Diets high in vitamin K should be encouraged.
• Risk of serious hemorrhage is high in anticoagulated persons older than age 70, especially individuals at risk for falls. You need to educate patients about the increased possibility of bleeding while taking anticoagulants and suggest strategies such as avoidance of razors and applying pressure when scratched or cut.

THINK LIKE A NURSE

Mrs. D. was diagnosed with pancreatic cancer and goes to an outpatient clinic laboratory weekly for blood draws to assist in medication management and assessment of the cancer progress. She knows how important the results are to her overall health.

1. List tests that are important for you to assess and review to monitor a patient with pancreatic or other gastrointestinal cancer.
2. Explain why you, as the LPN, need to review these laboratory values and screening tests.

• When PT or PTT values are abnormal, risk of bleeding or signs of bleeding such as hematuria, black tarry stools, hematemesis, bruising and petechiae, epistaxis, hemoptysis, continuous abdominal or head pain, faintness, or dizziness should be reviewed with the patient and the anticoagulant dose withheld. Notify the physician immediately.
• Periodic urinalyses and stool guaiac and liver function tests are carried out to detect hemorrhage or liver dysfunction.

COMPREHENSIVE METABOLIC PROFILE INDICATORS

Glucose, Plasma
Normal Reference Values
Fasting (no food or drink except water for 8 hours or more):
Normal: 70–99 mg/dL
Older adult: Increase of 1–2 mg/dL per decade
Prediabetes: 100–125 mg/dL
Note: 40% of adults 50 years or older have prediabetes.
Diabetes mellitus: >125 mg/dL
(Verify by glycolated hemoglobin [HbA1c] or two fasting blood glucose values.)

Glycolated Hemoglobin
Normal Reference Values
There is no information to show that the HbA1c changes with age.
Normal: <5.7%
Prediabetes: 5.7%–6.4%
Diabetes: >6.5%
Goal for diabetic patients: 7% or less

General Information
The **glycolated hemoglobin (HbA1c)** test measures the mean results of plasma glucose over a period of about 3 or 4 months. It is a good indicator of serum glucose and is a reliable test to show the absence or presence of diabetes as well as the prediabetes risk. In elderly people, the exact definition of abnormal glucose tolerance is unclear. The National Institute of Diabetes and Digestive and Kidney Diseases recommends serum glucose and HbA1c testing to screen for diabetes. There are three diagnostic categories of diabetes: type 1 diabetes, type 2 diabetes, and prediabetes inclusive of gestational diabetes and chronic marginally elevated fasting blood glucose. In the past, two elevated fasting serum or finger-stick values were suggested. Using the two separate laboratory values, a diagnosis of diabetes or prediabetes is

confirmed with the HbA1c when the blood glucose is high normal to slightly elevated over time. If the patient is pre-diabetic, lifestyle recommendations should be advised. Once the HbA1c is at 6% to 6.5% in families with a strong history of diabetes, diabetic medications are advised. Hemoconcentration can affect this result.

Hypoglycemia

1. Signs and symptoms of decreased blood plasma glucose or hypoglycemia include:
   Plasma blood glucose values: <70 mg/dL
   Weakness
   Restlessness
   Hunger
   Nervousness
   Sweating
   Rapidly decreasing mental alertness in an elderly person without the previously listed common symptoms
2. Hypoglycemia may be caused by:
   Beta blockers
   Ethanol
   Clofibrate
   Monoamine oxidase inhibitors
   Strenuous exercise
   Failure to refrigerate the blood sample and analyze it within a few hours of collection

Hyperglycemia

1. One sign and symptom of increased blood plasma glucose or hyperglycemia is plasma glucose levels that exceed 600 mg/dL. These levels can be life-threatening. Plasma glucose greater than 160–180 mg/dL is the average renal threshold, but can result in glucose presence in the urine, or glycosuria, in older adults. The following typical signs and symptoms of hyperglycemia may not be present or may be less pronounced in older adults:
   Urinary frequency
   Dehydration
   Weakness
2. Hyperglycemia may be caused by medications that can increase glucose levels such as:
   Chlorthalidone
   Thiazide diuretics
   Furosemide
   Oral contraceptives
   Benzodiazepines
   Phenytoin
   Phenothiazines
   Lithium
   Epinephrine
   Nicotinic acid
   Corticosteroids
   Recent illness or infection

Undetected or worsening hyperglycemia causes a mental status decrease that progresses more quickly to hyperosmolar coma in an older person with non-insulin-dependent diabetes mellitus.

Electrolytes

Normal values for electrolytes are the same for both younger and older individuals. Numerous conditions, medications, and dietary factors influence electrolyte values. Common electrolyte-related causes of weakness in elderly people are hypernatremia (high sodium), hyponatremia (low sodium), and hypokalemia (low potassium). In general, electrolyte values represent what is in the serum and not in the cells. Electrolytes are present in the cells and often determine cellular activity and health. The two main electrolytes are sodium and potassium.

Sodium is primarily present in extracellular fluid (outside cells), whereas potassium, magnesium, and phosphate are intracellular electrolytes. When a positive electrolyte moves from extracellular to intracellular areas, a negative electrolyte sodium, bicarbonate, or chloride follows. There is evidence to support that low magnesium level is a risk for diabetes or elevated glucose and increased lipoproteins (cholesterol and triglyceride).

Sodium, Serum
NORMAL REFERENCE VALUES
Normal: 136–145 mEq/L

GENERAL INFORMATION. Elderly people are at increased risk of serum sodium imbalance. Decreased sodium levels promote water excretion, and increased levels promote retention, primarily through stimulation or depression of aldosterone secretion. Loss of body water causes concentration of serum sodium (hypernatremia), whereas an increase in body water causes dilution of serum sodium (hyponatremia). Sodium also influences the acid-base balance, chloride or potassium levels, and neuromuscular function.

Safe, Effective Nursing Care

Goals for LPNs Related to Laboratory Testing in the Elderly

Evidence-based practice is essential for optimal specimen collection and monitoring. LPNs have accountability to patients related to managing the requested (ordered) interventions and laboratory assessments for patients they are assigned. Safe, Effective Nursing Care (SENC) includes a basic understanding of common laboratory tests and general implications for patient care. The LPN collaborates with registered nurses (RNs), physicians, and other health-care workers to influence healthcare outcomes through activities within their scope of practice. LPN responsibilities vary state by state and include supervision by an RN. One important role of the LPN is that of collecting information (laboratory data) and notifying those who need to know regarding pertinent results or changes to ensure safe effective nursing care and patient outcomes.

Often, you or a certified nursing assistant (CNA) whom you supervise will be responsible for obtaining any urine, stool, wound, or sputum specimens needed for laboratory testing. Your priority is to gather all specimens correctly according to standards and protocols. Sending a specimen to the laboratory that has been improperly collected increases the likelihood of an inaccurate result.

When an older adult is asked to give you a midstream urine specimen, the patient may not understand what that means. Not wanting to look "dumb," the patient may not ask for an explanation. As the patient's advocate, you need to determine whether the person understands the instructions by asking for responses about what you expect him or her to do and the reason for doing things in a specific way. When instructed to cleanse the urinary meatus before voiding for a clean-catch specimen, an older person may simply not do it because they are uncomfortable or unfamiliar with the procedure. When obtaining a sputum specimen, the LPN should ensure that specimen comes from a deep cough. Most people do not like mucus, and it may even be painful for the older person to cough deeply.

You need to plan ahead and be prepared with a strategy to obtain specimens as needed. As in all things you do, be patient and caring, because these are the hallmark behaviors of professionals in nursing. Nurses are essential to the success of patient care and as a collaborative interprofessional team member, you contribute to safe, effective nursing care.

HYPONATREMIA. A sodium concentration of less than 136 mEq/L occurs when there is an excess of water in relation to total sodium.

1. Symptoms include the following (although they may also be absent):
   Fatigue
   Headache
   Restlessness
   Decreased skin turgor
   Nausea
   Muscle cramps and tremors
   Disorientation
   Confusion
   Coma
   Seizures
   Death
2. Causes of hyponatremia include:
   Vomiting
   Diarrhea
   Renal disorders
   Diuretics
   Congestive heart failure
   Cirrhosis
   Overhydration
   Adrenal insufficiency
   Use of nutritional support formulas without additional sodium
   Syndrome of inappropriate antidiuretic hormone secretion associated with numerous drugs and diseases

HYPERNATREMIA. A sodium concentration greater than 146 mEq/L is a result of a deficit of body water relative to total sodium content and is usually caused by dehydration.

1. Symptoms include:
   Weakness
   Thirst
   Restlessness
   Dry, sticky mucous membranes

Flushed skin
Oliguria
Diminished reflexes
2. Causes of hypernatremia include:
   Inadequate fluid intake
   Diarrhea
   Polyuria associated with diabetes mellitus
   Diuretics
   Increased insensible water loss from fever
      and tachypnea
   Hypertension
   Dyspnea
   Edema
   Kidney disease owing to a lack of response to
      antidiuretic hormone
3. Causes of excess sodium concentration include:
   Increased dietary intake
   Aldosteronism
   Intravenous infusion of normal saline for
      treatment of fluid loss or shock

Potassium, Serum
NORMAL REFERENCE VALUES
Normal: 3.5–5.0 mEq/L

GENERAL INFORMATION. Potassium maintains cellular osmotic equilibrium and helps regulate muscle activity by maintaining electrical conduction within the cardiac and skeletal muscles. Potassium also helps regulate acid-base balance, enzyme activity, and kidney function. Potassium deficiency develops rapidly because the body has no effective way to conserve potassium.

HYPOKALEMIA
1. Signs and symptoms of hypokalemia include:
   Mental confusion
   Rapid, weak, irregular pulse
   Hypotension
   Anorexia
   Decreased reflexes
   Muscle weakness
   Paresthesia
2. Causes of hypokalemia include:
   Diuretics
   Diarrhea
   Vomiting
   Renal tubular acidosis
   Malnutrition
   Urinary potassium losses associated with
      glycosuria and ketonuria and with
      hyperaldosteronism

HYPERKALEMIA
1. Signs and symptoms of hyperkalemia include:
   Weakness
   Malaise
   Nausea
   Diarrhea
   Muscle irritability
   Oliguria
   Bradycardia
2. Causes of hyperkalemia include:
   Renal failure
   Cell damage from burns
   Injuries
   Chemotherapy
   Acidosis
   Addison's disease
   Diabetes mellitus
3. Medications affecting serum potassium level
   include:
   Spironolactone
   Triamterene
   NSAIDs
   Beta blockers
   Angiotensin-converting enzyme inhibitors
   Penicillin G
   Amphotericin B
   Methicillin
   Tetracycline

Calcium, Plasma
NORMAL REFERENCE VALUES
Normal: 9–10.5 mg/dL

GENERAL INFORMATION. Calcium absorption becomes less efficient with age in men and women. Inadequate dietary calcium is associated with the loss of bone that begins in the 40s. Calcium helps regulate and promote neuromuscular and enzyme activity, skeletal development, and blood coagulation. Parathyroid hormone, vitamin D, calcitonin, and adrenal steroids control calcium blood levels. Almost all of the body's calcium is stored in the bones and teeth. Serum calcium varies inversely with the body's phosphorus level. The body requires ingestion of about 1 g per day of dietary calcium because calcium is excreted in the urine and feces.

HYPOCALCEMIA
1. Signs and symptoms of hypocalcemia include:
   Circumoral and peripheral numbness and
      tingling

Muscle twitching
Facial muscle spasm
Muscle cramping
Seizures
Dysrhythmias
2. Causes of hypocalcemia include:
Insufficient activity of the parathyroid glands
Hypomagnesemia
Hyperphosphatemia owing to renal failure
Laxatives
Chemotherapy
Corticosteroids
Malabsorption
Acute pancreatitis
Diarrhea
Rickets (vitamin D deficiency)

HYPERCALCEMIA

1. Signs and symptoms of hypercalcemia include:
Hypertension
Bone pain
Muscle hypotonicity
Nausea
Vomiting
Dehydration
Mental confusion
Coma
Cardiac arrest
2. Causes of hypercalcemia include:
Hyperparathyroidism
Thiazide diuretics
Cancer
Addison's disease
Hyperthyroidism
Paget's disease
Immobilization
Excessive vitamin D intake
Calcium-containing antacids
Androgens
Progestins or estrogens
Lithium carbonate

Phosphate, Serum
NORMAL REFERENCE VALUES
Normal: 3–4.5 mg/dL

GENERAL INFORMATION. Phosphate helps regulate calcium levels, carbohydrate and lipid metabolism, and acid-base balance. Adequate levels of vitamin D are necessary for absorption of phosphates from the intestine. About 85% of the body's phosphate is found in bone. Calcium and phosphate have a reciprocal relationship. The kidneys regulate phosphate excretion to maintain a balance with serum calcium.

Chloride, Serum
NORMAL REFERENCE VALUES
Normal: 98–106 mEq/L

GENERAL INFORMATION. Chloride interacts with sodium to maintain the osmotic pressure of the blood. Chloride is important in maintaining the acid-base balance in the body and varies inversely with the bicarbonate level. It also is an important electrolyte for maintaining the body's osmotic pressure. Low chloride levels correspond to low sodium and potassium levels. Chloride is also an important electrolyte for maintaining the body's osmotic pressure. Renal disease can decrease chloride excretion and cause fluid accumulation.

End Products of Metabolism
BUN, Serum
NORMAL REFERENCE VALUES
Normal: 8–25 mg/dL

In elderly adults, BUN increases slightly as renal function decreases with aging. If the BUN is greater than 28–30 mg/dL, additional laboratory tests should be ordered. Generally, a 24-hour urine collection is recommended as the follow-up diagnostic lab test.

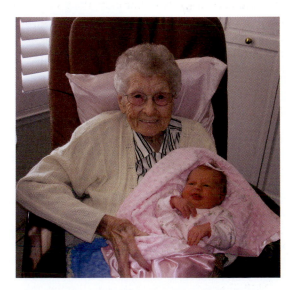

Family is this woman's greatest joy. She appreciates the monthly laboratory work that is done for her at the nursing home where she resides. She doesn't worry about the results because she knows the physician and nurses will manage the situation for her. That leaves her more time to be with her family.

GENERAL INFORMATION. Urea nitrogen is the main end product of protein metabolism. The BUN level measures the amount of urea nitrogen in the blood. It reflects protein intake, liver function, and kidney excretory capacity. The normal BUN value remains unchanged with age. Because protein intake is often low in older adults, BUN values may be normal even with impaired renal function. Elevation of BUN levels without serum creatinine elevation suggests dehydration.

There are usually no signs or symptoms of an increased BUN level other than the signs and symptoms associated with dehydration or other underlying renal disease. Likewise, with decreased BUN levels, the signs and symptoms are those of the underlying condition.

1. Causes of increased BUN levels include:
   Renal disease
   Reduced renal blood flow
   Urinary tract obstruction
   GI bleed
   Increased protein catabolism (starvation, burns)
   Drugs such as aminoglycosides, amphotericin B, and methicillin
2. Causes of decreased BUN levels include:
   Severe liver failure
   Malnutrition
   Overhydration
   Chloramphenicol use

Creatinine, Serum
NORMAL REFERENCE VALUES
Normal male: 0.6–1.5 mg/dL
Normal female: 0.6–1.1 mg/dL

In older adults, values decrease as muscle mass decreases and renal function changes. Levels greater than 5.0 mg/dL indicate a more than 50% decrease in nephron function.

GENERAL INFORMATION. There are no age adjustments in the normal reference value range for creatinine. It should be noted that lean body mass declines with age along with the total daily production of creatinine. As blood test values are not amended for older adults related to this serum marker, there can be an overestimate of actual renal function. Evaluating creatinine along with a standard urinalysis (protein) and BUN are recommended in older adults for optimal management.

Creatinine clearance declines by almost 10% per decade after 40 years of age and is a more reliable indicator of kidney function than BUN and serum creatinine values. In elderly people, creatinine clearance is important for determining the dosage for drugs that are cleared by the kidney to avoid drug toxicity. Creatinine levels change more slowly than BUN levels do, so monitoring the creatinine level is a better measure of kidney function in the elderly.

Causes of increased serum creatinine include:

Renal disease
Diabetic acidosis
Starvation
Muscle disease
Hyperthyroidism
Use of ascorbic acid (vitamin C)
Barbiturates
Diuretics

A high serum creatinine level with nonspecific symptoms may not indicate renal failure but rather may be the result of weight loss and reports of weakness. Because the kidneys easily excrete creatinine with minimal tubular reabsorption, serum creatinine levels are directly related to the GFR.

Bilirubin, Serum
NORMAL REFERENCE VALUES
Total: 0.1–1.0 mg/dL
Direct: 0.0–0.4 mg/dL
Indirect: 0.1–1.0 mg/dL

GENERAL INFORMATION. Bilirubin is the major product of hemoglobin breakdown and is excreted as a pigment in bile. The excretion of bilirubin depends on the normal production and destruction of RBCs and a functional hepatobiliary system, where bilirubin is conjugated and excreted. The direct bilirubin value increases with obstruction of the flow of bile through the biliary system, which causes uptake of direct bilirubin into the circulation. Levodopa may cause a false-positive increase in bilirubin. GI bleeding can contribute to an elevated bilirubin value.

Uric Acid, Serum
NORMAL REFERENCE VALUES
Men: 3.6–8.0 mg/dL
Women: 2.3–6.0 mg/dL
Older male: 2.0–8.5 mg/dL
Older female: 2.0–8.0 mg/dL

GENERAL INFORMATION. Uric acid, the major end metabolite of dietary and endogenous purines, is excreted through the kidneys. Cell breakdown and catabolism of nucleic acids, excessive production and destruction of cells, and inability to excrete uric acid are causes of hyperuricemia. An increase in serum uric acid is found in various conditions, including gout, impaired renal function, congestive heart failure, hemolytic anemia, polycythemia, neoplasms, and psoriasis. Uric acid level is influenced by foods high in purine, so dietary measures are part of the treatment for an elevated uric acid level. Gout is the most common symptom manifested when levels increase, and all joints can be affected; the joints of the foot are the most common site.

Serum uric acid levels greater than 8 mg/dL in men and greater than 6 mg/dL in women are often associated with symptoms of gout. Gout is an acute inflammation of a joint, commonly the metatarsophalangeal joint of the great toe, caused by uric acid crystal accumulation.

Causes of increased serum uric acid levels include:

Diuretics, especially thiazide diuretics
Starvation
High-purine/protein diet
Obesity
Dyslipidemia
Diabetes or other blood sugar disorders
Alcohol overuse and abuse
Chemotherapy
Menopause
Regular high-dose aspirin use
Levodopa, acetaminophen, ascorbic acid, and
   phenacetin may cause false elevations in uric
   acid. levels.

Liver Function Tests

Most liver function tests results do not change with increasing age. The alkaline phosphatase level is frequently elevated in older adults as bone degeneration and decreased bone remodeling occur. Total alkaline phosphatase (ALP) may increase due to Paget's disease, bone fracture, trauma, or osteoporosis. For people taking tacrine (Cognex) for Alzheimer's disease, it is important to monitor liver function tests.

Alanine Aminotransferase (ALT)
NORMAL REFERENCE VALUES
Normal: 10–56 U/L

A slight increase is noted in the seventh to ninth decade of life.

GENERAL INFORMATION. ALT, an enzyme necessary for tissue energy production, is present predominantly in the liver. It also is present in the kidney, heart, and skeletal muscles and is a relatively specific indicator of acute liver cell damage.

Causes of elevated ALT include:

Fatty liver disease
Tuberculosis
Liver disease (cirrhosis)
Various medications
Cholecystitis
Intrahepatic cholestasis
Pancreatitis
Hepatic congestion associated with heart failure
Acute myocardial infarction
Trauma
Lead ingestion

Falsely elevated ALT levels may be caused by barbiturate or narcotic analgesic use.

Aspartate Aminotransferase (AST) or Serum Glutamic-Oxaloacetic Transaminase (SGOT)
NORMAL REFERENCE VALUES
Normal: 5–41 U/L

GENERAL INFORMATION. AST is an enzyme found in cells of the liver, heart, muscles, kidneys, pancreas, and RBCs. Serum levels are highest during acute cellular damage and decrease during tissue repair. The AST level is useful in monitoring the progress of myocardial infarction (MI) and acute liver disease. Tuberculosis and its subsequent treatment are both reasons for a rise in AST.

Causes of AST elevation include:

MI
Liver disease
Extensive surgery resulting in muscle damage
Hemolytic anemia
Pulmonary emboli
Delirium tremens from alcohol withdrawal
Diseases of the brain, pancreas, spleen, lungs,
   and muscle

ALP
NORMAL REFERENCE VALUES
Adult male: 45–115 U/L
Adult female: 30–100 U/L

Increased values are seen with each decade after age 50 years. There are no parameters identified; age considerations and provider judgment are based on presentation of patient.

GENERAL INFORMATION. ALP is an enzyme that is active in bone calcification and in lipid and metabolite transport. Serum alkaline phosphatase levels are sensitive to biliary obstruction by space-occupying hepatic lesions, such as tumors or abscesses, and to metabolic bone disease. ALP isoenzymes may be used to differentiate hepatic and skeletal diseases. This test does not indicate the source of cellular or organ change. It is used less frequently today as a standalone diagnostic lab test for bone or liver disease. Decreases in the level of ALP can indicate malnutrition or excessive vitamin D intake. Anticonvulsant medications increase levels of this enzyme.

Causes of increased alkaline phosphatase include:

Obstructive gallbladder disease
Paget's disease
Bone metastasis
Hyperparathyroidism
Liver disease
Osteomalacia

Protein Assays
Creatinine Kinase (CK) or Creatinine Phosphokinase (CPK)
NORMAL REFERENCE VALUES
Normal male total: 60–400 U/L
Normal female total: 40–150 U/L
Isoenzyme Values:
CK-I (BB or brain): 0%–1%
CK-II (MB or heart): 3% or 0–7.5 ng/mL
CK-III (MM or muscle): 95%–100%

GENERAL INFORMATION. Creatinine kinase is important for energy and is integral for muscular tissue function and health. Values of this enzyme are elevated after any muscular injury or activity. Because of this, the enzyme is a useful marker for acute MI and to assess progressive muscular diseases or necrosis of muscle from trauma.

If CK-II is greater than 10 U/L, then a cardiac event has not occurred. If it is greater than 12 U/L, it is likely the patient had an MI or ischemic event other than angina. CK-II is present in the serum between 3 and 6 hours after acute MI. It peaks in about 24 hours and remains elevated for 3 days or less.

Troponins
NORMAL REFERENCE VALUES
Troponin I: >1.5 ng/mL positive for MI
Troponin T: >0.1–0.2 ng/mL positive for MI

GENERAL INFORMATION. Troponins are proteins found in muscle and increase with an acute MI. Troponin levels are often tested along with CK levels because they are present as early as 2 hours after the event and peak within 24 hours, as does the CK level. They remain elevated for up to 1 week and are therefore used for assessment and treatment of an elderly person. This test is especially important for aging women who often have different or vague heart attack symptoms and may not seek medical care as readily.

B-Natriuretic Peptide (BNP)
NORMAL REFERENCE VALUES
Normal reference: <100 pg/mL
Positive congestive heart failure: >100 pg/mL

GENERAL INFORMATION. This peptide is found in the ventricles of the heart and is useful for detecting early to late changes in cardiac function related to hypertrophy of the ventricles. It is useful for diagnosing congestive heart failure because it is a cardiac-specific peptide.

Prostate-Specific Antigen (PSA)
NORMAL REFERENCE VALUES
African American (Black)
    60–69 years: 0–4.50 ng/mL
    70–79 years: increases to 0–5.50 ng/mL
Asian
    60–69 years: 0–4.0 ng/mL
    70–79 years: increases to 0–5.0 ng/mL
Caucasian
    60–69 years: 0–4.50 ng/mL
    70–79 years: and increases to 0–6.50 ng/mL

GENERAL INFORMATION. PSA is a protein released from the prostate gland. It is measured in the serum. PSA was once considered a valuable serum-marker to determine the likelihood of prostate cancer. There is now controversy regarding the value of regular PSA screening as part of annual wellness exams. PSA is elevated during infection, after a rectal and prostate exam, and with benign prostatic hypertrophy (BPH) or prostate enlargement. African American (Black) males have a higher risk of developing prostate cancer than many of their male peers (Center for Disease Control and Prevention, 2018). Asian males are at lowest risk for prostate cancer (Feng et al., 2017).

Men with a family history of prostate cancer are generally screened more frequently than other men because of increased risk for prostate cancer (CDC,

2018). The decision to screen is based on patient preference and provider recommendation.

As men age, the prostate gland enlarges. An increase of 0.75 ng/mL annually indicates prostate enlargement from BPH or a benign or malignant tumor. The U.S. Preventive Services Task Force (USPSTF) does not recommend general PSA screening after age 70 for men at average risk of prostate cancer. The task force concluded that PSA screening at a younger age may lead to overdiagnosis and unnecessary interventions to determine whether benign asymptomatic prostate disease is actually cancer. Men at average risk who have a life expectancy of at least 10 years should be given the opportunity to discuss prostate cancer screening with their healthcare providers beginning at 50 years (Schieszer, 2018). Male patients should be provided information on the limited risks associated with slow-growing prostate tumors and potential harm from interventions or prostate surgery for optimal decision making. PSA results are most specific for cancer or prostate disease with serial measurements.

Thyroid Function Tests
NORMAL REFERENCE VALUES
TSH:
   0.4–4.0 mU/L
   0.5–3.0 mU/L (when treated for thyroid disorder)
Total triiodothyronine (free T3):
   100–200 ng/dL
Thyroxine (free T4):
   0.9–2.4 ng/dL

GENERAL INFORMATION. Proper function of the thyroid gland influences overall patient health. The thyroid gland secretes T3 and T4. TSH is released from the pituitary gland and controls the production of T3 and T4. Thyroid disease causes a variety of symptoms affecting quality of life. Approximately 5% to 10% of older adults have thyroid dysfunction without many of the normal symptoms. New onset of depression, atrial fibrillation, increasing apathy, and debilitation (frailty) may indicate abnormal thyroid hormone levels. As individuals age, some of these signs and symptoms are natural consequences of chronic disease and nutritional changes.

The level of TSH is inversely proportional to thyroid function: The higher the TSH level, the less active the thyroid gland.

Decreased TSH: **HYPERTHYROIDISM**
   (decreased TSH with increased free T4)

Graves' disease
Thyroid nodules
Thyroid adenoma
Multinodular goiter
Increased TSH: **HYPOTHYROIDISM** (increased TSH with decreased free T4)
Aging
Iodine insufficiency
Thyroiditis (Hashimoto's syndrome)
Autoimmune disease (increased prevalence if diagnosis of diabetes)
Thyroid surgery
Radiation therapy
Treatment for hypothyroidism
Pituitary disease (less common)

NUTRITIONAL INDICATORS

Older adults generally require and consume fewer total calories per day than younger adults. Carbohydrate intake often increases whereas fat and protein intakes generally decline in older people. This is associated with easy access to prepared carbohydrate products. Lean body mass and total body protein decrease, whereas the percentage of body fat increases with age.

It is crucial that the LPN recognizes that older adults are often at risk for malnutrition. This risk is due to decreased mobility; cognitive and sensory deficits; chewing and swallowing difficulties; and loss of appetite because of medications, illness, or the environment. The increased occurrence of wounds, infection, and dehydration creates additional nutritional demands on elderly persons; however, the most significant causes of poor nutrition in older people are poverty and chronic illness.

Because of these physiological and societal factors, it is important to have baseline laboratory values for the following indices of nutritional status and to understand their significance:

- Total serum proteins measure visceral protein stores.
- Serum albumin is the most widely used indicator of protein status.
- Serum transferrin is an indicator of protein stores.
- Serum cholesterol indicates lipid mass.
- Serum creatinine indicates lean body mass.

The hemoglobin, hematocrit, and lymphocyte count included in the CBC reflect the body's ability to transport nutrients and resist disease. Other

Focused Learning Chart: Elderly Persons Often are at Risk for Malnutrition. Possible Reasons are:

Physical	*Psychological*	*Environmental*
Chronic illness*	Depression	Poverty*
Decreased mobility	Cognitive deficits	Inability to travel to grocery store
Sensory deficits		
Loss of appetite due to medications		
Chewing and swallowing difficulties		

*The most significant causes of malnutrition in the elderly

common nutritional indicators are iron and micronutrients such as vitamins and minerals.

Nutritional deficiencies are often identified only when an associated problem, such as weight loss, poor wound healing, or weakness, occurs. Treating an underlying cause such as medication use or an illness may correct the deficiency. Otherwise, an increased dietary intake of the nutrient or vitamin and mineral supplements may be indicated.

Protein Indicators
Total Serum Protein
NORMAL REFERENCE VALUES
6.0–8.0 g/dL

GENERAL INFORMATION. The major blood proteins are serum albumin and the globulins, which together equal the total serum protein value. The measurement of total protein is performed by protein electrophoresis and aids in the diagnosis of protein deficiency; blood dyscrasia; and hepatic, GI, renal, and neoplastic diseases. In older adults, the lower the protein blood markers, the higher the likelihood the patient is frail. This marker indicates muscle mass, body stores, and overall skin and wound healing ability.

1. Low serum protein symptoms include:
   Dermatitis
   Hair thinning
   Muscle wasting
   Weakness
   Poor wound healing
2. Causes of increased total protein include:
   Dehydration
   Diabetic acidosis
   Infections
   Multiple myeloma

Monocytic leukemia
Chronic alcoholism
Chronic inflammatory disease
Edema
Tissue breakdown
Poor wound healing
3. Causes of decreased total protein include:
   Malnutrition
   Hepatic disease
   Renal disease
   GI disease
   Hodgkin's disease
   Trauma, such as burns, hemorrhage, and shock
   Hyperthyroidism
   Congestive heart failure

Albumin, Serum
Normal: 3.1–4.3 g/dL

GENERAL INFORMATION. Albumin values of less than 3.0 g/dL indicate protein malnutrition and are accompanied by an increased incidence of morbidity and mortality. Albumin maintains oncotic pressure and transports substances such as bilirubin, fatty acids, hormones, and drugs that are insoluble in water.

1. Albumin is increased in multiple myeloma and with dehydration.
2. Causes of decreased albumin include:
   Malnutrition
   Liver and/or renal disease
   Collagen diseases
   Rheumatoid arthritis
   Metastatic carcinoma
   Hyperthyroidism
   Essential hypertension
   Use of cytotoxic agents

Globulins, Serum
NORMAL REFERENCE VALUES
Normal: 2.6–4.1 g/dL

GENERAL INFORMATION. The four types of globulins identified by protein electrophoresis are found in differing quantities in various conditions. Alpha$_1$ globulin, alpha$_2$ globulin, and beta globulin are carrier proteins that transport lipids, hormones, and metals through the blood. Gamma globulin is an important component of the immune system.

Causes of increased globulins include:

Tuberculosis
Chronic syphilis
Subacute bacterial endocarditis
MI
Multiple myeloma
Collagen diseases
Rheumatoid arthritis
Diabetes mellitus
Hodgkin's disease

NURSING IMPLICATIONS. Because a consistent relationship between protein intake and serum albumin levels has not been established, a high-protein diet is not advised except for individuals with evidence of protein calorie malnutrition. Protein allowance is the same for older people as for younger people: 0.8 g/kg body weight. Protein should provide at least 12% of total calories for the healthy older person. The proteins from animal sources such as beef, poultry, fish, and dairy products are the most complete, whereas complementary vegetable proteins have less biological value. Some older people may need nutritional supplementation through oral, enteral, or parenteral routes if malnutrition is severe.

Iron Indicators
NORMAL REFERENCE VALUES
Iron, Serum
Male: 80–180 mg/dL
Female: 60–160 mg/dL

GENERAL INFORMATION. Iron appears in the plasma bound to the glycoprotein transferrin. Iron is essential in the production and function of hemoglobin and other compounds. Dietary iron is absorbed by the intestine and distributed in the body for synthesis, storage, and transport. The body has no mechanism for eliminating excessive iron; total body and bone marrow iron stores increase with advancing age, although serum iron may be depleted.

Serum iron values should be interpreted together with the total iron-binding capacity (TIBC) and serum ferritin. Bone marrow and liver biopsy and iron absorption or excretion studies may be necessary to obtain a definitive diagnosis in iron-related disease. A decrease in serum iron with an increased TIBC occurs in iron-deficiency anemia, which is most commonly caused in older adults by GI blood loss or malabsorption.

Ferritin, Serum
NORMAL REFERENCE VALUES
Normal: 20–400 ng/mL

GENERAL INFORMATION. Ferritin is an iron-storage protein. Serum ferritin level indicates the amount of available iron stored in the body. It is measured to distinguish between iron deficiency (decreased ferritin level) and chronic infection or inflammation (increased or normal ferritin level).

1. Causes of increased serum ferritin include:
   Liver disease
   Iron overload
   Leukemia
   Hodgkin's disease
   Chronic renal failure
   Hemolytic anemias
   Acute or chronic infection and inflammation
2. Ferritin is decreased only with chronic iron deficiency

TIBC (Transferrin), Serum
NORMAL REFERENCE VALUES
250–410 mg/dL

GENERAL INFORMATION. TIBC decreases with age and reflects the transferrin content of the serum. Transferrin, a beta globulin protein, transports circulating iron that is stored in various forms in the bone marrow, liver, and spleen. In protein-energy malnutrition, TIBC is less than 250 mg/dL (see previous discussion under serum iron).

Lipoproteins
NORMAL REFERENCE VALUES
Total plasma cholesterol:

Desired: <200 mg/dL
Borderline: 200–239 mg/dL
High: ≥240 mg/dL

High-density lipoprotein (HDL) cholesterol:

Desired: >35 mg/dL

Low-density lipoprotein (LDL) cholesterol:

Desired: 130 mg/dL
Borderline: 130–159 mg/dL
High: 160 mg/dL
Triglycerides: 160 mg/dL

GENERAL INFORMATION. Blood lipid and lipoprotein cholesterol levels, which are influenced by heredity, diet, and obesity, are directly related to atherosclerotic heart disease in elderly people. Higher HDL cholesterol, lower LDL cholesterol, and a decreased level of plasma triglycerides all are associated with decreased incidence of coronary heart disease.

In women, the increase in total plasma cholesterol with age is due primarily to an increase in LDL cholesterol. HDL cholesterol increases slightly in men older than 65 years but decreases in women of the same age. Without intervening therapy, the risk for coronary heart disease in elderly people gradually increases.

Total cholesterol and HDL cholesterol should be measured in screening tests for the elderly population. The findings of a high initial cholesterol value should be followed by two subsequent evaluations because there may be significant daily variations in values. Older persons may have a total cholesterol of less than 200 to 240 mg/dL but have elevated LDL cholesterol and decreased HDL cholesterol and so have an increased risk of coronary heart disease. Conversely, if HDL cholesterol is high, accounting for a total cholesterol level greater than 200 mg/dL, there is a reduced risk for coronary heart disease. Total cholesterol and HDL cholesterol may be obtained from non-fasting blood samples. Triglyceride levels are accurate only after a 12-hour fast. LDL cholesterol levels may be calculated after total cholesterol, HDL cholesterol, and triglycerides are known.

Lipid abnormalities are often genetic. Causes of secondary lipid elevation include:

Diets high in saturated fat or cholesterol
Excessive alcohol intake
Estrogen supplements
Thiazide diuretics
Beta blockers
Smoking
Uncontrolled diabetes
Hypothyroidism
Uremia

Corticosteroid use
Sedentary lifestyle
Morbid obesity

Cholesterol levels less than 120 to 156 mg/dL have been associated with increased mortality in nursing home residents. Causes of decreased cholesterol include:

Malnutrition
Hyperthyroidism
Chronic obstructive pulmonary disease

NURSING IMPLICATIONS
Weight control

• Increased physical activity
• Restriction of alcohol
• Cessation of smoking
• Restriction of dietary fat

Dietary restrictions should be cautiously initiated so that adequate calorie and protein intake is considered in the elderly. Drug therapy to control lipid levels may be beneficial in older persons with known coronary heart disease or high risk of disease.

DRUG MONITORING AND TOXICOLOGY

Drug monitoring is important when the margin of safety between therapeutic and toxic blood levels is narrow. Drug blood levels are useful guides in maintaining therapeutic levels and in identifying toxic levels of drugs. Not all drugs have a known therapeutic blood level even though toxic levels have been identified. Some drugs, such as amphetamines, are monitored through urine testing. Older adults metabolize and eliminate drugs more slowly than middle-aged adults, which heightens the importance of drug monitoring.

Three commonly monitored drugs—digoxin, theophylline, and phenytoin—are discussed because they require close observation by the LPN. Numerous classes of drugs are commonly checked for therapeutic or toxic levels. Review the list in Box 21.3. Refer to a basic laboratory manual for specific drug therapeutic and toxic values.

Digoxin Level, Serum
Normal Reference Values
Therapeutic: 0.5–2.0 ng/mL
Toxic: 2.5 ng/mL

Box 21.3
Commonly Monitored Medication Levels

Alcohol
Ethanol
Isopropanol (rubbing alcohol)
Methanol (antifreeze)

Amphetamines (Urine Testing)
Amphetamine
Dextroamphetamine
Methamphetamine (Desoxyn)
Phenmetrazine (Preludin)

Antiarrhythmics
Lidocaine (Xylocaine)
Procainamide (Pronestyl)
Propranolol (Inderal)
Quinidine (Quinaglute and others)
Verapamil (Calan, Isoptin)

Antibiotics
Kanamycin (Kantrex)
Netilmicin (Netromycin)
Tobramycin (Nebcin)
Vancomycin (Vanocin)

Anticonvulsants
Carbamazepine (Tegretol)
Ethosuximide (Zarontin)
Phenobarbital (Luminal)
Phenytoin (Dilantin)
Primidone (Mysoline)

Antidepressants
Amitriptyline
Nortriptyline (Pamelor, Aventyl)

Desipramine (Norpramin)
Doxepin (Sinequan and others)
Imipramine (Tofranil)
Lithium (Lithobid)

Barbiturates and Hypnotics
Pentobarbital (Nembutal)
Phenobarbital (Luminal)
Secobarbital (Seconal)

Bronchodilators
Aminophylline
Theophylline (Theo-Dur and others)

Cardiac Glycosides
Digoxin (Lanoxin) [Rarely used]

Hemoglobin Derivatives
Carboxyhemoglobin (Hg = CO)
Methemoglobin
Sulfhemoglobin

Non-narcotic Analgesics
Acetaminophen (Tylenol and others)
Salicylates (aspirin)

Phenothiazines
Chlorpromazine (Thorazine)
Prochlorperazine (Compazine)
Thioridazine (Mellaril)
Trifluoperazine (Stelazine)

General Information

Digoxin, used in the treatment of congestive heart failure and cardiac arrhythmias, has a prolonged half-life in elderly patients because of its reduced renal clearance. Serum digoxin level has a narrow therapeutic range, and digitalis toxicity is relatively common in older adults despite the availability of tests for serum drug levels.

Common side effects of digitalis toxicity include:

Visual changes
Headache
Nausea and vomiting
Weakness and fatigue

Weakness and fatigue are sometimes the only indicators of digitalis toxicity in an elderly person.

Quinidine significantly increases the serum level of digoxin. Consequently, the digoxin dosage must be reduced when both of these drugs are prescribed. Also, a change from tablet to elixir preparation of digoxin increases the absorption and serum level, so that the digoxin dose again needs to be reduced. Low serum potassium levels and high serum calcium levels increase the risk of serious arrhythmias in persons receiving digoxin therapy.

Nursing Implications

• Draw blood samples for determining serum digoxin levels at least 5 to 6 hours after the daily dose and preferably just before the next scheduled daily dose.
• Check the apical pulse for 1 full minute.

- Suspect digitalis toxicity when there is a sudden change in heart rhythm or pulse (especially a decrease).
- Withhold the medication and report to the physician when there is a sudden change in pulse or rhythm.
- Monitor the serum potassium level, especially if the person is taking diuretics.

Phenytoin (Dilantin), Serum

Normal Reference Values

Therapeutic: 10–20 µg/mL
Toxic: 30 µg/mL

General Information

Phenytoin, an anticonvulsant that also has antiarrhythmic properties, is metabolized by the liver and excreted in the bile and partially by the kidneys. Phenytoin has many potentially serious adverse reactions and side effects that necessitate monitoring of several parameters, including liver, kidney, thyroid, and hematologic functioning.

1. Potential adverse reactions and side effects include:
   Drowsiness
   Mental confusion
   Tremors
   Bradycardia
   Hypotension
   Photophobia
   Blurred vision
   Nausea
   Vomiting
   Epigastric pain
   Abnormal blood counts
   Fever
   Skin eruptions
   Pneumonitis
2. Acute kidney or liver dysfunction results in toxic drug levels.

3. Causes for decreased serum levels include:
   Chronic alcohol abuse
   Antacids
   Antihistamines
   Antineoplastics
   Barbiturates
   Excess of folic acid
   Rifampin
4. Causes for increased serum levels include:
   Acute intake of alcohol
   Anticoagulants
   Aminosalicylic acid
   Benzodiazepines
   Cimetidine
   Dexamethasone
   Estrogens
   Isoniazid
   Methylphenidate
   Phenothiazines
   Salicylates
   Sulfonamides
   Phenylbutazone

Nursing Implications

- Liver and thyroid function tests, blood counts, and urinalysis are recommended before the initiation of therapy, at monthly intervals during early therapy, and at regular intervals thereafter.
- Lower doses are given to older adults and individuals with liver or kidney impairment.
- When phenytoin is given intravenously, vital signs and cardiac function must be monitored closely.
- Serum concentrations of magnesium, folic acid, vitamin D, and vitamin K may be decreased with phenytoin therapy and should be monitored.
- Symptoms of low serum magnesium may mimic symptoms of phenytoin toxicity.

CASE STUDY SOLUTIONS

Discussion Question Solutions

1. What potential concerns do you have based on Mrs. J.'s history, physical exam, current health problems, and urinalysis results?
   Urinalysis results
   - Glucose in the urine
   - Trace protein
   - WBCs >10
   - Trace blood
   - Nitrites positive
   - Increased specific gravity
   - Amber color, not clear
   History, physical exam, and health problems:
   - Recent falls and osteoporosis
   - Concertation /consciousness / memory changes

CASE STUDY SOLUTIONS—cont'd

- Decreased appetite and fluid intake (hemoconcentration)
- Possible orthostatic hypotension because of her lower BP than on previous visits

2. What other laboratory tests might be ordered to assess Mrs. J.'s health status?
   - CBC to assess for anemia and infection
   - Vitamin D and calcium level
   - Protein or albumin level to assess nutritional status
   - Blood glucose to assess current level because of her diabetes
   - HbA1c to measure overall control of diabetes in recent months
   - A CMP could be ordered to include BUN and creatinine as well as Na and K to assess renal and electrolyte status
   - TSH with possible free T4 to determine if there is thyroid disease
   - A urine culture should be ordered based on pyuria.

3. What nursing actions or education might you provide for Mrs. J.?
   - Safety measures to prevent falls, such as having Mrs. J. call for assistance before getting up to go to the restroom while in the emergency department (ED). If hospitalized, she should have the nurse or CNA help her.
   - Advise her to change positions slowly from lying to sitting and then from sitting to standing.
   - Consider a bedside commode based on recent changes such as falling and level of consciousness changes.
   - Hydrate while in the ED (IV fluids or po fluids as directed).
   - If nausea occurs, notify the physician.
   - Withhold the BP medications based on low BP and hemoconcentration per physician orders in the ED.
   - Report BP to supervising RN, physician, or nurse practitioner.
   - Document stool(s) for occult blood because she is taking a nonsteroidal anti-inflammatory drug and aspirin (possible GI bleed). Describe consistency to determine constipation from decreased food and fluid intake.
   - If the CBC indicates iron-deficiency anemia, the physician will probably discontinue the NSAID and maybe the aspirin.

   Acetaminophen (Tylenol) may be used on a regular schedule to control joint pain.

   If anemic discuss medicines and foods appropriate for an older adult to increase iron level.

Key Points

- Laboratory tests are part of routine nursing care for older adults. Laboratory findings reflect the condition of an individual older adult and their specific circumstances. Abnormal laboratory values may indicate disease states or factors such as dehydration or medication side effects affecting older adult health and wellness. Nurses play a key role in obtaining quality lab specimens and monitoring lab results for their patients.
- Simple and common laboratory screening tests performed on elderly people include urinalysis; urine microalbumin; stool guaiac; RBC and WBC determination in the complete blood count (CBC); platelets; sedimentation rate; PT and INR; glucose and HbA1c; serum electrolytes; BUN and creatinine; uric acid; liver function tests (enzymes); thyroid function tests; nutritional indicators of total protein, albumin, and globulin; iron; lipids; and monitoring of drug levels.
- Urinalysis is one of the most common point-of-care and diagnostic lab tests performed for older adults to assess for a variety of potential health issues. The test involves a urine dipstick, assessment of urine characteristics such as color and odor, and urine microscopic examination.
- A two-step skin test is now the standard for tuberculosis screening. QuantiFERON TB is a new serum blood test effective for tuberculosis screening, especially for those who were previous health-care workers or who have lived in endemic areas.
- The CBC is the most common lab test to assess important information about cellular elements in the blood. It provides information about overall patient health. The CBC with differential

includes: RBC count, hemoglobin, hematocrit, RBC indices, WBC count, WBC types (neutrophils, eosinophils, basophils, lymphocytes, and monocytes), and platelets. It often includes a sedimentation rate, which is known to increase between the fifth and sixth decades of life.

- Vitamin D and folic acid levels are monitored in older adults because of frequent GI disease, malnutrition, and the effect of vitamin D on bone health.
- Coagulation tests include PT, PTT, and INR. PT is assessed more frequently in acute care settings. The INR is now the standard marker for assessing and managing anticoagulation therapy in the outpatient, extended care, or resident care organizations.
- Blood glucose is frequently measured as part of a comprehensive metabolic profile or as an individual finger stick value. HbA1c measures overall glycemic control for 3 to 4 months.
- Other components of a metabolic profile include assessment of serum electrolytes (Na, K, Ca, HCO, Mg, Cl, and HPO_4); BUN; creatinine; bilirubin; uric acid; and liver function tests (ALT, AST, and ALP).

- PSA is a protein marker useful in identifying prostate disease or cancer. It is no longer recommended as an annual screening test but still is an effective screening marker for specific men.
- TSH, total triiodothyronine (free T3), and thyroxine (free T4) are measured to assess thyroid metabolic regulation and optimal body function.
- Older adults are often at risk for nutritional deficits or changes for a variety of reasons (physiological, psychological, and socioeconomic). Side effects of medications may affect nutritional status. Serum assessment of total proteins, albumin, globulins, iron, ferritin, transferrin, and cholesterol (HDL and LDL) allow nurses to understand overall health status related to nutritional status.
- Monitoring the presence or absence of drugs as well as documenting levels of specified drugs allows health-care providers and nurses to manage patients effectively. Therapeutic levels of drugs are established to ensure safe effective interventions. Some drugs have small therapeutic ranges and toxicity is possible if drug levels are too high. Digoxin and phenytoin are two drugs that are frequently monitored in older adults.

Review Questions

1. All laboratory test results for older adults should be:
   1. Evaluated against younger clients.
   2. Evaluated against the other older adults on the unit.
   3. Evaluated against the client's total clinical situation.
   4. Evaluated against the person's CBC results.

2. With the incidence of tuberculosis (TB) increasing among elderly people, it is critical for the LPN to know that:
   1. TB skin tests are inaccurate on people older than age 65.
   2. When there is no initial reaction to the TB skin test in elderly people, it should be given again 1 week later.
   3. It is unnecessary and expensive to do TB screening on nursing home residents.
   4. Isoniazid is not an effective TB drug of choice for the elderly.

3. What two tests determine if an individual is on the right dose of warfarin (Coumadin)?
   1. PT and PTT.
   2. INR and PTT.
   3. BNP and INR.
   4. INR and PT.

4. Potassium deficiency develops:
   1. Slowly in the older adult.
   2. In the kidneys.
   3. Rapidly because there is no way to conserve potassium.
   4. Only when using diuretics.

5. Every elderly person with a low serum albumin level should be:
   1. Put on a high-protein diet.
   2. Put on bedrest.
   3. Put on a diet of 12% complete proteins.
   4. Put on vitamin supplements.

ANSWERS 1, 3; 2, 2; 3, 4; 4, 3; 5, 3

APPENDIX A
Sample Advance Directives: Living Will and Power of Attorney for Health Care

The following document is reproduced courtesy of Caring Info, 1731 King Street, Suite 100, Alexandria, VA 22314. It is a sample for the state of California. To get a similar document for your state, please go to Caring Info's Web site at www.caringinfo.org or call 800-658-8898.

INTRODUCTION TO YOUR CALIFORNIA ADVANCE HEALTH CARE DIRECTIVE

This packet contains a legal document, a **California Advance Health Care Directive,** that protects your right to refuse medical treatment you do not want, or to request treatment you do want, in the event you lose the ability to make decisions yourself. You may complete any or all of the first four parts, depending on your advance planning needs. You must complete part 5.

Part 1 is a **Power of Attorney for Health Care**. This part lets you name someone (an agent) to make decisions about your health care. Unless otherwise written in your advance directive, your power of attorney for health care becomes effective when your primary doctor determines that you lack the ability to understand the nature and consequences of your health care decisions or the ability to make and communicate your health care decisions. If you want your agent to make health care decisions for you now, even though you are still capable of making health care decisions, you can include this instruction in your power of attorney for health care designation.

Part 2 includes your **Individual Instructions**. This is your state's living will. It lets you state your wishes about health care in the event that you can no longer speak for yourself and you may limit the individual instructions to take effect only if a specified condition arises.

Part 3 allows you to express your wishes regarding organ donation.

Part 4 of this form lets you designate a physician to have primary responsibility for your health care.

Part 5 contains the signature and witnessing provisions so that your document will be effective.

This form does not expressly address mental illness. If you would like to make advance care plans regarding mental illness, you should talk to your physician and an attorney about an advance directive tailored to your needs.

Note: These documents will be legally binding only if the person completing them is a competent adult, who is 18 years of age or older, or an emancipated minor.

INSTRUCTIONS FOR YOUR CALIFORNIA ADVANCE HEALTH CARE DIRECTIVE

How do I make my advance health care directive legal?

You must sign and date your advance directive or direct an adult to do so for you if you are unable to sign it yourself.

Your signature must be witnessed by or you must acknowledge your signature before a notary public or two adult witnesses. Your two adult witnesses may not be
- your health care provider or an employee of your health care provider,
- the operator or an employee of a community care facility,
- the operator or an employee of a residential care facility for the elderly, or
- the person you have appointed as an agent, if you have appointed an agent.

In addition, one of your witnesses must be unrelated to you by blood, marriage, or adoption and not entitled to any portion of your estate.

If you are a patient in a skilled nursing facility when you execute your advance directive, one of your witnesses must be a patient advocate or ombudsman.

Whom should I appoint as my agent?

Your agent is the person you appoint to make decisions about your health care if you become unable to make those decisions yourself. Your agent may be a family member or a close friend whom you trust to make serious decisions. The person you name as your agent should clearly understand your wishes and be willing to accept the responsibility of making health care decisions for you.

Your agent cannot be
- your supervising health care provider,
- the operator of a community care facility or residential care facility where you are receiving care, or
- the employee of a health care institution where you are receiving care or employee of a community care facility or residential care facility where you are receiving care, unless:
    o the employee is related to you by blood, marriage, or adoption,
    o the employee is your registered domestic partner, or
    o the employee is your coworker at the facility or institution.

If you have a conservator appointed for you as part of involuntary commitment proceedings under the Lanterman-Petris-Short Act, that conservator cannot be appointed as your agent unless you are represented by a lawyer who signs a certificate stating that you have been advised of your rights. If this applies to you, you should talk with your lawyer about your rights, the applicable law, and the potential consequences involved.

On the other hand, you may include in your advance directive a nomination for the individual appointed as your conservator, if necessary. The court will consider your nomination in any protective proceeding.

You can appoint a second and third person as your alternate agents. An alternate agent will step in if the person(s) you name as agent is/are unable, unwilling or unavailable to act for you.

Should I add personal instructions to my advance directive?

One of the strongest reasons for naming an agent is to have someone who can respond flexibly as your medical situation changes and deal with situations that you did not foresee. If you add instructions to this document it may help your agent carry out your wishes, but be careful that you do not unintentionally restrict your agent's power to act in your best interest. In any event, be sure to talk with your agent about your future health care and describe what you consider to be an acceptable "quality of life."

What if I change my mind?

Except for the appointment of your agent, you may revoke any portion or this entire advance directive at any time and in any way that communicates your intent to revoke. This could be by telling your agent or physician that you revoke, by signing a revocation, or simply by tearing up your advance directive.

In order to revoke your agent's appointment, you must either tell your supervising health care provider of your intent to revoke or revoke your agent's appointment in a signed writing.

If you execute a new advance directive, it will revoke the old advance directive to the extent of any conflict between the two documents.

Unless you specify otherwise in Part 2, if you designate your spouse as your agent, that designation will automatically be revoked by divorce or annulment of your marriage.

What other important facts should I know?

Your agent, if you appoint one, does not have authority to authorize convulsive treatment, psychosurgery, sterilization, or abortion, or to have you committed or placed in a mental health treatment facility.

CALIFORNIA ADVANCE HEALTH CARE DIRECTIVE - PAGE 1 OF 13

Explanation

You have the right to give instructions about your own health care. You also have the right to name someone else to make health care decisions for you. This form lets you do either or both of these things. It also lets you express your wishes regarding donation of organs and the designation of your primary physician. If you use this form, you may complete or modify all or any part of it. You are free to use a different form.

Part 1 of this form is a **power of attorney for health care**. Part 1 lets you name another individual as agent to make health care decisions for you if you become incapable of making your own decisions or if you want someone else to make those decisions for you now even though you are still capable. You may name an alternate agent to act for you if your first choice is not willing, able, or reasonably available to make decisions for you. (Your agent may not be an operator or employee of a community care facility or a residential care facility where you are receiving care, or an employee of the health care institution where you are receiving care, unless your agent is related to you, is your registered domestic partner, or is a co-worker. Your supervising health care provider can never act as your agent.)

Unless the form you sign limits the authority of your agent, your agent may make all health care decisions for you. This form has a place for you to limit the authority of your agent. You need not limit the authority of your agent if you wish to rely on your agent for all health care decisions that may have to be made. If you choose not to limit the authority of your agent, your agent will have the right to:

(a)   Consent or refuse consent to any care, treatment, service, or procedure to maintain, diagnose, or otherwise affect a physical or mental condition;

(b)   Select or discharge health care providers and institutions;

(c)   Approve or disapprove diagnostic tests, surgical procedures and programs of medication;

(d)   Direct the provision, withholding, or withdrawal of artificial nutrition and hydration and all other forms of health care, including cardiopulmonary resuscitation; and

(e)   Make anatomical gifts, authorize an autopsy, and direct the disposition of your remains.

CALIFORNIA ADVANCE HEALTH CARE DIRECTIVE - PAGE 2 OF 13

Explanation Continued

Part 2 of this form lets you give specific **instructions** about any aspect of your health care, whether or not you appoint an agent. Choices are provided for you to express your wishes regarding the provision, withholding, or withdrawal of treatment to keep you alive, as well as the provision of pain relief. Space is provided for you to add to the choices you have made or for you to write out any additional wishes. If you are satisfied to allow your agent to determine what is best for you in making end-of-life decisions, you need not fill out part 2 of this form.

Part 3 of this form lets you express an intention to donate your bodily organs and tissues following your death.

Part 4 of this form lets you designate a physician to have primary responsibility for your health care.

After completing this form, sign and date the form in **Part 5**. The form must be signed by two qualified witnesses or acknowledged before a notary public. Give a copy of the signed and completed form to your physician, to any other health care providers you may have, to any health care institution at which you are receiving care, and to any health care agents you have named. You should talk to the person you have named as agent and alternate agent(s) to make sure that he or she understands your wishes and is willing to take the responsibility.

You have the right to revoke this advance health care directive or replace this form at any time.

CALIFORNIA ADVANCE HEALTH CARE DIRECTIVE — PAGE 3 OF 13

PART 1: POWER OF ATTORNEY FOR HEALTH CARE

INSTRUCTIONS

PRINT THE NAME,
HOME ADDRESS
AND HOME AND
WORK TELEPHONE
NUMBERS OF YOUR
PRIMARY
AGENT

PRINT THE NAME,
HOME ADDRESS
AND HOME AND
WORK TELEPHONE
NUMBERS OF YOUR
FIRST ALTERNATE
AGENT
(OPTIONAL)

PRINT THE NAME,
HOME ADDRESS
AND HOME AND
WORK TELEPHONE
NUMBERS OF YOUR
SECOND
ALTERNATE
AGENT
(OPTIONAL)

© 2005 National
Hospice and
Palliative Care
Organization
2017 Revised.

(1) DESIGNATION OF AGENT: I designate the following individual as my agent to make health care decisions for me:

_____

(Name of individual you choose as agent)

_____

(address)   (city) (state)   (zip code)

_____

(home phone)   (work phone)

OPTIONAL: If I revoke my agent's authority or if my agent is not willing, able, or reasonably available to make a health care decision for me, I designate as my first alternate agent:

_____

(Name of individual you choose as first alternate agent)

_____

(address)

_____

(city)   (state)   (zip code)

_____

(home phone)   (work phone)

OPTIONAL: If I revoke the authority of my agent and first alternate agent or if neither is willing, able, or reasonably available to make a health care decision for me, I designate as my second alternate agent:

_____

(Name of individual you choose as second alternate agent)

_____

(address)

_____

(city)   (state)   (zip code)

_____

(home phone)   (work phone)

CALIFORNIA ADVANCE HEALTH CARE DIRECTIVE — PAGE 4 OF 13

ADD INSTRUCTIONS HERE ONLY IF YOU WANT TO LIMIT THE POWER OF YOUR AGENT

(2) AGENT'S AUTHORITY: My agent is authorized to make all health care decisions for me, including decisions to provide, withhold, or withdraw artificial nutrition and hydration, and all other forms of health care to keep me alive, except as I state here:

_____

_____

_____

_____

(Add additional sheets if needed.)

(3) WHEN AGENT'S AUTHORITY BECOMES EFFECTIVE: My agent's authority becomes effective when my primary physician determines that I am unable to make my own health care decisions unless I mark the following box. If I mark this box [   ], my agent's authority to make health care decisions for me takes effect immediately.

INITIAL THE BOX IF YOU WISH YOUR AGENT'S AUTHORITY TO BECOME EFFECTIVE IMMEDIATELY

(4) AGENT'S OBLIGATION: My agent shall make health care decisions for me in accordance with this power of attorney for health care, any instructions I give in Part 2 of this form, and my other wishes to the extent known to my agent. To the extent my wishes are unknown, my agent shall make health care decisions for me in accordance with what my agent determines to be in my best interest. In determining my best interest, my agent shall consider my personal values to the extent known to my agent.

CROSS OUT AND INITIAL ANY STATEMENTS IN PARAGRAPHS 4, 5, OR 6 THAT DO NOT REFLECT YOUR WISHES

(5) AGENT'S POSTDEATH AUTHORITY: My agent is authorized to make anatomical gifts, authorize an autopsy, and direct disposition of my remains, except as I state here, in paragraph (2) above, or in Part 3 of this form:

_____

_____

_____

(6) NOMINATION OF CONSERVATOR: If a conservator of my person needs to be appointed for me by a court, I nominate the agent designated in this form. If that agent is not willing, able, or reasonably available to act as conservator, I nominate the alternate agents whom I have named, in the order designated.

CALIFORNIA ADVANCE HEALTH CARE DIRECTIVE — PAGE 5 OF 13

PART 2: INSTRUCTIONS FOR HEALTH CARE

If you fill out this part of the form, you may strike any wording you do not want.

(7) END-OF-LIFE DECISIONS: I direct that my health care providers and others involved in my care provide, withhold, or withdraw treatment in accordance with the choice I have marked below: (**Initial only one box**)

[   ] (a) **Choice NOT To Prolong Life**
I do not want my life to be prolonged if (1) I have an incurable and irreversible condition that will result in my death within a relatively short time, (2) I become unconscious and, to a reasonable degree of medical certainty, I will not regain consciousness, or (3) the likely risks and burdens of treatment would outweigh the expected benefits,

OR

[   ] (b) **Choice To Prolong Life**
I want my life to be prolonged as long as possible within the limits of generally accepted health care standards.

(8) RELIEF FROM PAIN: Except as I state in the following space, I direct that treatment for alleviation of pain or discomfort should be provided at all times even if it hastens my death:

_____

_____

_____

_____

_____

_____

_____

_____

INITIAL THE PARAGRAPH THAT BEST REFLECTS YOUR WISHES REGARDING LIFE-SUPPORT MEASURES

ADD INSTRUCTIONS HERE ONLY IF YOU WANT TO LIMIT PAIN RELIEF OR COMFORT CARE

CALIFORNIA ADVANCE HEALTH CARE DIRECTIVE — PAGE 6 OF 13

ADD OTHER
INSTRUCTIONS, IF
ANY, REGARDING
YOUR ADVANCE
CARE PLANS

THESE
INSTRUCTIONS CAN
FURTHER ADDRESS
YOUR HEALTH CARE
PLANS, SUCH AS
YOUR WISHES
REGARDING
HOSPICE
TREATMENT, BUT
CAN ALSO ADDRESS
OTHER ADVANCE
PLANNING ISSUES,
SUCH AS YOUR
BURIAL WISHES

ATTACH
ADDITIONAL PAGES
IF NEEDED

© 2005 National
Hospice and
Palliative Care
Organization
2017 Revised.

(9) OTHER WISHES: (If you do not agree with any of the optional choices above and wish to write your own, or if you wish to add to the instructions you have given above, you may do so here.) I direct that:

_____

_____

_____

_____

_____

_____

_____

_____

_____

_____

_____

_____

_____

_____

_____

(Add additional sheets if needed.)

CALIFORNIA ADVANCE HEALTH CARE DIRECTIVE — PAGE 7 OF 13

PART 3: DONATION OF ORGANS AT DEATH
(OPTIONAL)

ORGAN
DONATION
(OPTIONAL)

(10) Upon my death: (initial applicable box)

INITIAL THE BOX
THAT AGREES WITH
YOUR WISHES
ABOUT ORGAN
DONATION

[   ] (a) I do not give any of my organs, tissues, or parts and do
            not want my agent, conservator, or family to make a
            donation on my behalf,

[   ] (b) I give any needed organs, tissues, or parts,

OR

[   ] (c) I give the following organs, tissues, or parts only

_____
_____
_____

STRIKE THROUGH
ANY USES YOU DO
NOT AGREE TO

My gift is for the following purposes:
(strike any of the following you do not want)
        (1) Transplant
        (2) Therapy
        (3) Research
        (4) Education

CALIFORNIA ADVANCE HEALTH CARE DIRECTIVE — PAGE 8 OF 13

PART 4: PRIMARY PHYSICIAN
(OPTIONAL)

PRINT THE NAME, ADDRESS AND TELEPHONE NUMBER OF YOUR PRIMARY PHYSICIAN (OPTIONAL)

(11) I designate the following physician as my primary physician:

_____
(name of physician)

_____
(address)

_____
(city)   (state)   (zip code)

_____
(phone)

PRINT THE NAME, ADDRESS AND TELEPHONE NUMBER OF YOUR ALTERNATE PRIMARY PHYSICIAN (OPTIONAL)

OPTIONAL: If the physician I have designated above is not willing, able, or reasonably available to act as my primary physician, I designate the following physician as my primary physician:

_____
(name of physician)

_____
(address)

_____
(city)   (state)   (zip code)

_____
(phone)

(12) EFFECT OF COPY: A copy of this form has the same effect as the original.

© 2005 National Hospice and Palliative Care Organization 2017 Revised.

CALIFORNIA ADVANCE HEALTH CARE DIRECTIVE - PAGE 9 OF 13

PART 5: EXECUTION

This Health Care Directive will not be valid unless it is EITHER:

(A)   Signed by two (2) qualified adult witnesses who are personally known to you or to whom you have proven your identity by convincing evidence and who are present when you sign or acknowledge your signature. Your witnesses may not be
- your health care provider or an employee of your health care provider,
- the operator or an employee of a community care facility,
- the operator or an employee of a residential care facility for the elderly, or
- the person you have appointed as an agent, if you have appointed an agent.

In addition, one of your witnesses must be unrelated to you by blood, marriage, or adoption and not entitled to any portion of your estate. (Use Alternative 1, below, if you decide to have your signature witnessed.)

OR

(B)   Witnessed by a notary. (Use Alternative 2, below [page 12], if you decide to have your signature notarized.)

If you are a patient in a skilled nursing facility when you execute your advance directive, one of your witnesses must be a patient advocate or ombudsman. This witness must sign the statement on page 13, even if you have had your advance directive notarized.

CALIFORNIA ADVANCE HEALTH CARE DIRECTIVE - PAGE 10 OF 13

OPTION 1: Sign before a Witness

(date)	(sign your name)

(print your name)

(address)

(city)	(state)	(zip code)

SIGN AND DATE THE DOCUMENT AND THEN PRINT YOUR NAME AND ADDRESS

STATEMENT OF WITNESSES

I declare under penalty of perjury under the laws of California (1) that the individual who signed or acknowledged this advance health care directive is personally known to me, or that the individual's identity was proven to me by convincing evidence, (2) that the individual signed or acknowledged this advance directive in my presence, (3) that the individual appears to be of sound mind and under no duress, fraud, or undue influence, (4) that I am not a person appointed as an agent by this advance directive, and (5) that I am not the individual's health care provider, an employee of the individual's health care provider, the operator of a community care facility, an employee of an operator of a community care facility, the operator of a residential care facility for the elderly, nor an employee of an operator of a residential care facility for the elderly.

WITNESSING PROCEDURE

BOTH OF YOUR WITNESSES MUST AGREE WITH THIS STATEMENT

First Witness:

(date)	(signature of witness)

(printed name of witness)

(address)

(city)	(state)	(zip code)

ONE WITNESS MUST ALSO SIGN THE STATEMENT ON PAGE 11

Second Witness:

(date)	(signature of witness)

(printed name of witness)

(address)

(city)	(state)	(zip code)

HAVE YOUR WITNESSES SIGN AND DATE THE DOCUMENT AND THEN PRINT THEIR NAME AND ADDRESS

© 2005 National Hospice and Palliative Care Organization 2017 Revised.

CALIFORNIA ADVANCE HEALTH CARE DIRECTIVE - PAGE 11 OF 13

ONE OF YOUR WITNESSES MUST ALSO SIGN THIS STATEMENT

ADDITIONAL WITNESS STATEMENT
I further declare under penalty of perjury under the laws of California that I am not related to the individual executing this advance health care directive by blood, marriage, or adoption, and, to the best of my knowledge, I am not entitled to any part of the individual's estate upon his or her death under a will now existing or by operation of law.

_____   _____
             (date)   (signature of witness)

CALIFORNIA ADVANCE HEALTH CARE DIRECTIVE - PAGE 12 OF 13

ALTERNATIVE NO. 2: NOTARY PUBLIC

SIGN AND DATE
THE DOCUMENT
AND THEN PRINT
YOUR NAME AND
ADDRESS

_____   _____
(date)   (sign your name)

_____
(print your name)

_____
(address)

_____
(city)   (state)   (zip code)

A NOTARY PUBLIC
MUST FILL OUT
THIS PORTION OF
THE FORM

State of California   )
) SS.
County of _____)

On _____ before me,_____
                                       (insert name of notary public)
personally appeared _____,
                          (insert the name of principal)

Who proved to me on the basis of satisfactory evidence to be the
person(s) is/are subscribed to the within instrument and acknowledged to
me that he/she/they executed the same in his/her/their authorized
capacity(ies), and that by his/her their signature(s) on the instrument the
person(s), or the entity upon behalf of which the person(s) acted,
executed the instrument.

I certify under PENALTY OF PERJURY under the laws of the state of
California that the foregoing paragraph is true and correct.

WITNESS my hand and official seal.

NOTARY SEAL

_____
(signature of notary)

CALIFORNIA ADVANCE HEALTH CARE DIRECTIVE - PAGE 13 OF 13

THIS SECTION
MUST BE
COMPLETED
BY A PATIENT
ADVOCATE OR
OMBUDSMAN IF
YOU ARE A
RESIDENT IN A
SKILLED NURSING
FACILITY

STATEMENT OF PATIENT ADVOCATE OR OMBUDSMAN
I declare under penalty of perjury under the laws of California that I am
a patient advocate or ombudsman as designated by the State
Department of Aging and that I am serving as witness as required by
section 4675 of the Probate Code.

_____   _____
(date)   (signature)

_____
(printed name)

_____
(address)

_____
(city)   (state)   (zip code)

Courtesy of Caring Info
1731 King St., Suite 100, Alexandria, VA 22314
www.caringinfo.org, 800/658-8898

Glossary

Abuse: Cruel or inhumane treatment of an individual, often with repetition.

Activities of daily living (ADLs): The daily tasks performed by an individual that maintain independence, including hygiene, dressing, feeding, and mobility (Taber's Cyclopedic Medical Dictionary, 2017).

Acute condition: A condition characterized by an abrupt onset of symptoms that generally last less than one month.

Adult day services (ADS): Nonresidential facilities available in many communities that provide supervised activities for older adults during the day.

Advance directive: A legal document made and signed by a competent adult regarding life-sustaining issues and other concerns related to end-of-life care.

Adverse drug reaction (ADR): Any effect of a drug other than the intended therapeutic effect. Adverse drug reactions can range in severity from minor expected side effects to life-threatening effects.

Ageism: A systematic stereotyping of and discrimination against people simply because they are old.

Albumin: A group of simple proteins distributed in plant and animal tissues. Measurement of this metabolic profile substance indicates the body's ability to keep fluid from leaking into the tissues and maintain ideal osmotic pressure. Albumin levels indicate overall health and nutritional status.

Anxiety disorder: A mental health condition in which the individual feels worried, nervous, or uneasy, often accompanied with uncertainty.

Anxiety: Generalized unpleasant feeling of apprehension.

Assisted living environment: A residential facility that provides independent older adults assistance in performing activities of daily living and medication management.

Asymptomatic bacteriuria: Presence of bacteria in the urine without symptoms. It is sometimes associated with inflammation and bladder spasms.

Auscultation: Listening for sounds within the body (Taber's Cyclopedic Medical Dictionary, 2017).

Bullying: Consistent and repetitive actions and behaviors towards vulnerable individuals with the intention of intimidation, embarrassment, and isolation (Taber's Cyclopedic Medical Dictionary, 2017).

Care area assessment (CAA): Review of one or more of the 20 problem areas included in the minimum data set (MDS) that is initiated by certain responses on the MDS (CMS, 2017).

Care area trigger (CAT): A response on the MDS that indicates conditions or issues affecting residents (CMS, 2017).

Catheter-associated urinary tract infection: A urinary tract infection associated with long-term use of an indwelling urinary catheter.

Chronic condition: A condition that lasts longer than three months; may develop from an acute condition.

Chronic disease: A disease that generally lasts a long length of time (usually longer than three months).

Circadian rhythm: Synchronization of the body's processes to a 24-hour cycle.

Climate of caring: An approach to care that includes the people in the environment and the environmental tone and atmosphere.

Cognition: Thinking skills that include language use, calculation, perception, memory, awareness, judgment, reasoning, learning, intellect, social skills, and imagination (Taber's Cyclopedic Medical Dictionary, 2017).

Community-based care: Care provided to individuals in a community clinic, dialysis center, or physician's office usually under the supervision of a physician.

Complete protein: A protein that comes from an animal source.

Complex carbohydrate: A carbohydrate that breaks down slowly in the body.

Confidentiality: The maintenance of privacy by not sharing patient information to a third party.

Contracture: Fibrosis of connective tissue in skin, fascia, muscle, or a joint capsule that prevents normal mobility of the related tissue or joint.

Cultural sensitivity: Sensitivity to the cultural, philosophical, religious, and social preferences of people of varying ethnicities or nationalities.

Delegation: Assignment of any responsibility or authority to another person (normally from a manager to a subordinate) to carry out specific activities.

Delirium: Acute, reversible state of disorientation, inattention, and confusion (Taber's Cyclopedic Medical Dictionary, 2017).

Delusion: False, fixed idea, or belief.

Dementia: A progressive, irreversible decline in mental function (Taber's Cyclopedic Medical Dictionary, 2017).

Depression: Any of several mood disorders marked by loss of interest or pleasure in living (Taber's Cyclopedic Medical Dictionary, 2017).

Diagnostic tests: Tests performed to establish a diagnosis and are ordered based on the presence of specific symptom clusters and recent subjective/objective report of a positive screening test.

Disaster: A sudden event that can cause extreme damage or loss of life caused by an accident or natural causes.

Disorientation: State of not knowing what day or time it is, or not knowing where one is.

Elder abuse: Abuse of someone older than age 65 years. It may include physical violence, financial exploitation, intimidation, isolation, and neglect.

Emergency: An unexpected serious occurrence that may cause a great number of injuries, which usually require immediate attention.

End-of-life issues: Plans and processes for preparing for end of life, including treatment and care planning for how an individual wishes to spend his or her last days.

Environments of care model: A framework for care in which the patient environment is composed of three elements: the building or space in which care is given and how it is arranged; the equipment used to assist patients and facilitate work; and the people in the area where care is given, including workers and residents (The Joint Commission, 2015).

Essential amino acid: An amino acid that the body cannot make in sufficient quantities for metabolic needs and usually comes from the diet.

Ethics: The study of moral actions and values.

Evaluation: A rating or assessment.

Extrinsic factors: Environmental conditions that can lead to falls, such as inadequate lighting, rugs, or inadequate footwear.

Fat-soluble vitamin: A vitamin that is absorbed in the presence of fat.

Function: A term that refers to an older adult's ability to perform activities of daily living (ADLs) and independent activities of daily living (IADLs).

Functional protein: A protein that helps the body perform the activities that keep the body alive. Examples of functional proteins include hemoglobin and antibodies.

Functional status: The features of an individual's health history related to ability to care for oneself and used in goal setting.

Functionality: The ability to continue to live one's preferred lifestyle without disruption.

Geriatrics: The medical specialty that deals with the diagnosis and treatment of older adults.

Gerontology: The study of the complex world of human aging.

Gerotranscendence: A transition from a materialistic and rationalistic perspective to a more cosmic and transcendent view of life accompanying the process of aging. People experience a redefinition of time, place, life and death, and a redefinition of the self throughout the aging process (Tornstam, 2005).

Glycolated hemoglobin (HbA1c): A blood test used to monitor overall glycemic (glucose) control over a period of time of 100 to 120 days. It is a useful test indicating effectiveness of diabetes treatments and patient adherence to diet and lifestyle recommendations.

Grief: A normal and natural emotional reaction to loss or profound life change of any kind.

Hallucination: False sensory impression, often seeing or hearing something that is not there.

Health assessment: The process of evaluating a patient's condition that includes history, lab values, clinical data, and the patient's account of symptoms.

Health promotion: The process of improving one's health through the use of available programs, education, and activities.

Hemoconcentration: An increase in the number of red blood cells resulting from a decrease in the volume of plasma. It is often associated with tissue fluid loss or inadequate fluid intake.

Hepatitis C: An infection affecting the liver caused by the hepatitis C virus. In most people who do not receive treatment, the infection persists and may cause chronic liver disease.

Holism: The belief that individuals function as an entire unit and cannot be reduced to the sum of their parts.

Holistic assessment: An assessment that includes all aspects of the patient, not just information related to the particular problem expressed.

Holistic care: Caring for the body, mind, socialization, and spirit of an individual.

Holistic wellness: The achievement of balance in the spiritual, physical, and mental aspects of life in balance. It is not just the absence of disease but being in optimal health for that individual.

Home healthcare: Care that takes place in a person's home.

Hospice care: An interdisciplinary program of palliative care and supportive service that addresses the physical, spiritual, social, and economic needs of terminally ill patients and their families.

Hyperthermia: A very high core body temperature.

Hypothermia: A very low core body temperature.

Illusion: Misperception of a real event or object.

Immobility: Inability to move.

Immunization: The protection of individuals or groups from specific diseases by vaccination or the injection of immune globulins (Taber's Cyclopedic Medical Dictionary, 2017).

Impaired skin integrity: A state in which an individual has altered epidermis and/or dermis.

Incivility: One or more rude, discourteous, or disrespectful actions that may or may not have a negative intent behind them (ANA, n.d.).

Incomplete protein: A protein that comes from plant sources.

Informed consent: A process in which a patient or guardian is provided with comprehensive information about the benefits, risks, and alternatives of a treatment or procedure before agreeing to have the treatment or procedure.

Insomnia: A disruption in the amount and quality of sleep that impairs functioning.

Inspection: Visual examination of the external surfaces of the body (Taber's Cyclopedic Medical Dictionary, 2017).

Instrumental activities of daily living (IADLs): Living skills such as cooking, cleaning, shopping, and managing money, that are needed for life at home.

Interdisciplinary healthcare team (IDT): A team comprised of members of two or more healthcare professions who work together in a collaborative manner (Taber's Cyclopedic Medical Dictionary, 2017).

International normalized ratio (INR): Standardized measurement of oral anticoagulation that standardizes the PT results worldwide.

Intrinsic factors: Conditions inherent to the individual that can lead to falls, such as normal aging changes, immobility, or changes in mental status.

Law: Rules and regulations that guide society in a formal and binding manner.

Leader: A person who is able to move people forward toward a vision or goal.

Leukocyte esterase: An enzyme produced by white blood cells. In urinalysis, leukocyte esterase presence indicates an inflammatory response initiated by leukocytes (WBC) from either infection or irritation. Positive leukocyte esterase and nitrite test values are diagnostic for urinary tract infection (UTI).

Level of consciousness: State of arousal and awareness, ranging from fully awake and oriented to comatose (Taber's Cyclopedic Medical Dictionary, 2017).

Liability: Legal responsibility for an action taken.

Living will: An advance directive prepared by a competent person regarding instruction about end-of-life care.

Long-term care facility: A residential facility where care is provided for individuals unable to perform activities of daily living (ADLs) due to physical or cognitive decline.

Malnutrition: Inadequate or excessive exposure to nutrients.

Malpractice: Any action or omission by a healthcare provider during the course of treating a patient that fails to meet reasonable standards of care and that causes injury to a patient.

Manager: An individual who has a position of authority.

Medicaid: Federally funded but state-administered program for providing medical care to qualifying low-income individuals.

Medicare: A federally funded health insurance program for individuals 65 years of age and older, younger disabled individuals who qualify, and individuals with end-stage renal disease.

Medication compliance: The extent to which a person follows the medication regimen given by the prescriber. Medication compliance is affected by both ability and willingness of a person to follow the prescribed regimen.

Mental health: A state of psychological, emotional, and social well-being.

Minimum data set (MDS): A comprehensive computer-compatible assessment form that is used for assessment of Medicare- or Medicaid-certified nursing home residents (Taber's Cyclopedic Medical Dictionary, 2017).

Negligence: Failure of a reasonable person to provide care to another person in a given situation.

Nonessential amino acid: An amino acid that the body can make in adequate amounts to meet its needs.

North American Nursing Diagnosis Association (NANDA): A professional organization that standardizes nursing language and terminology that aid in care planning (NANDA, 2018).

Omission: Failure to do something that has a legal or moral obligation.

Palliative care: Care that works to relieve symptoms and improve quality of life for people of any age and at any stage in a serious illness, whether that illness is curable, chronic, or life-threatening.

Palpation: Examination of external surfaces with the fingers or hands (Taber's Cyclopedic Medical Dictionary, 2017).

Paranoia: A way of thinking that systematically interprets

others as being intentionally harmful.

Personal space: The distance from another person at which one feels comfortable when talking to or being next to that other person.

Pharmacokinetics: The movement of a medication through the body from the point of entrance to the point of exit. The four processes of pharmacokinetics are absorption, distribution, metabolism, and excretion.

Pharmacology: The study of drugs.

Pharmacotherapeutics: The use of drugs to treat diseases and health conditions.

Pneumococcal disease: Infections caused by the bacterium *Streptococcus pneumoniae.*

Post-traumatic stress disorder (PTSD): Mental health condition in which the individual experiences emotional stress resulting from extreme injury or shock, often accompanied with vivid and frequent recollection of the initial event(s).

Prejudice: A preconceived judgment or opinion formed without factual knowledge (Taber's Cyclopedic Medical Dictionary, 2017).

Pressure ulcer: Any lesion caused by unrelieved pressure that results in damage to the underlying tissue.

Progressively lowered stress threshold model: A model or reference to assist in understanding behaviors associated with dementia or Alzheimer's disease.

QuantiFERON TB: A blood test used to measure the presence of tubercle bacillus in an individual. It determines if an antigen/antibody reaction has occurred from exposure to the bacteria *Mycobacterium tuberculosis.*

Racism: Racial prejudice (Dahlkemper, 2018).

Rehabilitation: The process of teaching and training individuals to achieve their highest level of independent function.

Rehabilitation goal: A written statement of desired behavioral outcomes from which steps or strategies may be designed to achieve that desired end.

Religion: A defined system (may be cultural) of views, practices, or behaviors related to spiritual elements. Individuals may follow a certain religion and be spiritual, but an individual can be spiritual without following a religion.

Relocation stress syndrome: The stress experienced when moving from one environment to another. Symptoms can be physical and or psychosocial in nature and include disorientation, depression, anxiety, withdrawal, weight change, and change in eating patterns.

Resident assessment instrument (RAI): A tool that helps staff to gather assessment information about residents in various environments of care (CMS, 2017).

Restorative care: Care that helps individuals maintain their highest level of function over time.

Restraint: The use of pharmacological or physical means to prevent a patient from harming themselves or others.

Review of systems (ROS): A list of questions that addresses each system of the body to determine medical history.

Sarcopenia: Loss of muscle mass and strength (Taber's Cyclopedic Medical Dictionary, 2017).

Screening tests: Laboratory tests performed on people without signs and symptoms of a specific health problem or diagnosis to determine whether there is evidence to support risk for certain conditions (e.g., cervical cancer screening).

Seasonal influenza: An acute contagious respiratory infection that usually strikes during the winter months (Taber's Cyclopedic Medical Dictionary, 2017).

Self-care: The care an individual provides oneself to maintain physical, mental, and emotional health.

Self-transcendence: The ability to focus on things other than self, such as altruism or spirituality.

Sexism: Actions and attitudes that relegate individuals of either sex to an inferior status in society (Taber's Cyclopedic Medical Dictionary, 2017).

Sexual orientation: An individual's identity based on the person's enduring pattern of emotional, romantic, or sexual attraction to men, women, or both sexes.

Shingles: A painful, localized skin rash caused by the varicella-zoster virus.

Simple carbohydrate: A carbohydrate that is easy for the body to digest and provides a source of quick energy.

Sleep apnea: A sleep disorder characterized by episodes of stalled breathing.

Somatization: Extreme preoccupation with physical problems.

Spirituality: The belief in something more powerful than oneself.

Standard precautions: Guidelines to reduce the risk of the spread of infection. Precautions include handwashing and wearing personal protective equipment.

Stereotype: An assumption that all people of one culture or race have the same personal characteristics (Dahlkemper, 2018).

Stress: Any physical, physiological, or psychological force that disturbs equilibrium in the human body.

Stressors: Anything that causes stress to an individual. This can be physical, psychological, or emotional.

Structural protein: A protein that provides support for various body parts. Examples of structural proteins include keratin, collagen, and elastin.

Substance use disorder: The recurrent use of alcohol or drugs that causes health problems, disability, or inability to maintain personal responsibilities.

Territory: The space used by a person and seen as owned by the person.

Tetanus-diphtheria-pertussis (Tdap) vaccine: A vaccine given to children and adults to prevent tetanus, diphtheria, and pertussis.

Theory of Human Caring: A focus on the human component of caring and the interactions between the patient and the nurse. The focus is on the whole person and their relationship with the world around them and the person caring for them.

Therapeutic diet: A diet designed to control the intake of certain foods.

Transformational leadership: A style of leadership involving trust and respect that motivates and inspires staff to exceed expectations.

Transition: A change from what was established and familiar to something new and unfamiliar.

Transpersonal caring: The ability to provide care intentionally focused on caring and healing instead of the disease or illness.

Tuberculosis: An infectious disease caused by the tubercle bacillus *Mycobacterium tuberculosis* that most commonly affects the respiratory system.

Urinary incontinence: Involuntary loss of urine that is sufficient to be a problem to the patient.

Urine microalbumin: A test that measures the amount of albumin (a blood protein) in the urine. It is ordered to determine microvascular kidney damage in people with diabetes or hypertension who are at risk for developing kidney disease (especially if it is uncontrolled).

Water-soluble vitamin: A vitamin that is absorbed in the presence of water.

Index

Note: Page numbers followed by b refer to boxes, f refer to figures, t refer to tables.